Pathophysiology

A 2-in-1 Reference for Nurses

Pathophysiology

A 2-in-1 Reference for Nurses

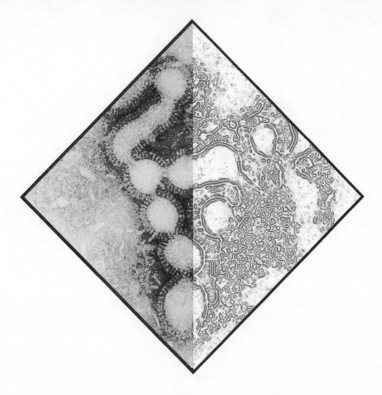

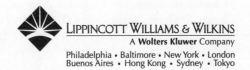

LIPPINCOTT WILLIAMS & WILKINS
A **Wolters Kluwer** Company

Philadelphia • Baltimore • New York • London
Buenos Aires • Hong Kong • Sydney • Tokyo

STAFF

Executive Publisher
Judith A. Schilling McCann, RN, MSN

Editorial Director
David Moreau

Clinical Director
Joan M. Robinson, RN, MSN

Senior Art Director
Arlene Putterman

Art Director
Elaine Kasmer

Editorial Project Manager
Tracy S. Diehl

Clinical Project Manager
Jana L. Sciarra, RN, MSN, CRNP

Editors
Carol Munson, Rob Traister

Clinical Editors
Maryann Foley, RN, BSN;
Karen A. Hamel, RN, BSN;
Ann Wray Clarke Marland, RN, BSN, BA

Copy Editors
Kimberly Bilotta (supervisor),
Scotti Cohn, Shana Harrington,
Dona Hightower Perkins, Dorothy P. Terry,
Pamela Wingrod

Designer
Susan L. Sheridan (project manager)

Digital Composition Services
Diane Paluba (manager), Joyce Rossi Biletz,
Donna S. Morris

Manufacturing
Patricia K. Dorshaw (director),
Beth Janae Orr

Editorial Assistants
Megan L. Aldinger, Tara L. Carter-Bell,
Linda K. Ruhf

Librarian
Wani Z. Larsen

Indexer
Karen C. Comerford

PA2IN1010404 — 041006

**Library of Congress
Cataloging-in Publication Data**
Pathophysiology : a 2-in-1 reference for nurses.
    p. ; cm.
Includes bibliographical references and index.
  1. Physiology, Pathological. 2. Nurses. I. Lippincott Williams & Wilkins.
  [DNLM: 1. Nursing Care—Handbooks. 2. Disease—Handbooks. 3. Pathology, Clinical—Handbooks. WY 49 P2965 2004]
RB113.P359 2004
616.07—dc22
ISBN13 978-1-58255-317-7
ISBN10 1-58255-317-3 (alk. paper)   2003023945

Contents

Contributors and consultants

Margaret Hamilton Birney, RN, PhD
Associate Professor
University of Delaware
Newark

Cheryl L. Brady, RN, MSN
Nursing Instructor
Mercy College
Youngstown, Ohio

Karen T. Bruchak, RN, MSN, MBA
*Oncology Product Marketing
    Administrator*
Siemens Corp.
Malvern, Pa.

Concha Carrillo, MS, APN, CGRN, CNP
Gastroenterology Nurse Practitioner
Sterling Rock Falls Clinic
Sterling, Ill.

Sandra H. Clark, RN, MSN
Assistant Professor
Armstrong Atlantic State University
Savannah, Ga.

Yvette P. Conley, PhD
Assistant Professor
University of Pittsburgh

Louise Diehl-Oplinger, RN, MSN,
    APRN, BC, CCRN, CLNC
Advanced Practice Nurse
Warren Hospital
Phillipsburg, N.J.

Shelba Durston, RN, MSN, CCRN
Staff Nurse
San Joaquin General Hospital
French Camp, Calif.
Faculty
San Joaquin Delta College
Stockton, Calif.

Ellie Z. Franges, RN, MSN, CNRN
Clinical Nurse Specialist, Neuroscience
St. Luke's Hospital and Health Network
Bethlehem, Pa.

Linda Fuhrman, MSN, ANP
Nurse Practitioner
San Francisco Veterans Administration

Julie A. Grant, BA, MSPA-C
*Physician Assistant, Division of Allergy-
    Immunology*
Department of Internal Medicine
University of Iowa Hospitals and
    Clinics
Iowa City

Nancy H. Haynes, RN, PhD(c), CCRN
Assistant Professor
Saint Luke's College
Kansas City, Mo.

Sally S. Russell, RN, MN, BC
Director, Education Services
Anthony J. Jannetti, Inc.
Pitman, N.J.

Mary Clare Schafer, RN, MS, ONC
*Infection Control Nurse/Osteoporosis
    Program Coordinator*
Tenet — Graduate Hospital
Philadelphia

Mary A. Stahl, RN, MSN, APRN, BC, CCRN
Clinical Nurse Specialist
Saint Luke's Hospital
Kansas City, Mo.

Tamara D. Thell, RN, BSN, PHN
Nurse Educator/Nursing Instructor
Anoka-Hennepin Technical College
Anoka, Minn.

David Toub, MD, FACOG
Medical Director
Med Cases, Inc.
Philadelphia

Foreword

Pathophysiology can be a confusing topic. The ability to understand the relationship between altered body system functions and normal anatomy and physiology is essential to successful nursing. *Pathophysiology: A 2-in-1 Reference for Nurses* delves into the important issues you need to know and helps you grasp the difficult topics.

This book communicates important clinical information available to health care providers in a clear, concise, and unique way: it offers nurses the opportunity to save time, a resource that's usually lacking in today's health care market.

Each page is arranged in a two-column format: comprehensive coverage in the inner column and condensed, bulleted information in the outer column. This innovative approach offers practicing nurses two ways to get the information they need. They can reach key, pertinent information quickly and have the opportunity to go back to the book later to obtain a more comprehensive understanding of the issue.

Opening chapters include fundamentals of pathophysiology, cancer, fluids and electrolytes, and genetics. Next, 11 chapters examine common pathologic changes associated with the major body systems — cardiovascular, respiratory, nervous, GI, musculoskeletal, hematologic, immune, endocrine, renal, integumentary, and reproductive. In addition, these chapters identify the signs and symptoms associated with these changes, relevant diagnostic tests, disease complications, and common treatments.

As an educator and a clinician, I must share evidence-based interventions with my patients as well as with my students, because it allows them to become active participants in the health care decision-making process. This book offers a clinically accurate understanding of the complex working of our bodies, in easy to understand language. To help simplify complex issues, the editors have provided flowcharts, diagrams, and illustrations throughout the book and logos that highlight clinical alerts and potentially life-threatening disorders.

Pathophysiology: A 2-in-1 Reference for Nurses is what the title claims — two books in one! Between its unique style and text that's chock-full of information, this book is a must-have in every health care provider's library!

Lisa Salamon, MSN, CNS, RNBC, ETN
Clinical Nurse Specialist
Cleveland Clinic Foundation

Fundamentals of pathophysiology

An understanding of pathophysiology requires a review of normal physiology — how the body functions day-to-day, minute-to-minute — at the levels of cells, tissues, organs, and as a whole organism.

HOMEOSTASIS

Every cell in the body is involved in maintaining a dynamic, steady state of internal balance called *homeostasis*. Any change or damage at the cellular level can affect the entire body. When homeostasis is disrupted by an external stressor — such as injury, lack of nutrients, or invasion by parasites or other organisms — illness may occur. Many external stressors affect the body's internal equilibrium throughout a person's life. Pathophysiology can be defined as what happens when normal defenses fail.

MAINTAINING BALANCE

Three structures in the brain are responsible for maintaining the body's homeostasis. The first is the *medulla oblongata,* which is the part of the brain stem associated with vital functions, such as respiration and circulation. The next is the *pituitary gland,* which regulates the function of other glands and thereby a person's growth, maturation, and reproduction. The third structure is the *reticular formation,* a network of nerve cells (nuclei) and fibers in the brain stem and spinal cord. The reticular formation helps control vital reflexes, such as cardiovascular function and respiration.

Homeostasis is maintained by self-regulating feedback mechanisms. These mechanisms have three components.

The first component, a *sensor,* detects disruptions in homeostasis that are caused by nerve impulses or by changes in hormone levels. The second component,

3 feedback components

+ Sensor: detects disruptions in homeostasis caused by nerve impulses or changes in hormone levels
+ CNS control center: receives signals from sensor and regulates the body's response to disruptions
+ Effector: restores homeostasis

Feedback mechanisms

+ Positive: moves the system away from homeostasis
+ Negative: works to restore homeostasis

Characteristics of disease and illness

Disease

+ Occurs when homeostasis isn't maintained
+ Influenced by genetic factors, unhealthy behaviors, attitudes, and disease perception
+ Idiopathic diseases have no known cause

Illness

+ Occurs when a person is no longer in "normal" health
+ Refers to subjective symptoms that may indicate disease

Disease pathogenesis

+ Unless treated, most diseases progress by symptom patterns
+ Usually detected by signs and symptoms
+ Manifestations include hypofunction, hyperfunction, or increased mechanical function
+ Response and resolution depend on many factors

a *central nervous system (CNS) control center,* receives signals from the sensor and regulates the body's response to the disruptions by initiating the effector mechanism. The third component, an *effector,* acts to restore homeostasis.

Feedback mechanisms exist in two varieties. A *positive* feedback mechanism moves the system away from homeostasis by enhancing a change in the system. For example, the heart pumps at increased rate and force when a person is in shock. If the shock progresses, the heart action may require more oxygen than is available. The result is heart failure. A *negative* feedback mechanism works to restore homeostasis by correcting a deficit in the system.

An effective negative feedback mechanism must sense a change in the body—such as a high blood glucose level—and attempt to return body functions to normal. In the case of a high blood glucose level, the effector mechanism triggers increased insulin production by the pancreas, returning blood glucose levels to normal and restoring homeostasis.

DISEASE AND ILLNESS

Although *disease* and *illness* are commonly used interchangeably, their meanings aren't synonymous. Disease occurs when homeostasis isn't maintained. Illness occurs when a person is no longer in a state of perceived "normal" health. For example, a person may have coronary artery disease, diabetes, or asthma but not be ill all the time because his body has adapted to the disease. In such a situation, a person can perform necessary activities of daily living. Illness usually refers to subjective symptoms that may indicate the presence of disease.

The course and outcome of a disease are influenced by genetic factors (such as a tendency toward obesity), unhealthy behaviors (such as smoking), attitudes (such as being a "Type A" personality), and even the person's perception of the disease (such as acceptance or denial). Diseases are dynamic and may be manifested in various ways, depending on the patient or his environment.

CAUSE

The cause of disease may be intrinsic or extrinsic. Inheritance, age, gender, infectious agents, or behaviors (such as inactivity, smoking, or abusing illegal drugs) can cause disease. Diseases that have no known cause are called *idiopathic.*

DEVELOPMENT

A disease's development is called its *pathogenesis.* Unless identified and successfully treated, most diseases progress according to a typical pattern of symptoms. Some diseases are self-limiting or resolve quickly with limited or no intervention; others are chronic and never resolve. Patients with chronic diseases may undergo periodic remissions and exacerbations.

A disease is usually detected when it causes a change in metabolism or cell division that causes signs and symptoms. Manifestations of disease may include hypofunction (such as constipation), hyperfunction (such as increased mucus production), or increased mechanical function (such as a seizure).

How the cells respond to disease depends on the causative agent and the affected cells, tissues, and organs. The resolution of disease depends on many factors functioning over time, such as the extent of disease and the presence of other diseases.

STAGES

Typically, diseases progress through various stages. An *exposure or injury* occurs, causing target tissue to be injured or exposed to a causative agent. During the second stage, the *latency or incubation period*, no signs or symptoms are evident. In the third stage, or *prodromal period*, signs and symptoms are usually mild and nonspecific. The disease reaches its full intensity in the *acute stage*, possibly resulting in complications. If the patient can still function as though the disease wasn't present, this stage is referred to as the *subclinical acute stage*. *Remission*, a second latent stage, occurs only in some diseases and is usually followed by another acute stage. During the next stage, *convalescence*, the patient progresses toward recovery after the disease's termination. During the last stage, *recovery*, the patient regains health or normal functioning, and no signs or symptoms of the disease remain.

STRESS AND DISEASE

When a stressor such as a life change occurs, a person can respond in one of two ways: by adapting successfully or by failing to adapt. A maladaptive response to stress may result in disease.

Hans Selye, a pioneer in the study of stress and disease, describes the following stages of adaptation to a stressful event: alarm, resistance, and recovery or exhaustion. (See *Physical response to stress*.) In the alarm stage, the body senses stress and

Stages of disease progression

+ Exposure or injury occurs
+ Latency or intubation period: no signs or symptoms are evident
+ Prodromal period: signs and symptoms are mild
+ Acute stage: disease reaches full intensity
+ Remission: occurs only in some diseases; usually followed by another acute stage
+ Convalescence: patient progresses toward recovery
+ Recovery: patient regains health or normal functioning; no signs or symptoms remain

Stages of stress

+ Physical or psychological stressor
+ Alarm reaction
+ Resistance
+ Recovery
+ Exhaustion

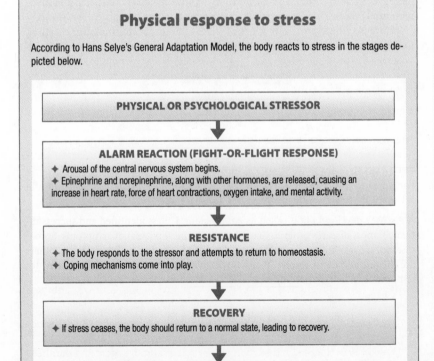

Physical response to stress

According to Hans Selye's General Adaptation Model, the body reacts to stress in the stages depicted below.

PHYSICAL OR PSYCHOLOGICAL STRESSOR

↓

ALARM REACTION (FIGHT-OR-FLIGHT RESPONSE)
+ Arousal of the central nervous system begins.
+ Epinephrine and norepinephrine, along with other hormones, are released, causing an increase in heart rate, force of heart contractions, oxygen intake, and mental activity.

↓

RESISTANCE
+ The body responds to the stressor and attempts to return to homeostasis.
+ Coping mechanisms come into play.

↓

RECOVERY
+ If stress ceases, the body should return to a normal state, leading to recovery.

↓

EXHAUSTION
+ The body can no longer produce hormones as it did in the alarm stage.
+ Organ damage begins.

The stress response

+ Controlled by events in the nervous and endocrine systems
+ Actions try to redirect energy to the organ most affected by stress
+ Physiologic (elicit harmful response) or psychological (may cause a maladaptive response)
+ Can exacerbate chronic illnesses
+ Reduced by coping strategies

Characteristics of cells

+ Made up of single cell or billions of cells
+ Highly specialized cells perform an identical function and are organized into tissue
+ Tissues form organs that are integrated into body systems
+ Normal cell's largest components are cytoplasm, nucleus, and cell membrane

Key facts about cytoplasm

+ Consists of cytosol: a semitransparent fluid
+ Suspended in cytosol are organelles
+ Organelles perform a function to maintain the cell's life

arouses the CNS. The body releases chemicals to mobilize the fight-or-flight response. In this dual effort, the sympathoadrenal medullary response causes the release of epinephrine and the hypothalamic pituitary adrenal axis causes the release of glucocorticoids. These systems work in concert to enable the body to respond to stressors. This release is the adrenaline rush associated with panic or aggression. In the resistance stage, the body either adapts and achieves homeostasis or it fails to adapt and enters the exhaustion stage, resulting in disease.

The stress response is controlled by actions that take place in the cells of the nervous and endocrine systems. These actions try to redirect energy to the organ that's most affected by the stress, such as the heart, lungs, or brain.

Stressors may be physiologic or psychological. Physiologic stressors such as exposure to a toxin may elicit a harmful response leading to an identifiable illness or set of signs and symptoms. Psychological stressors such as the death of a loved one may also cause a maladaptive response. Stressful events can exacerbate some chronic diseases, such as diabetes or multiple sclerosis. Effective coping strategies can prevent or reduce the harmful effects of stress.

CELL PHYSIOLOGY

The cell is the smallest living component of a living organism. Organisms may be made up of a single cell (such as bacteria) or billions of cells (such as human beings). In large organisms, highly specialized cells that perform an identical function are organized into tissue, such as epithelial tissue, connective tissue, nerve tissue, and muscle tissue. Tissues, in turn, form organs (skin, skeleton, brain, and heart), which are integrated into body systems, such as the CNS, cardiovascular system, and musculoskeletal system.

CELL COMPONENTS

Like organisms, cells are complex organizations of specialized components, each component having its own function. A normal cell's largest components are the cytoplasm, the nucleus, and the cell membrane, which surrounds the internal components and holds the cell together. (See *A look at cell components.*)

Cytoplasm

The gel-like cytoplasm consists primarily of cytosol, a viscous, semitransparent fluid that's 70% to 90% water plus various proteins, salts, and sugars. Suspended in the cytosol are many tiny structures called *organelles*.

Organelles are the cell's metabolic machinery. Each performs a function to maintain the cell's life. Organelles include mitochondria, ribosomes, endoplasmic reticulum, Golgi apparatus, lysosomes, peroxisomes, cytoskeletal elements, centrosomes, microfilaments, and microtubules.

+ *Mitochondria* are spherical or rod-shaped structures that produce most of the body's adenosine triphosphate (ATP). ATP contains high-energy phosphate chemical bonds that fuel many cellular activities. Mitochondria are the sites of cellular respiration—the metabolic use of oxygen to produce energy, carbon dioxide, and water.
+ *Ribosomes* are the sites of protein synthesis.
+ The *endoplasmic reticulum* is an extensive network of two varieties of membrane-enclosed tubules. The rough endoplasmic reticulum is covered with ribosomes. The smooth endoplasmic reticulum contains enzymes that synthesize lipids.

A look at cell components

The illustration below shows a cell's components and structures. Each part has a function in maintaining the cell's life and homeostasis.

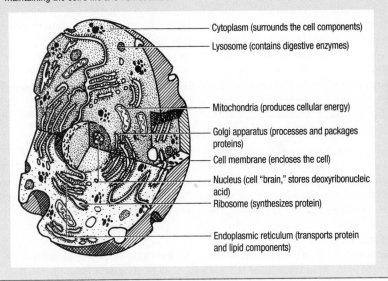

Cytoplasm (surrounds the cell components)

Lysosome (contains digestive enzymes)

Mitochondria (produces cellular energy)

Golgi apparatus (processes and packages proteins)

Cell membrane (encloses the cell)

Nucleus (cell "brain," stores deoxyribonucleic acid)

Ribosome (synthesizes protein)

Endoplasmic reticulum (transports protein and lipid components)

✦ The *Golgi apparatus* synthesizes carbohydrate molecules that combine with protein produced by the rough endoplasmic reticulum and lipids produced by the smooth endoplasmic reticulum to form such products as lipoproteins, glycoproteins, and enzymes.

✦ *Lysosomes* are digestive bodies that break down nutrient material as well as foreign or damaged material in cells. A membrane surrounding each lysosome separates its digestive enzymes from the rest of the cytoplasm. The enzymes digest nutrient matter brought into the cell by means of endocytosis, in which a portion of the cell membrane surrounds and engulfs matter to form a membrane-bound intracellular vesicle. The lysosome membrane fuses with the vesicle membrane surrounding the material that has undergone endocytosis. The lysosomal enzymes then digest the engulfed material. Lysosomes digest the foreign matter ingested by white blood cells (WBCs) by a similar process called *phagocytosis*.

✦ *Peroxisomes* contain oxidases, which are enzymes that chemically reduce oxygen to hydrogen peroxide and hydrogen peroxide to water.

✦ *Cytoskeletal elements* form a network of protein structures that maintain the cell's shape.

✦ *Centrosomes* contain centrioles, which are short cylinders adjacent to the nucleus that take part in cell division.

✦ *Microfilaments* and *microtubules* enable the movement of intracellular vesicles (allowing axons to transport neurotransmitters) and the formation of the mitotic spindle, the framework for cell division.

Types of organelles

Mitochondria
✦ Structures that produce ATP
✦ Site of cellular respiration

Ribosomes
✦ Site of protein synthesis

Endoplasmic reticulum
✦ Extensive network of membrane-enclosed tubules
✦ Two varieties: rough endoplasmic reticulum and smooth endoplasmic reticulum

Golgi apparatus
✦ Synthesizes carbohydrate molecules
✦ Forms lipoproteins, glycoproteins, and enzymes

Lysosomes
✦ Digestive bodies that break down nutrient material; endocytosis occurs
✦ Membrane fuses with the vesicle membrane surrounding the endocytosis material
✦ Lysosomes digest the foreign matter ingested by WBCs

Peroxisomes
✦ Contain oxidases

Cytoskeletal elements
✦ Form network of protein structures that maintain cell's shape

Centrosomes
✦ Contain centrioles; take part in cell division

Microfilaments and microtubules
✦ Enable movement of intracellular vesicles and formation of mitotic spindle
✦ Framework for cell division

Nucleus

The cell's control center is the nucleus, which plays a role in cell growth, metabolism, and reproduction. Within the nucleus, one or more nucleoli (dark-staining intranuclear structures) synthesize ribonucleic acid (RNA), a complex polynucleotide that controls protein synthesis. The nucleus also stores deoxyribonucleic acid (DNA), the double helix that carries genetic material and is responsible for cellular reproduction or division.

Cell membrane

The semipermeable cell membrane forms the cell's external boundary, separating it from other cells and from the external environment. Roughly 75Å (3/10 millionths of an inch) thick, the cell membrane consists of a double layer of phospholipids with protein molecules embedded in it. These protein molecules act as receptors, ion channels, or carriers for specific substances.

CELL DIVISION

Each cell must replicate itself for life to continue. Cells replicate by division in one of two ways: mitosis (division that results in two daughter cells with the same DNA and chromosome content as the mother cell) or meiosis (division that creates four gametocytes, each containing one-half of the number of chromosomes of the original cell). Most cells undergo mitosis; meiosis occurs only in reproductive cells.

Mitosis

Mitosis, the type of cell division that leads to tissue growth, creates an equal division of material in the nucleus (karyokinesis) followed by division of the cell body (cytokinesis). This process yields two duplicates of the original cell. (See chapter 5, Genetics, for a detailed discussion of mitosis and meiosis.)

CELL FUNCTIONS

A cell's basic functions are movement, conduction, absorption, secretion, excretion, respiration, and reproduction. In the human body, different cells are specialized to perform only one function; muscle cells, for example, are responsible for movement. However, respiration and reproduction occur in all cells.

Movement

Some cells, such as muscle cells, work together to produce movement of a specific body part, the contents within an organ, or the entire organism. Muscle cells attached to bone move the extremities. When muscle cells that envelop hollow organs or cavities contract, they produce movement of contents, such as the peristaltic movement of the intestines or the ejection of blood from the heart.

Conduction

Conduction is the transmission of a stimulus, such as a nerve impulse, heat, or sound wave, from one body part to another.

Absorption

The absorption process occurs as substances move through a cell membrane. For example, food is broken down into amino acids, fatty acids, and glucose in the digestive tract. Specialized cells in the intestine then absorb the nutrients and transport them to blood vessels, which carry them to other cells of the body. These target cells, in turn, absorb the substances, using them as energy sources or as building blocks to form or repair structural and functional cellular components.

Secretion

Some cells, such as those in the glands, release substances that are used in another part of the body. For example, the beta cells of the islets of Langerhans of the pancreas secrete insulin, which is transported by the blood to its target cells, where the insulin facilitates the movement of glucose across cell membranes.

Excretion

Cells excrete the waste generated by normal metabolic processes. This waste includes such substances as carbon dioxide and certain acids and nitrogen-containing molecules.

Respiration

Cellular respiration occurs in the mitochondria, where ATP is produced. The cell absorbs oxygen; it then uses the oxygen and releases carbon dioxide during cellular metabolism. The energy stored in ATP is used in other reactions that require energy.

Reproduction

New cells are needed to replace older cells for tissue and body growth. Most cells divide and reproduce through mitosis. However, some cells, such as nerve and muscle cells, typically lose their ability to reproduce after birth.

CELL TYPES

Each of the four types of tissue (epithelial, connective, nerve, and muscle) consists of several specialized cell types, which perform specific functions.

Epithelial cell

Epithelial cells line most of the body's internal and external surfaces, such as the skin's epidermis, internal organs, blood vessels, body cavities, glands, and sensory organs. The functions of epithelial cells include support, protection, absorption, excretion, and secretion.

Connective tissue cell

Connective tissue cells are found in skin, bones and joints, artery walls, fascia around organs, nerves, and body fat. The types of connective tissue cells include fibroblasts (such as collagen, elastin, and reticular fibers), adipose (fat) cells, mast cells (which release histamines and other substances during inflammation), and bone. The major functions of connective tissues are protection, metabolism, support, temperature maintenance, and elasticity.

Nerve cell

Two types of cells—neurons and neuroglial cells—comprise the nervous system. Neurons have a cell body, dendrites, and an axon. The dendrites carry nerve impulses to the cell body from the axons of other neurons. Axons carry impulses away from the cell body to other neurons or organs. A myelin sheath around the axon facilitates rapid conduction of impulses by keeping them within the nerve cell. Neurons' functions include generating electrical impulses, conducting electrical impulses, influencing other neurons, muscle cells, and cells of glands by transmitting those impulses.

Types of cell functions

Secretion
+ Cells release substances that are used in another part of the body

Excretion
+ Cells excrete waste generated by metabolic processes

Respiration
+ Occurs in the mitochondria
+ Cells absorb oxygen, then use it and release carbon dioxide

Reproduction
+ New cells replace old cells for tissue and body growth

Type of cells

Epithelial cells
+ Line most of the body's internal and external surfaces
+ Functions include support, protection, absorption, secretion, and excretion

Connective tissue cells
+ Found in skin, bones and joints, artery walls, fascia around organs, nerves, and body fat
+ Types include fibroblasts, adipose cells, mast cells, and bone
+ Functions include protection, metabolism, support, temperature maintenance, and elasticity

Nerve cells
+ Two types: neurons and neuroglial cells
+ Neurons have a cell body, dendrites, and an axon
+ Neurons' functions include generating and conducting electrical impulses
+ Four types of neuroglial cells: oligodendroglia, astrocytes, ependymal, and microglia
+ Neuroglial cells support, nourish, and protect neurons

There are four types of neuroglial cells; they support, nourish, and protect the neurons. Oligodendroglia produce myelin within the CNS; astrocytes provide essential nutrients to neurons and assist neurons in maintaining the proper bioelectrical potentials for impulse conduction and synaptic transmission; ependymal cells are involved in the production of cerebrospinal fluid; and microglia ingest and digest tissue debris when nerve tissue is damaged.

Muscle cell

Muscle cells contract to produce movement or tension. The intracellular proteins actin and myosin interact to form cross-bridges that result in muscle contraction. An increase in intracellular calcium is necessary for muscle to contract.

There are three basic types of muscle cells:

+ *Skeletal (striated) muscle cells* are long, cylindrical cells that extend along the entire length of the skeletal muscles. These muscles, which attach directly to the bone or are connected to the bone by tendons, are responsible for voluntary movement. By contracting and relaxing, striated muscle cells alter the muscle's length. Contraction shortens the muscle; relaxation permits the muscle to return to its resting length.

+ *Smooth (nonstriated) muscle cells* are present in the walls of hollow internal organs, such as the GI and genitourinary tracts, and of blood vessels and bronchioles. Unlike striated muscle, these spindle-shaped cells contract involuntarily. By contracting and relaxing, they change the hollow structure's luminal diameter and thereby move substances through the organ.

+ *Cardiac muscle cells* branch out across the smooth muscle of the heart's chambers and contract involuntarily. They produce and transmit cardiac action potentials, which cause cardiac muscle cells to contract. Impulses travel from cell to cell as though no cell membrane existed.

 CLINICAL ALERT In older adults, skeletal muscle cells become smaller and many are replaced by fibrous connective tissue. The result is loss of muscle strength and mass.

PATHOPHYSIOLOGIC CHANGES

The cell faces several challenges through its life. Stressors, changes in the body's health, disease, and other extrinsic and intrinsic factors can change the cell's normal functioning (homeostasis).

CELL ADAPTATION

Cells can generally continue functioning despite changing conditions or stressors. However, severe or prolonged stress or changes may injure or even destroy cells. When cell integrity is threatened—for example, by hypoxia, anoxia, chemical injury, infection, or temperature extremes—the cell reacts in one of two ways: by drawing on its reserves to keep functioning or by adaptive changes or cellular dysfunction.

If enough cellular reserve is available and the body doesn't detect abnormalities, the cell adapts by atrophy, hypertrophy, hyperplasia, metaplasia, or dysplasia. (See *Adaptive cell changes.*) If cellular reserve is insufficient, cell death (necrosis) occurs. Necrosis is usually localized and easily identifiable.

Adaptive cell changes

Cells adapt to changing conditions and stressors within the body in the ways shown below.

NORMAL CELLS

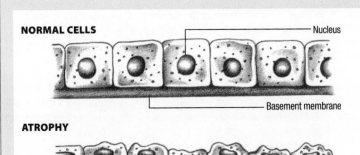

Nucleus

Basement membrane

ATROPHY

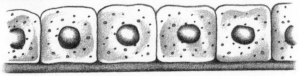

HYPERTROPHY

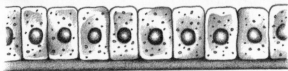

HYPERPLASIA

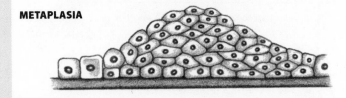

METAPLASIA

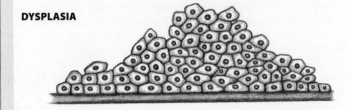

DYSPLASIA

Adaptive cell changes

Atrophy
+ Reduction in size of cell or organ
+ May occur when cells face reduced workload or disuse

Hypertrophy
+ Increase in size of cell or organ
+ Due to an increase in workload
+ Three types: physiologic, compensatory, pathologic

Hyperplasia
+ Increase in the number of cells
+ Caused by increased workload, hormonal stimulation, or decreased tissue density
+ Three types: physiologic, compensatory, pathologic

Metaplasia
+ Replacement of one cell type with another
+ Common cause is constant irritation or injury
+ New cell can better endure stress
+ Two types: physiologic, pathologic

Dysplasia
+ Abnormal differentiation of dividing cells causes abnormal size, shape, and appearance of cells
+ Not cancerous but may precede cancerous changes

Atrophy

Atrophy is a reduction in the size of a cell or organ that may occur when cells face reduced workload or disuse, insufficient blood flow, malnutrition, or reduced hormonal and nerve stimulation. Examples of atrophy include loss of muscle mass and tone after prolonged bed rest.

Hypertrophy

In contrast, hypertrophy is an increase in the size of a cell or organ due to an increase in workload. There are three basic types of hypertrophy: *physiologic hypertrophy* reflects an increase in workload that isn't caused by disease—for example, the increase in muscle size caused by hard physical labor or weight training; *compensatory hypertrophy* takes place when cell size increases to take over for nonfunctioning cells—for instance, one kidney will enlarge when the other isn't functioning or is removed; and *pathologic hypertrophy* is a response to disease—an example is thickening of the heart muscle as the muscle pumps against increasing resistance in patients with hypertension.

Hyperplasia

Hyperplasia is an increase in the number of cells caused by increased workload, hormonal stimulation, or decreased tissue density. Like hypertrophy, hyperplasia may be *physiologic*, *compensatory*, or *pathologic*.
+ *Physiologic hyperplasia* is an adaptive response to normal changes. An example is the monthly increase in number of uterine cells that occurs in response to estrogen stimulation of the endometrium after ovulation.
+ *Compensatory hyperplasia* occurs in some organs to replace tissue that has been removed or destroyed. For example, liver cells regenerate when part of the liver is surgically removed.
+ *Pathologic hyperplasia* is a response to either excessive hormonal stimulation or abnormal production of hormonal growth factors. Examples include acromegaly, in which excessive growth hormone production causes bones to enlarge, and endometrial hyperplasia, in which excessive secretion of estrogen causes heavy menstrual bleeding and, possibly, malignant changes.

Metaplasia

Metaplasia is the replacement of one cell type with another cell type (one that can better endure the change or stressor). A common cause of metaplasia is constant irritation or injury that initiates an inflammatory response. The new cell type can better endure the stress of chronic inflammation. Metaplasia may be either *physiologic* or *pathologic*.
+ *Physiologic metaplasia* is a normal response to changing conditions and is generally transient. For example, in the body's normal response to inflammation, monocytes that migrate to inflamed tissues transform into macrophages.
+ *Pathologic metaplasia* is a response to an extrinsic toxin or stressor and is generally irreversible. For example, after years of exposure to cigarette smoke, stratified squamous epithelial cells replace the normal ciliated columnar epithelial cells of the bronchi. Although the new cells can better withstand smoke, they don't secrete mucus nor do they have cilia to protect the airway. If exposure to cigarette smoke continues, the squamous cells can become cancerous.

Dysplasia

In dysplasia, abnormal differentiation of dividing cells results in cells that are abnormal in size, shape, and appearance. Although dysplastic cell changes aren't cancerous, they can precede cancerous changes. Common examples include dysplasia of epithelial cells of the cervix or the respiratory tract.

CELL INJURY

Injury to any cellular component can lead to illness as the cells lose their ability to adapt. One early indication of cell injury is a biochemical lesion that forms on the cell at the point of injury. For example, in a patient with chronic alcoholism, biochemical lesions on the cells of the immune system may increase the patient's susceptibility to infection, and cells of the pancreas and liver are affected in a way that prevents their reproduction. These cells can't return to normal functioning.

Causes of cell injury

Cell injury may result from any of several intrinsic or extrinsic causes. Toxic injuries may be caused by substances that originate in the body (endogenous factors) or outside the body (exogenous factors). Common endogenous toxins include products of genetically determined metabolic errors, gross malformations, and hypersensitivity reactions. Exogenous toxins include alcohol, lead, carbon monoxide, and drugs that alter cellular function. Examples of such drugs include chemotherapeutic agents used for cancer and immunosuppressants used to prevent rejection in organ transplant recipients.

Viruses, fungi, protozoa, and bacteria can cause infections, which can lead to cell injury or death. These organisms affect cell integrity, usually by interfering with cell division, producing nonviable, mutant cells. For example, human immunodeficiency virus alters the cell when the virus is replicated in the cell's RNA.

Physical injury results from a disruption in the cell or in the relationships of the intracellular organelles. Two major types of physical injury are thermal and mechanical. Causes of thermal injury include burns, radiation therapy for cancer, X-rays, and ultraviolet radiation. Causes of mechanical injury include surgery, trauma from motor vehicle accidents, and frostbite.

When a deficit of water, oxygen, or nutrients occurs, or if constant temperature and adequate waste disposal aren't maintained, a deficit injury occurs, and normal cellular metabolism can't take place. A lack of just one of these basic requirements can cause cell disruption or death. Causes of deficit include hypoxia (inadequate oxygen), ischemia (inadequate blood supply), and malnutrition.

Irreversible cell injury occurs when the cell membrane or the organelles can no longer function.

CELL DEGENERATION

Degeneration is a type of nonlethal cell damage that generally occurs in the cytoplasm and that doesn't affect the nucleus. Degeneration usually affects organs with metabolically active cells, such as the liver, heart, and kidneys, and is caused by various problems such as increased water in the cell or cellular swelling, fatty infiltrates, atrophy, autophagocytosis (the cell absorbs some of its own parts), pigmentation changes, calcification, hyaline infiltration, hypertrophy, dysplasia (related to chronic irritation), and hyperplasia.

When changes in cells are identified, prompt health care can slow degeneration and prevent cell death. An electron microscope can help identify cellular changes, and thus diagnose a disease, before the patient complains of any symptoms. Unfortunately, many cell changes remain unidentifiable even under a microscope, making early detection of disease impossible. An example of reversible degenerative

Key facts about cell aging

+ Atrophy may indicate loss of cell structure
+ Hypertrophy or hyperplasia is characteristic of lost cell function
+ Signs occur in all body systems
+ Cell aging process limits the human life span

Key facts about cell death

Apoptosis
+ Genetically programmed cell death

Liquefaction necrosis
+ Occurs when a lytic enzyme liquefies necrotic cells
+ Common in the brain

Caseous necrosis
+ Necrotic cells disintegrate; cellular pieces remain undigested
+ Occurs commonly in pulmonary tuberculosis

Fat necrosis
+ Lipases break down intracellular triglycerides into free fatty acids, which form soaps; tissue becomes opaque

Coagulative necrosis
+ Occurs when blood supply to any organ is interrupted
+ Affects the kidneys, heart, and adrenal glands

Gangrenous necrosis
+ Results from lack of blood flow
+ Complicated by overgrowth and invasion of bacteria
+ Can occur as dry (minimal bacterial invasion), moist (develops with liquefication necrosis), or gas (anaerobic bacteria of the genus *Clostridium* infect tissue)

change is cervical dysplasia. Examples of irreversible degenerative diseases include Huntington's disease and amyotrophic lateral sclerosis.

CELL AGING

During the normal process of aging, cells lose structure and function. Atrophy, a decrease in size or wasting away, may indicate loss of cell structure. Hypertrophy or hyperplasia is characteristic of lost cell function. (See *Factors that affect cell aging.*)

Signs of aging occur in all body systems. Examples include diminished elasticity of blood vessels, bowel motility, muscle mass, and subcutaneous fat. Cell aging can slow down or speed up, depending on the number and extent of injuries and the amount of wear and tear on the cell.

The cell aging process limits the human life span (of course, many people die from disease before they reach the maximum life span of about 110 years).

CELL DEATH

Like disease, cell death may be caused by internal (intrinsic) factors that limit the cell's life span or external (extrinsic) factors that contribute to cell damage and aging. When a stressor is severe or prolonged, the cell can no longer adapt and it dies.

Cell death, or necrosis, may manifest in different ways, depending on the tissues or organs involved.

+ *Apoptosis* is genetically programmed cell death. This accounts for the constant cell turnover in the skin's outer keratin layer and the eye's lens.
+ *Liquefaction necrosis* occurs when a lytic (dissolving) enzyme liquefies necrotic cells. This type of necrosis is common in the brain, which has a rich supply of lytic enzymes.
+ In *caseous necrosis,* the necrotic cells disintegrate but the cellular pieces remain undigested for months or years. This type of necrotic tissue gets its name from its crumbly, cheeselike (caseous) appearance. It commonly occurs in pulmonary tuberculosis.
+ In *fat necrosis,* enzymes called *lipases* break down intracellular triglycerides into free fatty acids. These free fatty acids combine with sodium, magnesium, or calcium ions to form soaps. The tissue becomes opaque and chalky white.
+ *Coagulative necrosis* commonly occurs when the blood supply to any organ (except the brain) is interrupted. It typically affects the kidneys, heart, and adrenal glands. Lytic (lysosomal) enzyme activity in the cells is inhibited, so that the necrotic cells maintain their shape, at least temporarily.
+ *Gangrenous necrosis,* a form of coagulative necrosis, typically results from a lack of blood flow and is complicated by an overgrowth and invasion of bacteria. It commonly occurs in the lower legs as a result of arteriosclerosis or in the GI tract. Gangrene can occur in one of three forms: *dry, moist (or wet),* or *gas.*

Dry gangrene occurs when bacterial invasion is minimal. It's marked by dry, wrinkled, dark brown or blackened tissue on an extremity. *Moist gangrene* develops with liquefaction necrosis that includes extensive lytic activity from bacteria and WBCs to produce a liquid center in an affected area. It can occur in the internal organs as well as the extremities. *Gas gangrene* develops when anaerobic bacteria of the genus *Clostridium* infect tissue. It's more likely to occur with severe trauma and may be fatal. The bacteria release toxins that kill nearby cells and the gas gangrene rapidly spreads. Release of gas bubbles from affected muscle cells indicates that gas gangrene is present.

Factors that affect cell aging

Cell aging can be affected by the intrinsic and extrinsic factors listed below.

INTRINSIC FACTORS
- Congenital
- Degenerative
- Immunologic
- Inherited
- Metabolic
- Neoplastic
- Nutritional
- Psychogenic

EXTRINSIC FACTORS
Physical agents
- Chemicals
- Electricity
- Force
- Humidity
- Radiation
- Temperature

Infectious agents
- Bacteria
- Fungi
- Insects
- Protozoa
- Viruses
- Worms

Necrotic changes

When a cell dies, enzymes inside the cell are released and start to dissolve cellular components. This triggers an acute inflammatory reaction in which WBCs migrate to the necrotic area and begin to digest the dead cells. At this point, the dead cells — primarily the nuclei — begin to change morphologically in one of three ways.

In *pyknosis*, the nucleus of the cell shrinks, becoming a dense mass of genetic material with an irregular outline. In *karyorrhexis,* the nucleus breaks up, strewing pieces of genetic material throughout the cell. Lastly, in *karyolysis,* hydrolytic enzymes released from intracellular structures called *lysosomes* dissolve the nucleus.

Types of necrotic changes

- Pyknosis: nucleus shrinks and becomes a dense mass of genetic material
- Karyorrhexis: nucleus breaks up, strewing pieces of genetic material throughout the cell
- Karyolysis: lysosomes dissolve in the nucleus

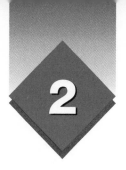

2

Cancer

Characteristics of cancer

✦ Refers to more than 100 diseases characterized by DNA damage
✦ Damage causes abnormal cell growth and development
✦ Malignant cells can no longer divide and differentiate normally and can invade surrounding tissues and travel to distant sites
✦ Accounts for more than one-half million deaths each year in the United States
✦ Most common cases in the United States are skin, prostate, breast, lung, and colorectal

Cancer, also called *malignant neoplasia*, refers to a group of more than 100 different diseases that are characterized by deoxyribonucleic acid (DNA) damage that causes abnormal cell growth and development. Malignant cells have two defining characteristics: they can no longer divide and differentiate normally, and they have acquired the ability to invade surrounding tissues and travel to distant sites.

In the United States, cancer accounts for more than one-half million deaths each year, second only to cardiovascular disease. However, a 1999 review of the Healthy People 2010 cancer objectives by the Department of Health and Human Services had encouraging results: a reversal of a 20-year trend of increasing cancer incidence and deaths. The rates for all cancers combined and for most of the top 10 cancer sites declined between 1990 and 1996.

Worldwide, the most common malignancies include skin cancer, leukemias, lymphomas, and cancers of the breast, bone, GI tract and associated structures, thyroid, lung, urinary tract, and reproductive tract. (See *Reviewing common cancers.*) In the United States, the most common forms of cancer are skin, prostate, breast, lung, and colorectal. Some cancers, such as ovarian germ-cell tumors and retinoblastoma, occur predominantly in younger patients; however, more than two-thirds of the patients who develop cancer are older than age 65.

HOW DOES CANCER HAPPEN?

Most of the numerous theories about carcinogenesis suggest that it involves three steps: initiation, promotion, and progression.

3 steps of cancer

✦ Initiation
✦ Promotion
✦ Progression

INITIATION

Initiation refers to the damage to or mutation of DNA that occurs when the cell is exposed to an initiating substance or event (such as a chemical, virus, or radiation) during DNA replication (transcription). Usually, enzymes detect errors in tran-

(*Text continues on page 24.*)

Reviewing common cancers

The chart below highlights the important signs and symptoms and diagnostic test results for some of the most common cancers.

TYPE AND FINDINGS	DIAGNOSTIC TEST RESULTS
Acute leukemia	
✦ Sudden onset of high fever resulting from bone marrow invasion and cellular proliferation within bone marrow ✦ Thrombocytopenia and abnormal bleeding secondary to bone marrow suppression ✦ Weakness and lassitude related to anemia from bone marrow invasion ✦ Pallor and weakness related to anemia ✦ Chills and recurrent infections related to proliferation of immature nonfunctioning white blood cells (WBCs) ✦ Bone pain from leukemic infiltration of bone ✦ Neurologic manifestations, including headache, papilledema, facial palsy, blurred vision, and meningeal irritation secondary to leukemic infiltration or cerebral bleeding ✦ Liver, spleen, and lymph node enlargement related to leukemic cell infiltration	✦ Bone marrow aspiration reveals proliferation of immature WBCs. ✦ Complete blood count (CBC) shows thrombocytopenia and neutropenia. ✦ Differential WBC count reveals cell type. ✦ Lumbar puncture reveals leukemic infiltration to cerebrospinal fluid (CSF).
Basal cell carcinoma	
✦ Noduloulcerative lesions usually on face (forehead, eyelid regions, and nasolabial folds) appearing as small, smooth, pinkish, and translucent papules with telangiectatic vessels crossing surface; occasionally pigmented; depressed centers; firm elevated borders with enlargement resulting from basal cell proliferation and local invasion in the deepest layer of epidermis ✦ Superficial basal cell epitheliomas, commonly on chest and back, appearing as oval or irregularly shaped, lightly pigmented scaly plaques with sharply defined, threadlike elevated borders resembling psoriasis or eczema resulting from basal cell proliferation ✦ Sclerosing basal cell epitheliomas occurring on the head and neck and appearing as waxy, sclerotic yellow to white plaques without distinct borders resulting from basal cell proliferation	✦ All types are diagnosed by clinical appearance, incisional or excisional biopsy, and histologic study.
Bladder cancer	
Early stages ✦ Commonly produces no symptoms *Later* ✦ Gross painless intermittent hematuria secondary to tumor invasion	✦ Cystoscopy and biopsy confirm cell type. ✦ Urinalysis reveals hematuria and malignant cytology. ✦ Excretory urography identifies large early stage tumor or infiltrating tumor. ✦ Retrograde cystography reveals changes in bladder structure and bladder wall integrity.

(continued)

Acute leukemia findings

✦ Sudden onset of high fever
✦ Thrombocytopenia and abnormal bleeding
✦ Weakness, lassitude, and pallor
✦ Chills and recurrent infections
✦ Bone pain
✦ Neurologic manifestations
✦ Liver, spleen, and lymph node enlargement

Basal cell carcinoma findings

✦ Noduloulcerative lesions, usually on the face
✦ Superficial basal cell epitheliomas
✦ Sclerosing basal cell epitheliomas occurring on the head and neck

Bladder cancer findings

✦ Early stages: commonly produces no symptoms
✦ Later stages: gross painless intermittent hematuria
✦ Suprapubic pain after voiding
✦ Bladder irritability and frequency

Bone cancer findings
+ May not produce symptoms
+ Bone pain, especially at night
+ Tender, swollen, palpable mass
+ Pathologic fractures
+ Hypercalcemia
+ Limited mobility (late in the disease)

Breast cancer findings
+ Hard stony mass in the breast
+ Change in symmetry of breast
+ Skin thickening or dimpling, scaly skin around nipple or changes in nipple, edema or ulceration
+ Warm, hot, pink area from inflammation and infiltration
+ Unusual discharge or drainage
+ Pain
+ Hypercalcemia or pathologic fractures

Reviewing common cancers *(continued)*

TYPE AND FINDINGS	DIAGNOSTIC TEST RESULTS
Bladder cancer *(continued)*	
+ Suprapubic pain after voiding from pressure exerted by the tumor or obstruction + Bladder irritability and frequency related to tumor compression and invasion	+ Pelvic arteriography confirms tumor invasion into bladder wall. + Computed tomography (CT) scan reveals thickened bladder wall and enlarged retroperitoneal lymph nodes. + Ultrasonography detects metastasis beyond bladder; differentiates presence of tumor from cyst.
Bone cancer	
+ May not produce symptoms + Bone pain especially at night from tumor disruption of normal structural integrity and pressure on surrounding tissues + Tender, swollen, possibly palpable mass resulting from tumor growth + Pathologic fractures secondary to tumor invasion and destruction of bone causing weakening + Hypercalcemia from ectopic parathyroid hormone production by the tumor or increased bone resorption + Limited mobility (late in the disease) from continued tumor growth and disruption of bone strength	+ Incisional or aspiration biopsy confirms cell type. + Bone X-ray, radioisotope bone scan, and CT scan reveal tumor size. + Serum alkaline phosphatase is elevated.
Breast cancer	
+ Hard stony mass in the breast related to cellular growth + Change in symmetry of breast secondary to growth of tumor on one side + Skin thickening or dimpling (peau d'orange), scaly skin around nipple or changes in nipple, edema or ulceration related to tumor cell infiltration of surrounding tissues + Warm, hot, pink area from inflammation and infiltration of surrounding tissues + Unusual discharge or drainage indicating tumor invasion and infiltration into the ductal system + Pain related to advancement of tumor and subsequent pressure + Hypercalcemia or pathologic fractures secondary to metastasis to bone	+ Breast examination reveals lump or mass in breast. + Mammography reveals presence of mass and location. + Needle or surgical biopsy confirms the cell type. + Ultrasonography reveals solid tumor differentiating it from a fluid-filled cyst. + Bone scan and CT scan reveal metastasis. + Elevated alkaline phosphatase levels, liver biopsy, and liver function studies reveal liver metastasis. + Hormonal receptor assay identifies tumor as hormone dependent.

Reviewing common cancers *(continued)*

TYPE AND FINDINGS	DIAGNOSTIC TEST RESULTS
Cervical cancer	
✦ No symptoms or other clinically apparent changes in preinvasive cervical cancer ✦ Abnormal vaginal bleeding with persistent vaginal discharge and postcoital pain and bleeding related to cellular invasion and erosion of the cervical epithelium ✦ Pelvic pain secondary to pressure on surrounding tissues and nerves from cellular proliferation ✦ Vaginal leakage of urine and feces from fistulas due to erosion and necrosis of cervix ✦ Anorexia, weight loss, and anemia related to the hypermetabolic activity of cellular proliferation and increased tumor growth needs	✦ Papanicolaou (Pap) smear reveals malignant cellular changes. ✦ Colposcopy identifies the presence and extent of early lesions. ✦ Biopsy confirms cell type. ✦ CT scan, nuclear imaging scan, and lymphangiography identify metastasis.
Chronic lymphocytic leukemia	
✦ Slow onset of fatigue related to anemia ✦ Splenomegaly secondary to increased numbers of lysed red blood cells being filtered ✦ Hepatomegaly and lymph node enlargement from infiltration by leukemic cells ✦ Bleeding tendencies secondary to thrombocytopenia ✦ Infections related to deficient humoral immunity	✦ CBC count reveals: – numerous abnormal lymphocytes with mild but persistently elevated WBC count – granulocytopenia common but WBC count increasing as disease progresses – hemoglobin levels below 11 g/dl – neutropenia (under 1,500/µl) – lymphocytosis (over 10,000/µl) – thrombocytopenia (under 150,000/µl). ✦ Serum globulin levels are decreased. ✦ Bone marrow aspiration and biopsy show lymphocytic invasion.
Colorectal cancer	
Tumor on right colon ✦ Black, tarry stools secondary to tumor erosion and necrosis of the intestinal lining ✦ Anemia secondary to increased tumor growth needs and bleeding resulting from necrosis and ulceration of mucosa ✦ Abdominal aching, pressure, or cramps secondary to pressure from tumor ✦ Weakness, fatigue, anorexia, and weight loss secondary to increased tumor growth needs ✦ As disease progresses, vomiting, related to possible obstruction *Tumor on left colon* ✦ Intestinal obstruction, including abdominal distention, pain, vomiting, cramps, and rectal pressure related to increasing tumor size and ulceration of mucosa ✦ Constipation, diarrhea, or "ribbon" or pencil-shaped stools as disease progresses ✦ Dark red or bright red blood in stools secondary to erosion and ulceration of mucosa	✦ Digital rectal examination reveals mass. ✦ Hemoccult test (guaiac) detects blood in stools. ✦ Proctoscopy or sigmoidoscopy reveals tumor mass. ✦ Colonoscopy visualizes tumor location up to the ileocecal valve. ✦ CT scan reveals areas of possible metastasis. ✦ Barium X-ray shows location and size of lesions not manually or visually detectable. ✦ Carcinoembryonic antigen (tumor marker) may be elevated.

(continued)

Cervical cancer findings

✦ No symptoms in preinvasive cervical cancer
✦ Abnormal vaginal bleeding with persistent vaginal discharge and postcoital pain and bleeding
✦ Pelvic pain
✦ Vaginal leakage of urine and feces from fistulas
✦ Anorexia, weight loss, and anemia

Chronic lymphocytic leukemia findings

✦ Slow onset of fatigue
✦ Splenomegaly
✦ Hepatomegaly and lymph node enlargement
✦ Bleeding tendencies
✦ Infections

Colorectal cancer findings

Tumor on right colon
✦ Black, tarry stools
✦ Anemia and bleeding
✦ Abdominal aching, pressure, or cramps
✦ Weakness, fatigue, anorexia, and weight loss
✦ Vomiting

Tumor on left colon
✦ Intestinal obstruction, including abdominal distention, pain, vomiting, cramps, and rectal pressure
✦ Constipation, diarrhea, or "ribbon" or pencil-shaped stools
✦ Dark red or bright red blood in stools

Esophageal cancer findings

+ Dysphagia
+ Weight loss, tumor growth and increasing obstruction and anorexia
+ Ulceration and hemorrhage
+ Fistula formation and aspiration

Hodgkin's disease findings

+ Painless swelling in a lymph node; history of upper respiratory infection
+ Persistent fever, night sweats, fatigue, weight loss, and malaise
+ Pruritus
+ Extremity pain, nerve irritation, or absence of pulses
+ Pericardial friction rub, pericardial effusion, and jugular vein engorgement
+ Enlargement of retroperitoneal nodes, spleen, and liver

Laryngeal cancer findings

+ Hoarseness persisting longer than 3 weeks
+ Lump in the throat or pain or burning when drinking citrus juice or hot liquids
+ Dysphagia
+ Dyspnea and cough
+ Enlargement of the cervical lymph nodes and pain radiating to ear

Reviewing common cancers (continued)

TYPE AND FINDINGS	DIAGNOSTIC TEST RESULTS
Esophageal cancer	
+ No early symptoms + Dysphagia secondary to tumor interfering with passageway + Weight loss resulting from dysphasia, tumor growth, and increasing obstruction and anorexia related to tumor growth needs + Ulceration and subsequent hemorrhage from erosive effects (fungating and infiltrative) of the tumor + Fistula formation and possible aspiration secondary to continued erosive tumor effects	+ Esophageal X-ray with barium swallow and motility studies reveals structural and filling defects and reduced peristalsis. + Endoscopic examination with punch and brush biopsies confirms cancer cell type.
Hodgkin's disease	
+ Painless swelling in a lymph node (usually the cervical region) with a history of upper respiratory infection + Persistent fever, night sweats, fatigue, weight loss, and malaise related to hypermetabolic state of cellular proliferation and defective immune function + Pruritus that becomes acute as the disease progresses + Extremity pain, nerve irritation, or absence of pulse due to rapid enlargement of lymph nodes + Pericardial friction rub, pericardial effusion, and jugular vein engorgement secondary to direct invasion from mediastinal lymph nodes + Enlargement of retroperitoneal nodes, spleen, and liver related to progression of disease and cellular infiltration	+ Lymph node biopsy confirms presence of Reed-Sternberg cells, nodular fibrosis, and necrosis. + Bone marrow, liver, mediastinal, lymph node, and spleen biopsies reveal histologic presence of cells. + Chest X-ray, abdominal CT scan, lung scan, bone scan, and lymphangiography detect lymph and organ involvement. + Hematologic tests show: – mild to severe normocytic anemia – normochromic anemia – elevated, normal, or reduced WBC count – differential with any combination of neutrophilia, lymphocytopenia, monocytosis, and eosinophilia. + Elevated serum alkaline phosphatase indicates bone or liver involvement.
Laryngeal cancer	
+ Hoarseness persisting longer than 3 weeks related to encroachment on the true vocal cord + Lump in the throat or pain or burning when drinking citrus juice or hot liquids related to tumor growth + Dysphagia secondary to increasing pressure and obstruction with tumor growth + Dyspnea and cough related to progressive tumor growth and metastasis + Enlargement of cervical lymph nodes and pain radiating to ear related to invasion of lymphatic system and subsequent pressure	+ Laryngoscopy shows presence of tumor. + Xeroradiography, biopsy, laryngeal tomography, CT scan, or laryngography identifies borders of the lesion. + Chest X-ray reveals metastasis.

Reviewing common cancers *(continued)*

TYPE AND FINDINGS	DIAGNOSTIC TEST RESULTS
Liver cancer	
✦ Mass in right upper quadrant, with a tender nodular liver on palpation, secondary to tumor cell growth ✦ Severe pain in epigastrium or right upper quadrant related to tumor size and increased pressure on surrounding tissue ✦ Bruit, hum, or rubbing sound if tumor involves a large part of the liver ✦ Weight loss, weakness, and anorexia related to increased tumor growth needs ✦ Dependent edema secondary to tumor invasion and obstruction of portal veins	✦ Needle or open biopsy of the liver confirms cell type. ✦ Serum glutamic-oxaloacetic transaminase, serum glutamic-pyruvic transaminase, alkaline phosphatase, lactic dehydrogenase, and bilirubin levels are elevated, indicating abnormal liver function. ✦ Alpha-fetoprotein levels are elevated. ✦ Chest X-ray reveals possible metastasis. ✦ Liver scan may show filling defects. ✦ Serum electrolyte studies reveal hypernatremia and hypercalcemia; serum laboratory studies reveal hypoglycemia, leukocytosis, or hypocholesterolemia.
Lung cancer	
✦ Cough, hoarseness, wheezing, dyspnea, hemoptysis, and chest pain related to local infiltration of pulmonary membranes and vasculature ✦ Fever, weight loss, weakness, and anorexia related to increased tumor growth needs from hypermetabolic state of cellular proliferation ✦ Bone and joint pain from cartilage erosion due to abnormal production of growth hormone ✦ Cushing's syndrome related to abnormal production of corticotropin ✦ Hypercalcemia related to abnormal production of parathyroid hormone or bone metastasis ✦ Hemoptysis, atelectasis, pneumonitis, and dyspnea from bronchial obstruction related to increasing growth ✦ Shoulder pain and unilateral paralysis of diaphragm due to phrenic nerve involvement ✦ Dysphagia related to esophageal compression ✦ Venous distention and facial, neck, and chest edema secondary to obstruction of vena cava ✦ Piercing chest pain, increasing dyspnea, and severe arm pain secondary to invasion of the chest wall	✦ Chest X-ray shows an advanced lesion, including size and location. ✦ Sputum cytology reveals possible cell type. ✦ CT scan of the chest delineates tumor size and relationship to surrounding structures. ✦ Bronchoscopy locates tumor; washings reveal malignant cell type. ✦ Needle lung biopsy confirms cell type. ✦ Mediastinal and supraclavicular node biopsies reveal possible metastasis. ✦ Thorancentesis shows malignant cells in pleural fluid. ✦ Bone scan, bone marrow biopsy, and CT scan of brain and abdomen reveal metastasis.
Malignant brain tumors	
✦ Headache, dizziness, vertigo, nausea and vomiting, and papilledema secondary to increased intracranial pressure from tumor invasion and compression of surrounding tissues ✦ Cranial nerve dysfunction secondary to tumor invasion or compression of cranial nerves	✦ Stereotactic tissue biopsy confirms cell type. ✦ Neurologic assessment reveals manifestations of lesion affecting specific lobe. ✦ Skull X-ray, CT scan, magnetic resonance imaging (MRI), and cerebral angiography identify location of mass.

(continued)

Liver cancer findings
✦ Mass in right upper quadrant
✦ Severe pain in epigastrium or right upper quadrant
✦ Bruit, hum, or rubbing sound
✦ Weight loss, weakness, and anorexia
✦ Dependent edema

Lung cancer findings
✦ Cough, hoarseness, wheezing, dyspnea, hemoptysis, and chest pain
✦ Fever, weight loss, weakness, and anorexia
✦ Bone and joint pain
✦ Cushing's syndrome
✦ Hypercalcemia
✦ Hemoptysis, atelectasis, pneumonitis, and dyspnea
✦ Shoulder pain and unilateral paralysis of diaphragm
✦ Dysphagia
✦ Venous distention and facial, neck, and chest edema
✦ Piercing chest pain, increasing dyspnea, and severe arm pain

Malignant brain tumor findings
✦ Headache, dizziness, vertigo, nausea and vomiting, and papilledema
✦ Cranial nerve dysfunction
✦ Focal deficits and sensory disturbances
✦ Disturbances of higher function
✦ Local: dementia, personality or behavioral changes, gait disturbances, seizures, or language disorders; sensory loss, hemianopia, cranial nerve dysfunction, ataxia, pupillary abnormalities, nystagmus, hemiparesis, and autonomic dysfunction

Melanoma findings

+ Enlargement of skin lesions or nevus accompanied by changes in color, inflammation, or soreness, itching, ulceration, bleeding or textural changes
+ Superficial spreading melanoma: red, white, and blue color over a brown or black background; irregular notched margin
+ Nodular melanoma: polypoidal nodule with uniformly dark discoloration; appearing as blackberry, but possibly flesh-colored
+ Lentigo maligna melanoma: large freckle of tan, brown, black, whitish, or slate color; irregularly scattered black nodules on surface

Multiple myeloma findings

+ Severe, constant back and rib pain that increases with exercise
+ Arthritic symptoms
+ Pathologic fractures
+ Azotemia and pyelonephritis
+ Anemia, bleeding, and infections
+ Thoracic deformities and increasing vertebral complaints
+ Loss of 5″ or more of body height

Reviewing common cancers *(continued)*

TYPE AND FINDINGS	DIAGNOSTIC TEST RESULTS
Malignant brain tumors *(continued)*	
+ Focal deficits including motor deficits (weakness, paralysis, or gait disorders) and sensory disturbances (anesthesia, paresthesia, or disturbances of vision or hearing) secondary to tumor invasion or compression of motor or sensory control areas of the brain + Disturbances of higher function including defects in cognition, learning, and memory *Local* + Dementia, personality or behavioral changes, gait disturbances, seizures, or language disorders + Sensory loss, hemianopia, cranial nerve dysfunction, ataxia, pupillary abnormalities, nystagmus, hemiparesis, and autonomic dysfunction depending on location of tumor	+ Brain scan reveals area of increased uptake in location of tumor. + Lumbar puncture shows increased pressure and protein levels, decreased glucose levels and, occasionally, tumor cells in CSF.
Melanoma	
+ Enlargement of skin lesion or nevus accompanied by changes in color, inflammation or soreness, itching, ulceration, bleeding, or textural changes secondary to malignant transformation of melanocytes in the basal layer of the epidermis or within the aggregated melanocytes of an existing nevus *Superficial spreading melanoma* + Red, white, and blue color over a brown or black background with an irregular, notched margin typically on areas of chronic irritation *Nodular melanoma* + Polypoidal nodule with uniformly dark discoloration appearing as a blackberry but possibly flesh-colored with flecks of pigment around base *Lentigo maligna melanoma* + Large flat freckle of tan, brown, black, whitish, or slate color with irregularly scattered black nodules on surface	+ Skin biopsy with histologic examination confirms cell type and tumor thickness. + Chest X-ray, CT scan of chest and abdomen or brain reveals metastasis. + Bone scan reveals bone metastasis.
Multiple myeloma	
+ Severe, constant back and rib pain that increases with exercise secondary to invasion of bone + Arthritic symptoms including aching, joint swelling, and tenderness, possibly from vertebral compression + Pathologic fractures resulting from invasion of bone causing loss of structural integrity and strength	+ CBC shows moderate to severe anemia; differential may show 40% to 50% lymphocytes but seldom more than 3% plasma cells. + Differential smear reveals rouleaux formation from elevated erythrocyte sedimentation rate. + Urine studies reveal Bence Jones protein and hypercalciuria.

Reviewing common cancers *(continued)*

TYPE AND FINDINGS	DIAGNOSTIC TEST RESULTS
Multiple myeloma (continued)	

✦ Azotemia secondary to tumor proliferation to the kidney and pyelonephritis due to subsequent tubular damage from large amounts of Bence Jones protein, hypercalcemia, and hyperuricemia
✦ Anemia, bleeding, and infections secondary to tumor effects on bone marrow cell production
✦ Thoracic deformities and increasing vertebral complaints secondary to extension of tumor and continued vertebral compression
✦ Loss of 5″ (12.7 cm) or more of body height due to vertebral collapse

✦ Bone marrow aspiration detects myelomatous cells (abnormal number of immature plasma cells).
✦ Serum electrophoresis shows elevated globulin spike that's electrophoretically and immunologically abnormal.
✦ Bone X-rays early reveal diffuse osteoporosis; in later stages, they show multiple sharply circumscribed osteolytic lesions, particularly in the skull, pelvis, and spine.

Non-Hodgkin's lymphoma

✦ Swelling of the lymph glands, enlarged tonsils and adenoids, and painless, rubbery nodes in the cervical supraclavicular areas from cellular proliferation
✦ Dyspnea and coughing related to lymphocytic infiltration of oropharynx
✦ Abdominal pain and constipation secondary to mechanical obstruction of surrounding tissues

✦ Lymph node biopsy reveals cell type.
✦ Biopsy of tonsils, bone marrow, liver, bowel, or skin reveals malignant cells.
✦ CBC may show anemia.
✦ Uric acid level may be elevated or normal.
✦ Serum calcium levels are elevated if bone lesions are present.
✦ Serum protein levels are normal.
✦ Bone and chest X-rays, lymphangiography, liver and spleen scans, abdominal CT scan, and excretory urography show evidence of metastasis.

Ovarian cancer

✦ Vague abdominal discomfort, dyspepsia and other mild GI complaints from increasing size of tumor exerting pressure on nearby tissues
✦ Urinary frequency and constipation from obstruction resulting from increased tumor size
✦ Pain from tumor rupture, torsion, or infection
✦ Feminizing or masculinizing effects secondary to cellular type
✦ Ascites related to invasion and infiltration of the peritoneum
✦ Pleural effusions related to pulmonary metastasis

✦ Pap test may be normal.
✦ Abdominal ultrasound, CT scan, or X-ray delineates tumor presence and size.
✦ CBC may show anemia.
✦ Excretory urography reveals abnormal renal function and urinary tract abnormalities or obstruction.
✦ Chest X-ray reveals pleural effusion with distant metastasis.
✦ Barium enema shows obstruction and size of tumor.
✦ Lymphangiography reveals lymph node involvement.
✦ Mammography is normal to rule out breast cancer as the primary site.
✦ Liver function studies are abnormal with ascites.
✦ Paracentesis fluid aspiration reveals malignant cells.
✦ Tumor markers, such as carcinoembryonic antigen and human chorionic gonadotropin, are positive.

Non-Hodgkin's lymphoma findings
✦ Swelling of the lymph glands, enlarged tonsils and adenoids, and painless, rubbery nodes in the cervical supraclavicular areas
✦ Dyspnea and coughing
✦ Abdominal pain and constipation

Ovarian cancer findings
✦ Vague abdominal discomfort, dyspepsia, and other mild GI complaints
✦ Urinary frequency and constipation
✦ Pain
✦ Feminizing or masculinizing effects
✦ Ascites
✦ Pleural effusions

(continued)

Pancreatic cancer findings

+ Jaundice with clay-colored stools and dark urine
+ Recurrent thrombophlebitis
+ Nausea and vomiting
+ Weight loss, anorexia, and malaise
+ Abdominal or back pain
+ Blood in the stools

Prostate cancer findings

+ Symptoms appearing only in late stages
+ Difficulty initiating a urine stream, dribbling, and urine retention
+ Hematuria (rare)

Renal cancer findings

+ Pain
+ Hematuria
+ Smooth, firm, nontender mass palpable over affected kidney
+ Possible fever
+ Hypertension
+ Polycythemia
+ Hypercalcemia
+ Urine retention
+ Pulmonary hypertension

Reviewing common cancers (continued)

TYPE AND FINDINGS	DIAGNOSTIC TEST RESULTS
Pancreatic cancer	
+ Jaundice with clay-colored stools and dark urine secondary to obstruction of bile flow from tumor in head of pancreas + Recurrent thrombophlebitis from tumor cytokines acting as platelet aggregating factors + Nausea and vomiting secondary to duodenal obstruction + Weight loss, anorexia, and malaise secondary to effects of increased tumor growth needs + Abdominal or back pain secondary to tumor pressure + Blood in the stools from ulceration of GI tract or ampulla of Vater	+ Laparotomy with biopsy confirms cell type. + Ultrasound identifies location of mass. + Angiography reveals vascular supply of the tumor. + Endoscopic retrograde cholangiopancreatography visualizes tumor area. + CT scan and MRI identify tumor location and size. + Serum laboratory tests reveal increased serum bilirubin, serum amylase, and serum lipase. + Prothrombin time (PT) is prolonged. + Elevations of aspartate aminotransferase and alanine aminotransferase indicate necrosis of liver cells. + Marked elevation of alkaline phosphatase indicates biliary obstruction. + Plasma insulin immunoassay shows measurable serum insulin in the presence of islet cell tumors. + Hemoglobin levels and hematocrit may show mild anemia. + Fasting blood glucose may reveal hypoglycemia or hyperglycemia.
Prostate cancer	
+ Symptoms appearing only in late stages + Difficulty initiating a urine stream, dribbling, urine retention secondary to obstruction of urinary tract from tumor growth + Hematuria (rare) from infiltration of bladder	+ Biopsy confirms cell type. + Digital rectal examination reveals a small hard nodule. + Prostate surface antigen is elevated. + Serum acid phosphatase levels are elevated. + MRI, CT scan, and excretory urography identify tumor mass. + Elevated alkaline phosphatase levels and positive bone scan indicate bone metastasis.
Renal cancer	
+ Pain resulting from tumor pressure and invasion + Hematuria secondary to tumor spreading to renal pelvis + Smooth, firm, nontender mass palpable over affected kidney due to tumor growth + Possible fever from hemorrhage or necrosis + Hypertension from compression of renal artery with renal parenchymal ischemia and renin excess + Polycythemia secondary to erythropoietin excess	+ CT scan, I.V. and retrograde pyelography, ultrasound, cystoscopy (to rule out associated bladder cancer) and nephrotomography, and renal angiography identify presence of tumor and help differentiate it from a cyst. + Liver function tests show increased levels of alkaline phosphatase, bilirubin, alanine aminotransferase, and aspartate aminotransferase and prolonged PT. + Urinalysis reveals gross or microscopic hematuria.

Reviewing common cancers *(continued)*

TYPE AND FINDINGS	DIAGNOSTIC TEST RESULTS
Renal cancer *(continued)*	
✦ Hypercalcemia from ectopic parathyroid hormone production by the tumor or bone metastasis ✦ Urine retention secondary to obstruction of urine flow ✦ Pulmonary embolism secondary to renal venous obstruction	✦ CBC shows anemia, polycythemia, and increased erythrocyte sedimentation rate. ✦ Serum calcium levels are elevated.
Squamous cell carcinoma	
✦ Lesions on skin of the face, ears, dorsa of hands and forearms from cell proliferation in sun-damaged areas ✦ Induration and inflammation as cell changes from nonmalignant to malignant cell ✦ Ulceration and invasion of underlying tissues from continued cell proliferation	✦ Excisional biopsy confirms cell type.
Stomach cancer	
✦ Chronic dyspepsia and epigastric discomfort related to tumor growth in gastric cells and destruction of mucosal barrier ✦ Weight loss, anorexia, feelings of fullness after eating, anemia, and fatigue secondary to increased tumor growth needs ✦ Blood in stools from erosion of gastric mucosa by tumor	✦ Barium X-ray with fluoroscopy shows tumor or filling defects in outline of stomach, loss of flexibility and distensibility, and abnormal mucosa with or without ulceration. ✦ Gastroscopy with fiberoptic endoscopy visualizes gastric mucosa including presence of gastric lesions for biopsy. ✦ CT scans, X-rays, liver and bone scans, and liver biopsy reveal metastasis.
Testicular cancer	
✦ Firm, painless, smooth testicular mass and occasional complaints of heaviness secondary to tumor growth ✦ Gynecomastia and nipple tenderness related to tumor production of chorionic gonadotropin or estrogen ✦ Urinary complaints related to ureteral obstruction ✦ Cough, hemoptysis, and shortness of breath from invasion of the pulmonary system	✦ Testicular palpation reveals detectable mass. ✦ Transillumination of the testicles reveals a tumor that doesn't transilluminate. ✦ Surgical excision and biopsy reveal cell type; inguinal exploration determines the extent of nodal involvement. ✦ Excretory urography detects ureteral deviation from para-aortic node involvement. ✦ Serum alpha-fetoprotein and beta human chorionic gonadotropin levels as tumor markers are elevated. ✦ Lymphangiography, ultrasound, and abdominal CT scan reveal mass and possible metastasis.

Squamous cell carcinoma findings

✦ Lesions on skin of face, ears, dorsa of hands and forearms
✦ Induration and inflammation
✦ Ulceration and invasion of underlying tissues

Stomach cancer findings

✦ Chronic dyspepsia and epigastric discomfort
✦ Weight loss, anorexia, feelings of fullness after eating, anemia, and fatigue
✦ Blood in stools

Testicular cancer findings

✦ Firm, painless, smooth testicular mass and occasional complaints of heaviness
✦ Gynecomastia and nipple tenderness
✦ Urinary complaints
✦ Cough, hemoptysis, and shortness of breath

(continued)

Thyroid cancer findings
◆ Painless or hard nodule
◆ Hoarseness, dysphagia, and dyspnea
◆ Hyperthyroidism
◆ Hypothyroidism

Uterine cancer findings
◆ Uterine enlargement
◆ Postmenopausal bleeding or persistent unusual pre-menopausal bleeding
◆ Pain and weight loss

Promotion and progression
Promotion
◆ Involves the mutated cell's exposure to factors that enhance its growth
◆ Exposure may occur after initiation or years later
◆ May be hormones, food additives, or drugs

Progression
◆ Late promotion phase
◆ Tumor invades, metastasizes, and becomes resistant to drugs
◆ Irreversible

Reviewing common cancers *(continued)*

TYPE AND FINDINGS	DIAGNOSTIC TEST RESULTS
Thyroid cancer	
◆ Painless nodule or hard nodule in an enlarged thyroid gland or palpable lymph nodes with thyroid enlargement reflecting tumor growth ◆ Hoarseness, dysphagia, and dyspnea from increased tumor growth and pressure on surrounding structures ◆ Hyperthyroidism from excess thyroid hormone production from tumor ◆ Hypothyroidism secondary to tumor destruction of the gland	◆ Thyroid scan reveals hypofunctional nodes or cold spots. ◆ Needle biopsy confirms cell type. ◆ CT scan, ultrasound, and chest X-ray reveal medullary cancer.
Uterine (endometrial) cancer	
◆ Uterine enlargement secondary to tumor growth ◆ Postmenopausal bleeding or persistent and unusual premenopausal bleeding from erosive effects of tumor growth ◆ Pain and weight loss related to progressive infiltration and invasion of tumor cells and continued cellular proliferation	◆ Endometrial, cervical, and endocervical biopsies are positive for malignant cells, revealing cell type. ◆ Dilatation and curettage identifies malignancy in patients whose biopsies were negative. ◆ Multiple cervical biopsies and endocervical curettage pinpoint cervical involvement. ◆ Schiller's test reveals cervix resistant to staining (indicating cancerous tissues). ◆ Chest X-ray and CT scan reveal metastasis. ◆ Barium enema identifies possible bladder or rectal involvement.

scription and remove or repair them. Sometimes, however, an error is missed. If regulatory proteins recognize the error and block further division, then the error may be repaired or the cell may self-destruct. If these proteins miss the error, it becomes a permanent mutation that's passed on to future generations of cells.

PROMOTION
Promotion involves the mutated cell's exposure to promoters (*factors*) that enhance its growth. This exposure may occur shortly after initiation or years later.

Promoters may be hormones such as estrogen, food additives such as nitrates, or drugs such as nicotine. Promoters can affect the mutated cell by altering the function of genes that control cell growth and duplication, the cellular response to growth stimulators or inhibitors, and intercellular communication.

PROGRESSION
Some investigators believe that progression is a late promotion phase in which the tumor invades, metastasizes, and becomes resistant to drugs. This step is irreversible.

CAUSES

The healthy body is well equipped to defend itself against cancer. Only when the immune system and other defenses fail does cancer prevail.

Current evidence suggests that cancer develops from a complex interaction of exposure to carcinogens and accumulated mutations in several genes. Researchers have identified approximately 100 cancer genes. Some cancer genes, called *oncogenes*, activate cell division and influence embryonic development. Other cancer genes, the *tumor-suppressor genes*, halt cell division. Normal human cells typically contain proto-oncogenes (oncogene precursors) and tumor-suppressor genes that remain dormant unless they're transformed by genetic or acquired mutation.

Common causes of acquired genetic damage are viruses, radiation, environmental and dietary carcinogens, and hormones. Other factors that interact to increase a person's risk of developing cancer are age, nutritional status, hormonal balance, and response to stress.

GENETICS

Some cancers and precancerous lesions may result from genetic predisposition, either directly or indirectly. Direct causation occurs when a single gene is responsible for the cancer, as in Wilms' tumor and retinoblastoma, for example. Indirect carcinogenesis is associated with inherited conditions, such as Down syndrome or immunodeficiency diseases. Common characteristics of genetically predisposed cancer include early onset of malignant disease, increased incidence of bilateral cancer in paired organs (breasts, adrenal glands, kidneys, and eighth cranial nerves [acoustic neuroma]), increased incidence of multiple primary cancers in nonpaired organs, and abnormal chromosome complement in tumor cells.

VIRUSES

Viral proto-oncogenes typically contain DNA that's identical to that of human oncogenes. In animal studies of viral ability to transform cells, some viruses that infect people have demonstrated the potential to cause cancer. For example, the Epstein-Barr virus, which causes infectious mononucleosis, has been linked to Burkitt's lymphoma and nasopharyngeal carcinoma.

FAILURE OF IMMUNOSURVEILLANCE

Research suggests that cancer cells develop continually, but the immune system recognizes these cells as foreign and destroys them. This defense mechanism, termed immunosurveillance, has two major components: *cell-mediated* immune response and *humoral* immune response. Together these two components interact to promote antibody production, cellular immunity, and immunologic memory. Researchers believe that an intact immune system is responsible for spontaneous regression of tumors. Thus, cancer development is a concern for patients who must take immunosuppressant medications.

Cell-mediated immune response

Cancer cells carry cell-surface antigens (specialized protein molecules that trigger an immune response) called tumor-associated antigens (TAAs) and tumor-specific antigens (TSAs). The cell-mediated immune response begins when T lymphocytes encounter a TAA or a TSA and become sensitized to it. After repeated contacts, the sensitized T cells release chemical factors called *lymphokines*, some of which begin

Causes

Acquired
- Viruses
- Radiation
- Environmental and dietary carcinogens
- Hormones

Increase risk
- Age
- Nutritional status
- Hormonal balance
- Response to stress

Key facts about genetics

- Direct causation: a single gene is responsible for cancer
- Indirect carcinogenesis: inherited conditions

Key facts about viruses

- Viral proto-oncogenes contain DNA identical to human oncogenes
- Some infectious viruses have the potential to cause cancer

Immunosurveilance

- A defense mechanism against cancer cells
- Cell-mediated immune response and humoral immune response
- Promotes antibody production, cellular immunity, and immunologic memory
- Intact immune system responsible for spontaneous tumor regression

26 CANCER

How the cell-mediated response occurs
- T lymphocytes encounter a TAA or TSA and become sensitized to it
- Sensitized T cells release lymphokines, triggering the transformation of T lymphocytes into "killer T lymphocytes"

How the humoral immune response occurs
- Reacts to TAA by triggering antibody release and destroying the antigen-bearing cells
- "Blocking antibody" may enhance tumor growth by protecting malignant cells

How a disruption of the immune response occurs
- Failure of immune system to recognize tumor cells as foreign
- Tumor cells suppress immune defenses
- Tumor antigens combine with humoral antibodies that hide the antigens
- Tumors may change antigenic appearance
- Prolonged exposure to tumor antigen depletes lymphocytes
- Suppressor T lymphocytes may be inadequate

Factors that disrupt immune response
- Aging cells
- Cytotoxic drugs or steroids
- Extreme stress or certain viral infections
- Suppression of immune system
- AIDS
- Cancer

to destroy the antigen. This reaction triggers the transformation of a different population of T lymphocytes into "killer T lymphocytes" targeted to cells carrying the specific antigen—in this case, cancer cells.

Humoral immune response
The humoral immune response reacts to a TAA by triggering the release of antibodies from plasma cells and activating the serum-complement system to destroy the antigen-bearing cells. However, an opposing immune factor, a "blocking antibody," may enhance tumor growth by protecting malignant cells from immune destruction.

Disruption of the immune response
Immunosurveillance isn't a fail-safe system. If the immune system fails to recognize tumor cells as foreign, the immune response won't activate. The tumor will continue to grow until it's beyond the immune system's ability to destroy it. In addition to this failure of surveillance, other mechanisms may come into play.

The tumor cells may suppress the immune defenses. The tumor antigens may combine with humoral antibodies to form complexes that essentially hide the antigens from the normal immune defenses. These complexes could also depress further antibody production. Tumors may also change their antigenic "appearance" or produce substances that impair usual immune defenses. The tumor growth factors not only promote the growth of the tumor, but also increase the person's risk of infection. Finally, prolonged exposure to a tumor antigen may deplete the patient's lymphocytes and further impair the ability to mount an appropriate response.

The patient's population of suppressor T lymphocytes may be inadequate to defend against malignant tumors. Suppressor T lymphocytes usually assist in regulating antibody production; they also signal the immune system when an immune response is no longer needed. Certain carcinogens, such as viruses or chemicals, may weaken the immune system by destroying or damaging suppressor T cells or their precursors, and subsequently allow for tumor growth.

Theoretically, cancer develops when any of several factors disrupts the immune response:
- *Aging cells.* As cells age, errors in copying genetic material during cell division may give rise to mutations. If the aging immune system doesn't recognize these mutations as foreign, the mutated cells may proliferate and form a tumor.
- *Cytotoxic drugs or steroids.* These agents decrease antibody production and destroy circulating lymphocytes.
- *Extreme stress or certain viral infections.* These conditions may depress the immune response, thus allowing cancer cells to proliferate.
- *Suppression of immune system.* Radiation, cytotoxic drug therapy, and lymphoproliferative and myeloproliferative diseases (such as lymphatic and myelocytic leukemia) depress bone marrow production and impair leukocyte function.
- *Acquired immunodeficiency syndrome.* This condition weakens the cell-mediated immune response.
- *Cancer.* The disease itself is immunosuppressive. Advanced disease exhausts the immune system, leading to anergy (the absence of immune reactivity).

RISK FACTORS
Many cancers are related to specific environmental and lifestyle factors that predispose a person to develop cancer. Accumulated data suggest that some of these risk

factors initiate carcinogenesis, other risk factors act as promoters, and some risk factors initiate and promote the disease process.

AIR POLLUTION

Air pollution has been linked to the development of cancer, particularly lung cancer. Persons living near industries that release toxic chemicals have a documented increased risk of cancer. Many outdoor air pollutants—such as arsenic, benzene, hydrocarbons, polyvinyl chlorides, and other industrial emissions as well as vehicle exhaust—have been studied for their carcinogenic properties.

Indoor air pollution, such as from cigarette smoke and radon, also poses an increased risk of cancer. In fact, indoor air pollution is considered to be more carcinogenic than outdoor air pollution.

TOBACCO

Cigarette smoking increases the risk of lung cancer more than tenfold over that of nonsmokers by late middle age. Tobacco smoke contains nitrosamines and polycyclic hydrocarbons, two carcinogens that are known to cause mutations. The risk of lung cancer from cigarette smoking correlates directly with the duration of smoking and the number of cigarettes smoked per day. Tobacco smoke is also associated with laryngeal cancer and is considered a contributing factor in cancer of the bladder, pancreas, kidney, and cervix. Research also shows that a person who stops smoking decreases his or her risk of lung cancer.

Although the risk associated with pipe and cigar smoking is similar to that of cigarette smoking, some evidence suggests that the effects are less severe. Smoke from cigars and pipes is more alkaline. This alkalinity decreases nicotine absorption in the lungs and is more irritating to the lungs, so that the smoker doesn't inhale as readily.

Inhalation of "secondhand" smoke, or passive smoking, by nonsmokers also increases the risk of lung and other cancers. Use of smokeless tobacco, in which the oral tissue directly absorbs nicotine and other carcinogens, is linked to an increase in oral cancers that seldom occur in persons who don't use the product.

ALCOHOL

Alcohol consumption, especially in conjunction with cigarette smoking, is commonly associated with cirrhosis of the liver, a precursor to hepatocellular cancer. The risk of breast and colorectal cancers also increases with alcohol consumption. Possible mechanisms for breast cancer development include impaired removal of carcinogens by the liver, impaired immune response, and interference with cell membrane permeability of the breast tissue. Alcohol stimulates rectal cell proliferation in rats, an observation that may help explain the increased incidence of colorectal cancer in humans.

Heavy use of alcohol and cigarette smoking synergistically increase the incidence of cancers of the mouth, larynx, pharynx, and esophagus. Alcohol probably acts as a solvent for the carcinogenic substances found in smoke, enhancing their absorption.

SEXUAL AND REPRODUCTIVE BEHAVIOR

Sexual practices have been linked to specific types of cancer. The age of first sexual intercourse and the number of sexual partners are positively correlated with a woman's risk of cervical cancer. Furthermore, a woman who has had only one sex-

Risk factors

Air pollution
- Linked to lung cancer
- Outdoor air pollutants include arsenic, benzene, hydrocarbons, and polyvinyl chlorides
- Indoor air pollutants include cigarette smoke and radon; more carcinogenic than outdoor air

Tobacco
- Cigarette smoking increases lung cancer risk tenfold
- Contains nitrosamines and polycyclic hydrocarbons
- Risk correlates with duration of smoking and number of cigarettes smoked per day
- Quitting smoking decreases lung cancer risk
- Pipe and cigar smoking may cause fewer health problems
- Secondhand smoke increases lung and other cancer risk
- Smokeless tobacco is linked to oral cancers

Alcohol
- Associated with cirrhosis of the liver
- Increases risk of breast and colorectal cancers
- Heavy use combined with cigarette smoking increases incidence of cancers of the mouth, larynx, pharynx, and esophagus

Sexual and reproductive behavior
- Age of first sexual intercourse and number of partners correlates with risk of cervical cancer
- Virus transmission of HPV is likely responsible

Risk factors

Occupation
+ Exposure to asbestos increases risk of mesothelioma
+ Involvement in the production of dyes, rubber, paint, and beta-naphthylamine causes increased risk of bladder cancer

Ultraviolet radiation
+ Exposure causes genetic mutation in P53 control gene
+ Sunlight releases tumor necrosis factor alpha in exposed skin, diminishing the immune response
+ Exposure amount correlates with type of cancer developed

Ionizing radiation
+ Associated with acute leukemia; thyroid, breast, lung, stomach, colon, and urinary tract cancers; and multiple myeloma
+ Enhances effects of genetic abnormalities
+ Compounding variables: part and percentage of body exposed, age, hormonal balance, prescribed drugs, preexisting conditions

Hormones
+ Implicated as promoters of breast, endometrial, ovarian, or prostate cancer
+ Estrogen promotes breast and endometrial cancers
+ Male sex hormones stimulate growth of prostatic tissue

ual partner is at higher risk if that partner has had multiple partners. The suspected underlying mechanism here involves virus transmission, most likely human papillomavirus (HPV). HPV types 6 and 11 are associated with genital warts. HPV is the most common cause of abnormal Papanicolaou smears, and cervical dysplasia is a direct precursor to squamous cell carcinoma of the cervix, both of which have been linked to HPV (especially types 16 and 31).

OCCUPATION

Because of exposure to specific substances, certain occupations increase the risk of cancer. People exposed to asbestos, such as insulation installers and miners, are at risk for a type of lung cancer called mesothelioma. Asbestos may also act as a promoter for other carcinogens. Workers involved in the production of dyes, rubber, paint, and beta-naphthylamine are at increased risk for bladder cancer.

ULTRAVIOLET RADIATION

Exposure to ultraviolet radiation, or sunlight, causes genetic mutation in the P53 control gene. Sunlight also releases tumor necrosis factor alpha in exposed skin, possibly diminishing the immune response. Ultraviolet sunlight is a direct cause of basal and squamous cell cancers of the skin. The amount of exposure to ultraviolet radiation also correlates with the type of cancer that develops. For example, cumulative exposure to ultraviolet sunlight is associated with basal and squamous cell skin cancer, and severe episodes of burning and blistering at a young age are associated with melanoma.

IONIZING RADIATION

Ionizing radiation (such as X-rays) is associated with acute leukemia; thyroid, breast, lung, stomach, colon, and urinary tract cancers; and multiple myeloma. Low doses can cause DNA mutations and chromosomal abnormalities, and large doses can inhibit cell division. This damage can directly affect carbohydrate, protein, lipid, and nucleic acids (macromolecules), or it can act on intracellular water to produce free radicals that damage the macromolecules.

Ionizing radiation can also enhance the effects of genetic abnormalities. For example, it increases the risk of cancer in people with a genetic abnormality that affects DNA repair mechanisms. Other compounding variables include the part and percentage of the body exposed, the person's age, hormonal balance, prescribed drugs, and preexisting or concurrent conditions.

HORMONES

Hormones — specifically the sex steroid hormones estrogen, progesterone, and testosterone — have been implicated as promoters of breast, endometrial, ovarian, or prostate cancer.

Estrogen, which stimulates the proliferation of breast and endometrial cells, is considered a promoter for breast and endometrial cancers. Prolonged exposure to estrogen, as in women with early menarche and late menopause, increases the risk of breast cancer. Likewise, long-term use of estrogen replacement without progesterone supplementation for menopausal symptoms increases a woman's risk of endometrial cancer. Progesterone may play a protective role, counteracting estrogen's stimulatory effects.

ACS guidelines:
Diet, nutrition, and cancer prevention

Because of the numerous aspects of diet and nutrition that may contribute to the development of cancer, the American Cancer Society (ACS) has developed a list of guidelines to reduce cancer risk in people age 2 and older.

◆ Choose most of the foods you eat from plant sources.
   – Eat five or more servings of fruits and vegetables each day.
   – Eat other foods from plant sources, such as breads, cereals, grain products, rice, pasta, or beans several times each day.
◆ Limit your intake of high-fat foods, particularly from animal sources.
   – Choose low-fat foods.
   – Limit consumption of meats, especially high-fat and red meats.

◆ Be physically active and achieve and maintain a healthy weight.
   – Be at least moderately active for 60 minutes or more on most days of the week.
   – Stay within your healthy weight range.
◆ Limit your consumption of alcoholic beverages, if you drink at all.

The male sex hormones stimulate the growth of prostatic tissue. However, research fails to show an increased risk of prostate cancer in men who take exogenous androgens.

DIET

Numerous aspects of diet are linked to an increase in cancer. For example, obesity in women is linked to a suspected increased risk of endometrial cancer. A high consumption of dietary fat is linked to endometrial, breast, prostatic, ovarian, and rectal cancers, whereas a high consumption of smoked foods, salted fish or meats, and foods containing nitrites may be linked to gastric cancer. Naturally occurring carcinogens (such as hydrazines and aflatoxin) in foods have been linked to an increased incidence in liver cancer, and carcinogens produced by microorganisms have been linked to stomach cancer. A low-fiber diet slows transport through the gut and has been linked to colorectal cancer.

The American Cancer Society (ACS) has developed specific nutritional guidelines for cancer prevention. (See *ACS guidelines: Diet, nutrition, and cancer prevention.*)

PATHOPHYSIOLOGIC CHANGES

Cancer's characteristic features are rapid, uncontrollable proliferation of cells and independent spread from a primary site (site of origin) to other tissues where it establishes secondary foci (metastasis). This spread occurs through circulation in the blood or lymphatic fluid, by unintentional transplantation from one site to another during surgery, and by local extension. Cancer cells have the ability to travel to distant tissues and organ systems. (See *Cancer cell characteristics*, page 30.)

CELL GROWTH

Typically, each of the billions of cells in the human body has an internal clock that tells the cell when it's time to reproduce. Mitotic reproduction occurs in a sequence

ACS diet guidelines

◆ Eat food from plant sources
◆ Limit high-fat foods
◆ Be physically active
◆ Limit consumption of alcoholic beverages

Risk factors

Diet
◆ Obesity linked to endometrial cancer
◆ High consumption of dietary fat linked to endometrial, breast, prostate, ovarian, and rectal cancer
◆ High consumption of smoked foods linked to gastric cancer
◆ Naturally occurring carcinogens linked to liver cancer
◆ Carcinogens produced by microorganisms in food linked to stomach cancer
◆ Low-fiber diet linked to colorectal cancer

Key facts about pathophysiologic changes

◆ Cancer features rapid, uncontrollable proliferation of cells and spreads from primary site to where it metastasizes
◆ Spread occurs through circulation in blood or lymphatic fluid, unintentional transplantation, or local extension
◆ Cells able to travel to distant tissues and organ systems

Key characteristics of cancer cells

✦ Vary in size and shape
✦ Function abnormally
✦ Can spread to other sites

Key facts about cell growth

✦ Cell cycle is mitotic reproduction
✦ Mechanism for controlling growth and differentiation is absent in cancer cells
✦ Cancer cells commonly found in the synthesis and mitosis phases of cell cycle
✦ Normal cells reproduce at a controlled rate
✦ Hormones, growth factors, and chemicals can control gene activity
✦ Substances released by injured or infected cells can affect cellular reproduction
✦ Cells close to one another communicate through gap junctions
✦ The control genes fail to function normally in cancer cells
✦ Cancer cells fail to recognize signals emitted by nearby cells regarding available tissue space
✦ Autonomy is the loss of control over normal growth

Cancer cell characteristics

Cancer cells, which undergo uncontrolled cellular growth and development, typically exhibit these characteristics:

✦ Vary in size and shape
✦ Undergo abnormal mitosis
✦ Function abnormally
✦ Don't resemble the cell of origin
✦ Produce substances not usually associated with the original cell or tissue
✦ Aren't encapsulated
✦ Can spread to other sites

---

called the cell cycle. Normal cell division occurs in direct proportion to cells lost, thus providing a mechanism for controlling growth and differentiation. These controls are absent in cancer cells, and cell production exceeds cell loss. Consequently, cancer cells enter the cell cycle more frequently and at different rates. They're most commonly found in the synthesis and mitosis phases of the cell cycle, and they spend very little time in the resting phase. Cancer cells differ from normal cells in terms of cell size, shape, number, differentiation, and purpose or function.

Normal cells reproduce at a rate controlled through the activity of specific control or regulator genes (called proto-oncogenes when they function normally). These genes produce proteins that act as "on" and "off" switches. There's no generalized control gene; different cells respond to specific control genes. The P53 and c-myc genes are two examples of control genes: P53 can stop DNA replication if the cell's DNA has been damaged; c-myc helps initiate DNA replication and if it senses an error in DNA replication, it can cause the cell to self-destruct.

GENE ACTIVITY

Hormones, growth factors, and chemicals released by neighboring cells or by immune or inflammatory cells can affect control gene activity. These substances bind to specific receptors on the cell membranes and send out signals causing the control genes to stimulate or suppress cell reproduction. Examples of hormones and growth factors that affect control genes include erythropoietin, which stimulates red blood cell (RBC) proliferation; epidermal growth factor, which stimulates epidermal cell proliferation; insulin-like growth factor, which stimulates fat and connective tissue proliferation; and platelet-derived growth factor, which stimulates connective tissue cell proliferation.

Substances released by injured or infected nearby cells or by cells of the immune system also affect cellular reproduction. For example, interleukin, released by immune cells, stimulates cell proliferation and differentiation, and interferon, released from virus-infected and immune cells, may affect the cell's rate of reproduction.

Additionally, cells that are close to one another appear to communicate with each other through gap junctions (channels through which ions and other small molecules pass). This communication provides information to the cell about the neighboring cell types and the amount of space available. The nearby cells send out physical and chemical signals that control the reproduction rate. For example, if the area is crowded, the nearby cells will signal the same type of cells to slow or cease reproduction, thus allowing the formation of only a single layer of cells. This feature is called *density-dependent growth inhibition*.

In cancer cells, the control genes fail to function normally. The control may be lost or the gene may become damaged. An imbalance of growth factors may occur, or the cells may fail to respond to the suppressive action of the growth factors. Any of these mechanisms may lead to uncontrolled cellular reproduction.

Understanding anaplasia

Anaplasia refers to the loss of differentiation, a common characteristic of cancer cells. As differentiation is lost, the cancer cells no longer demonstrate the appearance and function of the original cell.

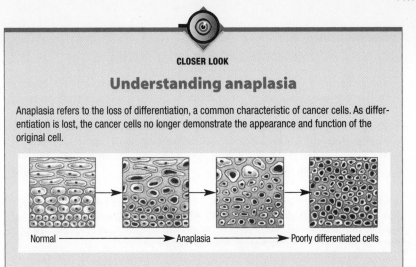

Normal ⟶ Anaplasia ⟶ Poorly differentiated cells

One striking characteristic of cancer cells is that they fail to recognize the signals emitted by nearby cells about available tissue space. Instead of forming only a single layer, cancer cells continue to accumulate in a disorderly array.

The loss of control over normal growth is termed *autonomy*. This independence is further evidenced by the ability of cancer cells to break off and travel to other sites.

DIFFERENTIATION

Usually, cells become specialized during development. That is, the cells develop highly individualized characteristics that reflect their specific structure and functions in their corresponding tissue. For example, all blood cells are derived from a single stem cell that differentiates into RBCs, white blood cells (WBCs), platelets, monocytes, and lymphocytes. As the cells become more specialized, their reproduction and development slow down. Eventually, highly differentiated cells become unable to reproduce and some, skin cells for example, are programmed to die and be replaced.

Cancer cells lose the ability to differentiate; that is, they enter a state, called *anaplasia*, in which they no longer appear or function like the original cell. (See *Understanding anaplasia.*)

Anaplasia occurs in varying degrees. The less the cells resemble the cell of origin, the more anaplastic they're said to be. As the anaplastic cells continue to reproduce, they lose the typical characteristics of the original cell.

Some anaplastic cells begin functioning as another type of cell, possibly becoming a site for hormone production. For example, oat-cell lung cancer cells typically produce antidiuretic hormone, which is produced by the hypothalamus but stored in and secreted by the posterior pituitary gland.

When anaplasia occurs, cells of the same type in the same site exhibit many different shapes and sizes. Mitosis is abnormal and chromosome defects are common.

INTRACELLULAR CHANGES

The abnormal and uncontrolled cell proliferation of cancer cells is associated with numerous changes within the cancer cell itself. These changes affect the cell membrane, cytoskeleton, and nucleus.

Key facts about differentiation

+ Cancer cells lose ability to differentiate; enter anaplasia state
+ No longer appear or function like original cell
+ Anaplasia occurs in varying degrees
+ Some anaplastic cells begin functioning as another type of cell
+ Cells of the same type in the same site exhibit different shapes and sizes

Cell membrane

This thin, dynamic semipermeable structure separates the cell's internal environment from its external environment. It consists of two layers of lipid molecules (called the lipid bilayer) with protein molecules attached to or embedded in each layer. The bilayer is composed of phospholipids, glycolipids, and other lipids such as cholesterol.

The protein molecules help stabilize the structure of the membrane and participate in the transport and exchange of material between the cell and its environment. Large glycoproteins, called fibronectin, are responsible for holding the cells in place and maintaining the specific arrangement of the receptors to allow for the exchange of material.

In the cancer cell, fibronectin is defective or is broken down as it's produced, thus affecting the organization, structure, adhesion, and migration of the cells. Some of the other proteins and glycolipids are also absent or altered. These changes affect the density of the receptors on the cell membrane and the cell's shape. Communication between the cells becomes impaired, response to growth factors is enhanced, and recognition of other cells is diminished. The result is uncontrolled growth.

Permeability of the cancer cell membrane is also altered. During its uncontrolled, rapid proliferation, the cancer cell has a much greater metabolic demand for nutrients to sustain its growth.

During normal development, cell division can occur only when the cells are anchored to nearby cells or to extracellular molecules via anchoring junctions. In cancer cells, anchoring junctions don't need to be present. Thus, they continue to divide and can metastasize.

Disruption or blockage of gap junctions interferes with intercellular communication. This may be the underlying mechanism by which cancer cells continue to grow and migrate, forming layers of undifferentiated cells, even in a crowded environment.

Cytoskeleton

The *cytoskeleton* is composed of protein filament networks including actin and microtubules. Usually, actin filaments exert a pull on the extracellular organic molecules that bind cells together. Microtubules control cell shape, movement, and division. In cancer cells, the functions of these components are altered. Additionally, cytoplasmic components are fewer and abnormally shaped. Less cellular work occurs because of a decrease in endoplasmic reticulum and mitochondria.

Nucleus

In cancer cells, nuclei are pleomorphic, meaning enlarged and of various shapes and sizes. They're also highly pigmented and have larger and more numerous nucleoli than normal. The nuclear membrane is typically irregular and commonly has projections, pouches, or blebs and fewer pores. Chromatin (uncoiled chromosomes) may clump along the outer areas of the nucleus. Breaks, deletions, translocations, and abnormal karyotypes (chromosome shape and number) are common changes in the chromosomes. The chromosome defects seem to stem from the increased mitotic rate in cancer cells. The appearance of the mitotic cancer cell under light microscopy is commonly described as atypical and bizarre.

TUMOR DEVELOPMENT AND GROWTH

Typically, a long time passes between the initiating event and the onset of the disease. During this time, the cancer cells continue to grow, develop, and replicate, each time undergoing successive changes and further mutations.

How fast a tumor grows depends on specific characteristics of the tumor itself and the host.

Tumor growth needs

For a tumor to grow, an initiating event or events must cause a mutation that will transform the normal cell into a cancer cell. After the initial event, the tumor continues to grow only if available nutrients, oxygen, and blood supply are adequate and the immune system fails to recognize or respond to the tumor.

Effects of tumor characteristics

Two important tumor characteristics affecting growth are tumor location and available blood supply. The location determines the originating cell type, which in turn determines the cell cycle time. For example, epithelial cells have a shorter cell cycle than connective tissue cells. Thus, tumors of epithelial cells grow more rapidly than do tumors of connective tissue cells.

Tumors need an available blood supply to provide nutrients and oxygen for continued growth and to remove wastes; however, a tumor larger than 1 to 2 mm has typically outgrown its available blood supply. Some tumors secrete tumor angiogenesis factors, which stimulate the formation of new blood vessels, to meet the demand.

The degree of anaplasia also affects tumor growth. Remember that the more anaplastic the tumor's cells, the less differentiated the cells and the more rapidly they divide.

Many cancer cells also produce their own growth factors. Numerous growth factor receptors are present on the cell membranes of rapidly growing cancer cells. This increase in receptors, in conjunction with the changes in the cell membranes, further enhances cancer cell proliferation.

Effects of host characteristics

Several important characteristics of the host affect tumor growth. These characteristics include age, gender, overall health status, and immune system function.

 CLINICAL ALERT Age is an important factor affecting tumor growth. Relatively few cancers are found in children. The incidence of cancer correlates directly with increasing age, suggesting that numerous or cumulative events are necessary for the initial mutation to continue, eventually forming a tumor.

Sex hormones influence tumor growth in the breast, endometrium, cervix, and prostate. Researchers believe that sex hormones sensitize the cell to the initial precipitating factor, thus promoting carcinogenesis.

Overall health status is also an important characteristic. As tumors obtain nutrients for growth from the host, they can alter normal body processes and cause cachexia. Conversely, if the person is nutritionally depleted, tumor growth may slow. Chronic tissue trauma also has been linked with tumor growth because healing involves increased cell division. The more rapidly cells divide, the greater the likelihood of mutations.

Development and growth of tumors
+ Initiating event occurs, causing a mutation that transforms normal cell into cancer cell
+ Tumor will grow if nutrients, oxygen, and blood supply are adequate and it goes unrecognized by immune system

Tumor effects
Location
+ Determines originating cell type which determines cell cycle time

Blood supply
+ Is needed to provide nutrients and oxygen to tumor
+ A 1 to 2 mm tumor has outgrown its available blood supply; stimulation of new blood vessels to meet demand occurs

Host characteristics affecting tumors
+ Age
+ Gender
+ Overall health status
+ Immune system functions

Alert!
+ Age is an important factor in tumor growth.
+ Cancer incidence correlates with increasing age.
+ Suggests that numerous events are necessary for the initial mutation to continue and form a tumor.

How cancer is spread

- After initial event, some mutated cells may die.
- Survivors reproduce until the tumor becomes 1 to 2 mm.
- New blood vessels form to support growth.
- Number of cancer cells exceeds normal cells.
- Tumor mass extends, invading surrounding tissue.
- Process is called *metastasis*.

Spread of various cancer cells

Dysplasia
- Change in size, shape, and organization of cells
- Not always sign of cancer
- Precancerous or dysplastic lesions can progress to cancer

Localized tumor
- Initial phase of all tumors
- Cells continue to grow and form masses; masses block blood supply, can cause neighboring cells to die

Invasive tumor
- Invasion is first step in metastasis
- Interaction of five mechanisms needed for invasion: cellular multiplication, mechanical pressure, lysis of nearby cells, reduced cell adhesion, and increased motility
- Loss of mechanical resistance causes cancer cells to spread
- Reduced cell adhesion occurs
- Proteolytic enzymes break through cell membrane letting in cancer cells
- Cancer cells secrete chemotactic factor that stimulates motility
- Pseudopodia facilitate cell movement

SPREAD OF CANCER

Between the initiating event and the emergence of a detectable tumor, some or all of the mutated cells may die. The survivors, if any, reproduce until the tumor reaches a diameter of 1 to 2 mm. New blood vessels form to support continued growth and proliferation. As the cells further mutate and divide more rapidly, they become more undifferentiated. The number of cancerous cells soon begins to exceed the number of normal cells. Eventually, the tumor mass extends, spreading into local tissues and invading the surrounding tissues. When the local tissue is blood or lymph, the tumor can gain access to the circulation. After access is gained, tumor cells that detach or break off travel to distant sites in the body, where tumor cells can survive and form a new tumor in that secondary site. This process is called *metastasis*.

Dysplasia

Not all cells that proliferate rapidly go on to become cancerous. Throughout a person's life span, various body tissues experience periods of benign rapid growth such as during wound healing. Sometimes changes in the size, shape, and organization of the cells leads to a condition called dysplasia.

Exposure to chemicals, viruses, radiation, or chronic inflammation causes dysplastic changes that may be reversed by removing the initiating stimulus or treating its effects. However, if the stimulus isn't removed, precancerous or dysplastic lesions can progress and give rise to cancer. For example, actinic keratoses, thickened patches on the skin of the face and hands of people exposed to sunlight, are associated with the development of skin cancer. Removal of the lesions and the use of sunblock help minimize the risk that the lesions will progress to skin cancer. Knowledge about precancerous lesions and promoter events provides the rationale for early detection and screening as important preventive measures.

Localized tumor

Initially, a tumor remains localized but because cancer cells communicate poorly with nearby cells, the cells continue to grow and enlarge, forming a mass or clumps of cells. The mass exerts pressure on the neighboring cells, blocking their blood supply and, subsequently, causing their death.

Invasive tumor

Invasion is growth of the tumor into surrounding tissues. It's the first step in metastasis. Five mechanisms are linked to invasion: cellular multiplication, mechanical pressure, lysis of nearby cells, reduced cell adhesion, and increased motility. Experimental data indicate that the interaction of all five mechanisms is necessary for invasion.

By their nature, cancer cells multiply rapidly (cellular multiplication). As they grow, they exert pressure on surrounding cells and tissues, which eventually die because their blood supply has been cut off or blocked (mechanical pressure). Loss of mechanical resistance leads the way for the cancer cells to spread along the lines of least resistance and occupy the space once filled by the dead cells.

Vesicles on the cancer cell surface contain a rich supply of receptors for laminin, a complex glycoprotein that's a major component of the basement membrane, a thin sheet of noncellular connective tissue upon which cells rest. These receptors permit the cancer cells to attach to the basement membrane, forming a bridgelike connection (lysis of nearby cells). Some cancer cells produce and excrete powerful proteolytic enzymes; other cancer cells induce normal host cells to produce them.

These enzymes, such as collagenases and proteases, destroy the normal cells and break through their basement membrane, enabling the cancer cells to enter.

Reduced cell adhesion is also seen with cancer cells. As discussed in the section on intracellular changes, reduced cell adhesion likely results when the cell-stabilizing glycoprotein fibronectin is deficient or defective. Cancer cells also secrete a chemotactic factor that stimulates motility. Thus, the cancer cells can move independently into adjacent tissues, into the circulation and, then, on to a secondary site. Finally, cancer cells develop fingerlike projections called pseudopodia that facilitate cell movement. These projections injure and kill neighboring cells and attach to vessel walls, enabling the cancer cells to enter.

Metastatic tumor

Metastatic tumors are those in which the cancer cells have traveled from the original or primary site to a second or more distant site. Most commonly, metastasis occurs through the blood vessels and lymphatic system. Tumor cells can also be transported from one body location to another by external means, such as carriage on instruments or gloves during surgery.

Hematogenous spread

Invasive tumor cells break down the basement membrane and walls of blood vessels, and the tumor sheds malignant cells into the circulation. Most of the cells die, but a few escape the host defenses and the turbulent environment of the bloodstream. From here, the surviving mass of tumor cells, called a *tumor cell embolus,* travels via the bloodstream or lymphatic system and commonly lodges in the first capillary bed it encounters.

When lodged, the tumor cells develop a protective coat of fibrin, platelets, and clotting factors to evade detection by the immune system. They then become attached to the epithelium, ultimately invading the vessel wall, interstitium, and the parenchyma of the target organ. (See *How cancer metastasizes,* page 36.) To survive, the new tumor develops its own vascular network and may ultimately spread again.

Lymphatic spread

The lymphatic system is the most common route for distant metastasis. Tumor cells enter the lymphatic vessels through damaged basement membranes and are transported to regional lymph nodes. In this case, the tumor becomes trapped in the first lymph node it encounters. The consequent enlargement, possibly the first evidence of metastasis, may be due to the increased tumor growth within the node or a localized immune reaction to the tumor. The lymph node may filter out or contain some of the tumor cells, limiting further spread. The cells that escape can enter the blood from the lymphatic circulation through plentiful connections between the venous and lymphatic systems.

Metastatic sites

Typically, the first capillary bed encountered by the circulating tumor mass determines the location of the metastasis. For example, because the lungs receive all of the systemic venous return, they're a frequent site for metastasis. In breast cancer, the axillary lymph nodes, which are close to the breast, are a common site of metastasis. Other types of cancer seem most likely to spread to specific organs. This organ tropism may be a result of growth factor or hormones secreted by the target organ or chemotactic factors that attract the tumor. (See *Common sites of metastasis,* page 37.)

Spread of various cancer cells

Metastatic tumor

✦ Hematogenous spread: invasive tumor cells break down the basement membrane of blood vessel walls; tumor sheds malignant cells into circulation; lodge in capillary bed and new tumor develops that may spread again

✦ Lymphatic spread: most common for distant metastasis; tumor becomes trapped in lymph node; enlargement occurs, as first evidence of the metastasis

✦ Metastatic sites: first capillary bed encountered by tumor mass determines location of metastasis; organ tropism may be result of growth factor or hormones secreted by the target organ

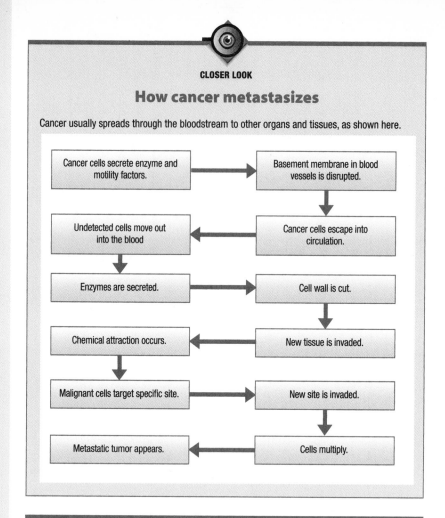

CLOSER LOOK

How cancer metastasizes

Cancer usually spreads through the bloodstream to other organs and tissues, as shown here.

Cancer cells secrete enzyme and motility factors.	Basement membrane in blood vessels is disrupted.
Undetected cells move out into the blood	Cancer cells escape into circulation.
Enzymes are secreted.	Cell wall is cut.
Chemical attraction occurs.	New tissue is invaded.
Malignant cells target specific site.	New site is invaded.
Metastatic tumor appears.	Cells multiply.

Key signs and symptoms

Fatigue

- Described as feeling of weakness
- Underlying mechanism unknown
- Believed to be the combined result of several pathophysiologic mechanisms
- Existence of tumor may contribute to fatigue; a malignant tumor needs oxygen and nutrients to grow
- Pain can be physically and emotionally draining
- Stress, anxiety, lack of energy for daily life can cause fatigue

SIGNS AND SYMPTOMS

In most patients, the earlier the cancer is found, the more effective the treatment is likely to be and the better the prognosis. Some cancers may be diagnosed on a routine physical examination, even before the person develops signs or symptoms. Others may display early warning signals. The ACS developed a mnemonic device to identify cancer's warning signs. (See *Cancer's seven warning signs,* page 38.)

Unfortunately, a person may not notice or heed the warning signs. These patients may present with some of the more common signs and symptoms of advancing disease, such as fatigue, cachexia, pain, anemia, leukopenia and thrombocytopenia, and infection. These signs and symptoms are nonspecific and can be attributed to many other disorders.

FATIGUE

Patients commonly describe fatigue as feelings of weakness, being tired, and lacking energy or the ability to concentrate. The underlying mechanism for fatigue isn't known, but it's believed to be the combined result of several pathophysiologic mechanisms.

Common sites of metastasis

The chart below lists some of the more common sites of metastasis for selected cancers.

CANCER TYPE	SITES FOR METASTASIS
Breast	Axillary lymph nodes, lung, liver, bone, brain
Colorectal	Liver, lung, peritoneum
Lung	Liver, brain, bone
Ovarian	Peritoneum, diaphragm, liver, lungs
Prostate	Bone
Testicular	Lungs, liver

The very existence of the tumor may contribute to fatigue. A malignant tumor needs oxygen and nutrients to grow. Thus, it depletes the surrounding tissues of blood and oxygen. For example, a vascular tumor can cause lethargy secondary to inadequate oxygen supply to the brain. Lung cancer can interfere with gas exchange and oxygen supply to the heart and peripheral tissues. Accumulating waste products and muscle loss from the release of toxic products of metabolism or other substances from the tumor further add to the fatigue.

Other factors also play a role in fatigue. Pain can be physically and emotionally draining. Stress, anxiety, and other emotional factors further compound the problem. If the person lacks the energy required for self-care, malnutrition, consequent lack of energy reserves, and anemia can contribute to complaints of fatigue.

CACHEXIA

Cachexia, a generalized wasting of fat and protein, is common in an individual with cancer. A person with cachexia typically appears emaciated and wasted, and experiences an overall deterioration in physical status. Cachexia is characterized by anorexia (loss of appetite), alterations in taste perception, early satiety, weight loss, anemia, marked weakness, and altered metabolism of proteins, carbohydrates, and lipids.

Anorexia may accompany pain or adverse reactions to chemotherapy or radiation therapy. Diminished perception of sweet, sour, or salty sensations also contributes to anorexia. Food that once seemed seasoned and palatable now tastes bland.

Protein-calorie malnutrition may cause hypoalbuminemia, edema (the lack of serum proteins, which usually keep fluid in the blood vessels, enables fluid to escape into the tissues), muscle wasting, and immunodeficiency.

The high metabolic activity of malignant tumor cells carries with it the need for nutrients above those required for normal metabolism. As cancer cells appropriate nutrients to fuel their growth, normal tissue becomes starved and depleted, and wasting begins. Under normal circumstances, when starvation occurs, the body spares protein, relying on carbohydrates and fats for energy production. However, cancer cells metabolize both protein and fatty acids to produce energy.

Key signs and symptoms

Cachexia
- ✦ Common in cancer patients
- ✦ Characterized by anorexia, taste perception alterations, early satiety, weight loss, anemia, marked weakness, altered metabolism
- ✦ May accompany pain or adverse reactions to chemotherapy or radiation therapy
- ✦ Protein-calorie malnutrition may cause hypoalbuminemia, edema, muscle wasting, and immunodeficiency
- ✦ Malignant tumor cells have high metabolic activity; normal tissue becomes starved and depleted

---

Cancer's seven warning signs

The American Cancer Society has developed an easy way to remember the seven warning signs of cancer. Each letter in the word CAUTION represents a possible warning sign that should urge an individual to see a physician.

Change in bowel or bladder habits

A sore that doesn't heal

Unusual bleeding or discharge

Thickening or lump in the breast or elsewhere

Indigestion or difficulty swallowing

Obvious change in a wart or mole

Nagging cough or hoarseness

Key signs and symptoms

Pain
+ Mild or absent in early stages of cancer
+ Increases as cancer progresses
+ Pressure on nerves, blood vessels, or tissue can cause tissue death
+ Occurs when viscera is stretched by a tumor
+ Cancer cells release proteolytic enzymes that destroy neighboring cells; inflammatory response occurs

Anemia
+ Caused by cancer of blood-forming cells, WBCs, or RBCs
+ Common in metastatic cancer

Leukopenia and thrombocytopenia
+ Occur when cancer invades bone marrow
+ Can be caused by chemotherapy and radiation therapy
+ Greatly increases patient's risk of infection and hemorrhage

The patient with cancer commonly feels sated after eating only a few bites of food. This feeling is believed to be the result of metabolites released from the tumor. In addition, tumor necrosis factor, produced by the body in response to cancer, also contributes to cachexia.

PAIN

In cancer's early stages, pain is typically absent or mild; as cancer progresses, however, the pain's severity usually increases. Generally, pain can be the result of one or more factors.

Pressure on or obstruction of nerves, blood vessels, or other tissues and organs leads to tissue hypoxia, accumulation of lactic acid, and possibly cell death. In areas where space for the tumor to grow is limited, such as in the brain or bone, compression is a common cause of pain. Additionally, pain occurs when the viscera, which is usually hollow, is stretched by a tumor as in GI cancer.

Cancer cells also release proteolytic enzymes that directly injure or destroy neighboring cells. This injury sets up a painful inflammatory response.

ANEMIA

Cancer of the blood-forming cells, WBCs, or RBCs may directly cause anemia. Anemia in patients with metastatic cancer is commonly the result of chronic bleeding, severe malnutrition, or chemotherapy or radiation.

LEUKOPENIA AND THROMBOCYTOPENIA

Typically, leukopenia and thrombocytopenia occur when cancer invades the bone marrow. Chemotherapy and radiation therapy to the bones can also cause leukopenia.

Leukopenia greatly increases the patient's risk of infection. The patient with thrombocytopenia is at risk for hemorrhage. Even when the platelet count is normal, platelet function may be impaired in certain hematologic cancers.

INFECTION

Infection is common in the patient with advanced cancer, particularly one with myelosuppression from treatment, direct invasion of the bone marrow, development of fistulas, or immunosuppression from hormonal release in response to chronic stress. Malnutrition and anemia further increase the patient's risk of infection. In addition, obstructions, effusions, and ulcerations may develop, creating a favorable environment for microbial growth.

DIAGNOSIS

A thorough history and physical examination should precede sophisticated diagnostic tests. The choice of diagnostic tests is determined by the patient's presenting signs and symptoms and the suspected body system involved. Diagnostic tests establish tumor presence and identify the stage and grade of the tumor. They help to determine the extent of disease and indicate possible sites of metastasis. These tests can also be used to evaluate affected and unaffected body systems.

Useful tests for early detection and staging of tumors include screening tests, X-rays, radioactive isotope scanning (nuclear medicine imaging), CT scanning, endoscopy, ultrasonography, MRI, and positron emission tomography (PET) scanning. The single most important diagnostic tool is the biopsy for direct histologic study of the tumor tissue.

SCREENING TESTS

Screening tests are perhaps the most important diagnostic tools in the prevention and early detection of cancer. They may provide valuable information about the possibility of cancer even before the patient develops signs and symptoms. The ACS has recommended specific screening tests to aid in the early detection of cancer. (See *ACS guidelines: Early cancer detection,* page 40.)

DIAGNOSIS BY IMAGING

X-rays

Most commonly, X-rays are ordered to identify and evaluate changes in tissue densities. The type and location of the X-ray is determined by the patient's signs and symptoms and the suspected location of the tumor or metastasis. For example, a chest X-ray may be indicated to identify lung cancer if the patient is an older, long-term smoker or to rule out lung metastasis in a patient with colorectal cancer.

Some X-rays such as those of the GI tract (barium enema) and the urinary tract (excretory urography) involve the use of contrast agents. Radiopaque substances can also be injected into the lymphatic system, and their flow can be monitored by lymphangiography. This specialized X-ray technique is helpful in evaluating tumors of the lymph nodes and determining the location of metastasis. Because lymphangiography is invasive and may be difficult to interpret, CT scans and MRIs have largely replaced it.

Radioactive isotope scanning

A specialized camera detects radioactive isotopes that are injected into the bloodstream or ingested. The radiologist evaluates their distribution (uptake) throughout tissues, organs, and organ systems. This type of scanning provides a view of organs and regions within an organ that can't be seen with a simple X-ray. The area of

Screening tests

Breast
+ Mammogram
+ Examination

Colon and rectum
+ FOBT
+ Flexible sigmoidoscopy
+ Colonoscopy
+ Double-contrast barium enema

Prostate
+ Prostate-specific antigen
+ Digital rectal examination

Cervix
+ Pap test

Endometrium
+ Tissue sampling

ACS guidelines: Early cancer detection

The following recommendations from the American Cancer Society (ACS) focus on five common cancers whose survival rates can be improved if the cancer is detected and treated early.

SCREENING AREA	RECOMMENDATIONS
Generalized cancer-related checkup (including health counseling and specific examinations for malignant and nonmalignant disorders)	+ Every 3 years for ages 20 to 40 + Every year for age 40 and older

Breast

+ Mammogram	+ Every year for age 40 and older
+ Clinical breast examination	+ Every year for age 40 and older; every 3 years for ages 20 to 39
+ Breast self-examination (BSE)	+ Optional; suggested monthly for age 20 and older**

Colon and rectum (one of the examinations below)

Men and women age 50 and older

+ Fecal occult blood test (FOBT)	+ Every year
+ Flexible sigmoidoscopy	+ Every 5 years
+ FOBT plus flexible sigmoidoscopy	+ Every year; every 5 years*
+ Colonoscopy	+ Every 10 years
+ Double-contrast barium enema	+ Every 5 years

Prostate

Men age 50 and older with life expectancy of at least 10 years and younger men at higher risk

+ Prostate-specific antigen	+ Annually
+ Digital rectal examination	+ Annually

Cervix

Sexually active females or females age 18 and older

+ Papanicolaou (Pap) test	+ Annually; females ages 30 to 70, with three or more consecutive satisfactory examinations with normal findings, every 2 to 3 years; females age 70 and older with three or more consecutive satisfactory examinations and no abnormal Pap tests in the last 10 years, screening may stop

Endometrium

For women at risk for hereditary nonpolyposis colon cancer

+ Tissue sampling	+ Annually, beginning at age 35

* Most clinicians prefer the combination of FOBT and flexible sigmoidoscopy to either of the two tests alone.
* Women in their 20s are to be instructed about the benefits and limitations of BSE; women have the option of not performing BSE or performing it only occassionally.

---

uptake is termed a hot spot or a cold spot (an area of decreased uptake). Typically, tumors are revealed as cold spots; the exception is the bone scan, in which hot spots indicate the presence of disease. Examples of organs commonly evaluated with radioactive isotope scanning include thyroid, liver, spleen, brain, and bone.

CT scanning

CT scanning evaluates successive layers of tissue by using narrow-beam X-ray to provide a cross-sectional view of the structure. It can also reveal different characteristics of tissues within a solid organ. CT scans are commonly obtained of the brain and head, chest, abdomen, and pelvis to evaluate for neurologic, pelvic, abdominal, and thoracic cancers.

Ultrasonography

Ultrasonography uses high-frequency sound waves to detect tissue density changes that are difficult or impossible to observe by radiology or endoscopy. Ultrasound helps differentiate cysts from solid tumors and is commonly used to provide information about abdominal and pelvic cancer.

MRI

MRI uses magnetic fields and radio frequencies to show a cross-sectional view of the body organs and structures. Like CT scanning, it's commonly used to evaluate neurologic, pelvic, abdominal, and thoracic cancers.

PET scanning

PET scans use radioisotope technology to create a picture of the body in action. PET scans use computers to construct images from the emission of positive electrons (positrons) by radioactive substances administered to the patient. Unlike other diagnostic methods that simply create images of how the body looks, PET scans provide real-time imaging of the body while it functions. Using PET scans to study the spread of cancer involves injecting the cancer patient with a small amount of radioactive glucose. Cancerous cells metabolize sugar more quickly than healthy cells, and this can be seen in the image. The three-dimensional PET scan pictures show malignancies as having a greater concentration of sugar.

ENDOSCOPY

Endoscopy provides a direct view of a body cavity or passageway to detect abnormalities. Common endoscopic sites include the upper and lower GI tract and the bronchial tree. During endoscopy, the physician can excise small tumors, aspirate fluid, or obtain tissue samples for histologic examination.

BIOPSY

A *biopsy*, the removal of a portion of suspicious tissue, is the only definitive method to diagnose cancer. Biopsy tissue samples can be taken by curettage, fluid aspiration (pleural effusion), fine-needle aspiration (breast), dermal punch (skin or mouth), endoscopy (rectal polyps and esophageal lesions), and surgical excision (visceral tissue and nodes). The specimen then undergoes laboratory analysis for cell type and characteristics to provide information about the grade and stage of the cancer.

TUMOR CELL MARKERS

Some cancer cells release substances that usually aren't present in the body or are present only in small quantities. These substances, called tumor markers or biologic markers, are produced by the cancer cell's genetic material during growth and development or by other cells in response to the presence of cancer. (See *Common tumor cell markers*, pages 43 and 44.) Markers may be found on the tumor's cell membrane or in the blood, cerebrospinal fluid, or urine. Tumor cell markers in-

Imaging diagnostics

CT scanning
✦ Uses narrow-beam X-ray to provide cross-sectional view
✦ Used commonly to evaluate neurologic, pelvic, abdominal, and thoracic cancers

Ultrasonography
✦ Detects tissue density changes difficult to observe by radiology or endoscopy via sound waves
✦ Used to provide information on abdominal and pelvic cancer

MRI
✦ Uses magnetic fields and radio frequencies
✦ Provides cross-sectional view of body organs and structures
✦ Used to evaluate neurologic, pelvis, abdominal, and thoracic cancers

PET scanning
✦ Uses radioisotope technology to create a picture of the body in action; real-time imaging of the body while it functions
✦ Detects the rate at which sugar is metabolized (cancer cells metabolize it quicker)

Endoscopy facts
✦ Provides direct view of a body cavity or passageway
✦ Tumors or tissue samples can be excised

Biopsy facts
✦ Removal of suspicious tissue
✦ Only definitive method to diagnose cancer
✦ Laboratory analysis determines cell type and characteristics

Tumor cell markers facts

+ Produced by cancer cell's genetic material
+ Found on tumor's cell membrane, in blood, CSF, or urine

Advantages
+ Allow clinicians to screen people with a high cancer risk, diagnose a type of cancer, monitor effectiveness of therapy, and detect recurrence

Disadvantages
+ By the time it's detected, it may be too advanced to treat
+ Most aren't specific enough to identify one type of cancer
+ Absence doesn't mean the person is free from cancer

Classifying tumors

Benign
+ Well differentiated
+ Grow slowly, displacing but not infiltrating surrounding tissue
+ Cause only slight damage
+ Don't metastasize

Malignant
+ Undifferentiated to varying degrees
+ Seldom encapsulated and poorly delineated
+ Expand rapidly, causing damage when infiltrating tissue
+ Most metastasize
+ Further classified by tissue type, grading, and staging

clude hormones, enzymes, genes, antigens, and antibodies. They allow clinicians to screen people who are at high risk for cancer, diagnose a specific type of cancer in conjunction with clinical manifestations, monitor the effectiveness of therapy, and detect recurrence.

Although they provide a method for detecting and monitoring the progression of certain types of cancer, there are several disadvantages to using tumor cell markers. For example, tumor cell marker levels rise over time and by the time an elevated level is detected the disease may be too far advanced to treat. In addition, most tumor cell markers aren't specific enough to identify one type of cancer, and some nonmalignant diseases, such as pancreatitis or ulcerative colitis, are also associated with tumor cell markers. Although an important piece of the diagnostic puzzle, these disadvantages preclude the use of tumor cell markers as independent diagnostic tools.

Perhaps the worst drawback is that the absence of a tumor cell marker doesn't mean that a person is free from cancer. For example, mucinous ovarian cancer tumors typically don't express the ovarian cancer marker CA 125, so that a negative test doesn't eliminate the possibility of ovarian malignancy.

TUMOR CLASSIFICATION

Tumors are initially classified as benign or malignant depending on the specific features exhibited by the tumor. Typically, benign tumors are well differentiated; that is, their cells closely resemble those of the tissue of origin. Commonly encapsulated with well-defined borders, benign tumors grow slowly, usually displacing but not infiltrating surrounding tissues and, therefore, causing only slight damage. Benign tumors don't metastasize.

Conversely, most malignant tumors are undifferentiated to varying degrees, having cells that may differ considerably from those of the tissue of origin. They're seldom encapsulated and are commonly poorly delineated. They rapidly expand in all directions, causing extensive damage as they infiltrate surrounding tissues. Most malignant tumors metastasize through the blood or lymph to secondary sites.

Malignant tumors are further classified by tissue type, degree of differentiation (grading), and extent of the disease (staging). High-grade tumors are poorly differentiated and are more aggressive than low-grade tumors. Early-stage cancers carry a more favorable prognosis than later-stage cancers that have spread to nearby or distant sites.

TISSUE TYPE

Histologically, the type of tissue in which the growth originates classifies malignant tumors. Three cell layers form during the early stages of embryonic development; they include the ectoderm, the mesoderm, and the endoderm. The *ectoderm* primarily forms the external embryonic covering and the structures that will come into contact with the environment; the *mesoderm* forms the circulatory system, muscles, supporting tissue, and most of the urinary and reproductive system; and the *endoderm* gives rise to the internal linings of the embryo, such as the epithelial lining of the pharynx and respiratory and GI tracts.

Carcinomas are tumors of epithelial tissue. They may originate in the endodermal tissues, which develop into internal structures, such as the stomach and intestine, or in ectodermal tissues, which develop into external structures such as the skin. Tumors arising from glandular epithelial tissue are commonly called adenocarcinomas.

Common tumor cell markers

Tumor cell markers may be used to detect, diagnose, or treat cancer. Alone, however, they aren't sufficient for a diagnosis. Tumor cell markers may also be associated with other benign (nonmalignant) conditions. The chart below highlights some of the more commonly used tumor cell markers and their associated malignant and nonmalignant conditions.

MARKER	MALIGNANT CONDITIONS	NONMALIGNANT CONDITIONS
Alpha-fetoprotein	✦ Endodermal sinus tumor ✦ Liver cancer ✦ Ovarian germ cell cancer ✦ Testicular germ cell cancer (specifically embryonal cell carcinoma)	✦ Ataxia-telangiectasia ✦ Cirrhosis ✦ Hepatitis ✦ Pregnancy ✦ Wiskott-Aldrich syndrome
Carcinoembryonic antigen	✦ Bladder cancer ✦ Breast cancer ✦ Cervical cancer ✦ Colorectal cancer ✦ Kidney cancer ✦ Liver cancer ✦ Lung cancer ✦ Lymphoma ✦ Melanoma ✦ Ovarian cancer ✦ Pancreatic cancer ✦ Stomach cancer ✦ Thyroid cancer	✦ Inflammatory bowel disease ✦ Liver disease ✦ Pancreatitis ✦ Tobacco use
CA 15-3	✦ Breast cancer (usually advanced) ✦ Lung cancer ✦ Ovarian cancer ✦ Prostate cancer	✦ Benign breast disease ✦ Benign ovarian disease ✦ Endometriosis ✦ Hepatitis ✦ Lactation ✦ Pelvic inflammatory disease ✦ Pregnancy
CA 19-9	✦ Bile duct cancer ✦ Colorectal cancer ✦ Pancreatic cancer ✦ Stomach cancer	✦ Cholecystitis ✦ Cirrhosis ✦ Gallstones ✦ Pancreatitis
CA 27-29	✦ Breast cancer ✦ Colon cancer ✦ Kidney cancer ✦ Liver cancer ✦ Lung cancer ✦ Ovarian cancer ✦ Pancreatic cancer ✦ Stomach cancer ✦ Uterine cancer	✦ Benign breast disease ✦ Endometriosis ✦ Kidney disease ✦ Liver disease ✦ Ovarian cysts ✦ Pregnancy (first trimester)

Tumor cell markers commonly used

✦ Alpha-fetoprotein
✦ Carcinoembryonic antigen
✦ CA 15-3
✦ CA 19-9
✦ CA 27-29
✦ CA 125
✦ Human chorionic gonadotropin
✦ Lactate dehydrogenase
✦ Neuron-specific enolase
✦ Prostatic acid phosphatase
✦ Prostate-specific antigen

(continued)

Common tumor cell markers *(continued)*

MARKER	MALIGNANT CONDITIONS	NONMALIGNANT CONDITIONS
CA 125	✦ Colorectal cancer ✦ Gastric cancer ✦ Ovarian cancer ✦ Pancreatic cancer	✦ Endometriosis ✦ Liver disease ✦ Menstruation ✦ Pancreatitis ✦ Pelvic inflammatory disease ✦ Peritonitis ✦ Pregnancy
Human chorionic gonadotropin	✦ Choriocarcinoma ✦ Embryonal cell carcinoma ✦ Gestational trophoblastic disease ✦ Liver cancer ✦ Lung cancer ✦ Pancreatic cancer ✦ Specific dysgerminomas of the ovary ✦ Stomach cancer ✦ Testicular cancer	✦ Marijuana use ✦ Pregnancy
Lactate dehydrogenase	✦ Almost all cancers ✦ Ewing's sarcoma ✦ Leukemia ✦ Non-Hodgkin's lymphoma ✦ Testicular cancer	✦ Anemia ✦ Heart failure ✦ Hypothyroidism ✦ Liver disease ✦ Lung disease
Neuron-specific enolase	✦ Kidney cancer ✦ Melanoma ✦ Neuroblastoma ✦ Pancreatic cancer ✦ Small-cell lung cancer ✦ Testicular cancer ✦ Thyroid cancer ✦ Wilms' tumor	✦ Unknown
Prostatic acid phosphatase	✦ Prostate cancer	✦ Benign prostatic conditions
Prostate-specific antigen	✦ Prostate cancer	✦ Benign prostatic hyperplasia ✦ Prostatitis

Type of tissue

✦ Three cell layers: ectoderm, mesoderm, and endoderm
✦ Carcinomas are tumors of epithelial tissue; originate in endodermal or ectodermal tissues
✦ Adenocarcinomas: tumors arising from glandular epithelial tissue
✦ Sarcomas originate in mesodermal tissues; may be further classified based on specific cells involved

Sarcomas originate in the mesodermal tissues, which develop into supporting structures, such as the bone, muscle, fat, or blood. Sarcomas may be further classified based on the specific cells involved. For example, malignant tumors arising from pigmented cells are called melanomas; from plasma cells, myelomas; and from lymphatic tissue, lymphomas.

Understanding TNM staging

The TNM (tumor, node, and metastasis) system developed by the American Joint Committee on Cancer provides a consistent method for classifying malignant tumors based on the extent of the disease. It also offers a convenient structure to standardize diagnostic and treatment protocols. Differences in classification may occur, depending on the primary cancer site.

T FOR PRIMARY TUMOR
The anatomic extent of the primary tumor depends on its size, depth of invasion, and surface spread. Tumor stages progress from TX to T4 as follows:
TX — Primary tumor can't be assessed
T0 — No evidence of primary tumor
Tis — Carcinoma in situ
T1, T2, T3, T4 — Increasing size or local extent (or both) of primary tumor

N FOR NODAL INVOLVEMENT
Nodal involvement reflects the tumor's spread to the lymph nodes as follows:
NX — Regional lymph nodes can't be assessed
N0 — No evidence of regional lymph node metastasis
N1, N2, N3 — Increasing involvement of regional lymph nodes

M FOR DISTANT METASTASIS
Metastasis denotes the extent (or spread) of disease. Levels range from MX to M4 as follows:
MX — Distant metastasis can't be assessed
M0 — No evidence of distant metastasis
M1 — Single, solitary distant metastasis
M2, M3, M4 — Multiple foci or multiple organ metastasis

TNM staging terms
✦ T — Tumor
✦ N — Nodal involvement
✦ M — Metastasis

Tumor grading
✦ Grade 1: well differentiated; cells resemble tissue of origin and maintain some function
✦ Grade 2: moderately well differentiated; cells vary in size and shape
✦ Grade 3: poorly differentiated; cells vary widely in size and shape; mitosis is greatly increased
✦ Grade 4: malignancies are undifferentiated; cells exhibit no similarity to tissue of origin

GRADING

Histologically, malignant tumors are classified by their degree of differentiation. The greater their differentiation, the greater the tumor cells' similarity to the tissue of origin. Typically, a malignant tumor is graded on a scale of 1 to 4, in order of increasing clinical severity.

Grade 1 tumors are well differentiated. The cells closely resemble the tissue of origin and maintain some specialized function. Grade 2 malignancies are moderately well differentiated. The cells vary somewhat in size and shape with increased mitosis. A Grade 3 tumor is poorly differentiated with cells varying widely in size and shape with little resemblance to the tissue of origin; mitosis is greatly increased. Grade 4 malignancies are undifferentiated with cells that exhibit no similarity to tissue of origin.

STAGING

Malignant tumors are staged (classified anatomically) by the extent of the disease. The most commonly used method for staging is the TNM staging system, which evaluates **T**umor size, **N**odal involvement, and **M**etastatic progress. This classification system provides an accurate tumor description that's adjustable as the disease progresses. TNM staging enables reliable comparison of treatments and survival rates among large population groups; it also identifies nodal involvement and metastasis to other areas. (See *Understanding TNM staging*.)

Tumor staging
✦ TNM system provides accurate tumor description that's adjustable
✦ Enables reliable comparison of treatments and survival rates
✦ Identifies nodal involvement and metastasis to other areas

Treatment

+ Types include surgery, radiation therapy, chemotherapy, biotherapy, and hormone therapy; each used alone or in combination
+ Four goals: cure and eradicate the cancer; control or arrest tumor growth; provide palliation to alleviate symptoms; provide prophylaxis or treatment when no tumor is detectible, but patient is at high risk
+ Adverse effects to treatment include fluid and electrolyte imbalances, bone marrow suppression, hypercalcemia, and pain
+ Some treatment complications are life-threatening

Surgical options

+ Typically combined with other therapies
+ Biopsy is diagnostic surgery
+ Surgery as primary treatment attempts to remove the entire tumor, along with surrounding tissues and lymph nodes
+ Wide and local excision used to removing small tumor mass
+ Radical or modified radical excision removes the primary tumor and lymph nodes; results in disfigurement and altered functioning
+ Palliative surgery relieves complications
+ Prophylactic surgery removes nonvital tissues or organs with high potential for developing cancer; very controversial

TREATMENT

Cancer treatments include surgery, radiation therapy, chemotherapy, immunotherapy (also called *biotherapy*), and hormone therapy. Each may be used alone or in combination (called *multimodal therapy*), depending on the tumor's type, stage, localization, and responsiveness and on limitations imposed by the patient's clinical status.

Cancer treatment has four goals. The first is to cure and eradicate the cancer and promote long-term patient survival. The second is to control or to arrest tumor growth. The third goal is to provide palliation to alleviate symptoms when the disease is beyond control. The final goal is to provide prophylaxis or treatment when no tumor is detectable, but the patient is known to be at high risk for tumor development or recurrence.

Cancer treatment is further categorized by type according to when it's used. Primary treatment is used to eradicate the disease. Adjuvant therapy is used in addition to primary treatment in order to eliminate microscopic disease and promote cure or improve the patient's response. When the goal is to manage recurrent disease, salvage or palliative therapy is employed.

As with any treatment regimen, complications may arise. Indeed, many complications of cancer are related to the adverse effects of treatment, such as fluid and electrolyte imbalances secondary to anorexia, vomiting, or diarrhea; bone marrow suppression, including anemia, leukopenia, thrombocytopenia, and neutropenia; and infection. Hypercalcemia is the most common metabolic abnormality experienced by cancer patients. Pain, which accompanies all progressing cancers, can reach intolerable levels.

Certain complications are life-threatening and require prompt intervention. These oncologic emergencies may result from the tumor's effects or its byproducts, secondary involvement of other organs due to disease spread, or adverse effects of treatment. (See *Common cancer emergencies.*)

SURGERY

Surgery, once the mainstay of cancer treatment, is now typically combined with other therapies. It may be performed to diagnose the disease, initiate primary treatment, or achieve palliation and is occasionally done for prophylaxis. The surgical biopsy procedure is diagnostic surgery; continuing surgery then removes the bulk of the tumor. When used as a primary treatment method, surgery is an attempt to remove the entire tumor (or as much as possible, by a procedure called debulking), along with surrounding tissues, including lymph nodes.

A common method of surgical removal of a small tumor mass is called wide and local excision. The tumor mass is removed along with a small or moderate amount of easily accessible surrounding tissue that's normal. A radical or modified radical excision removes the primary tumor along with lymph nodes, nearby involved structures, and surrounding structures that may be at high risk for disease spread. Typically a radical excision results in some degree of disfigurement and altered functioning. Today's less radical surgical procedures such as a lumpectomy instead of mastectomy are more acceptable to the patient. The health care professional and the patient should discuss the type of surgery. Ultimately the choice belongs to the patient.

Palliative surgery is used to relieve complications, such as pain, ulceration, obstruction, hemorrhage, or pressure. Examples include a cordotomy to relieve intractable pain and bowel resection or ostomy to remove a bowel obstruction. Addi-

Common cancer emergencies

The following chart lists certain oncologic emergencies that may arise and the associated malignancy.

EMERGENCY AND CAUSE	ASSOCIATED MALIGNANCY
Cardiac tamponade	
✦ Fluid accumulation around pericardial space or pericardial thickening secondary to radiation therapy	✦ Breast cancer ✦ Leukemia ✦ Lymphoma ✦ Melanoma
Hypercalcemia	
✦ Increased bone resorption due to bone destruction or tumor-related elevation of parathyroid hormone, osteoclast-activating factor, or prostaglandin levels	✦ Breast cancer ✦ Lung cancer ✦ Multiple myeloma ✦ Renal cancer
Disseminated intravascular coagulation	
✦ Widespread clotting in arterioles and capillaries and simultaneous hemorrhage	✦ Hematologic malignancies ✦ Mucin-producing adenocarcinomas
Malignant peritoneal infusion	
✦ Seeding of tumor into the peritoneum, excess intraperitoneal fluid production or release of humoral factors by the tumor	✦ Ovarian cancer
Malignant pleural effusion	
✦ Implantation of cancer cells on pleural surface, tumor obstruction of lymphatic channels on pulmonary veins, shedding of necrotic tumor cells into the pleural space or thoracic duct perforation	✦ Breast cancer ✦ GI tract cancer ✦ Leukemia ✦ Lung cancer (most common) ✦ Lymphoma ✦ Testicular cancer
Spinal cord compression	
✦ Encroachment on spinal cord or cauda equina due to metastasis or vertebral collapse and displacement of bony elements	✦ Cancer of lung, breast, kidney, GI tract, prostate, or cervix ✦ Melanoma
Superior vena cava syndrome	
✦ Impaired venous return secondary to occlusion of vena cava	✦ Breast cancer ✦ Lung cancer ✦ Lymphoma
Syndrome of inappropriate antidiuretic hormone	
✦ Ectopic production by tumor; abnormal stimulation of hypothalamus-pituitary axis; mimicking or enhanced effects on kidney; may be induced by chemotherapy	✦ Bladder cancer ✦ GI tract cancer ✦ Hodgkin's disease ✦ Prostate cancer ✦ Sarcomas ✦ Small-cell lung cancer

(continued)

Common cancer emergencies

✦ Cardiac tamponade
✦ Hypercalcemia
✦ Disseminated intravascular coagulation
✦ Malignant peritoneal infusion
✦ Malignant pleural effusion
✦ Spinal cord compression
✦ Superior vena cava syndrome
✦ Syndrome of inappropriate antidiuretic hormone
✦ Tumor lysis syndrome

Common cancer emergencies *(continued)*

EMERGENCY AND CAUSE	ASSOCIATED MALIGNANCY
Tumor lysis syndrome	
✦ Rapid cell destruction and turnover caused by chemotherapy or rapid tumor growth	✦ Leukemias ✦ Lymphomas

tionally, surgery may be performed to remove hormone-producing glands, thereby limiting the growth of a hormone-sensitive tumor.

Prophylactic surgery may be done if a patient has personal or familial risk factors for a particular type of cancer. This treatment involves the removal of nonvital tissues or organs with a high potential for developing cancer. One example is prophylactic mastectomy. Much controversy exists over this type of surgery because of the possible long-term physiologic and psychological effects, although potential benefits may significantly outweigh the downside.

RADIATION THERAPY

Radiation therapy involves the use of high-energy radiation to treat cancer. Used alone or in conjunction with other therapies, it aims to destroy dividing cancer cells while damaging normal cells as little as possible. Two types of radiation are used to treat cancer: ionizing radiation and particle beam radiation. Both target the cellular DNA. Ionizing radiation deposits energy that damages the genetic material inside the cancer cells. Normal cells are also affected but can recover. Particle beam radiation uses a special machine and fast-moving particles to treat the cancer. The particles can cause more cell damage than ionizing radiation does.

The guiding principle for radiation therapy is that the dose administered be large enough to eradicate the tumor, but small enough to minimize the adverse effects to the surrounding normal tissue. How well the treatment meets this goal is known as the *therapeutic ratio*.

Radiation interacts with oxygen in the nucleus to break strands of DNA and interacts with water in body fluids (including intracellular fluid) to form free radicals, which also damage the DNA. If this damage isn't repaired, the cells die, immediately or when they attempt to divide. Radiation may also render tumor cells unable to enter the cell cycle. Thus, cells most vulnerable to radiation therapy are those that undergo frequent cell division, for example, cells of the bone marrow, lymph, GI epithelium, and gonads.

Therapeutic radiation may be delivered by external beam radiation or by intracavitary or interstitial implants. Use of implants requires an inpatient stay. Anyone who comes in contact with the patient while the internal radiation implants are in place must wear radiation protection. High-dose-rate remote brachytherapy, a temporary form of radiation implantation (it's in place for only a few minutes), delivers powerful radiation directly to the tumor through several hollow catheters, while minimizing damage to the surrounding tissues. This therapy is typically done on an outpatient basis. It has been used to treat breast, cervical, esophageal, lung, pancreatic, and prostatic cancers.

Normal and malignant cells respond to radiation differently, depending on blood supply, oxygen saturation, previous irradiation, and immune status. Generally, normal cells recover from radiation faster than malignant cells. Success of treat-

Key facts about radiation therapy

- ✦ Uses high-energy radiation
- ✦ Aims to destroy dividing cancer cells while minimizing damage to normal cells
- ✦ Two types: ionizing radiation and particle beam radiation
- ✦ Therapeutic ratio: how well treatment meets the goal of administering large enough dose to eradicate tumor, but minimizing adverse effects to normal tissue
- ✦ Interacts with oxygen to break strands of DNA
- ✦ Interacts with body fluid water to form free radicals
- ✦ May be delivered by external beam radiation or intracavitary or interstitial implants
- ✦ Normal and malignant cells respond to radiation differently
- ✦ Normal cells recover from radiation faster than malignant cells
- ✦ Protracted schedule allows time for normal tissue to recover between doses

ment and damage to normal tissue also vary with the radiation's intensity. Although a large, single dose of radiation has greater cellular effects than fractions of the same amount delivered sequentially, a protracted schedule allows time for normal tissue to recover between doses.

Radiation may be used palliatively to relieve pain, obstruction, malignant effusions, cough, dyspnea, ulcerations, and hemorrhage. It can also promote healing of pathologic fractures after surgical stabilization and delay metastasis.

Combining radiation and surgery can minimize the need for radical surgery, prolong survival, and preserve anatomic function. For example, preoperative doses of radiation shrink a large tumor to operable size while preventing further spread of the disease during surgery. After the wound heals, postoperative doses prevent residual cancer cells from multiplying or metastasizing.

Adverse effects

Radiation therapy has local and systemic adverse effects, because it affects normal and malignant cells. Systemic adverse effects, such as weakness, fatigue, anorexia, nausea, vomiting, and anemia may respond to antiemetics, steroids, frequent small meals, fluid maintenance, and rest. They're seldom severe enough to require discontinuing radiation but they may mandate a dosage adjustment. (For localized adverse effects, see *Radiation's adverse effects,* page 50.)

Patients receiving radiation therapy must have frequent blood counts, particularly of WBCs and platelets if the target site involves areas of bone marrow production. Radiation also requires special skin care measures, such as covering the irradiated area with loose cotton clothing to protect it from light and avoiding deodorants, colognes, and other topical agents during treatment.

CHEMOTHERAPY

Chemotherapy includes a wide range of antineoplastic drugs, which may induce regression of a tumor and its metastasis. It's particularly useful in controlling residual disease and as an adjunct to surgery or radiation therapy. It can induce long remissions and sometimes effect cure, especially in a patient with childhood leukemia, Hodgkin's disease, choriocarcinoma, or testicular cancer. As a palliative treatment, chemotherapy aims to improve the patient's quality of life by temporarily relieving pain and other symptoms.

Every dose of a chemotherapeutic agent destroys only a percentage of tumor cells. Therefore, regression of the tumor requires repeated doses of drugs. The goal is to eradicate enough of the tumor so that the immune system can destroy the remaining malignant cells.

Tumor cells that are in the active phase of cell division (called the *growth fraction*) are the most sensitive to chemotherapeutic agents. Nondividing cells are the least sensitive and thus are the most potentially dangerous. They must be destroyed to eradicate a malignancy. Therefore, repeated cycles of chemotherapy are used to destroy nondividing cells as they enter the cell cycle to begin active proliferation.

Depending on the type of cancer, one or more different categories of chemotherapeutic agents may be used. The most commonly used types of chemotherapeutic agents are:

✦ Alkylating agents and nitrosoureas inhibit cell growth and division by reacting with DNA at any phase of the cell cycle. They prevent cell replication by breaking and cross-linking DNA.

✦ Antimetabolites prevent cell growth by competing with metabolites in the production of nucleic acid, substituting themselves for purines and pyrimidines which

Key facts about chemotherapy

✦ Includes range of antineoplastic drugs

✦ Useful in controlling residual disease and as adjunct to surgery or radiation therapy

✦ Can induce long remissions

✦ Each dose destroys only a percentage of tumor cells; repeated doses are required

✦ Tumor cells in the growth fraction are the most sensitive

✦ Nondividing cells must be destroyed to eradicate a malignancy

Adverse effects of radiation therapy

- Alopecia
- Mucositis
- Xerostomia
- Dental caries
- Lung tissue irritation
- Pericarditis
- Myocarditis
- Esophagitis
- Anemia
- Azotemia
- Edema
- Headache
- Hypertensive nephropathy
- Lassitude
- Nephritis
- Cramps
- Diarrhea

Radiation's adverse effects

Radiation therapy can cause local adverse effects depending on the area irradiated. This chart highlights some of the more commonly seen local effects and the measures to manage them.

AREA IRRADIATED	ADVERSE EFFECT	MANAGEMENT
Head and neck	• Alopecia	• Gentle combing and grooming of scalp • Soft head cover
	• Mucositis	• Cool carbonated drinks • Ice, ice pops • Soft, nonirritating diet • Nonalcohol-based mouthwash with viscous lidocaine • Soft toothbrushes or swabs
	• Xerostomia (dry mouth)	• Good oral hygiene • Oral saliva replacement
	• Dental caries	• Gingival care • Prophylactic fluoride to teeth
Chest	• Lung tissue irritation	• Avoidance of persons with upper respiratory infections • Humidifier if necessary • Steroid therapy
	• Pericarditis • Myocarditis	• Antiarrhythmic drugs
	• Esophagitis	• Analgesia • Fluid maintenance • Total parenteral nutrition
Kidneys	• Anemia • Azotemia • Edema • Headache • Hypertensive nephropathy • Lassitude • Nephritis	• Fluid and electrolyte maintenance • Monitoring for signs of renal failure
Abdomen and pelvis	• Cramps • Diarrhea	• Fluid and electrolyte maintenance • Loperamide and diphenoxylate with atropine • Low-residue diet

are essential for DNA and ribonucleic acid (RNA) synthesis. They exert their effect during the S phase of the cell cycle.

✦ Antitumor antibiotics block cell growth by binding with DNA and interfering with DNA-dependent RNA synthesis. Acting in any phase of the cell cycle, they bind to DNA and generate toxic oxygen free radicals that break one or both strands of DNA.

✦ Plant (Vinca) alkaloids prevent cellular reproduction by disrupting mitosis. Acting primarily in the M phase of the cell cycle, they interfere with the formation of the mitotic spindle by binding to microtubular proteins.

✦ Hormones and hormone antagonists impair cell growth by one or both of two mechanisms. They may alter the cell environment, thereby affecting the cell membrane's permeability, or they may inhibit the growth of hormone-susceptible tumors by changing their chemical environment. These agents include adrenocorticosteroids, androgens, gonadotropin inhibitors, and aromatase inhibitors.

Other chemotherapeutic agents include podophyllotoxins and taxanes which, like plant alkaloids, interfere with formation of the mitotic spindle, and miscellaneous agents, such as hydroxyurea and L-asparaginase, which seem to be cell-cycle-specific agents but whose mode of action is unclear. (See *Chemotherapy's action in the cell cycle,* page 52.)

A combination of drugs from different categories may be used to maximize the tumor cell kill. Combination therapy typically includes drugs with different toxicities and synergistic actions. Use of combination therapy also helps prevent the development of drug-resistant mechanisms by the tumor cells.

Adverse effects

Chemotherapy causes numerous adverse effects that reflect the drugs' mechanism of action. Although antineoplastic agents are toxic to cancer cells, they can also cause transient changes in normal tissues, especially those with proliferating cells. For example, antineoplastic agents typically cause anemia, leukopenia, and thrombocytopenia because they suppress bone marrow function; vomiting because they irritate the GI epithelial cells; and alopecia and dermatitis because they destroy hair follicles and skin cells.

Many antineoplastic agents are given I.V., and they can cause venous sclerosis and pain when administered. If extravasated, they may cause deep cutaneous necrosis, requiring debridement and skin grafting. To minimize the risk of extravasation, most drugs with the potential for direct tissue injury are now given through a central venous catheter.

The pharmacologic action of a given drug determines whether it's administered orally, subcutaneously, I.M., I.V., intracavitary, intrathecally, or by arterial infusion. Dosages are calculated according to the patient's body surface area, with adjustments for general condition, previous reactions to the drug, and degree of myelosuppression.

Many patients approach chemotherapy apprehensively. They need to be allowed to express their concerns and be provided with simple and truthful information. Explanations about what to expect, including possible adverse effects, can help minimize fear and anxiety.

HORMONAL THERAPY

Hormonal therapy is based on studies showing that certain hormones can inhibit the growth of certain cancers. For example, the luteinizing hormone-releasing hormone analogue, leuprolide, is used to treat prostate cancer. With long-term use, this hormone inhibits testosterone release and tumor growth. Tamoxifen, an antiestrogen hormonal agent, blocks estrogen receptors in breast tumor cells that require estrogen to thrive. Additionally, tamoxifen can be given prophylactically to women at high risk for breast cancer. Adrenocortical steroids are effective in treating leukemias and lymphomas because they suppress lymphocytes.

Commonly used chemotherapeutic agents

✦ Alkylating agents
✦ Antimetabolites
✦ Antitumor antibiotics
✦ Vinca alkaloids
✦ Hormones and hormone antagonists
✦ Podophyllotoxins and taxanes

Adverse effects of chemotherapy

✦ Anemia
✦ Leukopenia
✦ Thrombocytopenia
✦ Vomiting
✦ Alopecia
✦ Dermatitis
✦ Venous sclerosis
✦ Pain
✦ Cutaneous necrosis

Key facts about hormonal therapy

✦ Certan hormones can inhibit growth of certain cancers
✦ Adverse effects include hot flashes, sweating, impotence, decreased libido, nausea and vomiting, and blood dyscrasias

FOCUS ON TREATMENT

Chemotherapy's action in the cell cycle

Some chemotherapeutic agents are cell-cycle specific, impairing cellular growth by causing changes in the cell during specific phases of the cell cycle. Other agents are cell-cycle nonspecific, affecting the cell at any phase during the cell cycle. This illustration shows where the cell-cycle-specific agents work to disrupt cancer cell growth.

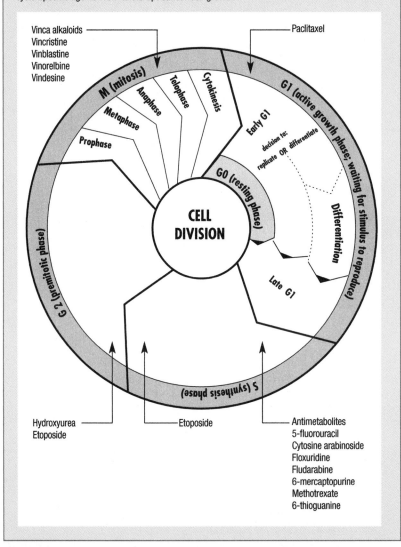

Adverse effects of these hormonal agents include hot flashes, sweating, impotence, decreased libido, nausea and vomiting, and blood dyscrasias (with tamoxifen).

BIOTHERAPY

Biotherapy (also known as *immunotherapy*) relies on treatment agents known as *biological response modifiers*. Biological agents are usually combined with chemotherapeutic drugs or radiation therapy. Much of the work done in biotherapy is still experimental. However, the Food and Drug Administration has approved several new drugs, which are providing promising results. For example, rituximab — a monoclonal antibody — is effective to treat relapsed or refractory B-cell non-Hodgkin's lymphoma.

The main biotherapy agent classifications include interferons, interleukins, hematopoietic growth factors, and monoclonal antibodies. Interferons have antiviral, antiproliferative, and immunomodulary effects. The interleukins exert their effects on the T lymphocytes. Monoclonal antibodies such as rituximab provide the most tumor-specific therapy for cancer by selectively binding to tumor cell surfaces.

Although not used to treat cancer directly, hematopoietic growth factors are used to increase the patient's blood counts when chemotherapy or radiation causes a decrease.

Adverse effects of biotherapeutic agents mimic the body's normal immune response, with flulike symptoms being the most common.

Key facts about biotherapy

◆ Also known as *immunotherapy*
◆ Relies on biological response modifiers
◆ FDA has approved several new drugs, including rituximab
◆ Main agent classifications include interferons, interleukins, hemapoietic growth factors, and monoclonal antibodies
◆ Adverse effects mimic the body's normal immune response; flulike symptoms are most common

Infection

The twentieth century encompassed astonishing advances in treating and preventing infection such as potent antibiotics, complex immunizations, and modern sanitation, yet infection remains the most common cause of human disease. Even in countries with advanced medical care, infectious disease remains a major cause of serious illness. In developing countries, infection is one of the most critical health problems.

Characteristics of infections

+ Invasion and multiplication of microorganisms in or on body tissue
+ Produce signs and symptoms as well as an immune response
+ Severity of infection varies with the pathogenicity, number of invading microorganisms, and strength of host defenses
+ For transmission: causative agent, infections reservoir with a portal of transmission, a portal of entry into the host, and a susceptible host must be present

WHAT IS INFECTION?

Infection is the invasion and multiplication of microorganisms in or on body tissue that produce signs and symptoms as well as an immune response. Such reproduction injures the host by causing cell damage from microorganism-produced toxins or from intracellular multiplication or by competing with host metabolism. Infectious diseases range from relatively mild illnesses to debilitating and lethal conditions: from the common cold through chronic hepatitis to acquired immunodeficiency syndrome. The severity of the infection varies with the pathogenicity and number of the invading microorganisms and the strength of host defenses. The very young, the very old, and the immunosuppressed are especially susceptible.

For infection to be transmitted, the following must be present: causative agent, infectious reservoir with a portal of exit, mode of transmission, a portal of entry into the host, and a susceptible host.

RISK FACTORS

A healthy person can usually ward off infections with the body's own built-in defense mechanisms, including intact skin; the normal flora that inhabit the skin and various organs (see *How microbes interact with the body*); lysozymes (enzymes that can kill microorganisms or microbes) secreted by eyes, nasal passages, glands,

How microbes interact with the body

Microbes interact with their host in various ways.

DOUBLE BENEFIT
Some of the microorganisms of the normal human flora interact with the body in ways that mutually benefit both parties. *Escherichia coli* organisms, part of the normal intestinal flora, obtain nutrients from the human host; in return, they secrete vitamin K, which the human body needs for blood clotting.

SINGLE BENEFIT
Other microbes of the normal flora have a commensal interaction with the human body—an interaction that benefits one party (in this case, the microbes) without affecting the other.

PARASITIC INTERACTION
Some pathogenic microbes such as helminths (worms) are parasites. This means that they harm the host while they benefit from their interaction with the host.

3 ways microbes interact with the body
- Single benefit
- Double benefit
- Parasitic interaction

stomach, and genitourinary organs; defensive structures such as the cilia that sweep foreign matter from the airways; and a healthy immune system.

However, if an imbalance develops, the potential for infection increases. Risk factors for the development of infection include weakened defense mechanisms, environmental and developmental factors, and pathogen characteristics.

WEAKENED DEFENSE MECHANISMS

The body has many defense mechanisms for resisting entry and multiplication of microbes. However, a weakened immune system makes it easier for these pathogens to invade the body and launch an infectious disease. This weakened state is referred to as *immunodeficiency* or *immunocompromise.*

Impaired function of white blood cells (WBCs) and low levels of T and B cells characterize immunodeficiencies. An immunodeficiency may be congenital (caused by a genetic defect and present at birth) or acquired (developed after birth). Acquired immunodeficiency may result from infection, malnutrition, chronic stress, or pregnancy. Diabetes, renal failure, and cirrhosis can suppress the immune response, as can drugs such as corticosteroids and chemotherapy.

Regardless of cause, the result of immunodeficiency is the same. The body's ability to recognize and fight pathogens is impaired. People who are immunodeficient are more susceptible to all infections, are more acutely ill when they become infected, and require a much longer time to heal.

Weakened defense mechanisms
- Immunodeficiency or immunocompromise
- Impaired WBCs and low level of T and B cells characterize immunodeficiency
- May be congenital or acquired
- Body's ability to recognize and fight pathogens is impaired

ENVIRONMENTAL FACTORS

Other conditions that may weaken a person's immune defenses include poor hygiene, malnutrition, inadequate physical barriers, emotional and physical stressors, chronic diseases, medical and surgical treatments, and inadequate immunization.

Good hygiene promotes normal host defenses; poor hygiene increases the risk of infection. Unclean skin harbors microbes and offers an environment for them to colonize, and untended skin is more likely to allow invasion. Frequent washing removes surface microbes and maintains an intact barrier to infection, but it may damage the skin. To maintain skin integrity, lubricants and emollients may be used to prevent cracks and breaks.

The body needs a balanced diet to provide the nutrients, vitamins, and minerals that an effective immune system needs. Protein malnutrition inhibits the production of antibodies, without which the body can't mount an effective attack against

Environmental factors
- Poor hygiene
- Malnutrition
- Inadequate physical barriers
- Emotional and physical stressors
- Chronic diseases
- Medical and surgical treatments
- Inadequate immunization

Development factors

✦ Young children are at high risk for infection: immune system isn't fully developed

✦ Older adults are at risk also: risk of declining immune system

Characteristics of pathogens

✦ Sufficient quantities of microbes must be present to cause a disease

✦ Severity of infection depends on microbe's pathogenicity

Factors affecting pathogenicity

✦ Specificity: range of hosts to which microbe is attracted

✦ Invasiveness: microbe's ability to invade and multiply

✦ Quantity: number of microbes that successfully invade and reproduce

✦ Virulence: severity of disease produced

✦ Toxigenicity: pathogen's potential to damage tissues

✦ Adhesiveness: ability to attach to the host

✦ Antigenicity: degree to which pathogen can induce an immune response

✦ Viability: ability to survive outside host

microbe invasion. Malnutrition is directly related to incidence of nosocomial infections. Along with a balanced diet, the body needs adequate vitamins and minerals to use ingested nutrients.

Dust can facilitate transportation of pathogens. For example, dust-borne spores of the fungus *aspergillus* transmit the infection. If the inhaled spores become established in the lungs, they're notoriously difficult to expel. Fortunately, persons with intact immune systems can usually resist infection with *aspergillus,* which is usually dangerous only in the presence of severe immunosuppression.

DEVELOPMENTAL FACTORS

The very young and very old are at higher risk for infection. The immune system doesn't fully develop until about age 6 months. An infant exposed to an infectious agent usually develops an infection. The most common type of infection in toddlers affects the respiratory tract. When young children put toys and other objects in their mouths, they increase their exposure to various pathogens.

Exposure to communicable diseases continues throughout childhood, as children progress from day-care facilities to schools. Skin diseases such as impetigo and lice infestation commonly pass from one child to the next at this age. Accidents are common in childhood as well, and broken or abraded skin opens the way for bacterial invasion. Lack of immunization also contributes to incidence of childhood diseases.

Advancing age, on the other hand, is associated with a declining immune system, partly as a result of decreasing thymus function. Chronic diseases, such as diabetes and atherosclerosis, can weaken defenses by impairing blood flow and nutrient delivery to body systems.

PATHOGEN CHARACTERISTICS

A microbe must be present in sufficient quantities to cause a disease in a healthy human. The number needed to cause a disease varies from one microbe to the next and from host to host, and may be affected by the mode of transmission. The severity of an infection depends on several factors, including the microbe's pathogenicity, that is, the likelihood that it will cause pathogenic changes or disease. Factors that affect pathogenicity include the microbe's specificity, invasiveness, quantity, virulence, toxigenicity, adhesiveness, antigenicity, and viability. (See *Chain of infection.*)

✦ *Specificity* is the range of hosts to which a microbe is attracted. Some microbes may be attracted to a wide range of humans and animals, whereas others select only human or only animal hosts.

✦ *Invasiveness* (sometimes called *infectivity*) is a microbe's ability to invade and multiply in the host tissues. Some microbes can enter through intact skin; others can enter only if the skin or mucous membrane is broken. Some microbes produce enzymes that enhance their invasiveness.

✦ *Quantity* refers to the number of microbes that succeed in invading and reproducing in the body.

✦ *Virulence* is the severity of the disease a pathogen can produce. Virulence can vary depending on the host defenses; any infection can be life-threatening in an immunodeficient patient. Infection with a pathogen known to be particularly virulent requires early diagnosis and treatment.

✦ *Toxigenicity* is related to virulence. It describes a pathogen's potential to damage host tissues by producing and releasing toxins.

Chain of infection

An infection can occur only if the six components depicted here are present. Removing one link in the chain prevents infection.

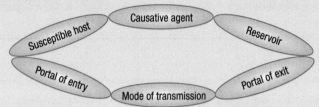

CAUSATIVE AGENT

A *causative agent* for infection is any microbe that can produce disease.

RESERVOIR

The *reservoir* is the environment or object in or on which a microbe can survive and, in some cases, multiply. Inanimate objects, human beings, and other animals can all serve as reservoirs, providing the essential requirements for a microbe to survive at specific stages in its life cycle.

PORTAL OF EXIT

The *portal of exit* is the path by which an infectious agent leaves its reservoir. Usually, this portal is the site where the organism grows. Common portals of exit associated with human reservoirs include the respiratory, genitourinary, and GI tracts; the skin and mucous membranes; and the placenta (in transplacental disease transmission from mother to fetus). Blood, sputum, emesis, stools, urine, wound drainage, and genital secretions also serve as portals of exit. The portal of exit varies from one infectious agent to the next.

MODE OF TRANSMISSION

The *mode of transmission* is the means by which the infectious agent passes from the portal of exit in the reservoir to the susceptible host. Infections can be transmitted through one of four modes: contact, airborne, enteric, and vector-borne. Some organisms use more than one transmission mode to get from the reservoir to a new host. As with portals of exit, the transmission mode varies with the specific microbe.

Contact transmission is subdivided into direct contact, indirect contact, and droplet spread (contact with droplets that enter the environment).

Direct contact refers to person-to-person spread of organisms through physical contact.

Indirect contact occurs when a susceptible person comes in contact with a contaminated object.

Droplet spread results from contact with contaminated respiratory secretions. It differs from airborne transmission in that the droplets don't remain suspended in the air but settle to surfaces.

Airborne transmission occurs when fine microbial particles containing pathogens remain suspended in the air for a prolonged period, and then are spread widely by air currents and inhaled.

Enteric (oral-fecal) transmission occurs when infecting organisms found in feces are ingested by susceptible victims, in many cases, through fecally contaminated food or water.

Vector-borne transmission occurs when an intermediate carrier, or vector, such as a flea or mosquito, transfers a microbe to another living organism. Vector-borne transmission is of most concern in tropical areas, where insects commonly transmit disease.

PORTAL OF ENTRY

Portal of entry refers to the path by which an infectious agent invades a susceptible host. Usually, this path is the same as the portal of exit.

SUSCEPTIBLE HOST

A *susceptible host* is also required for the transmission of infection to occur. The human body has many defense mechanisms for resisting the entry and multiplication of pathogens. When these mechanisms function normally, infection doesn't occur. However, in a weakened host, an infectious agent is more likely to invade the body and launch an infectious disease.

6 components of the chain of infection

✦ Causative agent
✦ Reservoir
✦ Portal of exit
✦ Mode of transmission
✦ Portal of entry
✦ Susceptible host

◆ *Adhesiveness* is the ability of the pathogen to attach to host tissue. Some pathogens secrete a sticky substance that helps them adhere to tissue while protecting them from the host's defense mechanisms.

◆ *Antigenicity* is the degree to which a pathogen can induce a specific immune response. Microbes that invade and localize in tissue initially stimulate a cellular response; those that disseminate quickly throughout the host's body generate an antibody response.

◆ *Viability* is the ability of a pathogen to survive outside its host. Most microbes can't live and multiply outside a reservoir.

4 stages of infection
◆ Incubation
◆ Prodromal stage
◆ Acute illness
◆ Convalescent stage

STAGES OF INFECTION

Development of an infection usually proceeds through four stages. The first stage, *incubation*, may be almost instantaneous or last for years. During this time, the pathogen is replicating, and the infected person is contagious and can transmit the disease. The *prodromal stage* (stage two) follows incubation, and the still-contagious host makes vague complaints of feeling unwell. In stage three, *acute illness*, microbes are actively destroying host cells and affecting specific host systems. The patient recognizes which area of the body is affected and voices complaints that are more specific. Finally, the *convalescent stage* (stage four) begins when the body's defense mechanisms have confined the microbes and the healing of damaged tissue is progressing.

INFECTION-CAUSING MICROBES

Microorganisms that are responsible for infectious diseases include bacteria, viruses, fungi, parasites, mycoplasmas, rickettsia, and chlamydiae.

BACTERIA

Bacteria are simple one-celled microorganisms with a cell wall that protects them from many of the human body's defense mechanisms. Although they lack a nucleus, bacteria possess all the other mechanisms they need to survive and rapidly reproduce.

Characteristics of bacteria
◆ One-celled microorganisms
◆ Cell wall protects them from the human body's defense mechanisms
◆ Classified according to shape, need for oxygen, mobility, and tendency to form protective capsules or spores
◆ Damage tissue by interfering with essential cell function or by releasing exotoxins or endotoxins

Bacteria can be classified according to shape—spherical cocci, rod-shaped bacilli, and spiral-shaped spirilla. (See *Comparing bacterial shapes.*) Bacteria can also be classified according to their need for oxygen (aerobic or anaerobic), their mobility (motile or nonmotile), and their tendency to form protective capsules (encapsulated or nonencapsulated) or spores (sporulating or nonsporulating).

Bacteria damage body tissues by interfering with essential cell function or by releasing exotoxins or endotoxins, which cause cell damage. (See *How bacteria damage tissue,* page 60.) During bacterial growth, the cells release exotoxins, enzymes that damage the host cell, altering its function or killing it. Enterotoxins are a specific type of exotoxin secreted by bacteria that infect the GI tract; they affect the vomiting center of the brain and cause gastroenteritis. Exotoxins also can cause diffuse reactions in the host, such as inflammation, bleeding, clotting, and fever. Endotoxins are contained in the cell walls of gram-negative bacteria, and they're released during lysis of the bacteria.

Examples of bacterial infection include staphylococcal wound infection, cholera, and streptococcal pneumonia. (See *Gram-positive and gram-negative bacteria,* page 61.)

Comparing bacterial shapes

Bacteria exist in three basic shapes: rods (bacilli), spheres (cocci), and spirals (spirilla).

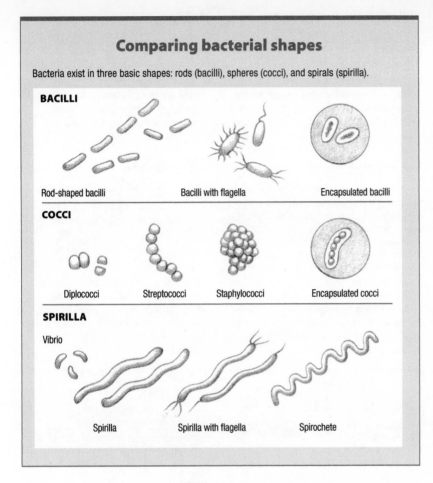

BACILLI

Rod-shaped bacilli   Bacilli with flagella   Encapsulated bacilli

COCCI

Diplococci   Streptococci   Staphylococci   Encapsulated cocci

SPIRILLA

Vibrio

Spirilla   Spirilla with flagella   Spirochete

VIRUSES

Viruses are subcellular organisms made up only of a ribonucleic acid (RNA) nucleus or a deoxyribonucleic acid (DNA) nucleus covered with proteins. They're the smallest known organisms, so tiny that only an electron microscope can make them visible. (See *How viruses size up,* page 62.) Independent of the host cells, viruses can't replicate. Rather, they invade a host cell and stimulate it to participate in forming additional virus particles. Some viruses destroy surrounding tissue and release toxins. (See *Viral infection of a host cell,* page 63.) Viruses lack the genes necessary for energy production. They depend on the ribosomes and nutrients of infected host cells for protein production. The estimated 400 viruses that infect humans are classified according to their size, shape, and means of transmission (respiratory, fecal, oral, or sexual).

Most viruses enter the body through the respiratory, GI, and genital tracts. A few, such as human immunodeficiency virus (HIV), are transmitted through blood, broken skin, and mucous membranes. Viruses can produce a wide variety of illnesses, including the common cold, herpes simplex, herpes zoster, chickenpox, infectious mononucleosis, hepatitis B and C, and rubella. Signs and symptoms depend on the host cell's status, the specific virus, and whether the intracellular environment provides good living conditions for the virus.

Characteristics of viruses

✦ Subcellular organisms made up of RNA and DNA
✦ Can't replicate outside of host cells
✦ Depend on ribosomes and nutrients of infected host cells for protein production
✦ Classified according to shape, size, and means of transmission
✦ Enter through respiratory, GI, and genital tracts, or by blood, broken skin, and mucous membranes
✦ Signs and symptoms depend on the host cell's status, specific virus, and whether intracellular environment provides good conditions for the virus
✦ Retroviruses carry genetic code to RNA; RNA viruses change viral RNA to DNA; host cell incorporates DNA into its own genetic material

Pathophysiology of bacteria

+ Bacteria enter a host
+ Bacteria adversely affect biochemical reactions in cells
+ Disruption of normal cell function or cell death occurs

CLOSER LOOK

How bacteria damage tissue

Bacteria and other infectious organisms constantly infect the human body. Some, such as the intestinal bacteria that produce vitamins, are beneficial. Others are harmful, causing illnesses ranging from the common cold to life-threatening septic shock.

To infect a host, bacteria must first enter it. They do this by adhering to the mucosal surface and directly invading the host cell or by attaching to epithelial cells and producing toxins, which invade host cells. To survive and multiply within a host, bacteria or their toxins adversely affect biochemical reactions in cells. The result is a disruption of normal cell function or cell death (see illustration below). For example, the diphtheria toxin damages heart muscle by inhibiting protein synthesis. In addition, as some organisms multiply, they extend into deeper tissue and eventually gain access to the bloodstream.

Some toxins cause blood to clot in small blood vessels. The tissues supplied by these vessels may be deprived of blood and damaged (see illustration below).

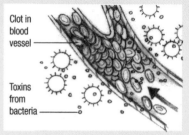

Other toxins can damage the cell walls of small blood vessels, causing leakage. This fluid loss results in decreased blood pressure, which in turn impairs the heart's ability to pump enough blood to vital organs (see illustration below).

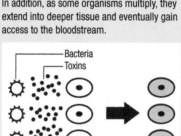

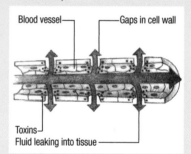

Retroviruses are a unique type of virus that carries its genetic code in RNA rather than the more common carrier, DNA. These RNA viruses contain the enzyme reverse transcriptase, which changes viral RNA into DNA. The host cell then incorporates the alien DNA into its own genetic material. The most notorious retrovirus today is HIV.

FUNGI

Characteristics of fungi

+ Occur as yeast or molds, or both
+ Live on organic matter in water, soil and on plants and animals
+ Can live inside or outside host

Fungi have rigid walls and nuclei that are enveloped by nuclear membranes. They occur as yeast (single-cell, oval-shaped organisms) or molds (organisms with hyphae, or branching filaments). Depending on the environment, some fungi may occur in both forms. Found almost everywhere on earth, fungi live on organic matter, in water and soil, on animals and plants, and on a wide variety of unlikely materials. They can live inside and outside their host. Superficial fungal infections cause athlete's foot and vaginal infections. *Candida albicans* is part of the body's normal flora; however, under certain circumstances it can cause yeast infections of virtually any part of the body, especially the mouth, skin, vagina, and GI tract. For example,

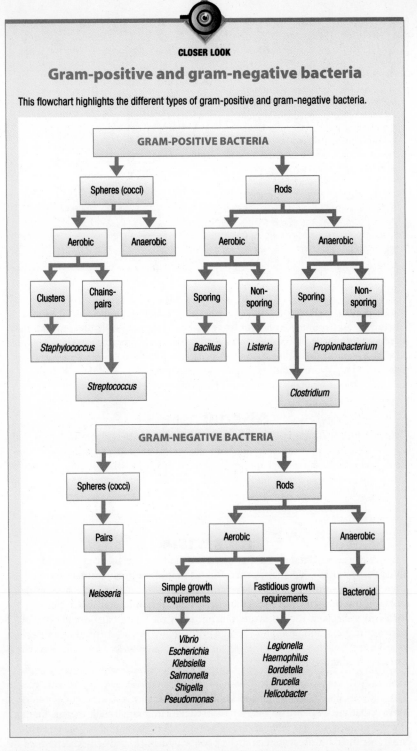

CLOSER LOOK

Gram-positive and gram-negative bacteria

This flowchart highlights the different types of gram-positive and gram-negative bacteria.

antibiotic treatment or a change in the pH of the susceptible tissues (because of a disease such as diabetes or the use of certain drugs such as hormonal contraceptives) can wipe out the normal bacteria that keep the yeast population in check.

How viruses size up

Viruses vary in size, appearance, and behavior. This illustration compares the sizes of selected viruses with the size of a typical bacterium, *Escherichia coli* (*E. coli*).

E. COLI BACTERIUM

- Poxvirus
- Rhabdovirus
- Herpesvirus
- Adenovirus
- Parvovirus

1,000 nm

Characteristics of parasites

✦ Unicellular or multicellular organisms
✦ Live on or within organism and are nourished by the host
✦ Usually don't kill their hosts

Characteristics of mycoplasmas

✦ Bacteria-like organisms
✦ Can live outside host cell or be parasitic
✦ Can assume different shapes
✦ Resilient to penicillin and antibiotics that inhibit cell wall synthesis

Characteristics of rickettsia

✦ Can cause life-threatening illnesses
✦ Require a host cell for replication
✦ Transmitted by bites of arthropods

Characteristics of chlamydiae

✦ Depend on host cells for replication
✦ Susceptible to antibiotics
✦ Transmitted by direct contact

PARASITES

Parasites are unicellular or multicellular organisms that live on or within another organism and obtain nourishment from the host. They take only the nutrients they need and usually don't kill their hosts. Examples of parasites that can produce an infection if they cause cellular damage to the host include helminths, such as pinworms and tapeworms, and arthropods, such as mites, fleas, and ticks. Helminths can infect the human gut; arthropods commonly cause skin and systemic disease.

MYCOPLASMAS

Mycoplasmas are bacteria-like organisms, the smallest of the cellular microbes that can live outside a host cell, although some may be parasitic. Lacking cell walls, they can assume many different shapes ranging from coccoid to filamentous. The lack of a cell wall makes them resistant to penicillin and other antibiotics that work by inhibiting cell wall synthesis. Mycoplasmas can cause primary atypical pneumonia and many secondary infections.

RICKETTSIA

Rickettsia are small, gram-negative, bacteria-like organisms that can cause life-threatening illness. They may be coccoid, rod-shaped, or irregularly shaped. Because they're live viruses, rickettsia require a host cell for replication. They have no cell wall, and their cell membranes are leaky; thus, they must live inside another, better-protected cell. Rickettsia are transmitted by the bites of arthropod carriers, such as lice, fleas, and ticks, and through exposure to their waste products. Rickettsial infections that occur in the United States include Rocky Mountain spotted fever, typhus, and Q fever.

CHLAMYDIAE

Chlamydiae are smaller than rickettsia and bacteria but larger than viruses. They depend on host cells for replication and are susceptible to antibiotics. Chlamydiae are transmitted by direct contact such as contact during sexual activity. They're a common cause of infections of the urethra, bladder, fallopian tubes, and prostate gland.

CLOSER LOOK

Viral infection of a host cell

The virion (A) attaches to receptors on the host-cell membrane and releases enzymes (called *absorption*) (B) that weaken the membrane and enable the virion to penetrate the cell. The virion removes the protein coat that protects its genetic material (C), replicates (D), and matures, and then escapes from the cell by budding from the plasma membrane (E). The infection then can spread to other host cells.

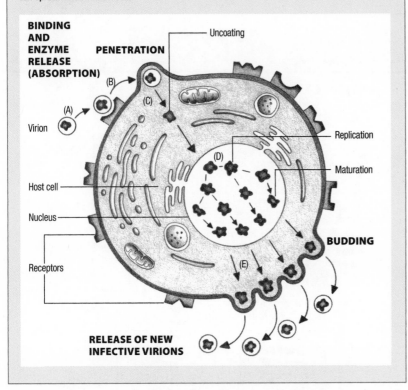

BINDING AND ENZYME RELEASE (ABSORPTION)
PENETRATION
Uncoating
(B)
(C)
(A)
Virion
Replication
(D)
Maturation
Host cell
Nucleus
BUDDING
Receptors
(E)
RELEASE OF NEW INFECTIVE VIRIONS

PATHOPHYSIOLOGIC CHANGES

Clinical expressions of infectious disease vary, depending on the pathogen involved and the organ system affected. Most of the signs and symptoms result from host responses, which vary from host to host. During the prodromal stage, a person will complain of common, nonspecific signs and symptoms, such as fever, muscle aches, headache, and lethargy. In the acute stage, signs and symptoms that are more specific provide evidence of the microbe's target. However, some illnesses produce no symptoms and are discovered only by laboratory tests.

INFLAMMATION

The inflammatory response is a major reactive defense mechanism in the battle against infective agents. Inflammation may be the result of tissue injury, infection, or allergic reaction. Acute inflammation has two stages: vascular and cellular. In the

Characteristics of pathophysiologic changes

Prodromal stage
✦ Fever
✦ Muscle aches
✦ Headache
✦ Lethargy

Acute stages
✦ More specific symptoms

Blocking inflammation

Several substances act to control inflammation. The flowchart below shows the progression of inflammation and the points ☼ at which drugs can reduce inflammation and pain.

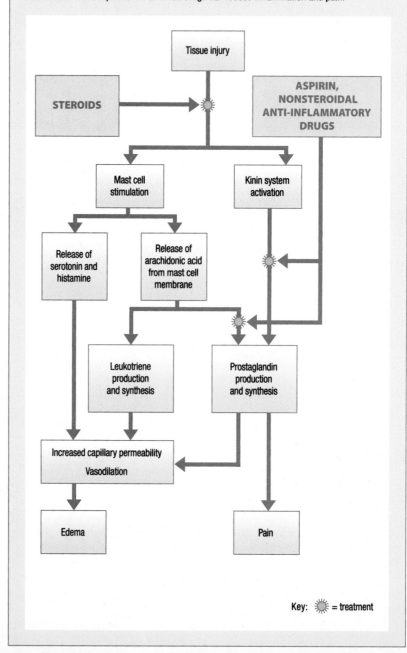

vascular stage, arterioles at or near the injury's site briefly constrict and then dilate, causing fluid pressure to increase in the capillaries. The consequent movement of plasma into the interstitial space causes edema. At the same time, inflammatory cells release histamine and bradykinin, which further increase capillary permeability. Red blood cells and fluid flow into the interstitial space, contributing to edema. The extra fluid arriving in the inflamed area dilutes microbial toxins.

During the cellular stage of inflammation, WBCs and platelets move toward the damaged cells. Phagocytosis of the dead cells and microorganisms begins. Platelets control any excess bleeding in the area, and mast cells arriving at the site release heparin to maintain blood flow to the area. (See *Blocking inflammation.*)

SIGNS AND SYMPTOMS

Acute inflammation is the body's immediate response to cell injury or cell death. The cardinal signs of inflammation include redness, heat, pain, edema, and decreased function of a body part.

✦ *Redness (rubor)* results when arterioles dilate and circulation to the site increases. Filling of previously empty or partially distended capillaries causes a localized blush.

✦ *Heat (calor)* in the area results from local vasodilation, fluid leakage into the interstitial spaces, and increased blood flow to the area.

✦ *Pain (dolor)* occurs when pain receptors are stimulated by swollen tissue, local pH changes, and chemicals excreted during the inflammatory process.

✦ *Edema (tumor)* is caused by local vasodilation, leakage of fluid into interstitial spaces, and the blockage of lymphatic drainage to help wall off the inflammation.

✦ *Loss of function (functio laesa)* occurs primarily as a result of edema and pain at the site.

 CLINICAL ALERT Localized infections produce a rapid inflammatory response with obvious signs and symptoms. Disseminated infections have a slow inflammatory response and take longer to identify and treat, thereby increasing morbidity and mortality.

FEVER

Fever occurs with the introduction of an infectious agent. An elevated temperature helps fight an infection because many microorganisms can't survive in a hot environment. When the body temperature rises too high, body cells can be damaged, particularly those of the nervous system.

Diaphoresis is the body's method of cooling itself and returning the temperature to "normal" for that individual. Artificial methods to reduce a slight fever can impair the body's defenses against infection.

LEUKOCYTOSIS

The body responds to the introduction of pathogens by increasing the number and types of circulating WBCs. This process is called *leukocytosis*. In the acute or early stage, the neutrophil count increases. Bone marrow begins to release immature leukocytes because existing neutrophils can't meet the body's demand for defensive cells. The immature neutrophils (called "bands" in the differential WBC count) can't serve any defensive purpose.

Key facts about leukocytosis
(continued)

◆ Neutrophils, monocytes, and macrophages begin phagocytosis of dead tissue and bacteria
◆ They identify the foreign antigen and kill the microorganism
◆ Elevated monocyte count is common during resolution of injury or chronic infections

Key facts about chronic infection

◆ Infection lasting longer than 2 weeks
◆ May follow acute process
◆ Permanent scarring and loss of tissue function may occur

Diagnosis

◆ Obtain patient's medical history
◆ Perform thorough examination
◆ Order appropriate tests
◆ WBC count is first test; recognizes only that something has stimulated an immune response
◆ Erythrocyte sedimentation rate test reveals occurrence of inflammatory process
◆ Gram stain identifies bacteria; silver stains identify fungi
◆ Cultures confirm pathogens

As the acute phase comes under control and the damage is isolated, the next stage of the inflammatory process takes place. Neutrophils, monocytes, and macrophages begin the process of phagocytosis of dead tissue and bacteria. Neutrophils and monocytes, attracted to the site of infection by chemotaxis, identify the foreign antigen and attach to it. Then they engulf, kill, and degrade the microorganism that carries the antigen on its surface. Macrophages, a mature type of monocyte, arrive at the site later and remain in the area of inflammation longer than the other cells. Besides phagocytosis, macrophages play several other key roles at the site, such as preparing the area for healing and processing antigens for a cellular immune response. An elevated monocyte count is common during resolution of an injury and in chronic infections.

CHRONIC INFLAMMATION

An inflammation reaction lasting longer than 2 weeks is referred to as chronic inflammation. It may follow an acute process, such as a poorly healed wound or an unresolved infection. The body may encapsulate a pathogen that it can't destroy in order to isolate it. An example of such a pathogen is *Mycobacterium tuberculosis,* the cause of tuberculosis; encapsulated mycobacteria appear in X-rays as identifiable spots in the lungs. With chronic inflammation, permanent scarring and loss of tissue function can occur.

DIAGNOSIS

Accurate assessment helps identify infectious diseases, appropriate treatment, and avoidable complications. It begins with obtaining the patient's complete medical history, performing a thorough physical examination, and performing or ordering appropriate diagnostic tests. Tests that can help identify and gauge the extent of infection include laboratory studies, radiographic tests, and scans.

Typically, the first test is a WBC count and a differential. Elevation in the overall number of WBCs is a positive result. The differential count is the relative number of each of five types of WBCs — neutrophils, eosinophils, basophils, lymphocytes, and monocytes. It's obtained by classifying 100 or more WBCs in a stained film of peripheral blood. Multiplying the percentage value of each type by the total WBC count gives the absolute number of each type of WBC. This test recognizes only that something has stimulated an immune response. Bacterial infection usually causes an elevation in the counts; viruses may cause no change or a decrease in normal WBC level.

An erythrocyte sedimentation rate test may be done to reveal that an inflammatory process is occurring within the body.

The next step is to obtain a stained smear from a specific body site to determine the causative agent. Stains may be used to visualize the microorganism. Gram stains identify gram-negative or gram-positive bacteria, acid-fast stains identify mycobacteria and *Nocardia,* and silver stains identify fungi, *Legionella*, and *Pneumocystis.*

Although stains provide rapid and valuable diagnostic information, they only tentatively identify a pathogen. Confirmation requires culturing. Any body substance can be cultured; however, enough growth to identify the microbe may occur in as few as 8 hours (streptococcal) or as long as several weeks, depending on how rapidly the microbe replicates. Types of cultures that may be ordered are blood, urine, sputum, throat, nasal, wound, skin, stool, and cerebrospinal fluid.

A specimen obtained for culture must not be contaminated with any other substance. For example, a urine specimen must not contain debris from the perineum or vaginal area. If obtaining a clean urine specimen isn't possible, the patient must be catheterized to make sure that only the urine is being examined. Contaminated specimens may mislead and prolong treatment.

Additional tests that may be requested include magnetic resonance imaging to locate infection sites, chest X-rays to search the lungs for respiratory changes, and gallium scans to detect abscesses.

TREATMENTS

Treatment of infections can vary widely. Vaccines may be administered to induce a primary immune response under conditions that won't cause disease. If infection occurs, treatment is tailored to the specific causative organism. Drug therapy should be used only when it's appropriate. Supportive therapy can play an important role in fighting infections.

◆ Antibiotics work in various ways, depending on the antibiotic class. Their action is bactericidal (killing the bacteria) or bacteriostatic (preventing the bacteria from multiplying). Antibiotics may inhibit cell wall synthesis, protein synthesis, bacterial metabolism, or nucleic acid synthesis or activity, or they may increase cell membrane permeability. (See *Antimicrobial drugs and chemicals,* page 68.)

◆ Antifungal drugs destroy the invading microbe by increasing cell membrane permeability. The antifungal binds sterols in the cell membrane, resulting in leakage of intracellular contents, such as potassium, sodium, and nutrients.

◆ Antiviral drugs stop viral replication by interfering with DNA synthesis.

The overuse of antimicrobials has created widespread resistance to some drugs. Some pathogens that were once well controlled by medicines are again surfacing with increased virulence. One such pathogen (known to cause tuberculosis) is *Mycobacterium tuberculosis.*

Some diseases, including most viral infections, don't respond to available drugs. Supportive care is the only recourse while the host defenses repel the invader. To help the body fight an infection, the patient should use standard precautions such as handwashing to avoid spreading the infection, drink plenty of fluids, get plenty of rest, and avoid people who may have other illnesses.

To alleviate symptoms, the patient may take appropriate over-the-counter medications. He should do so only with full knowledge about dosage, actions, and possible adverse effects or reactions. When taking prescription drugs, the patient should always follow the physician's orders exactly and be sure to finish the entire prescription. It's also important for the patient to understand that prescription drugs should never be shared with others.

Diagnosis
(continued)

◆ MRI to locate infection sites
◆ Chest X-ray to search the lungs for respiratory changes
◆ Gallium scans to detect abscesses

Treatment

◆ Administer vaccines to induce a primary immune response that won't cause disease
◆ Use drug therapy only when appropriate
◆ Supportive therapy can play a role
◆ Antibiotics kill bacteria and prevent it from multiplying
◆ Antifungal drugs destroy invading microbes by increasing cell membrane permeability
◆ Antiviral drugs stop viral replication
◆ Overuse of medications has created resistance to these drugs
◆ Some diseases don't respond to available drugs; standard precautions to avoid spreading the infection should be taken
◆ Over-the-counter medications can alleviate symptoms

Antimicrobial actions
- Inhibit cell wall synthesis
- Damage cytoplasmic membrane
- Metabolize nucleic acid
- Synthesize protein
- Modify energy metabolism

Antimicrobial drugs and chemicals

The following drugs or chemicals prevent growth of microorganisms or destroy them by a specific action.

MECHANISMS OF ACTION	AGENT
Inhibition of cell wall synthesis	Bacitracin
	Carbapenems
	Cephalosporins
	Cycloserine
	Fosfomycin
	Monobactams
	Penicillins
	Vancomycin
Damage to cytoplasmic membrane	Imidazoles
	Polyene antifungals
	Polymyxins
Metabolism of nucleic acid	Nitrofurans
	Nitroimidazoles
	Quinolones
	Rifampin
Protein synthesis	Aminoglycosides
	Chloramphenicol
	Clindamycin
	Macrolides
	Mupirocin
	Spectinomycin
	Tetracyclines
Modification of energy metabolism	Dapsone
	Isoniazid
	Sulfonamides
	Trimethoprim

INFECTIONS

Infection can strike any part of the body. The accompanying chart describes various infections along with their signs and symptoms and appropriate diagnostic tests. (See *Reviewing common infections.*)

Reviewing common infections

INFECTION AND FINDINGS	DIAGNOSIS

Bacterial infections

Anthrax

Cutaneous anthrax
+ Small, elevated, itchy lesion that resembles an insect bite, develops into a vesicle, and finally becomes a small, painless ulcer with a necrotic (black) center
+ Enlarged lymph glands

+ Isolation of *Bacillus anthracis* from cultures of the blood, skin lesions, or sputum confirms the diagnosis.
+ Specific antibodies may be detected in the blood.

Inhalational anthrax
+ Initial flulike symptoms, such as malaise, fever, headache, myalgia, and chills
+ Progression to severe respiratory difficulties, such as dyspnea, stridor, chest pain, and cyanosis
+ Onset of shock

Intestinal anthrax
+ Nausea and vomiting
+ Decreased appetite
+ Fever
+ Progression to abdominal pain, vomiting blood, and severe diarrhea

Botulism
+ Initial signs and symptoms include dry mouth, sore throat, weakness, dizziness, vomiting, and diarrhea
+ Cardinal sign: acute symmetrical cranial nerve impairment (ptosis, diplopia, and dysarthria)
+ Descending weakness or paralysis of muscles in the extremities or trunk
+ Dyspnea from respiratory muscle paralysis

+ Identification of the offending toxin in the patient's serum, stools, gastric content, or the suspected food confirms the diagnosis.
+ Electromyogram showing diminished muscle action potential after a single supramaximal nerve stimulus is also diagnostic.

Infant botulism
+ Generalized muscle weakness, hypotonia, and feeble cry
+ Constipation
+ Depressed gag reflex and inability to suck
+ Flaccid facial expression, ptosis, and ophthalmoplegia due to cranial nerve deficits
+ Areflexia and loss of head control

Chlamydial infections

Cervicitis
+ Cervical erosion
+ Dyspareunia
+ Mucopurulent discharge
+ Pelvic pain

+ Swab from site of infection establishes a diagnosis of urethritis, cervicitis, salpingitis, endometritis, or proctitis.
+ Culture of aspirated material establishes a diagnosis of epididymitis.
+ Antigen-detection methods are the diagnostic tests of choice for identifying chlamydial infection.
+ Polymerase chain reaction test is highly sensitive and specific.

Endometritis or salpingitis
+ Pain and tenderness of the lower abdomen, cervix, uterus, and lymph nodes
+ Chills and fever
+ Breakthrough bleeding, bleeding after intercourse, and vaginal discharge
+ Dysuria

(continued)

Key signs of anthrax

Cutaneous
+ Lesion that resembles insect bite
+ Enlarged lymph glands

Inhalational
+ Initial flulike symptoms
+ Respiratory difficulties
+ Shock

Intestinal
+ Nausea and vomiting
+ Decreased appetite
+ Fever
+ Abdominal pain, vomiting blood, severe diarrhea

Key signs of botulism
+ Acute symmetrical cranial nerve impairment
+ Dyspnea

Infants
+ Constipation
+ Depressed gag reflex and inability to suck
+ Loss of head control

Key signs of chlamydial infections

Cervicitis
+ Cervical erosion
+ Pelvic pain

Endometritis
+ Pain and tenderness in lower abdomen, cervix, uterus, and lymph nodes
+ Breakthrough bleeding

Key signs of chlamydial infections

Urethral syndrome
+ Dysuria and pyuria
+ Urinary frequency

Urethritis
+ Dysuria
+ Pruritus and urethral discharge

Epididymitis
+ Painful scrotal swelling

Prostatitis
+ Urinary frequency
+ Painful ejaculation

Proctitis
+ Pruritus
+ Diffuse or discrete ulceration

Key signs of conjunctivitis
+ Discharge
+ Itching and burning

Key signs of gonorrhea

Males
+ Urethritis

Females
+ Inflammation
+ Greenish-yellow discharge from cervix

Males and females
+ Tonsillitis
+ Rectal burning
+ Vary according to site involved

Reviewing common infections *(continued)*

INFECTION AND FINDINGS	DIAGNOSIS

Bacterial infections (continued)

Chlamydial infections *(continued)*
Urethral syndrome
+ Dysuria, pyuria, and urinary frequency
Urethritis
+ Dysuria, erythema, and tenderness of the urethral meatus
+ Urinary frequency
+ Pruritus and urethral discharge (copious and purulent or scant and clear or mucoid)

Epididymitis
+ Painful scrotal swelling
+ Urethral discharge

Prostatitis
+ Lower back pain
+ Urinary frequency, nocturia, and dysuria
+ Painful ejaculation

Proctitis
+ Diarrhea
+ Tenesmus
+ Pruritus
+ Bloody or mucopurulent discharge
+ Diffuse or discrete ulceration in the rectosigmoid colon

Conjunctivitis
+ Hyperemia of the conjunctiva
+ Discharge
+ Tearing
+ Pain
+ Photophobia (with corneal involvement)
+ Itching and burning
  Note: Conjunctivitis may also result from viral infection.

+ Culture from the conjunctiva identifies the causative organism.
+ In stained smears, predominance of lymphocytes indicates viral infection; of neutrophils, bacterial infection; of eosinophils, an allergy-related infection.

Gonorrhea
Males
+ May not produce symptoms
+ Urethritis, including dysuria and purulent urethral discharge, with redness and swelling at the site of infection

Females
+ May not produce symptoms
+ Inflammation and a greenish yellow discharge from the cervix

Males or females
+ Pharyngitis or tonsillitis
+ Rectal burning, itching, and bloody mucopurulent discharge

+ Culture from the site of infection, grown on a Thayer-Martin or Transgrow medium, establishes the diagnosis by isolating *Neisseria gonorrhoeae.*
+ Gram stain shows gram-negative diplococci.
+ Complement fixation and immunofluorescent assays of serum reveal antibody titers four times the normal rate.

Reviewing common infections *(continued)*

INFECTION AND FINDINGS	DIAGNOSIS

Bacterial infections *(continued)*

Gonorrhea *(continued)*
Clinical features vary according to the site involved
✦ Urethra: dysuria, urinary frequency and incontinence, purulent discharge, itching, and red and edematous meatus
✦ Vulva: occasional itching, burning, and pain due to exudate from an adjacent infected area
✦ Vagina: engorgement, redness, swelling, and profuse purulent discharge
✦ Liver: right upper quadrant pain
✦ Pelvis: severe pelvic and lower abdominal pain, muscle rigidity, tenderness, and abdominal distention; nausea, vomiting, fever, and tachycardia (may develop in patients with salpingitis or pelvic inflammatory disease)

Listeriosis
✦ Commonly causes asymptomatic carrier state
✦ Malaise
✦ Chills
✦ Fever
✦ Back pain

Fetuses
✦ Abortion
✦ Premature delivery or stillbirth
✦ Organ abscesses

Neonates
✦ Meningitis, resulting in tense fontanels
✦ Irritability
✦ Lethargy
✦ Seizures
✦ Coma

✦ *Listeria monocytogenes* is identified by its diagnostic tumbling motility on a wet mount of the culture.
✦ Positive culture of blood, spinal fluid, drainage from cervical or vaginal lesions, or lochia from a mother with an infected infant.

Lyme disease
Stage 1
✦ Erythema chronicum migrans (ECM): red macule or papule, commonly on the site of a tick bite, which grows to over 50 cm, feels hot and itchy, and resembles a bull's eye or target; after a few days, more lesions erupt and a migratory, ringlike rash appears
✦ Conjunctivitis
✦ Diffuse urticaria
✦ Lesions are replaced by small red blotches in 3 to 4 weeks
✦ Malaise and fatigue
✦ Intermittent headache
✦ Neck stiffness
✦ Fever, chills, and aching
✦ Regional lymphadenopathy

✦ Because *Borrelia burgdorferi* is unusual in humans and indirect immunofluorescent antibody tests are marginally sensitive, diagnosis is usually based on the characteristic ECM lesion and related clinical findings.
✦ Serology reveals mild anemia and elevated erythrocyte sedimentation rate, white blood cell (WBC) count, serum immunoglobulin (Ig) M level, and aspartate aminotransferase.
✦ Cerebrospinal fluid (CSF) analysis reveals presence of antibodies to *B. burgdorferi* if the disease has affected the central nervous system (CNS).

Key signs of listeriosis
✦ Malaise
✦ Back pain

Fetuses
✦ Abortion
✦ Premature delivery

Neonates
✦ Meningitis
✦ Coma

Key signs of lyme disease

Stage 1
✦ ECM
✦ Malaise and fatigue
✦ Neck stiffness

(continued)

Key signs of lyme disease

Stage 2
+ Neurologic abnormalities
+ Facial palsy

Stage 3
+ Arthritis
+ Ophthalmic manifestations

Key signs of meningitis
+ Fever and chills
+ Lethargy
+ Coma
+ Bradycardia
+ Occasional rash

Key signs of otitis media
+ Ear pain
+ Lethargy
+ Vertigo
+ Tinnitus

Reviewing common infections *(continued)*

INFECTION AND FINDINGS	DIAGNOSIS
Bacterial infections (continued)	

Lyme disease *(continued)*
Stage 2
+ Neurologic abnormalities: fluctuating meningoen-cephalitis with peripheral and cranial neuropathy; begins weeks to months later
+ Facial palsy
+ Cardiac abnormalities: brief, fluctuating atrioventricular heart block, left ventricular dysfunction, and cardiomegaly

Stage 3
+ Arthritis with marked swelling begins weeks or years later
+ Neuropsychiatric symptoms such as psychotic behavior, memory loss, dementia, and depression
+ Encephalopathic symptoms, such as headache, confusion, and difficulty concentrating
+ Ophthalmic manifestations such as iritis, keratitis, renal vasculitis, and optic neuritis

---

Meningitis
+ Fever
+ Chills
+ Headache
+ Nuchal rigidity
+ Vomiting
+ Photophobia
+ Lethargy
+ Coma
+ Positive Brudzinski's and Kernig's signs
+ Exaggerated and symmetrical deep tendon reflexes and opisthotonos
+ Wide pulse pressure
+ Bradycardia
+ Occasional rash
  Note: Meningitis may also result from viral, protozoal, or fungal infection.

+ Lumbar puncture isolates the infecting organism (usually *Neisseria meningitidis, Haemophilus influenzae* [in children and young adults], or *Streptococcus pneumoniae* [in adults]) from CSF and shows increased CSF cell count and protein level and decreased CSF glucose level.
+ Blood culture isolates the infecting organism.

Otitis media
+ Ear pain
+ Ear drainage
+ Hearing loss
+ Fever
+ Lethargy
+ Irritability
+ Vertigo
+ Signs of upper respiratory tract infection (such as sneezing and coughing)
+ Tinnitus

+ Otoscopy reveals obscured or distorted bony landmarks of the tympanic membrane.
+ Pneumatoscopy can show decreased tympanic membrane mobility.
+ Culture of the ear drainage identifies the causative organism.

Reviewing common infections *(continued)*

INFECTION AND FINDINGS	DIAGNOSIS

Bacterial infections (continued)

Peritonitis

✦ Sudden, severe, and diffuse abdominal pain that tends to intensify and localize in the area of the underlying disorder with associated rebound tenderness
✦ Weakness and pallor
✦ Excessive sweating
✦ Cold skin
✦ Decreased intestinal motility and paralytic ileus
✦ Intestinal obstruction causes nausea, vomiting, and abdominal rigidity
✦ Hypotension
✦ Tachycardia
✦ Fever
✦ Abdominal distention

✦ Abdominal X-ray shows edematous and gaseous distention of the small and large bowel or in the case of visceral organ perforation, air lying under the diaphragm.
✦ Chest X-ray may show elevation of the diaphragm.
✦ Blood studies show leukocytosis.
✦ Paracentesis reveals bacteria, exudate, blood, pus, or urine.
✦ Laparotomy may be necessary to identify the underlying cause.

Plague

Bubonic plague
✦ Malaise and fever
✦ Pain or tenderness in regional lymph nodes, possibly associated with swelling
✦ Painful, inflamed, and possibly suppurative buboes; classic sign is an excruciatingly painful bubo
✦ Hemorrhagic areas that become necrotic; such areas appear dark (hence the name "black death")
✦ Restlessness, disorientation, delirium, toxemia, and staggering gait

Primary pneumonic plague
✦ Acute onset of high fever, chills, severe headache, tachycardia, tachypnea, and dyspnea
✦ Productive cough (first mucoid sputum, later frothy pink or red)
✦ Severe prostration, respiratory distress, and usually death

Secondary pneumonic plague
✦ Pulmonary extension of the bubonic form
✦ Cough producing bloody sputum
✦ Severe prostration, respiratory distress, and usually death

Septicemic plague
✦ Toxicity, hyperpyrexia, seizures, prostration, shock, and disseminated intravascular coagulation
✦ Widespread nonspecific tissue damage

✦ Characteristic buboes and a history of exposure to rodents are strongly suggestive of diagnosis.
✦ Stained smears and cultures of *Yersinia pestis* obtained from a needle aspirate of a small amount of fluid from skin lesions confirm the diagnosis.
✦ Other laboratory findings include elevated WBC count with increased polymorphonuclear leukocytes and hemoagglutination reaction (antibody titer) studies.
✦ In pneumonic plague, chest X-ray shows fulminating pneumonia and stained smear and culture of sputum identify *Y. pestis.*
✦ In septicemic plague, stained smear and blood culture containing *Y. pestis* are diagnostic.
✦ For a presumptive diagnosis of plague, a fluorescent antibody test may be ordered.

Key signs of peritonitis
✦ Abdominal pain; localized and intense
✦ Intestinal obstruction
✦ Abdominal distention

Key signs of plague

Bubonic
✦ Malaise and fever
✦ Lymph node pain or tenderness
✦ Hemorrhagic areas that become nectrotic

Primary pneumonic
✦ Acute onset of high fever and chills
✦ Severe prostration and respiratory distress

Secondary pneumonic
✦ Pulmonary extension of the bubonic form
✦ Bloody sputum produced by cough

Septicemic
✦ Toxicity
✦ Widespread nonspecific tissue damage

(continued)

Key signs of pneumonia

- High temperature
- Dyspnea
- Crackles
- Chills

Key signs of salmonellosis

- Fever
- Abdominal pain

Typhoidal infection

- Increasing fever
- Constipation

Key signs of shigellosis

Children

- High fever
- Diarrhea with tenesmus
- Dehydration and weight loss

Adults

- Rectal irritability
- Tenesmus
- Headache and prostration

Reviewing common infections *(continued)*

INFECTION AND FINDINGS	DIAGNOSIS
Bacterial Infections *(continued)*	
Pneumonia ◆ High temperature ◆ Cough with purulent, yellow or bloody sputum ◆ Dyspnea ◆ Crackles and decreased breath sounds ◆ Pleuritic pain ◆ Chills ◆ Malaise ◆ Tachypnea *Note:* Pneumonia may also result from fungal or protozoal infection.	◆ Chest X-rays confirm the diagnosis by disclosing infiltrates. ◆ Sputum specimen, Gram stain and culture, and sensitivity tests help differentiate the type of infection and the drugs that are effective. ◆ WBC count indicates leukocytosis in bacterial pneumonia, and a normal or low count in viral or mycoplasmal pneumonia. ◆ Blood cultures reflect bacteremia and are used to determine the causative organism. ◆ Arterial blood gas levels vary, depending on severity of pneumonia and underlying lung state. ◆ Bronchoscopy or transtracheal aspiration allows the collection of material for culture. ◆ Pulse oximetry may show a reduced oxygen saturation level.
Salmonellosis ◆ Fever ◆ Abdominal pain, severe diarrhea with enterocolitis *Typhoidal infection* ◆ Headache ◆ Increasing fever ◆ Constipation	◆ Blood cultures isolate the organism in typhoid fever, paratyphoid fever, and bacteremia. ◆ Stool cultures isolate the organism in typhoid fever, paratyphoid fever, and enterocolitis. ◆ Cultures of urine, bone marrow, pus, and vomitus may show the presence of *Salmonella*.
Shigellosis *Children* ◆ High fever ◆ Diarrhea with tenesmus ◆ Nausea, vomiting, and abdominal pain and distention ◆ Irritability ◆ Drowsiness ◆ Stools may contain pus, mucus, or blood ◆ Dehydration and weight loss *Adults* ◆ Sporadic, intense abdominal pain ◆ Rectal irritability ◆ Tenesmus ◆ Headache and prostration ◆ Stools may contain pus, mucus, and blood	◆ Microscopic examination of fresh stools may reveal mucus, red blood cells (RBCs), and polymorphonuclear leukocytes; direct immunofluorescence with specific antisera may reveal *Shigella*. ◆ Severe infection increases hemagglutinating antibodies. ◆ Sigmoidoscopy or proctoscopy may reveal typical superficial ulcerations.

Reviewing common infections *(continued)*

INFECTION AND FINDINGS	DIAGNOSIS

Bacterial infections (continued)

Syphilis

Primary syphilis
+ Chancres (small, fluid-filled lesions) on the anus, fingers, lips, tongue, nipples, tonsils, or eyelids
+ Regional lymphadenopathy

Secondary syphilis
+ Symmetrical mucocutaneous lesions
+ General lymphadenopathy
+ Rash may be macular, papular, pustular, or nodular
+ Headache
+ Malaise
+ Anorexia, weight loss, nausea, and vomiting
+ Sore throat and slight fever
+ Alopecia
+ Brittle and pitted nails

Late syphilis
+ Benign—gumma lesion found on any bone or organ
+ Gastric pain, tenderness, and enlarged spleen
+ Anemia
+ Involvement of the upper respiratory tract, perforation of the nasal septum or palate, and destruction of bones and organs
+ Fibrosis of elastic tissue of the aorta
+ Aortic insufficiency
+ Aortic aneurysm
+ Meningitis
+ Paresis
+ Personality changes
+ Arm and leg weakness

+ Dark field examination of a lesion identifies *Treponema pallidum*.
+ A fluorescent treponemal antibody absorption test identifies antigens of *T. pallidum* in tissue, ocular fluid, CSF, tracheobronchial secretions, and exudates from lesions.
+ Venereal Disease Research Laboratory (VDRL) slide test and rapid plasma reagin test detect nonspecific antibodies.

Tetanus

Localized
+ Spasm and increased muscle tone near the wound

Systemic
+ Marked muscle hypertonicity
+ Hyperactive deep tendon reflexes
+ Tachycardia
+ Profuse sweating
+ Low-grade fever
+ Painful, involuntary muscle contractions

+ Diagnosis may rest on clinical features, a history of trauma, and no previous tetanus immunization.
+ Blood cultures and tetanus antibody tests are commonly negative; only one-third of patients have a positive wound culture.
+ CSF pressure may rise above normal.

Key signs of syphilis

Primary
+ Chancres
+ Regional lymphadenopathy

Secondary
+ Symmetrical mucocutaneous lesions
+ Alopecia
+ Brittle and pitted nails

Late
+ Benign—gumma lesion
+ Aortic insufficiency
+ Meningitis
+ Arm and leg weakness

Key signs of tetanus

Localized
+ Spasm or increased muscle tone near the wound

Systemic
+ Marked muscle hypertonicity
+ Tachycardia
+ Painful, involuntary muscle contractions

(continued)

Key signs of toxic shock syndrome

+ Fever over 104° F
+ Vomiting and diarrhea
+ Decreased LOC
+ Severe hypotension

Key signs of tuberculosis

+ Fever and night sweats
+ Productive cough lasting longer than 3 weeks
+ Weight loss
+ Pleuritic chest pain

Key signs of urinary tract infections

Cystitis

+ Dysuria
+ Cloudy, malodorous, and possibly bloody urine

Acute pyelonephritis

+ Fever and shaking chills
+ Tachycardia
+ Generalized muscle tenderness

Urethritis

+ Dysuria, frequency, and pyuria

Reviewing common infections *(continued)*

INFECTION AND FINDINGS	DIAGNOSIS
Bacterial infections *(continued)*	

Toxic shock syndrome

+ Intense myalgia
+ Fever over 104° F (40° C)
+ Vomiting and diarrhea
+ Headache
+ Decreased level of consciousness (LOC)
+ Rigor
+ Conjunctival hyperemia
+ Vaginal hyperemia and discharge
+ Deep red rash (especially on the palms and soles) that later desquamates
+ Severe hypotension

+ Diagnosis is based on clinical findings and body system involvement.
+ *Staphylococcus aureus* is isolated from vaginal discharge or lesions.
+ Negative results on blood tests for Rocky Mountain spotted fever, leptospirosis, and measles help rule out these disorders.

Tuberculosis

+ Fever and night sweats
+ Productive cough lasting longer than 3 weeks
+ Hemoptysis
+ Malaise
+ Adenopathy
+ Weight loss
+ Pleuritic chest pain
+ Symptoms of airway obstruction from lymph node involvement

+ Chest X-ray shows nodular lesions, patchy infiltrates (mainly in upper lobes), cavity formation, scar tissue, and calcium deposits.
+ Tuberculin skin test reveals infection at some point, but doesn't indicate active disease.
+ Stains and cultures of sputum, CSF, urine, drainage from abscesses, or pleural fluid show heat-sensitive, nonmotile, aerobic, acid-fast bacilli.
+ Computed tomography (CT) scans or magnetic resonance imaging (MRI) allows the evaluation of lung damage and may confirm a difficult diagnosis.
+ Bronchoscopy shows inflammation and altered lung tissue. It may also be performed to obtain sputum if the patient can't produce an adequate sputum specimen.

Urinary tract infections

Cystitis
+ Dysuria, frequency, urgency, and suprapubic pain
+ Cloudy, malodorous, and possibly bloody urine
+ Fever
+ Nausea and vomiting
+ Costovertebral angle tenderness

+ Urine culture reveals microorganism.
+ Urinary microscopy is positive for pyuria, hematuria, or bacteriuria.

Acute pyelonephritis
+ Fever and shaking chills
+ Nausea, vomiting, and diarrhea
+ Symptoms of cystitis may be present
+ Tachycardia
+ Generalized muscle tenderness

Urethritis
+ Dysuria, frequency, and pyuria

Reviewing common infections *(continued)*

INFECTION AND FINDINGS	DIAGNOSIS

Bacterial infections (continued)

Whooping cough (Pertussis)
+ Irritating, hacking cough characteristically ending in a loud, crowing, inspiratory whoop that may expel tenacious mucus
+ Anorexia
+ Sneezing
+ Listlessness
+ Infected conjunctiva
+ Low-grade fever

+ Classic clinical findings suggest the disease.
+ Nasopharyngeal swabs and sputum cultures show *Bordetella pertussis.*
+ Fluorescent antibody screening of nasopharyngeal smears is less reliable than cultures.
+ Serology shows an elevated WBC count.

Viral infections

Chickenpox (Varicella)
+ Pruritic rash of small, erythematous macules that progresses to papules and then to clear vesicles on an erythematous base
+ Slight fever
+ Malaise and anorexia
+ Congenital varicella: hypoplastic deformity and scarring of a limb, retarded growth, and CNS and eye manifestations
+ An immunocompromised patient with progressive varicella: lesions and a high fever for over 7 days

+ Characteristic clinical signs suggest the virus.
+ Isolation of virus from vesicular fluid helps confirm the virus; Giemsa stain distinguishes varicella-zoster from vaccinia and variola viruses.

Cytomegalovirus infection
+ Mild, nonspecific complaints
+ Immunodeficient population: pneumonia, chorioretinitis, colitis, encephalitis, abdominal pain, diarrhea, or weight loss
+ Infants ages 3 to 6 months appear asymptomatic but may develop hepatic dysfunction, hepatosplenomegaly, spider angiomas, pneumonitis, and lymphadenopathy
+ Congenital infection: jaundice, petechial rash, hepatosplenomegaly, thrombocytopenia, and hemolytic anemia

+ Virus is isolated in urine, saliva, throat, cervix, WBCs, and biopsy specimens. Complement fixation studies, hemagglutination inhibition antibody tests, and indirect immunofluorescent test for cytomegalovirus immunoglobulin M (IgM) antibody (congenital infections) aid diagnosis.

Herpes simplex
Type 1
+ Fever
+ Sore, red, swollen throat
+ Submaxillary lymphadenopathy
+ Increased salivation, halitosis, and anorexia
+ Severe mouth pain
+ Edema of the mouth
+ Vesicles (on the tongue, gingiva, and cheeks, or anywhere in or around the mouth) on a red base that eventually rupture, leaving a painful ulcer and then yellow crusting

+ Tzanck test shows multinucleated giant cells.
+ Herpes simplex virus culture is positive.
+ Virus is isolated from local lesions.
+ A tissue biopsy aids in the diagnosis.
+ Elevated antibodies and increased WBC count indicate primary infection.

(continued)

Key signs of herpes simplex

Type 2
✦ Tingling in the area involved
✦ Leukorrhea
✦ Dyspareunia

Key signs of herpes zoster

✦ Pain within the dermatome affected
✦ Small, red, nodular skin lesions that change to pus or fluid-filled vesicles

Key signs of HIV infection

✦ Rapid weight loss
✦ Recurring fever or profuse night sweats
✦ Swollen lymph glands
✦ White spots or unusual blemishes in the mouth
✦ Pneumonia

Key signs of infectious mononucleosis

✦ Sore throat
✦ Cervical lymphadenopathy
✦ Temperature fluctuations with an evening peak
✦ Splenomegaly
✦ Stomatitis

Reviewing common infections *(continued)*

INFECTION AND FINDINGS	DIAGNOSIS
Viral Infections (continued)	

Herpes simplex *(continued)*
Type 2
✦ Tingling in the area involved
✦ Malaise
✦ Dysuria
✦ Dyspareunia (painful intercourse)
✦ Leukorrhea (white vaginal discharge containing mucus and pus cells)
✦ Localized, fluid-filled vesicles that are found on the cervix, labia, perianal skin, vulva, vagina, glans penis, foreskin, and penile shaft, mouth or anus; inguinal swelling may be present

---

Herpes zoster
✦ Pain within the dermatome affected
✦ Fever
✦ Malaise
✦ Pruritus
✦ Paresthesia or hyperesthesia in the trunk, arms, or legs may also occur
✦ Small, red, nodular skin lesions on painful areas (nerve specific) that change to pus or fluid-filled vesicles

✦ Staining antibodies from vesicular fluid and identification under fluorescent light differentiates herpes zoster from localized herpes simplex.
✦ Examination of vesicular fluid and infected tissue shows eosinophilic intranuclear inclusions and varicella virus.
✦ Lumbar puncture shows increased pressure; CSF shows increased protein levels and possibly pleocytosis.

Human immunodeficiency virus (HIV) infection
✦ Rapid weight loss
✦ Dry cough
✦ Recurring fever or profuse night sweats
✦ Profound and unexplained fatigue
✦ Swollen lymph glands in the armpits, groin, or neck
✦ Diarrhea that lasts for more than a week
✦ White spots or unusual blemishes on the tongue, in the mouth, or in the throat
✦ Pneumonia
✦ Red, brown, pink, or purplish blotches on or under the skin or inside the mouth, nose, or eyelids
✦ Memory loss, depression, and other neurologic disorders

✦ Two enzyme-linked immunosorbent assays (ELISA) are positive.
✦ Western blot test is positive.

Infectious mononucleosis
✦ Headache
✦ Malaise and fatigue
✦ Sore throat
✦ Cervical lymphadenopathy
✦ Temperature fluctuations with an evening peak
✦ Splenomegaly
✦ Hepatomegaly

✦ Monospot test is positive.
✦ WBC count is abnormally high (10,000 to 20,000/mm^2) during the second and third weeks of illness. From 50% to 70% of the total count consists of lymphocytes and monocytes, and 10% of the lymphocytes are atypical.

Reviewing common infections *(continued)*

INFECTION AND FINDINGS	DIAGNOSIS
Viral infections *(continued)*	

Infectious mononucleosis *(continued)*
- ✦ Stomatitis
- ✦ Exudative tonsillitis or pharyngitis
- ✦ Maculopapular rash

- ✦ Heterophil antibodies in serum, drawn during the acute phase and at 3- to 4-week intervals, increase to four times normal.
- ✦ Indirect immunofluorescence shows antibodies to Epstein-Barr virus and cellular antigens.

Monkeypox
- ✦ Rash (macular, papular, vesicular, or pustular; generalized or local)
- ✦ Chills and sweats
- ✦ Headache and backache
- ✦ Lymphadenopathy
- ✦ Sore throat
- ✦ Cough
- ✦ Shortness of breath

- ✦ Isolation of monkeypox virus (which, along with variola [smallpox virus], belongs to the orthopoxvirus group of viruses) or demonstration of monkeypox virus deoxyribonucleic acid (DNA) from skin lesion (or fluid), throat, blood, or serum specimens confirms diagnosis.
- ✦ Demonstration of a virus of the same structure and form as an orthopoxvirus, or the presence of orthopoxvirus in tissue, without exposure to another orthopoxvirus, also confirms diagnosis.

Mumps
- ✦ Myalgia
- ✦ Malaise and fever
- ✦ Headache
- ✦ Earache aggravated by chewing
- ✦ Parotid gland tenderness and swelling, and pain when chewing or when drinking sour or acidic liquids
- ✦ Swelling of the other salivary glands

- ✦ Virus is isolated from throat washings, urine, blood, or spinal fluid.
- ✦ Serologic antibody testing shows a rise in paired antibodies.
- ✦ Clinical signs and symptoms, especially parotid gland enlargement are characteristic.

Rabies

Prodromal symptoms
- ✦ Local or radiating pain or burning and a sensation of cold, pruritus, and tingling at the bite site
- ✦ Malaise and fever
- ✦ Headache
- ✦ Nausea
- ✦ Sore throat and persistent loose cough
- ✦ Nervousness, anxiety, irritability, hyperesthesia, and sensitivity to light and loud noises
- ✦ Excessive salivation, tearing, and perspiration

- ✦ Virus is isolated from saliva or throat.
- ✦ Fluorescent rabies antibody test is positive.
- ✦ WBC count is elevated.
- ✦ Histologic examination of brain tissue from human rabies victims shows perivascular inflammation of the gray matter, degeneration of neurons, and characteristic minute bodies, called *Negri bodies*, in the nerve cells.

Key signs of monkeypox
- ✦ Rash
- ✦ Chills and sweats
- ✦ Lymphadenopathy
- ✦ Shortness of breath

Key signs of mumps
- ✦ Myalgia
- ✦ Parotid gland tenderness and swelling
- ✦ Swelling of other salivary glands

Key signs of rabies
Prodromal symptoms
- ✦ Local or radiating pain or burning
- ✦ Nausea
- ✦ Sore throat and persistent loose cough
- ✦ Excessive salivation, tearing, and perspiration

(continued)

Key signs of rabies

Excitation phase
+ Shallow respirations
+ Altered LOC
+ Forceful, painful pharyngeal muscle spasms that expel fluids from the mouth
+ Swallowing problems
+ Nuchal rigidity

Terminal phase
+ Paralysis
+ Coma and death

Key signs of respiratory syncytial virus infection

Mild disease
+ Nasal congestion
+ Sore throat
+ Earache

Bronchitis, bronchiolitis, pneumonia
+ Wheezes, rhonchi, crackles
+ Weakness, irritability

Key signs of rubella

+ Itchy rash that begins on the face and spreads to extremities
+ Small, red macules on the soft palate
+ Sore throat
+ Cough

Reviewing common infections *(continued)*

INFECTION AND FINDINGS	DIAGNOSIS

Viral Infections (continued)

Rabies *(continued)*
Excitation phase
+ Intermittent hyperactivity, anxiety, and apprehension
+ Shallow respirations
+ Altered LOC
+ Ocular palsies
+ Strabismus
+ Asymmetrical pupillary dilation or constriction
+ Absence of corneal reflexes
+ Facial muscle weakness
+ Forceful, painful pharyngeal muscle spasms that expel fluids from the mouth, resulting in dehydration
+ Swallowing problems cause frothy drooling and soon the sight, sound, or thought of water triggers uncontrollable pharyngeal muscle spasms and excessive salivation
+ Nuchal rigidity
+ Cardiac arrhythmias
+ Seizures

Terminal phase
+ Gradual, generalized, flaccid paralysis
+ Peripheral vascular collapse
+ Coma and death

Respiratory syncytial virus infection
Mild disease
+ Nasal congestion
+ Coughing and wheezing
+ Malaise
+ Sore throat
+ Earache
+ Dyspnea
+ Fever

+ Cultures of nasal and pharyngeal secretions may reveal the virus; however, this infection is so labile that cultures aren't always reliable.
+ Serum antibody titers may be elevated.
+ Recently developed serologic techniques are the indirect immunofluorescent and ELISA methods.
+ Chest X-rays help detect pneumonia.

Bronchitis, bronchiolitis, pneumonia
+ Nasal flaring, retraction, cyanosis, and tachypnea
+ Wheezes, rhonchi, and crackles
+ Such signs as weakness, irritability, and nuchal rigidity of CNS infection may be observed

Rubella
+ Maculopapular, mildly itchy rash that usually begins on the face and then spreads rapidly, usually covering the trunk and extremities
+ Small, red macules on the soft palate (Forschheimer spots)
+ Low-grade fever
+ Headache
+ Malaise
+ Anorexia
+ Sore throat
+ Cough
+ Postauricular, suboccipital, and posterior cervical lymph node enlargement

+ Clinical signs and symptoms are usually sufficient to make a diagnosis.
+ Cell cultures of the throat, blood, urine, and CSF, along with convalescent serum that shows a fourfold rise in antibody titers, confirms the diagnosis.

Reviewing common infections *(continued)*

INFECTION AND FINDINGS	DIAGNOSIS

Viral infections (continued)

Rubeola
+ Fever
+ Photophobia
+ Malaise
+ Anorexia
+ Conjunctivitis, puffy red eyes, and rhinorrhea
+ Coryza
+ Hoarseness and a hacking cough
+ Koplik's spots (tiny, bluish white specks surrounded by a red halo), pruritic macular rash that becomes papular and erythematous

+ Diagnosis rests on distinctive clinical features.
+ Measles virus may be isolated from the blood, nasopharyngeal secretions, and urine during the febrile stage.
+ Serum antibodies appear within 3 days.

Severe acute respiratory syndrome (SARS)
+ Fever greater than 100.4° F (38° C)
+ Headache
+ Malaise and body aches
+ Respiratory signs and symptoms after 2 to 7 days (cough, shortness of breath, difficultly breathing, and hypoxia)

+ Detection of an antibody to SARS-associated coronavirus (SARS-COV), detection of SARS-COV ribonucleic acid (RNA), or isolation of SARS-COV from blood or respiratory specimens confirms diagnosis.

Smallpox
+ Abrupt onset of chills (and possible seizures in children)
+ High fever (above 104° F [40° C])
+ Headache, backache, severe malaise, vomiting (especially in children), and marked prostration
+ Occasionally, violent delirium, stupor, or coma
+ Sore throat and cough as well as lesions on the mucous membranes of the mouth, throat, and respiratory tract
+ Skin lesions progressing from macular to papular, vesicular, and pustular, with eventual desquamation causing intense pruritus and permanently disfiguring scars
+ In fatal cases, death typically resulting from encephalitic manifestations, extensive bleeding from orifices, or secondary bacterial infections

+ Most conclusive laboratory test is culture of variola virus isolated from an aspirate of vesicles and pustules.
+ Microscopic examination of smears from lesion scrapings and complement fixation are used to detect virus or antibodies to the virus in the patient's blood.

Fungal infections

Histoplasmosis
Primary acute histoplasmosis
+ May not produce symptoms or may cause symptoms of a mild respiratory illness similar to a severe cold or influenza
+ Fever
+ Malaise
+ Headache
+ Myalgia
+ Anorexia
+ Cough
+ Chest pain
+ Anemia, leukopenia, or thrombocytopenia
+ Oropharyngeal ulcers

+ Culture or histology reveals the organism.
+ Stained biopsies using Gomori's stains or periodic acid-Schiff reaction give a fast diagnosis of the disease.
+ Positive histoplasmin skin test or urine antigen test indicates exposure to histoplasmosis.
+ Rising complement fixation and agglutination titers (more than 1:32) strongly suggest histoplasmosis.

Key signs of rubeola
+ Fever
+ Photophobia
+ Coryza
+ Koplik's spots

Key signs of SARS
+ Fever greater than 100.4° F
+ Respiratory signs and symptoms after 2 to 7 days

Key signs of smallpox
+ High fever: above 104° F
+ Sore throat and cough; lesions on the mucous membranes of the mouth and throat
+ Skin lesions

Key signs of histoplasmosis
Primary acute histoplasmosis
+ Symptoms of a mild respiratory illness
+ Myalgia
+ Anemia, leukopenia, or thrombocytopenia
+ Oropharyngeal ulcers

(continued)

Key signs of histoplasmosis

Progressive disseminated histoplasmosis
✦ Hepatosplenomegaly
✦ Anorexia and weight loss

Chronic pulmonary histoplasmosis
✦ Productive cough, dyspnea, and occasional hemopytsis
✦ Breathlessness and cyanosis

African histoplasmosis
✦ Cutaneous nodules, papules, and ulcers
✦ Lesions of the skull and long bones

Key signs of malaria

Benign
✦ Chills
✦ Fever
✦ Headache and myalgia

Acute attacks
✦ High fever; up to 107° F
✦ Profuse sweating
✦ Hemolytic anemia

Life-threatening form
✦ Persistent high fever
✦ RBC sludging that leads to capillary obstruction
✦ Delirium and coma
✦ Abdominal pain, diarrhea, and melena

Reviewing common infections (continued)

INFECTION AND FINDINGS	DIAGNOSIS

Fungal Infections (continued)

Histoplasmosis (continued)
Progressive disseminated histoplasmosis
✦ Hepatosplenomegaly
✦ General lymphadenopathy
✦ Anorexia and weight loss
✦ Fever and, possibly, ulceration of the tongue, palate, epiglottis, and larynx, with resulting pain, hoarseness, and dysphagia

Chronic pulmonary histoplasmosis
✦ Productive cough, dyspnea, and occasional hemoptysis
✦ Weight loss
✦ Extreme weakness
✦ Breathlessness and cyanosis

African histoplasmosis
✦ Cutaneous nodules, papules, and ulcers
✦ Lesions of the skull and long bones
✦ Lymphadenopathy and visceral involvement without pulmonary lesions

Protozoal infections

Malaria
Benign form
✦ Chills
✦ Fever
✦ Headache and myalgia

Acute attacks (occur when erythrocytes rupture)
✦ Chills and shaking
✦ High fever (up to 107° F [41.7° C])
✦ Profuse sweating
✦ Hepatosplenomegaly
✦ Hemolytic anemia

Life-threatening form
✦ Persistent high fever
✦ Orthostatic hypotension
✦ RBC sludging that leads to capillary obstruction at various sites
✦ Hemiplegia
✦ Seizures
✦ Delirium and coma
✦ Hemoptysis
✦ Vomiting
✦ Abdominal pain, diarrhea, and melena
✦ Oliguria, anuria, and uremia

✦ Peripheral blood smears of RBCs identify the parasite.
✦ Indirect fluorescent serum antibody tests are unreliable in the acute phase.
✦ Hemoglobin levels are decreased.
✦ Leukocyte count is normal to decreased.
✦ Protein and leukocytes are present in urine sediment.

Reviewing common infections *(continued)*

INFECTION AND FINDINGS	DIAGNOSIS

Protozoal infections (continued)

Schistosomiasis
+ Transient pruritic rash at the site of cercariae penetration
+ Fever
+ Myalgia
+ Cough

Later signs and symptoms
+ Hepatomegaly, splenomegaly, and lymphadenopathy

Schistosoma mansoni *and* S. japonicum
+ Irregular fever
+ Malaise and weakness
+ Weight loss
+ Diarrhea
+ Ascites and hepatosplenomegaly
+ Portal hypertension
+ Fistulas and intestinal stricture

S. haematobium
+ Terminal hematuria and dysuria
+ Ureteral colic

+ Typical symptoms and a history of travel to endemic areas suggest the diagnosis.
+ Ova in the urine or stools or a mucosal lesion biopsy confirm diagnosis.
+ WBC count shows eosinophilia.

Toxoplasmosis
Ocular toxoplasmosis
+ Chorioretinitis
+ Yellow-white elevated cotton patches
+ Blurred vision
+ Scotoma
+ Pain
+ Photophobia

Acquired toxoplasmosis
+ Malaise, myalgia, and headache
+ Fatigue
+ Sore throat
+ Fever
+ Cervical lymphadenopathy
+ Maculopapular rash

Congenital
+ Hydrocephalus or microcephalus
+ Seizures
+ Jaundice
+ Purpura and rash

+ Identification of *Toxoplasma gondii* in an appropriate tissue specimen confirms diagnosis.
+ CT scans and MRI disclose lesions in patients with toxoplasmosis encephalitis.

Key signs of schistosomiasis
+ Transient pruritic rash at the site of cercariae penetration
+ Fever
+ Hepatomegaly, splenomegaly, and lymphadenopathy (later)

Schistosoma mansoni* and *S. japonicum
+ Irregular fever
+ Ascites and hepatosplenomegaly
+ Portal hypertension

S. haematobium
+ Terminal hematuria and dysuria
+ Ureteral colic

Key signs of toxoplasmosis
Ocular
+ Chorioretinitis
+ Yellow-white elevated cotton patches
+ Photophobia

Acquired
+ Sore throat
+ Cervical lymphadenopthy
+ Maculopapular rash

Congenital
+ Seizures
+ Jaundice

(continued)

Key signs of trichinosis

Stage 1
✦ Anorexia
✦ Abdominal pain and cramps

Stage 2 and Stage 3
✦ Edema (eyelids or face)
✦ Muscle pain
✦ Skin lesions
✦ Fever

Reviewing common infections *(continued)*

INFECTION AND FINDINGS	DIAGNOSIS
Protozoal Infections (continued)	

Trichinosis

Stage 1 (enteric phase)
✦ Anorexia
✦ Nausea, vomiting, and diarrhea
✦ Abdominal pain and cramps

Stage 2 (systemic phase) and Stage 3 (muscular encystment phase)
✦ Edema (especially of the eyelids or face)
✦ Muscle pain
✦ Itching and burning skin
✦ Sweating
✦ Skin lesions
✦ Fever
✦ Delirium and lethargy in severe respiratory, cardiovascular, or CNS infection

✦ Stools may contain mature worms and larvae during the invasion stage.
✦ Skeletal muscle biopsies can show encysted larvae 10 days after ingestion.
✦ Skin testing may show a positive histamine-like reactivity.
✦ Elevated acute and convalescent antibody titers confirm the diagnosis.
✦ Serology results indicate elevated aspartate aminotransferase, alanine aminotransferase, creatine kinase, and lactate dehydrogenase levels during the acute stages and an elevated eosinophil count.
✦ Lumbar puncture demonstrates CNS involvement with normal or elevated CSF lymphocytes and increased protein levels.

Fluids and electrolytes

The body is mostly liquid — various electrolytes dissolved in water. Electrolytes are ions (electrically charged versions) of essential elements — predominantly sodium (Na^+), chloride (Cl^-), hydrogen (H^+), bicarbonate (HCO_3^-), calcium (Ca^{2+}), potassium (K^+), sulfate (SO_4^{2-}), and phosphate (PO_4^{3-}). Only ionic forms of elements can dissolve or combine with other elements. Electrolyte balance must remain in a narrow range for the body to function. The kidneys maintain chemical balance throughout the body by producing and eliminating urine. They regulate the volume, electrolyte concentration, and acid-base balance of body fluids; detoxify and eliminate wastes; and regulate blood pressure by regulating fluid volume. The skin and lungs also play a role in fluid and electrolyte balance. Sweating results in loss of sodium and water; every breath contains water vapor.

FLUID BALANCE

The kidneys maintain fluid balance in the body by regulating the amount and components of fluid inside and around the cells.

INTRACELLULAR FLUID

The fluid inside each cell is called *intracellular fluid* (ICF). Each cell has its own mixture of components in the ICF, but the amounts of these substances are similar in every cell. ICF contains large amounts of potassium, magnesium, and phosphate ions.

EXTRACELLULAR FLUID

The fluid in the spaces outside the cells, called *extracellular fluid* (ECF), is constantly moving. Normally, ECF includes blood plasma and interstitial fluid (the fluid between the cells in tissues); in some pathologic states it accumulates in a so-called *third space,* the space around the organs in the chest or abdomen.

ECF is rapidly transported through the body by circulating blood and between blood and tissue fluids by fluid and electrolyte exchange across the capillary walls. ECF contains large amounts of sodium, chloride, and bicarbonate ions, plus substances needed for cellular function, such as oxygen, glucose, fatty acids, and amino acids. It also contains carbon dioxide, which is transported from the cells to the lungs for excretion, and other cellular products, which are transported from the cells to the kidneys for excretion.

The kidneys maintain the volume and composition of ECF and, to a lesser extent, ICF by continually exchanging water and ionic solutes, such as hydrogen, sodium, potassium, chloride, bicarbonate, sulfate, and phosphate ions, across the cell membranes of the renal tubules.

FLUID EXCHANGE

Two sets of forces determine the exchange of fluid between blood plasma and interstitial fluid. All four forces act to equalize concentrations of fluids, electrolytes, and proteins on both sides of the capillary wall.

Forces that tend to move fluid from the vessels to the interstitial fluid include hydrostatic pressure of blood (the outward pressure of plasma against the capillary walls) and osmotic pressure of tissue fluid (the tendency of ions to move across a semipermeable membrane — the capillary wall — from an area of greater concentration to one of lower concentration).

Forces that tend to move fluid into vessels include oncotic pressure of plasma proteins (similar to osmosis, but because proteins can't cross the vessel wall, they attract fluid into the area of greater concentration) and hydrostatic pressure of interstitial fluid (inward pressure against the capillary walls).

Hydrostatic pressure at the arteriolar end of the capillary bed is greater than at the venular end. Oncotic pressure of plasma increases slightly at the venular end as fluid escapes. When the endothelial barrier (capillary wall) is normal and intact, fluid escapes at the arteriolar end of the capillary bed and is returned at the venular end. The small amount of fluid lost from the capillaries into the interstitial tissue spaces is drained through the lymphatic system and returned to the bloodstream.

ACID-BASE BALANCE

Regulation of the ECF environment involves the ratio of acid to base, measured clinically as pH (a measurement of effective hydrogen ion concentration). In physiology, all positively charged ions are acids and all negatively charged ions are bases.

To regulate acid-base balance, the kidneys secrete hydrogen ions (acid), reabsorb sodium ions (acid) and bicarbonate ions (base), acidify phosphate salts, and produce ammonium ions (acid). This keeps the blood at its normal pH of 7.35 to 7.45. A pH of less than 6.8 or greater than 7.8 is incompatible with life. Cell function is seriously impaired with a pH of less than 7.2 or greater than 7.55; acidosis occurs with a pH less than 7.35 and alkalosis occurs with a pH greater than 7.45.

PATHOPHYSIOLOGIC CHANGES IN ELECTROLYTE IMBALANCE

The regulation of intracellular and extracellular electrolyte concentrations depends on the balance between the intake of substances containing electrolytes and the output of electrolytes in urine, feces, and sweat. It also depends on the transport of fluid and electrolytes between ECF and ICF.

Fluid imbalance occurs when regulatory mechanisms can't compensate for abnormal intake and output at any level from the cell to the organism. Fluid and electrolyte imbalances include edema, isotonic alterations, hypertonic alterations, hypotonic alterations, and electrolyte imbalances. Disorders of fluid volume or osmolarity (concentration of electrolytes in the fluid) result. Many conditions also affect capillary exchange, resulting in fluid shifts.

EDEMA

Despite almost constant interchange through the endothelial barrier, the body maintains a steady state of extracellular water balance between the plasma and interstitial fluid. Increased fluid volume in the interstitial spaces is called *edema*. It's classified as localized or systemic. Obstruction of the veins or lymphatic system or increased vascular permeability typically causes localized edema in the affected area such as the swelling around an injury. Systemic, or generalized edema may be due to heart failure or renal disease. Massive systemic edema is called *anasarca*.

Edema results from abnormal expansion of the interstitial fluid or the accumulation of fluid in a third space, such as the peritoneum (ascites), pleural cavity (hydrothorax), or pericardial sac (pericardial effusion). (See *Causes of edema*, page 88.)

TONICITY

Many fluid and electrolyte disorders are classified according to how they affect osmotic pressure, or tonicity. Tonicity describes the relative concentrations of electrolytes (osmotic pressure) on both sides of a semipermeable membrane (the cell wall or the capillary wall). The word *normal* in this context refers to the usual electrolyte concentration of physiologic fluids. Normal saline solution has a sodium chloride concentration of 0.9%. Isotonic solutions have the same electrolyte concentration and therefore the same osmotic pressure as ECF. Hypertonic solutions have a greater-than-normal concentration of some essential electrolyte, usually sodium. Hypotonic solutions have a lower-than-normal concentration of some essential electrolyte, also usually sodium.

Isotonic alterations

Isotonic alterations or disorders don't make the cells swell or shrink. They occur when ICF and ECF have equal osmotic pressure, but there's a dramatic change in total body fluid volume. Examples include blood loss from penetrating trauma or expansion of fluid volume if a patient receives too much normal saline solution.

Hypertonic alterations

Hypertonic alterations occur when the ECF is more concentrated than the ICF. Water flows out of the cell through the semipermeable cell membrane, causing cell shrinkage. This can occur when a patient is given hypertonic (greater than 0.9%) saline solution, when severe dehydration causes hypernatremia (high sodium concentration in blood), or when renal disease causes sodium retention.

Main causes of edema
+ Increased hydrostatic pressure
+ Hypoproteinemia
+ Lymphatic obstruction
+ Sodium retention
+ Increased endothelial permeability

Causes of edema

Edema results when excess fluid accumulates in the interstitial spaces. This chart shows the causes and effects of this fluid accumulation.

CAUSE	UNDERLYING CONDITION
Increased hydrostatic pressure	Heart failure Constrictive pericarditis Venous thrombosis Cirrhosis
Hypoproteinemia	Cirrhosis Malnutrition Nephrotic syndrome Gastroenteropathy
Lymphatic obstruction	Cancer Inflammatory scarring Radiation
Sodium retention	Excessive salt intake Increased tubular reabsorption of sodium Reduced renal perfusion
Increased endothelial permeability	Inflammation Burns Trauma Allergic or immunologic reactions

Hypotonic alterations
When the ECF becomes hypotonic, osmotic pressure forces some ECF into the cells, causing them to swell. Overhydration is the most common cause; as water dilutes the ECF, it becomes hypotonic with respect to the ICF. Water moves into the cells until balance is restored. In extreme hypotonicity, cells may swell until they burst and die.

ALTERATIONS IN ELECTROLYTE BALANCE
The major electrolytes are the cations (positively charged ions) sodium, potassium, calcium, and magnesium and the anions (negatively charged ions) chloride, phosphate, and bicarbonate. The body continuously attempts to maintain intracellular and extracellular equilibrium of electrolytes. Too much or too little of an electrolyte will affect most body systems.

Sodium and potassium
Sodium is the major cation in ECF, and potassium is the major cation in ICF. Especially in nerves and muscles, communication within and between cells involves changes (repolarization and depolarization) in the surface charge on the cell membrane. During repolarization, an active transport mechanism in the cell membrane, called the *sodium-potassium pump,* continually shifts sodium into and potassium out of cells; during depolarization, the process is reversed.

Alterations in electrolyte balance

Sodium and potassium
+ Positively charged cations and negatively charged anions are major electrolytes in the body
+ Sodium is the major cation in ECF; potassium in ICF; aid in cellular communication

Physiologic roles of sodium cations include maintaining tonicity of ECF and regulating acid-base balance by renal reabsorption of sodium ion (base) and excretion of hydrogen ion (acid).

Sodium cations also maintain water balance and facilitate nerve conduction, neuromuscular function, and glandular secretion. Physiologic roles of potassium include maintaining cell electrical neutrality and acid-base balance as well as facilitating cardiac muscle contraction, electrical conductivity, and neuromuscular transmission of nerve impulses.

Chloride

Chloride is mainly an extracellular anion; it accounts for two-thirds of all serum anions. Secreted by the stomach mucosa as hydrochloric acid, it provides an acid medium for digestion and enzyme activation. Chloride also helps maintain acid-base and water balances, influences the tonicity of ECF, facilitates the exchange of oxygen and carbon dioxide in red blood cells (RBCs), and helps activate salivary amylase, which triggers the digestive process.

Calcium

Calcium is indispensable in cell permeability, bone and tooth formation, blood coagulation, nerve impulse transmission, and normal muscle contraction. Hypocalcemia can cause tetany and seizures; hypercalcemia can cause cardiac arrhythmias and coma.

Magnesium

Magnesium is present in smaller quantities, but physiologically it's as significant as the other major electrolytes. The major function of magnesium is to enhance neuromuscular communication. Other functions include stimulating parathyroid hormone secretion, which regulates intracellular calcium; activating many enzymes in carbohydrate and protein metabolism; facilitating cell metabolism; facilitating sodium, potassium, and calcium transport across cell membranes; and facilitating protein transport.

Phosphate

The phosphate anion is involved in cellular metabolism as well as in neuromuscular regulation and hematologic function. Phosphate reabsorption in the renal tubules is inversely related to calcium levels, which means that an increase in urinary phosphorous triggers calcium reabsorption and vice versa.

Effects of electrolyte imbalance

Electrolyte imbalances can affect all body systems. Too much or too little potassium or too little calcium or magnesium can increase the excitability of the cardiac muscle, causing arrhythmias. Multiple neurologic symptoms may result from electrolyte imbalance, ranging from disorientation or confusion to a completely depressed central nervous system (CNS). Too much or too little sodium or too much potassium can cause oliguria. Blood pressure may be increased or decreased. (See *Fluid and electrolyte implications of blood pressure findings,* page 90.)

The GI tract is particularly susceptible to electrolyte imbalance. Too much potassium results in abdominal cramps, nausea, and diarrhea while too little potassium results in paralytic ileus. Too much magnesium results in nausea, vomiting, and diarrhea while too much calcium results in nausea, vomiting, and constipation.

Alterations in electrolyte balance

Chloride
+ Aids in digestion
+ Helps maintain acid and water balances
+ Influences tonicity of ECF
+ Aids in cell respiration

Calcium
+ Maintains cell permeability, bone and tooth formation, blood coagulation, impulse transmission and muscle contraction

Magnesium
+ Enhances neuromuscular communication, hormone secretion

Phosphate
+ Involved in cellular metabolism
+ Helps balance calcium absorption

Electrolyte imbalance
+ Imbalances affect all body systems
+ Multiple neurologic symptoms may result
+ GI tract especially susceptible

Fluid and electrolyte implications of blood pressure findings

Blood pressure reflects changes in fluid and electrolyte status.

BLOOD PRESSURE	FLUID AND ELECTROLYTE STATUS
Normal	✦ Hemodynamic stability ✦ Initial hemodynamic instability
Hypotension	✦ Fluid volume deficit ✦ Potassium imbalance ✦ Calcium imbalance ✦ Magnesium imbalance ✦ Acidosis
Hypertension	✦ Fluid volume excess ✦ Hypernatremia

Characteristics of hypovolemia

✦ Disorder of fluid and electrolyte imbalance—the isotonic loss of body fluids
✦ Also known as *ECF volume deficit*
✦ Usually occurs in first 10 years of life

Alert!

✦ Infants are at higher risk because their bodies need to have a higher proportion of water to total body weight.

Causes

✦ Excessive fluid loss
✦ Reduced fluid intake
✦ Third-space fluid shift

HYPOVOLEMIA

Hypovolemia is a disorder of fluid and electrolyte balance. Water content of the human body progressively decreases from birth to old age. In the neonate, as much as 75% of body weight is water. In adults, about 60% of body weight is water; in the elderly, about 55% is water.

Most of the decrease occurs in the first 10 years of life. Hypovolemia, or ECF volume deficit, is the isotonic loss of body fluids; that is, relatively equal losses of sodium and water. (See *Electrolyte imbalances.*)

 CLINICAL ALERT Infants are at risk for hypovolemia because their bodies need to have a higher proportion of water to total body weight.

CAUSES

Excessive fluid loss, reduced fluid intake, third-space fluid shift, or a combination of these factors can cause ECF volume loss.

Possible causes of fluid loss include hemorrhage, excessive perspiration, renal failure with polyuria, abdominal surgery, vomiting or diarrhea, nasogastric drainage, diabetes mellitus with polyuria, diabetes insipidus, fistulas, excessive use of laxatives, excessive diuretic therapy, and fever.

Possible causes of reduced fluid intake include dysphagia, coma, environmental conditions preventing fluid intake, and psychiatric illness.

Fluid shift may be related to burns (during the initial phase), acute intestinal obstruction, acute peritonitis, pancreatitis, crushing injury, pleural effusion, and hip fracture (1.5 to 2 L of blood may accumulate in tissues around the fracture).

PATHOPHYSIOLOGY

Hypovolemia is an isotonic disorder. Fluid volume deficit decreases capillary hydrostatic pressure and fluid transport. Cells are deprived of normal nutrients that serve as substrates for energy production, metabolism, and other cellular functions. Decreased renal blood flow triggers the renin-angiotensin system to increase sodi-

Electrolyte imbalances

Signs and symptoms of electrolyte imbalance are often subtle. Blood chemistry tests help diagnose and evaluate electrolyte imbalances.

ELECTROLYTE IMBALANCE	SIGNS AND SYMPTOMS	DIAGNOSTIC TEST RESULTS
Hyponatremia	✦ Muscle twitching and weakness due to osmotic swelling of cells ✦ Lethargy, confusion, seizures, and coma due to altered neurotransmission ✦ Hypotension and tachycardia due to decreased extracellular circulating volume ✦ Nausea, vomiting, and abdominal cramps due to edema affecting receptors in the brain or vomiting center of the brain stem ✦ Oliguria or anuria due to renal dysfunction	✦ Serum sodium < 135 mEq/L ✦ Decreased urine specific gravity ✦ Decreased serum osmolality ✦ Urine sodium > 100 mEq/24 hours ✦ Increased red blood cell count
Hypernatremia	✦ Agitation, restlessness, fever, and decreased level of consciousness due to altered cellular metabolism ✦ Hypertension, tachycardia, pitting edema, and excessive weight gain due to water shift from intracellular to extracellular fluid ✦ Thirst, increased viscosity of saliva, rough tongue due to fluid shift ✦ Dyspnea, respiratory arrest, and death from dramatic increase in osmotic pressure	✦ Serum sodium > 145 mEq/L ✦ Urine sodium < 40 mEq/24 hours ✦ High serum osmolality
Hypokalemia	✦ Dizziness, hypotension, arrhythmias, electrocardiogram (ECG) changes, and cardiac arrest due to changes in membrane excitability ✦ Nausea, vomiting, anorexia, diarrhea, decreased peristalsis, and abdominal distention due to decreased bowel motility ✦ Muscle weakness, fatigue, and leg cramps due to decreased neuromuscular excitability	✦ Serum potassium < 3.5 mEq/L ✦ Coexisting low serum calcium and magnesium levels not responsive to treatment for hypokalemia usually suggest hypomagnesemia ✦ Metabolic alkalosis ✦ ECG changes include flattened T waves, elevated U waves, depressed ST segment

Key signs and symptoms of hyponatremia

✦ Muscle twitching and weakness
✦ Lethargy
✦ Hypotension and tachycardia

Key signs and symptoms of hypernatremia

✦ Agitation, restlessness, and fever
✦ Hypertension, tachycardia, and pitting edema
✦ Thirst

Key signs and symptoms of hypokalemia

✦ Dizziness, hypotension, ECG changes, and cardiac arrest
✦ Nausea and vomiting
✦ Muscle weakness, leg cramps

(continued)

Key signs and symptoms of hyperkalemia

◆ Tachycardia, ECG changes, and cardiac arrest
◆ Nausea, diarrhea, and abdominal cramps

Key signs and symptoms of hypochloremia

◆ Muscle hypertonicity and tetany
◆ Shallow, depressed breathing

Key signs and symptoms of hyperchloremia

◆ Deep, rapid breathing
◆ Weakness

Key signs and symptoms of hypocalcemia

◆ Anxiety, irritability, and seizures
◆ Hypotension and arrhythmias

Key signs and symptoms of hypercalcemia

◆ Drowsiness, lethargy, and headaches
◆ Weakness and muscle flaccidity
◆ Heart block
◆ Anorexia, nausea, vomiting, constipation, and dehydration

Electrolyte imbalances *(continued)*

ELECTROLYTE IMBALANCE	SIGNS AND SYMPTOMS	DIAGNOSTIC TEST RESULTS
Hyperkalemia	◆ Tachycardia changing to bradycardia, ECG changes, and cardiac arrest due to hypopolarization and alterations in repolarization ◆ Nausea, diarrhea, and abdominal cramps due to decreased gastric motility ◆ Muscle weakness and flaccid paralysis due to inactivation of membrane sodium channels	◆ Serum potassium > 5 mEq/L ◆ Metabolic acidosis ◆ ECG changes include tented and elevated T waves, widened QRS complex, prolonged PR interval, flattened or absent P waves, depressed ST segment
Hypochloremia	◆ Muscle hypertonicity and tetany ◆ Shallow, depressed breathing ◆ Usually associated with hyponatremia and its characteristic symptoms, such as muscle weakness and twitching	◆ Serum chloride < 98 mEq/L ◆ Serum pH > 7.45 (supportive value) ◆ Serum CO_2 > 32 mEq/L (supportive value)
Hyperchloremia	◆ Deep, rapid breathing ◆ Weakness ◆ Diminished cognitive ability, possibly leading to coma	◆ Serum chloride > 108 mEq/L ◆ Serum pH < 7.35 ◆ Serum CO_2 < 22 mEq/L (supportive values)
Hypocalcemia	◆ Anxiety, irritability, twitching around the mouth, laryngospasm, seizures, positive Chvostek's and Trousseau's signs due to enhanced neuromuscular irritability ◆ Hypotension and arrhythmias due to decreased calcium influx	◆ Serum calcium < 8.5 mg/dl ◆ Low platelet count ◆ ECG shows lengthened QT interval, prolonged ST segment, arrhythmias ◆ Possible changes in serum protein because half of serum calcium is bound to albumin
Hypercalcemia	◆ Drowsiness, lethargy, headaches, irritability, confusion, depression, or apathy due to decreased neuromuscular irritability (increased threshold) ◆ Weakness and muscle flaccidity due to depressed neuromuscular irritability and release of acetylcholine at the myoneural junction ◆ Bone pain and pathological fractures due to calcium loss from bones ◆ Heart block due to decreased neuromuscular irritability ◆ Anorexia, nausea, vomiting, constipation, and dehydration due to hyperosmolarity ◆ Flank pain due to renal calculi formation	◆ Serum calcium > 10.5 mg/dl ◆ ECG shows signs of heart block and shortened QT interval ◆ Azotemia ◆ Decreased parathyroid hormone level ◆ Sulkowitch urine test shows increased calcium precipitation

Electrolyte imbalances *(continued)*

ELECTROLYTE IMBALANCE	SIGNS AND SYMPTOMS	DIAGNOSTIC TEST RESULTS
Hypomagnesemia	✦ Nearly always coexists with hypokalemia and hypocalcemia ✦ Hyperirritability, tetany, leg and foot cramps, positive Chvostek's and Trousseau's signs, confusion, delusions, and seizures due to alteration in neuromuscular transmission ✦ Arrhythmias, vasodilation, and hypotension due to enhanced inward sodium current or concurrent effects of calcium and potassium imbalance	✦ Serum magnesium < 1.5 mEq/L ✦ Coexisting low serum potassium and calcium levels
Hypermagnesemia	✦ Hypermagnesemia is uncommon, caused by decreased renal excretion (renal failure) or increased intake of magnesium ✦ Diminished reflexes, muscle weakness to flaccid paralysis due to suppression of acetylcholine release at the myoneural junction, blocking neuromuscular transmission and reducing cell excitability ✦ Respiratory distress secondary to respiratory muscle paralysis ✦ Heart block, bradycardia due to decreased inward sodium current ✦ Hypotension due to relaxation of vascular smooth muscle and reduction of vascular resistance by displacing calcium from the vascular wall surface	✦ Serum magnesium > 2.5 mEq/L ✦ Coexisting elevated potassium and calcium levels
Hypophosphatemia	✦ Muscle weakness, tremor, and paresthesia due to deficiency of adenosine triphosphate ✦ Peripheral hypoxia due to 2,3-diphosphoglycerate deficiency	✦ Serum phosphate < 2.5 mg/dl ✦ Urine phosphate > 1.3 g/24 hours
Hyperphosphatemia	✦ Usually produces no symptoms unless leading to hypocalcemia, with tetany and seizures	✦ Serum phosphate > 4.5 mg/dl ✦ Serum calcium < 9 mg/dl ✦ Urine phosphorus < 0.9 g/24 hours

Key signs and symptoms of hypomagnesemia
✦ Coexists with hypokalemia and hypocalcemia
✦ Hyperirritability, tetany, leg and foot cramps, and delusions

Key signs and symptoms of hypermagnesemia
✦ Diminished reflexes and muscle weakness
✦ Respiratory distress
✦ Heart block
✦ Hypotension

Key signs and symptoms of hypophosphatemia
✦ Muscle weakness and tremor
✦ Peripheral hypoxia

Key signs and symptoms of hyperphosphatemia
✦ Produces no symptoms
✦ May lead to hypocalcemia, with tetany and seizures

um and water reabsorption. The cardiovascular system compensates by increasing heart rate, cardiac contractility, venous constriction, and systemic vascular resistance, thus increasing cardiac output and mean arterial pressure (MAP). Hypovolemia also triggers the thirst response, releasing more antidiuretic hormone (ADH) and producing more aldosterone.

How it happens

+ Fluid deficit decreases capillary hydrostatic pressure and fluid transport; cells lose nutrients
+ Decreased renal blood flow triggers renin-angiotensin system to increase sodium and water retention
+ Cardiac output increases
+ If compensation fails, hypovolemic shock occurs

Key signs and symptoms

+ Depends on amount of fluid loss
+ Orthostatic hypertension
+ Tachycardia
+ Thirst
+ Flattened jugular veins

Alert!

+ In hypovolemic infants younger than 4 months, the posterior and anterior fontanels are sunken when palpated.
+ Between 4 and 18 months, the posterior fontanel is normally closed, but the anterior fontanel is sunken.

Complications

+ Shock
+ Acute renal failure
+ Death

Diagnosis

+ Increased BUN level
+ Elevated serum creatinine level
+ Increased serum protein, hemoglobin, and hematocrit
+ Rising blood glucose level
+ Elevated serum osmolality

When compensation fails, hypovolemic shock occurs. In hypovolemic shock, vascular fluid volume loss causes extreme tissue hypoperfusion. Inadequate vascular volume leads to decreased venous return, which reduces preload, decreases stroke volume, and reduces cardiac output. The resulting drop in MAP activates the body's compensatory mechanisms in an attempt to increase vascular volume and tissue perfusion. If the mechanisms fail, the decreased oxygen and nutrient delivery to the cells will result in multiple-organ-dysfunction syndrome and, eventually, death.

SIGNS AND SYMPTOMS

Signs and symptoms depend on the amount of fluid loss. (See *Assessing fluid loss.*) These may include orthostatic hypotension due to increased systemic vascular resistance and decreased cardiac output, tachycardia induced by the sympathetic nervous system to increase cardiac output and MAP, and thirst to prompt ingestion of fluid (increased ECF osmolality stimulates the thirst center in the hypothalamus).

Physical signs include flattened jugular veins due to decreased circulating blood volume, sunken eyeballs due to decreased volume of total body fluid and consequent dehydration of connective tissue and aqueous humor, dry mucous membranes due to decreased body fluid volume (glands that produce fluids to moisten and protect the vascular mucous membranes fail, so they dry rapidly), diminished skin turgor due to decreased fluid in the dermal layer (making skin less pliant), rapid weight loss due to acute loss of body fluid, decreased urine output due to decreased renal perfusion from renal vasoconstriction, and prolonged capillary refill time due to increased systemic vascular resistance.

 CLINICAL ALERT In hypovolemic infants younger than 4 months, the posterior and anterior fontanels are sunken when palpated. Between 4 and 18 months, the posterior fontanel is normally closed, but the anterior fontanel is sunken in hypovolemic infants.

COMPLICATIONS

Possible complications of hypovolemia include shock, acute renal failure, and death.

DIAGNOSIS

No single diagnostic finding confirms hypovolemia, but certain test results are suggestive. These include increased blood urea nitrogen (BUN) level (early sign); elevated serum creatinine level (late sign); increased serum protein, hemoglobin, and hematocrit (unless caused by hemorrhage, when loss of blood elements causes subnormal values); rising blood glucose level; and elevated serum osmolality (except in hyponatremia, where serum osmolality is low). Serum electrolyte and arterial blood gas (ABG) analysis may reflect associated clinical problems due to the underlying cause of hypovolemia or to the treatment regimen.

If the patient has no underlying renal disorder, typical urinalysis findings include urine specific gravity greater than 1.030, increased urine osmolality, and urine sodium level less than 50 mEq/L.

TREATMENT

Oral fluids may be adequate in mild hypovolemia if the patient is alert enough to swallow and can tolerate it. Parenteral fluids supplement or replace oral therapy in moderate to severe hypovolemia. The choice of parenteral fluid depends on the type of fluids lost, the severity of hypovolemia, and the patient's cardiovascular,

Assessing fluid loss

These assessment parameters indicate the severity of fluid loss.

MINIMAL FLUID LOSS
Intravascular fluid loss is regarded as minimal if the patient exhibits the following signs and symptoms:
+ slight tachycardia
+ normal supine blood pressure
+ positive postural vital signs, including a decrease in systolic blood pressure more than 10 mm Hg or an increase in pulse rate more than 20 beats/minute
+ increased capillary refill time (> 3 seconds)
+ urine output greater than 30 ml/hour
+ cool, pale skin on arms and legs
+ anxiety.

MODERATE FLUID LOSS
Intravascular fluid loss is regarded as moderate if the patient exhibits the following signs and symptoms:
+ rapid, thready pulse

+ supine hypotension
+ cool truncal skin
+ urine output of 10 to 30 ml/hour
+ severe thirst
+ restlessness, confusion, or irritability.

SEVERE FLUID LOSS
Intravascular fluid loss is regarded as severe if the patient exhibits the following signs and symptoms:
+ marked tachycardia
+ marked hypotension
+ weak or absent peripheral pulses
+ cold, mottled, or cyanotic skin
+ urine output less than 10 ml/hour
+ unconsciousness.

electrolyte, and acid-base status. Fluid resuscitation for severe volume depletion can be achieved by rapid I.V. administration; typically, depending on the patient's condition, 100 to 500 ml of fluid over 15 minutes to 1 hour although fluid bolus may be given more quickly if needed.

Other possible treatments may include blood or blood products (with hemorrhage), antidiarrheals or antiemetics as needed, I.V. dopamine (Intropin) or norepinephrine (Levophed) to increase cardiac contractility and renal perfusion (if the patient remains symptomatic after fluid replacement), oxygen therapy to ensure sufficient tissue perfusion, and autotransfusion in those patients with hypovolemia caused by trauma.

NURSING CONSIDERATIONS

+ I.V. infusions should be started with the shortest, largest-bore catheters possible because they offer less resistance to fluid flow than long, thin catheters.
+ The patient's mental status and vital signs should be monitored closely, including orthostatic blood pressure measurements when appropriate.
+ If the blood pressure doesn't respond to interventions as expected, the patient should be reassessed for a bleeding site that may have been missed. (Remember, a patient can lose a large amount of blood internally from a fractured hip or pelvis.)

HYPERVOLEMIA

The expansion of ECF volume, called *hypervolemia,* may involve the interstitial or intravascular space. A disorder of fluid and electrolyte balance, hypervolemia develops when excess sodium and water are retained in about the same proportions. It's

Treatment
+ Oral or parenteral fluids
+ 100 to 500 ml of I.V. fluid for severe volume depletion
+ Blood or blood products
+ Antidiarrheals and antiemetics
+ I.V. dopamine or norepinephrine
+ Oxygen therapy

Key nursing actions
+ Start I.V. infusions with the shortest, largest-bore catheters possible.
+ Monitor the patient's mental status and vital signs closely.
+ Reassess for a missed bleeding site if blood pressure doesn't respond to intervention.

Characteristics of hypervolemia
+ Excess sodium and water retention in relatively same proportions
+ Also known as *expansion of ECF volume*
+ Body can usually compensate and restore fluid balance

Causes

+ Heart failure
+ Cirrhosis of the liver
+ Nephrotic syndrome
+ Corticosteroid therapy
+ Low dietary protein intake
+ Renal failure

How it happens

+ Increased ECF volume causes circulatory overload, increased cardiac contractility, and MAP
+ Increased capillary hydrostatic pressure shifts fluid to interstitial space and edema
+ Urine output increases
+ If severe or prolonged, compensatory mechanisms fail and heart failure or pulmonary edema occurs

Key signs and symptoms

+ Rapid breathing
+ Dyspnea
+ Crackles
+ Rapid, bounding pulse
+ Hypertension
+ Distended jugular veins

Complications

+ Skin breakdown
+ Acute pulmonary edema

always secondary to an increase in total body sodium content, which causes water retention. In most instances, the body can compensate and restore fluid balance.

CAUSES

Conditions that increase the risk for sodium and water retention include heart failure, cirrhosis of the liver, nephrotic syndrome, corticosteroid therapy, low dietary protein intake, and renal failure.

Sources of excessive sodium and water intake include parenteral fluid replacement with normal saline or lactated Ringer's solution, blood or plasma replacement, and dietary intake of water, sodium chloride, or other salts.

Fluid shift to the ECF may follow remobilization of fluid after burn treatment or administration of such hypertonic fluids as mannitol (Osmitrol) or hypertonic saline solution, and colloid oncotic fluids such as albumin.

PATHOPHYSIOLOGY

An increased ECF volume causes circulatory overload and increased cardiac contractility and MAP. Increased capillary hydrostatic pressure leads to a shift of fluid to the interstitial space and edema.

Elevated MAP inhibits the secretion of ADH and aldosterone and consequently increases urinary elimination of water and sodium. These compensatory mechanisms usually restore normal intravascular volume. If hypervolemia is severe or prolonged or if the patient has a history of cardiovascular dysfunction, compensatory mechanisms may fail, and heart failure and pulmonary edema may ensue.

SIGNS AND SYMPTOMS

Signs and symptoms of hypervolemia include rapid breathing due to fewer RBCs per milliliter of blood (dilution causes a compensatory increase in respiratory rate to increase oxygenation), dyspnea (labored breathing) due to increased fluid volume in pleural spaces, crackles (gurgling or bubbling sounds on auscultation) due to elevated hydrostatic pressure in pulmonary capillaries, and a rapid, bounding pulse due to increased cardiac contractility (from circulatory overload).

Other possible signs and symptoms include hypertension (unless heart is failing) due to circulatory overload (causes increased MAP), distended jugular veins due to increased blood volume and increased preload, and moist skin (compensatory to increase water excretion through perspiration).

Patients may notice an acute weight gain due to an increased volume of total body fluid from circulatory overload (the best indicator of ECF volume excess) or edema (increased MAP leads to increased capillary hydrostatic pressure, causing fluid shift from plasma to interstitial spaces). Auscultation reveals an S_3 gallop caused by rapid filling and volume overload of the ventricles during diastole.

COMPLICATIONS

Hypervolemia can produce skin breakdown and acute pulmonary edema with hypoxemia.

DIAGNOSIS

No single diagnostic test confirms the disorder.

Hypervolemia is indicated by decreased serum potassium and BUN levels due to hemodilution (increased serum potassium and BUN levels usually indicate renal failure or impaired renal perfusion), decreased hematocrit due to hemodilution, normal serum sodium (unless associated sodium imbalance is present), and low urine sodium excretion (usually less than 10 mEq/day) because the edematous patient is retaining sodium.

Hemodynamic values include increased pulmonary artery, pulmonary artery wedge, and central venous pressures.

TREATMENT

Possible treatments for hypervolemia include restricted sodium and water intake and preload reduction agents, such as morphine, furosemide (Lasix), and nitroglycerin (Nitro-Bid), and afterload reduction agents, such as hydralazine (Apresoline) and captopril (Capoten) for pulmonary edema.

 CLINICAL ALERT Carefully monitor I.V. fluid administration rate and patient response, especially in elderly patients or those with impaired cardiac or renal function, who are particularly vulnerable to acute pulmonary edema.

For severe hypervolemia or renal failure, the patient may undergo renal replacement therapy, including hemodialysis or peritoneal dialysis, continuous arteriovenous hemofiltration (allows removal of excess fluid from critically ill patients who may not need dialysis; the patient's arterial pressure serves as a natural pump, driving blood through the arterial line), or continuous venovenous hemofiltration (similar to arteriovenous hemofiltration, but a mechanical pump is used when MAP is less than 60 mm Hg).

Supportive measures include oxygen administration, use of antiembolism stockings to help mobilize edematous fluid, bed rest, and treatment of the underlying condition that caused or contributed to hypervolemia.

NURSING CONSIDERATIONS

✦ If the patient is prone to hypervolemia, an infusion pump should be used with any infusions to prevent the administration of too much fluid.
✦ The patient's vital signs and hemodynamic status should be assessed to note his response to therapy. Signs of hypovolemia indicate overcorrection. Elderly, pediatric, and otherwise compromised patients are at higher risk for complications with therapy.
✦ If the hypervolemic patient isn't responding to diuretic therapy, his kidney function may be impaired. Dialysis is typically the next step. If the patient can't tolerate dialysis, continuous arteriovenous hemofiltration may be used.

PATHOPHYSIOLOGIC CHANGES IN ACID-BASE IMBALANCE

Acid-base balance is essential to life. Conditions related to imbalance include acidemia, acidosis, alkalemia, alkalosis, and compensation.

ACIDEMIA

Acidemia is an arterial pH of less than 7.35, which reflects a relative excess of acid in the blood. The hydrogen ion content in ECF increases, and the hydrogen ions move to the ICF. To keep the ICF electrically neutral, an equal amount of potassium leaves the cell, creating a relative hyperkalemia.

Key facts about pathophysiologic changes in acid-base imbalance

Acidosis

✦ Systemic increase in hydrogen ion concentration

✦ Occurs when lung can't eliminate CO_2, or if diarrhea causes loss of bicarbonate anions or if the kidneys fail to reabsorb bicarbonate or secrete hydrogen ions

Alkalemia

✦ Arterial blood pH > 7.45 — excess base in the blood

✦ Potassium moves into cells to neutralize, causing hypokalemia

Alkalosis

✦ Bodywide decrease in hydrogen ion concentration

✦ Caused by hyperventilation and loss of nonvital acids during vomiting or from excessive ingestion of base

Compensation

✦ Lungs, kidneys, other chemical buffer systems work together to maintain normal plasma pH range

✦ Buffer systems consist of a weak acid and corresponding base

✦ Four major buffers or buffer systems work to restore normal pH

✦ The kidneys normalize pH by altering handling of hydrogen and bicarbonate ions

✦ Responds in hours or days to respiratory alteration of pH

ACIDOSIS

Acidosis is a systemic increase in hydrogen ion concentration. If the lungs fail to eliminate carbon dioxide or if volatile (carbonic) or nonvolatile (lactic) acid products of metabolism accumulate, hydrogen ion concentration rises. Acidosis can also occur if persistent diarrhea causes loss of basic bicarbonate anions or if the kidneys fail to reabsorb bicarbonate or secrete hydrogen ions.

ALKALEMIA

Alkalemia is arterial blood pH greater than 7.45, which reflects a relative excess of base in the blood. In alkalemia, an excess of hydrogen ions in the ICF forces them into the ECF. To keep the ICF electrically neutral, potassium moves from the ECF to the ICF, creating a relative hypokalemia.

ALKALOSIS

Alkalosis is a bodywide decrease in hydrogen ion concentration. An excessive loss of carbon dioxide during hyperventilation, loss of nonvolatile acids during vomiting, or excessive ingestion of base may decrease hydrogen ion concentration.

COMPENSATION

The lungs and kidneys, along with a number of chemical buffer systems in the intracellular and extracellular compartments, work together to maintain plasma pH in the range of 7.35 to 7.45 (compensation). For a description of acid-base values and compensatory mechanisms, see *Interpreting ABG values*.

Buffer systems

A buffer system consists of a weak acid (one that doesn't readily release free hydrogen ions) and a corresponding base, such as sodium bicarbonate. These buffers resist or minimize a change in pH when an acid or base is added to the buffered solution. Buffers work in seconds.

There are four major buffers or buffer systems. The carbonic acid–bicarbonate system, the most important, works in the lungs. The hemoglobin–oxyhemoglobin system works in RBCs where hemoglobin binds free hydrogen; the blood then flows through lungs where the hydrogen combines with carbon dioxide. Other protein buffers are located in the ECF and ICF; the phosphate system operates primarily in ICF.

When primary disease processes alter either the acid or the base component of the ratio, the lungs or kidneys (whichever isn't affected by the disease process) act to restore the ratio and normalize pH. Because the body mechanisms that regulate pH occur in stepwise fashion over time, the body tolerates gradual changes in pH better than abrupt ones.

Compensation by the kidneys

If a respiratory disorder causes acidosis or alkalosis, the kidneys respond by altering their handling of hydrogen and bicarbonate ions to return the pH to normal. Renal compensation begins hours to days after a respiratory alteration in pH. Despite this delay, renal compensation is powerful.

In acidemia, the kidneys excrete excess hydrogen ions, which may combine with phosphate or ammonia to form titratable acids in the urine. The net effect is to *raise* the concentration of bicarbonate ions in the ECF and thereby restore acid-base balance.

Interpreting ABG values

This chart compares abnormal arterial blood gas (ABG) values and their significance for patient care. By comparison, normal values are pH 7.35 to 7.45, $Paco_2$ 35 to 45 mm Hg, HCO_3^- 22 to 26 mEq/L.

DISORDER	pH	Paco₂ (MM HG)	HCO₃⁻ (MEQ/L)	COMPENSATION
Respiratory acidosis	< 7.35	> 45	✦ Acute: may be normal ✦ Chronic: > 26	✦ Renal: increased secretion and excretion of acid; compensation takes 24 hours to begin ✦ Respiratory: rate increases to expel CO₂
Respiratory alkalosis	> 7.45	< 35	✦ Acute: may be normal ✦ Chronic: < 22	✦ Renal: decreased H+ secretion and active secretion of HCO₃⁻ into urine
Metabolic acidosis	< 7.35	< 35	< 22	✦ Respiratory: lungs expel more CO₂ by increasing rate and depth of respirations
Metabolic alkalosis	> 7.45	> 45	> 26	✦ Respiratory: hypoventilation is immediate but limited because of ensuing hypoxemia ✦ Renal: more effective but slow to excrete less acid and more base

In alkalemia, the kidneys excrete excess bicarbonate ions, usually with sodium ions. The net effect is to *reduce* the concentration of bicarbonate ions in the ECF and thereby restore acid-base balance.

Compensation by the lungs

If acidosis or alkalosis results from a metabolic or renal disorder, the respiratory system regulates the respiratory rate to return the pH to normal. The partial pressure of arterial carbon dioxide ($Paco_2$) reflects carbon dioxide levels proportionate to blood pH. As the concentration of the gas increases, so does its partial pressure. Within minutes after the slightest change in $Paco_2$, central chemoreceptors in the medulla that regulate the rate and depth of ventilation detect the change. Acidemia increases respiratory rate and depth to eliminate carbon dioxide Alkalemia decreases respiratory rate and depth to retain carbon dioxide.

RESPIRATORY ACIDOSIS

Respiratory acidosis is an acid-base disturbance characterized by reduced alveolar ventilation. The patient's pulmonary system can't clear enough carbon dioxide from the body. This leads to hypercapnia ($Paco_2$ greater than 45 mm Hg) and acidosis (pH less than 7.35). Respiratory acidosis can be acute (due to a sudden failure

Key facts about pathophysiologic changes in acid-base imbalance *(continued)*
✦ Compensation by the lungs regulates respiratory rate to adjust pH; respiration increases or decreases to raise or lower Paco₂ levels

Characteristics of respiratory acidosis
✦ Characterized by alveolar ventilation
✦ Patient can't clear enough CO₂ from the body
✦ Paco₂ buildup causes hypercapnia (Paco₂ > 45 mm Hg) and acidosis
✦ May be acute or chronic

Causes

+ Opioids
+ General anesthetics
+ Hypnotics
+ Injury to the medulla
+ Reduced cardiac output
+ Neuromuscular or respiratory disease
+ Sleep apnea

How it happens

+ Pulmonary ventilation decreases, $Paco_2$ increases, and CO_2 levels rise in all tissues
+ Respiration increases; pH falls
+ Respiratory mechanisms fail; kidney buffer mechanisms take over, then fail
+ Electrolyte imbalances critically depress neurologic and cardiac functions

Key signs and symptoms

+ Restlessness
+ Confusion
+ Apprehension
+ Somnolence
+ Asterixis
+ Coma
+ Headache
+ Dyspnea and tachypnea
+ Papilledema

in ventilation) or chronic (in long-term pulmonary disease). A compromise in the essential components of breathing — ventilation, perfusion, and diffusion — may cause respiratory acidosis.

Prognosis depends on the severity of the underlying disturbance as well as the patient's general clinical condition. The prognosis is least optimistic for a patient with a debilitating disorder.

CAUSES

Opioids, general anesthetics, hypnotics, alcohol, and sedatives (including some of the new "designer" drugs such as "ecstasy") decrease the sensitivity of the respiratory center. In addition, injury to the medulla may impair ventilatory drive and chronic metabolic alkalosis may occur when respiratory compensatory mechanisms try to normalize pH by decreasing alveolar ventilation. In ventilation therapy, the use of high-flow oxygen in patients with chronic respiratory disorders suppresses the patient's hypoxic drive to breathe; high positive end-expiratory pressure (PEEP) in the presence of reduced cardiac output may cause hypercapnia due to large increases in alveolar dead space.

Other factors leading to respiratory acidosis include neuromuscular diseases, such as myasthenia gravis, Guillain-Barré syndrome, and poliomyelitis (respiratory muscles can't respond properly to respiratory drive); airway obstruction or parenchymal lung disease (interferes with alveolar ventilation); chronic obstructive pulmonary disease (COPD) or asthma; severe acute respiratory distress syndrome (reduced pulmonary blood flow and poor exchange of carbon dioxide and oxygen between the lungs and blood); chronic bronchitis; large pneumothorax; extensive pneumonia; pulmonary edema; cardiac arrest; and sleep apnea.

PATHOPHYSIOLOGY

When pulmonary ventilation decreases, $Paco_2$ is increased, and the carbon dioxide level rises in all tissues and fluids, including the medulla and cerebrospinal fluid. Retained carbon dioxide combines with water to form carbonic acid. The carbonic acid dissociates to release free hydrogen and bicarbonate ions. Increased $Paco_2$ and free hydrogen ions stimulate the medulla to increase respiratory drive and expel carbon dioxide.

As pH falls, 2,3-diphosphoglycerate accumulates in RBCs, where it alters hemoglobin so it releases oxygen. This reduced hemoglobin, which is strongly alkaline, picks up hydrogen ions and carbon dioxide and removes them from the serum.

As respiratory mechanisms fail, rising $Paco_2$ stimulates the kidneys to retain bicarbonate and sodium ions and excrete hydrogen ions. As a result, more sodium bicarbonate is available to buffer free hydrogen ions. Some hydrogen is excreted in the form of ammonium ions, neutralizing ammonia, which is an important CNS toxin.

As the hydrogen ion concentration overwhelms compensatory mechanisms, hydrogen ions move into the cells and potassium ions move out. Without enough oxygen, anaerobic metabolism produces lactic acid. Electrolyte imbalances and acidosis critically depress neurologic and cardiac functions.

SIGNS AND SYMPTOMS

Clinical features vary according to the severity and duration of respiratory acidosis, the underlying disease, and the presence of hypoxemia. Carbon dioxide and hydrogen ions dilate cerebral blood vessels and increase blood flow to the brain, causing cerebral edema and depressing CNS activity.

Possible signs and symptoms include restlessness, confusion, apprehension, somnolence, fine or flapping tremor (asterixis), coma, headaches, dyspnea and tachypnea, papilledema, depressed reflexes, and hypoxemia, unless the patient is receiving oxygen.

Respiratory acidosis may also cause cardiovascular abnormalities, including tachycardia, hypertension, atrial and ventricular arrhythmias, and hypotension with vasodilation (bounding pulses and warm periphery, in severe acidosis).

COMPLICATIONS

Possible complications include profound CNS and cardiovascular deterioration due to dangerously low blood pH (less than 7.15), myocardial depression (leading to shock and cardiac arrest), and elevated $Paco_2$ despite optimal treatment (in chronic lung disease).

DIAGNOSIS

ABG analysis confirms respiratory acidosis when $Paco_2$ is greater than 45 mm Hg; pH is typically less than 7.35 to 7.45 and bicarbonate levels are normal in the acute stage and elevated in the chronic stage. Chest X-ray commonly reveals such causes as heart failure, pneumonia, COPD, and pneumothorax.

Other diagnostic tests may indicate potassium greater than 5 mEq/L, low serum chloride, and an acidic urine pH (as the kidneys excrete hydrogen ions to return blood pH to normal). Drug screening may confirm suspected drug overdose.

TREATMENT

Effective treatment of respiratory acidosis requires correction of the underlying source of alveolar hypoventilation. Treatment of pulmonary causes of respiratory acidosis includes removing a foreign body from the airway, creating an artificial airway through endotracheal intubation or tracheotomy, using mechanical ventilation (if the patient can't breathe spontaneously), increasing the partial pressure of arterial oxygen to at least 60 mm Hg, maintaining a pH greater than 7.2 to prevent cardiac arrhythmias, and administering aerosolized or I.V. bronchodilators to open constricted airways.

Other treatment choices are antibiotics to treat pneumonia, chest tubes to correct pneumothorax, PEEP to prevent alveolar collapse, thrombolytic or anticoagulant therapy for massive pulmonary emboli, and bronchoscopy to remove excessive retained secretions.

Treatment for patients with COPD includes bronchodilators, oxygen at low flow rates (more oxygen than the person's normal level removes the hypoxic drive, further reducing alveolar ventilation), corticosteroids, and gradual reduction in $Paco_2$ to baseline to provide sufficient chloride and potassium ions to enhance renal excretion of bicarbonate (in chronic respiratory acidosis).

Additional treatments include drug therapy for such conditions as myasthenia gravis, dialysis or charcoal to remove toxic drugs, correction of metabolic alkalosis, and careful administration of I.V. sodium bicarbonate.

NURSING CONSIDERATIONS

✦ Be alert for critical changes in the patient's respiratory, CNS, and cardiovascular functions. Report such changes as well as variations in ABG levels or electrolyte status immediately. Also, maintain adequate hydration.

Complications
✦ Profound CNS and cardiovascular deterioration
✦ Myocardial depression
✦ Elevated $Paco_2$ levels

Diagnosis
✦ ABG confirms when $Paco_2$ > 45 mm Hg
✦ pH typically < 7.35
✦ Chest X-ray may reveal causes
✦ Potassium > 5 mEq/L
✦ Low serum chloride
✦ Acidic urine pH

Treatment
✦ Remove airway obstructions
✦ Create artificial airway if necessary
✦ Mechanical ventilation
✦ Increasing arterial oxygen to 60 mm Hg
✦ Bronchodilators
✦ Antibiotics
✦ Chest tubes
✦ PEEP
✦ Thrombolytic or anticoagulant therapy
✦ Bronchoscopy
✦ Drug therapy

Key nursing actions

+ Be alert for and immediately report critical changes in respiratory, CNS, and cardiovascular functions.
+ Maintain the patient's airway and perform adequate humidification if on ventilation.
+ Perform tracheal suctioning regularly and chest physiotherapy.

Characteristics of respiratory alkalosis

+ $Paco_2$ < 35 mm Hg and blood pH > 7.45
+ Poor prognosis when severe

Causes

+ Pulmonary — pneumonia, interstitial lung disease, pulmonary vascular disease, and acute asthma
+ Nonpulmonary — anxiety, fever, aspirin toxicity, metabolic acidosis, CNS disease, sepsis, hepatic failure, and pregnancy

How it happens

+ Pulmonary ventilation increases to maintain normal CO_2 levels, leading to higher pH
+ Increased ECF hydrogen combines with bicarbonate to form acid, raising pH level
+ Heart rate increases, blood to brain decreases, and autonomic nervous system overexcites
+ Continued low $Paco_2$ and vasoconstriction increase hypoxia
+ Alkalosis overwhelms CNS and heart

✦ Maintain a patent airway and provide adequate humidification if acidosis requires mechanical ventilation. Perform tracheal suctioning regularly and vigorous chest physiotherapy if ordered. Continuously monitor ventilator settings and respiratory status.
✦ To prevent respiratory acidosis, closely monitor patients with COPD and chronic carbon dioxide retention for signs of acidosis. Also, administer oxygen at low flow rates.
✦ Closely monitor all patients who receive opioids and sedatives. Instruct the patient who has received a general anesthetic to turn, cough, and perform deep-breathing exercises frequently to prevent the onset of respiratory acidosis.

RESPIRATORY ALKALOSIS

Respiratory alkalosis is an acid-base disturbance characterized by a $Paco_2$ less than 35 mm Hg and blood pH greater than 7.45; alveolar hyperventilation is the cause. Hypocapnia (below normal $Paco_2$) occurs when the lungs eliminate more carbon dioxide than the cells produce.

Respiratory alkalosis is the most common acid-base disturbance in critically ill patients and, when severe, has a poor prognosis.

CAUSES

Causes of respiratory alkalosis fall into two categories: pulmonary and nonpulmonary. Severe hypoxemia, pneumonia, interstitial lung disease, pulmonary vascular disease, and acute asthma fall into the pulmonary category. Anxiety, fever, aspirin toxicity, metabolic acidosis, CNS disease (inflammation or tumor), sepsis, hepatic failure, and pregnancy fall into the nonpulmonary category.

PATHOPHYSIOLOGY

When pulmonary ventilation increases more than needed to maintain normal carbon dioxide levels, excessive amounts of carbon dioxide are exhaled. The consequent hypocapnia leads to a chemical reduction of carbonic acid, excretion of hydrogen and bicarbonate ions, and a rising pH.

In defense against the increasing serum pH, the hydrogen–potassium buffer system pulls hydrogen ions out of the cells and into the blood in exchange for potassium ions. The hydrogen ions entering the blood combine with available bicarbonate ions to form carbonic acid, and the pH falls.

Hypocapnia stimulates the carotid and aortic bodies as well as the medulla, increasing the heart rate (which hypokalemia can further aggravate) but not the blood pressure. At the same time, hypocapnia causes cerebral vasoconstriction and decreased cerebral blood flow. It also overexcites the medulla, pons, and other parts of the autonomic nervous system. When hypocapnia lasts more than 6 hours, the kidneys secrete more bicarbonate and less hydrogen. Full renal adaptation to respiratory alkalosis requires normal volume status and renal function, and it may take several days.

Continued low $Paco_2$ and the vasoconstriction it causes increases cerebral and peripheral hypoxia. Severe alkalosis inhibits calcium ionization; as calcium ions become unavailable, nerves and muscles become progressively more excitable. Eventually, alkalosis overwhelms the CNS and heart.

SIGNS AND SYMPTOMS

The cardinal sign of respiratory alkalosis is deep, rapid breathing (possibly more than 40 breaths/minute) much like the Kussmaul's respirations that characterize diabetic acidosis.

Such hyperventilation usually leads to CNS and neuromuscular disturbances, including light-headedness or dizziness due to decreased cerebral blood flow, agitation, circumoral and peripheral paresthesia, carpopedal spasms, twitching (possibly progressing to tetany), and muscle weakness.

COMPLICATIONS

Complications of severe respiratory alkalosis include cardiac arrhythmias that may not respond to conventional treatment as the hemoglobin–oxyhemoglobin buffer system becomes overwhelmed, hypocalcemic tetany, seizures, and periods of apnea if pH remains high and $PaCO_2$ remains low.

DIAGNOSIS

ABG analysis confirms respiratory alkalosis and rules out compensation for metabolic acidosis. $PaCO_2$ falls below 35 mm Hg; blood pH increases in proportion to a decrease in $PaCO_2$ in the acute stage but drops toward normal in the chronic stage. The bicarbonate level is normal in the acute stage but below normal in the chronic stage.

Serum electrolyte studies detect metabolic disorders causing compensatory respiratory alkalosis; a low chloride level is detected in severe respiratory alkalosis. Electrocardiogram (ECG) findings may indicate cardiac arrhythmias. A toxicology screening may reveal salicylate poisoning. A basic urine pH is detected as kidneys excrete bicarbonate to raise blood pH.

TREATMENT

Possible treatments to correct the underlying condition include removal of ingested toxins, such as salicylates, by inducing emesis or using gastric lavage; treatment of fever or sepsis; oxygen administration for acute hypoxemia; and treatment of CNS disease. For hyperventilation caused by severe anxiety, the patient should breathe into a paper bag to increase carbon dioxide levels and help relieve anxiety. Based on ABG analysis results, tidal volume and minute ventilation of patients on mechanical ventilation are adjusted to prevent hyperventilation.

NURSING CONSIDERATIONS

✦ Watch for and report changes in neurologic, neuromuscular, or cardiovascular functions.
✦ Remember that twitching and cardiac arrhythmias may be associated with alkalemia and electrolyte imbalances. Monitor ABG and serum electrolyte levels closely, reporting variations immediately.
✦ Explain all diagnostic tests and procedures to the patient to reduce his anxiety.

METABOLIC ACIDOSIS

Metabolic acidosis is an acid-base disorder characterized by excess acid and deficient bicarbonate caused by an underlying nonrespiratory disorder. A primary decrease in

Characteristics of metabolic acidosis

+ Characterized by excess acid and deficient bicarbonate
+ Can occur with increased production or decreased clearance of nonvolatile acid, or loss of bicarbonate; can be fatal

Alert!

+ More prevalent in children, who are more vulnerable to acid-base imbalances.

Causes

+ Excessive fat metabolism in absence of usable carbohydrates
+ Cardiac pump failure
+ Pulmonary or hepatic disease
+ Anemia
+ Renal insufficiency or failure
+ Aspirin overdose
+ Addison's disease
+ Hypoaldosteronism

How it happens

+ Excess hydrogen ions decrease blood pH and respiration increases
+ $PaCO_2$ fall frees hydrogen ions to bind with bicarbonate
+ Respiration can't compensate
+ Kidneys try to compensate by secreting excess hydrogen into renal tubules
+ Excess hydrogen ions in ECF diffuse into cells; cells release potassium ions
+ Imbalance impairs neural excitability

plasma bicarbonate causes pH to fall. It can occur with increased production of a nonvolatile acid (such as lactic acid), decreased renal clearance of a nonvolatile acid (as in renal failure), or loss of bicarbonate (as in chronic diarrhea). Symptoms result from action of compensatory mechanisms in the lungs, kidneys, and cells.

 CLINICAL ALERT Metabolic acidosis is more prevalent among children, who are vulnerable to acid-base imbalance because their metabolic rates are rapid and their ratios of water to total body weight are low.

Severe or untreated metabolic acidosis can be fatal. The prognosis improves with prompt treatment of the underlying cause and rapid reversal of the acidotic state.

CAUSES

Metabolic acidosis commonly results from excessive fat metabolism in the absence of usable carbohydrates. This can be caused by diabetic ketoacidosis, chronic alcoholism, malnutrition, or a low-carbohydrate, high-fat diet — all of which produce more ketoacids than the metabolic process can handle.

Other conditions may also be responsible for metabolic acidosis. In anaerobic carbohydrate metabolism, decreased tissue oxygenation or perfusion — as in cardiac pump failure after myocardial infarction, pulmonary or hepatic disease, shock, or anemia — forces a shift from aerobic to anaerobic metabolism, causing a corresponding increase in lactic acid level. Underexcretion of metabolized acids or an inability to conserve base due to renal insufficiency and failure (renal acidosis) results in excess acid accumulation or deficient base bicarbonate. Diarrhea, intestinal malabsorption, or loss of sodium bicarbonate from the intestines (as in ureteroenterostomy and Crohn's disease) causes the bicarbonate buffer system to shift to the acidic side. Salicylate intoxication (overuse of aspirin), exogenous poisoning or, less frequently, Addison's disease (increased excretion of sodium and chloride and retention of potassium) may produce acid-base imbalance. Hypoaldosteronism, or the use of potassium-sparing diuretics, inhibit distal tubular secretion of acid and potassium.

PATHOPHYSIOLOGY

As acid (hydrogen) starts to accumulate in the body, chemical buffers (plasma bicarbonate and proteins) in the cells and ECF bind the excess hydrogen ions.

Excess hydrogen ions that the buffers can't bind decrease blood pH and stimulate chemoreceptors in the medulla to increase respiration. The consequent fall of $PaCO_2$ frees hydrogen ions to bind with bicarbonate. Respiratory compensation occurs in minutes but isn't sufficient to correct the acidosis.

Healthy kidneys try to compensate by secreting excess hydrogen ions into the renal tubules. These ions are buffered by phosphate or ammonia and excreted into the urine in the form of weak acid. For each hydrogen ion secreted into the renal tubules, the tubules reabsorb and return to the blood one sodium and one bicarbonate ion.

The excess hydrogen ions in ECF passively diffuse into cells. To maintain the balance of charge across the membranes, the cells release potassium ions. Excess hydrogen ions change the normal balance of potassium, sodium, and calcium ions and thereby impair neural excitability.

SIGNS AND SYMPTOMS

In mild acidosis, symptoms of the underlying disease may hide the direct clinical evidence.

Metabolic acidosis typically begins with headache and lethargy progressing to drowsiness, CNS depression, Kussmaul's respirations (as the lungs attempt to compensate by blowing off carbon dioxide), hypotension, stupor, and (if the condition is severe and untreated) coma and death. Associated GI distress usually produces anorexia, nausea, vomiting, diarrhea and, possibly, dehydration. As acidosis grows more severe, ensuing shock is indicated by warm, flushed skin due to a pH-sensitive decrease in vascular response to sympathetic stimuli. Underling diabetes mellitus may cause fruity-smelling breath from fat catabolism and excretion of accumulated acetone through the lungs.

COMPLICATIONS

Metabolic acidosis depresses the CNS and, if untreated, may lead to weakness, flaccid paralysis, coma, ventricular arrhythmias and, possibly, cardiac arrest.

In metabolic acidosis caused by chronic renal failure, bicarbonate is drawn from bone to buffer hydrogen ions. The results include growth retardation in children and bone disorders such as renal osteodystrophy.

DIAGNOSIS

Arterial pH less than 7.35 (as low as 7.10 in severe acidosis) confirms metabolic acidosis. In addition, $PaCO_2$ may be normal or less than 34 mm Hg as respiratory compensatory mechanisms take hold and bicarbonate levels may be below 22 mEq/L.

Urine pH less than 4.5 in the absence of renal disease (as the kidneys excrete acid to raise blood pH), serum potassium greater than 5.5 mEq/L (from chemical buffering), and glucose levels greater than 150 mg/dl support the diagnosis of metabolic acidosis. Serum ketone bodies are elevated in diabetes and plasma lactic acid levels are elevated in lactic acidosis.

An anion gap of 14 mEq/L or greater indicates high-anion gap metabolic acidosis, lactic acidosis, ketoacidosis, aspirin overdose, alcohol poisoning, renal failure, or other conditions characterized by accumulation of organic acids, sulfates, or phosphates. An anion gap of 12 mEq/L or less indicates normal anion gap metabolic acidosis from bicarbonate loss, GI or renal loss, increased acid load (hyperalimentation fluids), rapid I.V. saline administration, or other conditions characterized by loss of bicarbonate.

TREATMENT

Treatment aims to correct the acidosis as quickly as possible by addressing both the symptoms and the underlying cause. Measures may include administration of sodium bicarbonate I.V. for severe high anion gap to neutralize blood acidity in patients with pH less than 7.20 and bicarbonate loss. Plasma electrolytes, especially potassium, are monitored during sodium bicarbonate therapy (potassium level may fall as pH rises). I.V. lactated Ringer's solution may be administered to correct normal anion gap metabolic acidosis and ECF volume deficit. Other treatment measures include careful evaluation and correction of electrolyte imbalances and, ultimately, correction of the underlying cause (for example, in diabetic ketoacidosis, continuous low-dose I.V. insulin infusion).

In addition, mechanical ventilation may be employed to maintain respiratory compensation if needed; antibiotic therapy is used to treat the infection, dialysis is performed for patients with renal failure or certain drug toxicities, and antidiarrheal agents are administered for diarrhea-induced bicarbonate loss.

Key signs and symptoms
- Headache
- Lethargy
- Drowsiness
- CNS depression
- Kussmaul's respirations
- Hypotension
- Stupor

Complications
- Weakness
- Flaccid paralysis
- Coma
- Ventricular arrhythmias
- Cardiac arrest
- Growth retardation in children
- Bone disorders

Diagnosis
- Arterial pH < 7.35
- $PaCO_2$ < 34 mm Hg
- Bicarbonate levels < 22 mEq/L
- Urine pH < 4.5 in absence of renal disease
- Serum potassium > 5.5 mEq/L
- Glucose levels > 150 mg/dl
- Anion gap: ≤ 12 mEq/L indicates normal anion gap metabolic acidosis; ≥ 14 mEq/L indicates high-anion gap metabolic acidosis

Treatment
- Address underlying cause
- Sodium bicarbonate I.V.
- I.V. lactated Ringer's solution
- Mechanical ventilation
- Antibiotic therapy
- Dialysis
- Antidiarrheal administration

Key nursing actions

+ Keep sodium bicarbonate ampules handy for emergencies.
+ Position the patient to prevent aspiration in case of vomiting.
+ Teach diabetic patients how to test urine; encourage adherence to hypoglycemic therapy.

NURSING CONSIDERATIONS

+ Keep sodium bicarbonate ampules handy for emergency administration. Frequently monitor vital signs, laboratory results, and level of consciousness because changes can occur rapidly.
+ In diabetic acidosis, monitor for secondary changes due to hypovolemia such as decreasing blood pressure.
+ Record intake and output accurately to monitor renal function. Watch for signs of excessive serum potassium — weakness, flaccid paralysis, and arrhythmias, possibly leading to cardiac arrest. After treatment, check for overcorrection to hypokalemia.
+ Because metabolic acidosis commonly causes vomiting, position the patient to prevent aspiration. Prepare for possible seizures with seizure precautions.
+ Provide good oral hygiene. Use sodium bicarbonate rinses to neutralize mouth acids, and lubricate the patient's lips with lemon-glycerin swabs.
+ To prevent metabolic acidosis, carefully observe patients receiving I.V. therapy or those who have intestinal tubes in place as well as patients with shock, hyperthyroidism, hepatic disease, circulatory failure, or dehydration.
+ Teach the patient with diabetes how to routinely test urine for glucose and acetone, and encourage strict adherence to insulin or oral hypoglycemic therapy.

Characteristics of metabolic alkalosis

+ Low acid or high bicarbonate levels cause metabolic, respiratory, and renal responses, producing characteristic symptoms
+ Always secondary to underlying cause
+ Prognosis good with prompt diagnosis and treatment
+ Can lead to coma and death

METABOLIC ALKALOSIS

Metabolic alkalosis occurs when low levels of acid or high bicarbonate levels cause metabolic, respiratory, and renal responses, producing characteristic symptoms (most notably, hypoventilation). This condition is always secondary to an underlying cause. With early diagnosis and prompt treatment, prognosis is good, but untreated metabolic alkalosis may lead to coma and death.

CAUSES

Metabolic alkalosis results from loss of acid, retention of base, or renal mechanisms associated with low serum levels of potassium and chloride.

Causes of critical acid loss include chronic vomiting, nasogastric tube drainage or lavage without adequate electrolyte replacement, fistulas, use of steroids and certain diuretics (furosemide [Lasix], thiazides, and ethacrynic acid [Edecrin]), massive blood transfusions, Cushing's disease, primary hyperaldosteronism, and Bartter's syndrome, which lead to sodium and chloride retention and urinary loss of potassium and hydrogen.

Excessive bicarbonate retention causing chronic hypercapnia can result from excessive intake of bicarbonate of soda or other antacids (usually for treatment of gastritis or peptic ulcer), excessive intake of absorbable alkali (as in milk-alkali syndrome, often seen in patients with peptic ulcers), excessive amounts of I.V. fluids with high concentrations of bicarbonate or lactate, and respiratory insufficiency.

Alterations in extracellular electrolyte levels that can cause metabolic alkalosis include low chloride (as chloride diffuses out of the cell, hydrogen diffuses into the cell) and low plasma potassium causing increased hydrogen ion excretion by the kidneys.

Causes

+ Loss of acid, retention of base, or renal mechanisms associated with low serum levels of potassium and chloride
+ Chronic vomiting
+ NG tube drainage or lavage without adequate electrolyte replacement
+ Fistulas
+ Use of steroids
+ Massive blood transfusions
+ Cushing's disease

PATHOPHYSIOLOGY

Chemical buffers in the ECF and ICF bind bicarbonate that accumulates in the body. Excess unbound bicarbonate raises blood pH, which depresses chemoreceptors in the medulla, inhibiting respiration and raising $Paco_2$. Carbon dioxide combines with water to form carbonic acid. Low oxygen levels limit respiratory compensation.

When the blood bicarbonate level rises to 28 mEq/L or more, the amount filtered by the renal glomeruli exceeds the reabsorptive capacity of the renal tubules. Excess bicarbonate is excreted in the urine, and hydrogen ions are retained. To maintain electrochemical balance, sodium ions and water are excreted with the bicarbonate ions.

When hydrogen ion levels in ECF are low, hydrogen ions diffuse passively out of the cells and, to maintain the balance of charge across the cell membrane, extracellular potassium ions move into the cells. As intracellular hydrogen ion levels fall, calcium ionization decreases, and nerve cells become more permeable to sodium ions. As sodium ions move into the cells, they trigger neural impulses, first in the peripheral nervous system and then in the CNS.

SIGNS AND SYMPTOMS

Clinical features of metabolic alkalosis result from the body's attempt to correct the acid-base imbalance, primarily through hypoventilation. Manifestations include irritability, picking at bedclothes (carphology), twitching, confusion due to decreased cerebral perfusion, nausea, vomiting, and diarrhea (which aggravate alkalosis). Cardiovascular abnormalities due to hypokalemia and respiratory disturbances (such as cyanosis and apnea) and slow, shallow respirations also occur. Diminished peripheral blood flow during repeated blood pressure checks may provoke carpopedal spasm in the hand (Trousseau's sign, a possible sign of impending tetany).

COMPLICATIONS

Uncorrected metabolic alkalosis may progress to seizures and coma.

DIAGNOSIS

Blood pH greater than 7.45 and bicarbonate level greater than 26 mEq/L confirm diagnosis. $Paco_2$ greater than 45 mm Hg indicates attempts at respiratory compensation. Serum electrolyte studies show low levels of potassium (less than 3.5 mEq/L), calcium (less than 8.9 mg/dl), and chloride (less than 98 mEq/L). Other characteristic findings are urine pH about 7; alkaline urine after the renal compensatory mechanism begins to excrete bicarbonate. ECG may show a low T wave, merging with a P wave, and atrial or sinus tachycardia.

TREATMENT

The goal of treatment is to correct the underlying cause of metabolic alkalosis. *Cautious* use of ammonium chloride I.V. (rarely) or hydrochloric acid can restore ECF hydrogen and chloride levels; potassium chloride and normal saline solution (except in heart failure) are usually sufficient to replace losses from gastric drainage. Discontinuation of diuretics and supplementary potassium chloride corrects metabolic alkalosis from potent diuretic therapy.

Oral or I.V. acetazolamide (Diamox), which enhances renal bicarbonate excretion, may be prescribed to correct metabolic alkalosis without rapid volume expansion. It also enhances potassium excretion, so potassium may be given before acetazolamide.

How it happens

- Excess unbound bicarbonate raises blood pH, inhibiting respiration and raising $Paco_2$
- Blood bicarbonate rises to > 28 mEq/L, is excreted into urine; hydrogen is retained
- Hydrogen in ECF drops and moves out of ICF to maintain balance; potassium moves into ICF
- Calcium ionization decreases; sodium moves into cells
- Neural impulses triggered in peripheral nervous system and CNS

Key signs and symptoms

- Irritability
- Confusion
- Nausea
- Vomiting
- Diarrhea

Diagnosis

- Blood pH > 7.45 and bicarbonate level > 26 mEq/L
- $Paco_2$ > 45 mm Hg
- Potassium < 3.5 mEq/L
- Calcium < 8.9 mg/dl
- Chloride < 98 mEq/L

Treatment

- Cautious use of ammonium chloride I.V. or hydrochloric acid
- I.V. potassium chloride and normal saline
- Discontinue diuretics and administer supplementary potassium chloride
- Oral or I.V. acetazolamide

Key nursing actions

+ Monitor patient's status.
+ Dilute potassium for I.V. fluids containing potassium salts.
+ Don't give ammonium chloride to patients with renal or hepatic disease.
+ Watch for muscle weakness, tetany, or decreased activity.
+ Irrigate NG tubes with isotonic saline solution.

NURSING CONSIDERATIONS

+ Structure the care plan around cautious I.V. therapy, keen observation, and strict monitoring of the patient's status.
+ Dilute potassium when giving I.V. fluids containing potassium salts. Monitor the infusion rate to prevent damage to blood vessels; watch for signs of phlebitis. When administering ammonium chloride 0.9%, limit the infusion rate to 1 L in 4 hours; faster administration may cause hemolysis of RBCs. Avoid overdosage because it may cause overcorrection to metabolic acidosis. Don't give ammonium chloride to a patient with signs of hepatic or renal disease; instead, use hydrochloric acid.
+ Watch closely for signs of muscle weakness, tetany, or decreased activity.
+ Monitor vital signs frequently, and record intake and output to evaluate respiratory, fluid, and electrolyte status. Remember, respiratory rate usually decreases in an effort to compensate for alkalosis. Hypotension and tachycardia may indicate electrolyte imbalance, especially hypokalemia.
+ Observe seizure precautions.
+ To prevent metabolic alkalosis, warn patients against overusing alkaline agents. Irrigate nasogastric tubes with isotonic saline solution instead of plain water to prevent loss of gastric electrolytes. Monitor I.V. fluid concentrations of bicarbonate or lactate. Teach patients with ulcers to recognize signs of milk-alkali syndrome: a distaste for milk, anorexia, weakness, and lethargy.

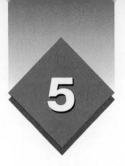

Genetics

Genetics is the study of heredity—the transmission of physical, biochemical, and physiologic traits from biological parents to their children. In this transmission, disorders can be passed on and mistakes or mutations can result in disability or death.

Genetic information is carried in genes, which are strung together on the deoxyribonucleic acid (DNA) double helix to form chromosomes. Every normal human cell (except reproductive cells) has 46 chromosomes, 22 paired chromosomes called *autosomes,* and 2 sex chromosomes (a pair of X's in females and an X and a Y in males). A representation of a person's individual set of chromosomes is called his *karyotype.* (See *Normal human karyotype,* page 110.)

The human genome has been under intense study for about 15 years to determine the structure of each gene in the genome and its location within each of the 23 chromosomes constituting the set of human chromosomes. In June 2000, two teams of scientists announced the completion of the "rough draft" of the entire genome sequence. The sequence consists of more than 3.1 billion pairs of chemicals. Decoding the genome will enable scientists to know who's likely to get a specific inherited disease and may enable researchers to eradicate or improve the treatment of many diseases. (See *The genome at a glance,* page 111.)

A word of warning at the outset: For a wide variety of reasons, not every gene that might be expressed actually is. Thus, this chapter may seem to contain a great many "hedge" words—may, perhaps, some. Genetic principles are based on studies of thousands of individuals. Those studies have led to generalities that are usually true, but exceptions occur. Genetics is an inexact science.

GENETIC COMPONENTS

Each of the two strands of DNA in a chromosome consists of thousands of combinations of four nucleotides—adenine (A), thymine (T), cytosine (C), and guanine (G). Some of our DNA is arranged into genes, which are composed of complemen-

---

Genetics
+ Study of inherited traits
+ Genetic information passed from parent to offspring through DNA in genes
+ DNA double helix forms chromosomes; normal cells contain 46 chromosomes, 22 paired autosomes, and 2 sex chromosomes
+ Males have XY sex chromosomes; females, XX
+ Representation of chromosomes called a *karyotype*
+ Sequence of genomes consists of 3.1 billion pairs of chemicals
+ Decoding the genome helps researchers treat or eradicate genetic conditions

109

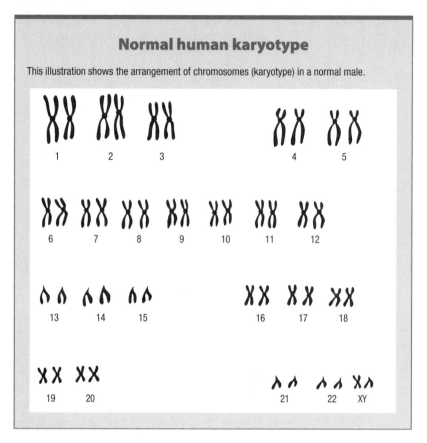

Normal human karyotype

This illustration shows the arrangement of chromosomes (karyotype) in a normal male.

Key facts about genetic components

- ✦ DNA strands in a chromosome consist of thousands of combinations of four nucleotides — A, T, C, G
- ✦ Some DNA is arranged into genes — complementary triplet pairs called *codons*
- ✦ Strands are held together by loose chemical bonds between adenine and thymine or cytosine and guanine
- ✦ Genes carry codes for each inheritable trait
- ✦ DNA controls formation of essential substances throughout the life of every cell in the body
- ✦ Genes control hereditary traits, cell reproduction and daily functions of all cells

Key facts about trait transmission

- ✦ Germ cells, or gametes (ovum and sperm), are one of two classes of cells in the body
- ✦ Germ cells contain 23 chromosomes in nucleus
- ✦ Ovum and sperm unite; corresponding chromosomes pair up to form 23 pairs of chromosomes in resulting fetus cells

tary triplet pairs called *codons.* The strands are loosely held together by chemical bonds between adenine and thymine or cytosine and guanine — for example, a triplet ACT on one strand is linked to the triplet TGA on the other. The looseness of the bonds allows the strands to separate easily during cell division. (See *DNA duplication: Two double helices from one,* page 112.) The genes carry a code for each trait a person inherits, from blood type to eye color to body shape and myriad other traits.

DNA ultimately controls the formation of essential substances throughout the life of every cell in the body. It does this through the genetic code, the precise sequence of AT and CG pairs on the DNA molecule. Genes not only control hereditary traits, transmitted from parents to offspring, but also cell reproduction and the daily functions of all cells. Genes control cell function by controlling the structures and chemicals that are synthesized within the cell. (See *How genes control cell function,* page 113.) For example, they control the formation of ribonucleic acid, which in turn controls the formation of specific proteins, most of which are enzymes that catalyze chemical reactions in the cells.

TRAIT TRANSMISSION

Germ cells, or gametes (ovum and sperm), are one of two classes of cells in the body; each germ cell contains 23 chromosomes (called the *haploid* number) in its nucleus. All the other cells in the body are somatic cells, which are *diploid,* meaning they contain 23 *pairs* of chromosomes.

The genome at a glance

In 1998, an international consortium of radiation hybrid mapping laboratories released a gene map containing more than 30,000 distinct cDNA-based markers. The particular makeup of an individual organism is called its *genome,* which is made up of the alleles (or different versions of the genes) it possesses.

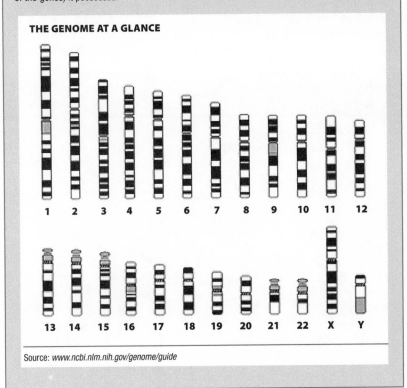

THE GENOME AT A GLANCE

Source: *www.ncbi.nlm.nih.gov/genome/guide*

When ovum and sperm unite, the corresponding chromosomes pair up so that the fertilized cell and every somatic cell of the new person has 23 pairs of chromosomes in its nucleus.

GERM CELLS

The body produces germ cells through a type of cell division called *meiosis.* Meiosis occurs only when the body is creating haploid germ cells from their diploid precursors. Each of the 23 pairs of chromosomes in the germ cell separates so that, when the cell then divides, each new cell (ovum or sperm) contains one set of 23 chromosomes.

Most of the genes on one chromosome are identical or almost identical to the gene on its mate. (As we discuss later, each chromosome may carry a different version of the same gene.) The location (or locus) of a gene on a chromosome is specific and doesn't vary from person to person. This allows each of the thousands of genes on a strand of DNA in an ovum to join the corresponding gene in a sperm when the chromosomes pair up at fertilization.

Key facts about germ cells

✦ Produced through meiosis; creating haploid germ cells from their diploid precursors

✦ Each of the 23 pairs of chromosomes in the germ cell separates

DNA duplication: Two double helices from one

The nucleotide, the basic structural unit of deoxyribonucleic acid (DNA), contains a phosphate group, deoxyribose, and a nitrogen base made of adenine (A), thymine (T), cytosine (C), and guanine (G). A DNA molecule's double helix forms from the twisting of nucleotide strands (shown here).

During duplication, a DNA chain separates and new complementary chains form and link to the separated originals (parents). The result is two identical double helices — parent and daughter.

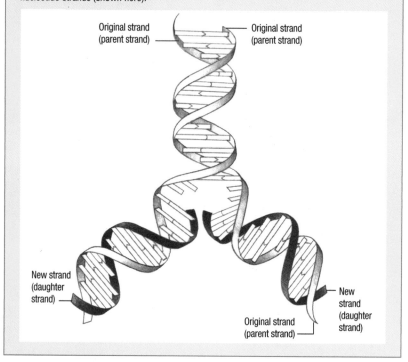

Original strand (parent strand)

Original strand (parent strand)

New strand (daughter strand)

New strand (daughter strand)

Original strand (parent strand)

How chromosomes determine sex

+ Only pair 23 of cell chromosome is involved in determining sex
+ Females: X chromosomes; males: X and Y
+ Each gamete produced by a male contains either an X or a Y chromosome
+ When a sperm with an X chromosome fertilizes an ovum, the offspring is female (two X chromosomes)
+ When a sperm with a Y chromosome fertilizes an ovum, the offspring is male (one X and one Y chromosome)
+ Errors can produce viable zygotes with XO, XXY, XXX, or XYY karyotype
+ Most other errors in sex chromosome division not viable

Determining sex

Only one pair of chromosomes in each cell — pair 23 — is involved in determining a person's sex. These are the sex chromosomes; the other 22 numbered chromosome pairs are called *autosomes*. Females have two X chromosomes; males have one X and one Y chromosome.

Each gamete produced by a male contains either an X or a Y chromosome. When a sperm with an X chromosome fertilizes an ovum, the offspring is female (two X chromosomes); when a sperm with a Y chromosome fertilizes an ovum, the offspring is male (one X and one Y chromosome). Very rare errors in cell division can result in a germ cell that has no sex chromosome or two sex chromosomes. After fertilization, with a gamete that contains an abnormal number of sex chromosomes, the zygote may have an XO, XXY, XXX, or XYY karyotype and still survive. Most other errors in sex chromosome division are incompatible with life.

How genes control cell function

This simplified diagram outlines how the genetic code directs formation of specific proteins. Some proteins are the building blocks of cell structure. Others, called *enzymes,* direct intracellular chemical reactions. Together, structural proteins and enzymes direct cell function.

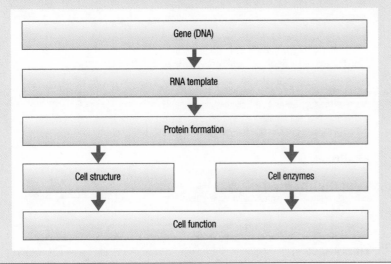

MITOSIS

The fertilized ovum—now called a *zygote*—undergoes a type of cell division called *mitosis.* Before a cell divides, its chromosomes duplicate. During this process, the double helix of DNA separates into two chains; each chain serves as a template for constructing a new chain. Individual DNA nucleotides are linked into new strands with bases complementary to those in the originals. In this way, two identical double helices are formed, each containing one of the original strands and a newly formed complementary strand. These double helices are duplicates of the original DNA chain.

Mitotic cell division occurs in five phases: an inactive phase (interphase) and four active phases (prophase, metaphase, anaphase, and telophase). (See *Five phases of mitosis,* page 114.) The result of every mitotic cell division is two new daughter cells, each genetically identical to the original and to each other. The two resulting cells likewise divide, and so on, eventually forming a multicellular human embryo. Thus, each cell in a person's body (except ovum or sperm) contains an identical set of 46 chromosomes that are unique to that person.

Key facts about mitosis

✦ Before a cell divides, chromosomes duplicate
✦ Double helix of DNA separates into two chains; each chain is a template for a new chain
✦ DNA nucleotides link into new strands with bases complementary to those in the originals
✦ Two identical double helices are formed—duplicates of the original DNA chain
✦ Occurs in five phases: interphase (inactive), and prophase, metaphase, anaphase, and telophase (active)
✦ Result is two new daughter cells genetically identical to the original and each other

5 phases of mitosis
- ✦ Interphase
- ✦ Prophase
- ✦ Metaphase
- ✦ Anaphase
- ✦ Telophase

Key facts about trait predominance
- ✦ Each parent contributes one set of chromosomes
- ✦ Some traits determined by one gene
- ✦ Polygenic traits require the interaction of one or more genes
- ✦ Environmental factors may affect how a gene or genes are expressed
- ✦ Variations in a particular gene called alleles
- ✦ Identical alleles on each chromosome are homozygous; if different, heterozygous

CLOSER LOOK

Five phases of mitosis

In mitosis (used by all cells except gametes), the nuclear contents of a cell reproduce and divide, resulting in the formation of two daughter cells. The five steps, or phases, of this process are illustrated here.

INTERPHASE
During interphase, the nucleus and nuclear membrane are well defined and the nucleolus is prominent. Chromosomes replicate, each forming a double strand that remains attached at the center of each chromosome by a structure called the *centromere;* they appear as an indistinguishable matrix within the nucleus. Centrioles (in animal cells only, not plant cells) appear outside the nucleus.

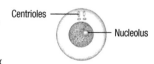

PROPHASE
During prophase, the nucleolus disappears and chromosomes become distinct. Halves of each duplicated chromosome (chromatids) remain attached by a centromere. Centrioles move to opposite sides of the cell and radiate spindle fibers.

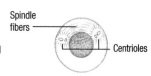

METAPHASE
During metaphase, chromosomes line up randomly in the center of the cell between the spindles, along the metaphase plate. The centromere of each chromosome replicates.

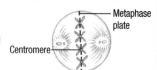

ANAPHASE
During anaphase, centromeres move apart, pulling the separate chromatids (now called *chromosomes*) to opposite ends of the cell. In human cells, each end of the cell now contains 46 chromosomes. The number of chromosomes at each end of the cell equals the original number.

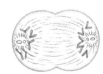

TELOPHASE
During telophase, a nuclear membrane forms around each end of the cell, and the spindle fibers disappear. The cytoplasm compresses and divides the cell in half. Each new cell contains the diploid number (46 in humans) of chromosomes.

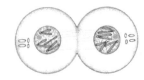

TRAIT PREDOMINANCE

Each parent contributes one set of chromosomes (and therefore one set of genes) so every offspring has two genes for every locus on the autosomal chromosomes.

Some characteristics, or traits, are determined by one gene that may have many variants such as eye color. Others, called *polygenic traits,* require the interaction of one or more genes. Environmental factors may affect how a gene or genes are expressed.

Variations in a particular gene — such as brown, blue, or green eye color — are called *alleles.* A person who has identical alleles on each chromosome is homozygous for that gene; if the alleles are different, they're heterozygous.

AUTOSOMAL INHERITANCE

For unknown reasons, one allele on autosomal chromosomes may be more influential than the other in determining a specific trait. The more powerful, or *dominant,* gene is more likely to be expressed in the offspring than the less influential, or *recessive,* gene. Offspring will express a dominant allele when one or both chromosomes in a pair carry it. A recessive allele won't be expressed unless both chromosomes carry recessive alleles. For example, a child may receive a gene for brown eyes from one parent and a gene for blue eyes from the other parent. The gene for brown eyes is dominant, and the gene for blue eyes is recessive. Because the dominant gene is more likely to be expressed, the child is more likely to have brown eyes.

SEX-LINKED INHERITANCE

The X and Y chromosomes aren't truly a pair because the X chromosome is much larger than the Y. The male has less genetic material than the female, which means he has only one copy of most genes on the X chromosome. Inheritance of those genes is called *X-linked.* A man will transmit one copy of each X-linked gene to his daughters and none to his sons. A woman will transmit one copy to each child, male or female.

Inheritance of genes on the X chromosomes is different in another way. Some recessive genes on the X chromosomes act like dominants in females. Due to X-inactivation, one recessive allele will be expressed in some somatic cells and another in other somatic cells. The most common example occurs not in people but in cats. Only female cats have calico (tricolor) coat patterns. Hair color in the cat is carried on the X chromosome. Some hair cells in females express the brown allele, others the white, and still others a third color.

MULTIFACTORIAL INHERITANCE

Environmental factors can affect the expression of some genes; this is called *multifactorial inheritance.* Height is a classic example of a multifactorial trait. In general, the height of offspring will be in a range between the height of the two parents. But nutritional patterns, health care, and other environmental factors also influence development. The better-nourished, healthier children of two short parents may be taller than either. Some diseases have genetic predisposition but multifactorial inheritance; that is, the gene for the disease is expressed only under certain environmental conditions.

Factors that may contribute to multifactorial inheritance include maternal age; use of drugs, alcohol, or hormones by either parent; maternal or paternal exposure to radiation; maternal infection during pregnancy or existing diseases in the mother; nutritional factors; and other factors, including high altitude, maternal smoking, maternal-fetal blood incompatibility, and inadequate prenatal care.

PATHOPHYSIOLOGIC CHANGES

Autosomal, sex-linked, and multifactorial disorders originate from damage to genes or chromosomes. Some defects arise spontaneously, whereas others may be caused by environmental teratogens.

Key facts about autosomal inheritance
- One allele on autosomal chromosomes may be more influential than the other
- Dominant gene is more likely to be expressed in offspring
- Dominant allele expressed when one or both chromosomes in a pair carry it
- Recessive allele not expressed unless both chromosomes carry recessive alleles

Key facts about sex-linked inheritance
- X chromosome is larger than Y
- Male has less genetic material than the female
- Inheritance of those genes called *X-linked*
- Males transmit one copy of each X-linked gene to daughters and none to sons
- Females transmit one copy to each child, male or female

Key facts about multifactorial inheritance
- Environmental factors can affect expression of some genes
- Diseases can have genetic predisposition
- Contributing factors include general maternal or paternal health, maternal smoking, maternal-fetal blood incompatibility, and inadequate prenatal care

Pathophysiologic changes
- Originate from damage to genes or chromosomes
- Can arise spontaneously or by environmental teratogens

Key facts about gene errors

✦ Permanent change in genetic material: mutation
✦ Occurs spontaneously or after exposure to radiation, chemicals, or viruses
✦ Can occur anywhere in the genome
✦ May produce different trait that is transmitted to offspring during reproduction

Key facts about autosomal disorders

✦ Error occurs at a single gene site on the DNA strand
✦ Inherited in identifiable patterns
✦ Cause most hereditary disorders
✦ Affects genders equally
✦ If one parent is affected, each child has 50% chance of being affected
✦ If both parents are affected, all offspring will be affected

Key facts about sex-linked disorders

✦ Genetic disorders caused by genes located on the sex chromosomes
✦ Passed mainly on the X chromosome as recessive traits
✦ Most who express X-linked recessive traits are males with unaffected parents

GENE ERRORS

A permanent change in genetic material is called a *mutation*. It may occur spontaneously or after exposure of a cell to radiation, certain chemicals, or viruses. Mutations can occur anywhere in the genome — the person's entire inventory of genes.

Every cell has built-in defenses against genetic damage. However, if a mutation isn't identified or repaired, the mutation may produce a trait different from the original trait that will be transmitted to offspring during reproduction. The mutation initially causes the cell to produce an abnormal protein that makes the cell different from its ancestors. Some mutations may have no effect, while others may change expression of a trait; others change the way a cell functions. Some mutations can cause serious or deadly defects, such as cancer or congenital anomalies.

Autosomal disorders

In single-gene disorders, an error occurs at a single gene site on the DNA strand. A mistake may occur in the copying and transcribing of a single codon (nucleotide triplet) through additions, deletions, excessive repetitions, or base changes.

Single-gene disorders are inherited in clearly identifiable patterns that are the same as those seen in the inheritance of normal traits. Because every person has 22 pairs of autosomes and only 1 pair of sex chromosomes, most hereditary disorders are caused by autosomal defects.

Autosomal dominant transmission usually affects male and female offspring equally. If one parent is affected, each child has one chance in two of being affected. If both parents are affected, they have affected or unaffected children. An example of this occurs in Marfan syndrome. (See *Autosomal dominant inheritance.*)

Autosomal recessive inheritance also usually affects male and female offspring equally. If both parents are affected, all of their offspring will be affected. If both parents are unaffected but are heterozygous for the trait (carriers of the defective gene), each child has one chance in four of being affected. If only one parent is affected, and the other isn't a carrier, none of their offspring will be affected, but all will carry the defective gene. If one parent is affected and the other is a carrier, their offspring will have a 50% chance of being affected. (See *Autosomal recessive inheritance.*) Autosomal recessive disorders may occur when there's no family history of the disease.

Sex-linked disorders

Genetic disorders caused by genes located on the sex chromosomes are termed *sex-linked disorders*. Most sex-linked disorders are passed on the X chromosome, usually as recessive traits. Because males have only one X chromosome, a single X-linked recessive gene can cause disease to be exhibited in a male. Females receive two X chromosomes, so they can be homozygous for a disease allele, homozygous for a normal allele, or heterozygous (a carrier).

Most people who express X-linked recessive traits are males with unaffected parents. In rare cases, the father is affected and the mother is a carrier. All daughters of an affected male will be carriers. Sons of an affected male will be unaffected, and the unaffected sons aren't carriers. Unaffected male children of a female carrier don't transmit the disorder. Hemophilia is an example of an X-linked inheritance disorder. (See *X-linked recessive inheritance,* page 118.)

Characteristics of X-linked dominant inheritance include evidence of the inherited trait in the family history. A person with the abnormal trait must have one affected parent. If the father has an X-linked dominant disorder, all of his daughters and none of his sons will be affected. If a mother has an X-linked dominant disorder, each of her children has 50% chance of being affected. (See *X-linked dominant inheritance,* page 118.)

Autosomal dominant inheritance

This diagram shows the inheritance pattern of an abnormal trait when one parent has recessive normal genes (aa) and the other has a dominant abnormal gene (Aa). Each child has a 50% chance of inheriting A.

		Affected parent	
		A	a
Normal parent	a	Aa Affected	aa Normal
	a	Aa Affected	aa Normal

Autosomal recessive inheritance

This diagram shows the inheritance pattern of an abnormal trait when both unaffected parents are heterozygous (Aa) for a recessive abnormal gene (a) on an autosome. As shown, each child has a one-in-four chance of being affected (aa), a one-in-four chance of having two normal genes (AA) and no chance of transmittal, and a 50% chance of being a carrier (Aa) who can transmit the gene.

		Heterozygous parent Aa	
		A	a
Heterozygous parent Aa	A	AA Normal	Aa Carrier
	a	Aa Carrier	aa Affected

Multifactorial disorders

Most multifactorial disorders result from the effects of several different genes and an environmental component. In polygenic inheritance, each gene has a small additive effect; the effect of a combination of genetic errors in a person is unpredictable. Multifactorial disorders can result from a less-than-optimum expression of many different genes, not from a specific error.

Some multifactorial disorders are apparent at birth, such as cleft lip, cleft palate, congenital heart disease, anencephaly, clubfoot, and myelomeningocele. Others don't become apparent until later, such as type II diabetes mellitus, hypertension, hyperlipidemia, most autoimmune diseases, and many cancers. Multifactorial disorders that develop during adulthood are often believed to be strongly related to environmental factors, not only in incidence but also in the degree of expression.

Environmental teratogens

Teratogens are environmental agents that can harm the developing fetus by causing congenital structural or functional defects. Teratogens may also cause spontaneous miscarriage, complications during labor and delivery, hidden defects in later development (such as cognitive or behavioral problems), or neoplastic transformations. (See *Teratogens and associated disorders,* pages 119 and 120.)

Key facts about multifactorial disorders

+ Most result from effects of several different genes and an environmental component
+ Polygenic inheritance — each gene has a small additive effect; combination of genetic errors unpredictable
+ Result from improper expression of many different genes, not a specific error
+ Some apparent at birth; others become apparent later
+ Development in adulthood often believed strongly related to environmental factors in incidence and degree of expression

X-linked recessive inheritance

This diagram shows the children of a normal parent and a parent with a recessive gene on the X chromosome (shown by an open dot). All daughters of an affected male will be carriers. The son of a female carrier may inherit a recessive gene on the X chromosome and be affected by the disease. Unaffected sons can't transmit the disorder.

		Normal mother	
		X	X
Affected father	X̶	X̶X Carrier daughter	XX̶ Carrier daughter
	Y	XY Normal son	XY Normal son

		Carrier mother	
		X̶	X
Normal father	X	X̶X Carrier daughter	XX Normal daughter
	Y	X̶Y Affected son	XY Normal son

X-linked dominant inheritance

This diagram shows the children of a normal parent and a parent with an abnormal, X-linked dominant gene on the X chromosome (shown by the dot on the X). When the father is affected, only his daughters have the abnormal gene. When the mother is affected, both sons and daughters may be affected.

		Normal mother	
		X	X
Affected father	X⋅	X⋅X Affected daughter	X⋅X Affected daughter
	Y	XY Normal son	XY Normal son

		Affected mother	
		X⋅	X
Normal father	X	X⋅X Affected daughter	XX Normal daughter
	Y	X⋅Y Affected son	XY Normal son

Key facts about environmental teratogens

✦ Environmental agents that can harm developing fetus, causing congenital structural or functional defects
✦ May cause spontaneous miscarriage, abortion, and delivery complications, hidden defects, neoplastic transformations
✦ Environmental factors of maternal or paternal origin
✦ Exposure to teratogens usually kills the embryo
✦ Exposure during fetal period can cause intrauterine growth retardation, cognitive abnormalities, or structural defects

Environmental factors of maternal or paternal origin include the use of chemicals (such as drugs, alcohol, or hormones), exposure to radiation, general health, and age. Maternal factors include infections during pregnancy, existing diseases, nutritional factors, exposure to high altitude, maternal-fetal blood incompatibility, and poor prenatal care.

The embryonic period—the first 8 weeks after fertilization—is a vulnerable time when specific organ systems are actively differentiating. Exposure to teratogens usually kills the embryo. During the fetal period, organ systems are formed and continue to mature. Exposure during this time can cause intrauterine growth retardation, cognitive abnormalities, or structural defects.

Teratogens and associated disorders

This chart lists common teratogens and their associated disorders.

TERATOGENS	ASSOCIATED DISORDERS
Infections	
Toxoplasmosis Rubella Cytomegalovirus Herpes simplex Other infections (syphilis, hepatitis B, mumps, gonorrhea, parvovirus, varicella)	✦ Growth deficiency ✦ Mental retardation ✦ Hepatosplenomegaly ✦ Hearing loss ✦ Cardiac and ocular defects ✦ Active infection ✦ Carrier state
Maternal disorders	
Diabetes mellitus	✦ Abnormalities of the spine, lower extremities, heart, kidney, or external genitalia
Phenylketonuria	✦ Mental retardation ✦ Microcephaly ✦ Congenital heart defects ✦ Intrauterine growth retardation
Hyperthermia	✦ Intrauterine growth retardation ✦ Central nervous system (CNS) and neural tube defects ✦ Facial defects
Drugs, chemicals, and physical agents	
Alcohol	✦ Fetal alcohol syndrome ✦ Learning disabilities
Anticonvulsants	✦ Intrauterine growth retardation ✦ Mental deficiency ✦ Facial abnormalities ✦ Cardiac defects ✦ Cleft lip and palate ✦ Malformed ears ✦ Genital defects
Cocaine	✦ Premature delivery ✦ Abruptio placentae ✦ Intracranial hemorrhage ✦ GI and genitourinary (GU) abnormalities
Diethylstilbestrol	✦ Clear-cell adenocarcinoma of vagina ✦ Structural and functional defects of female GU tract
Lithium	✦ Congenital heart disease

(continued)

Common teratogens and disorders

Infections
✦ Toxoplasmosis
✦ Rubella
✦ Cytomegalovirus
✦ Herpes simplex
✦ Other infections

Maternal disorders
✦ Diabetes mellitus
✦ Phenylketonuria
✦ Hyperthermia

Drugs, chemicals, and physical agents
✦ Alcohol
✦ Anticonvulsants
✦ Cocaine
✦ Diethylstilbestrol
✦ Lithium
✦ Methotrexate
✦ Radiation
✦ Tetracycline
✦ Vitamin A derivatives
✦ Warfarin

Key facts about chromosome defects

◆ Called *congenital anomalies* or *birth defects*
◆ Aberration may be loss, addition, or rearrangement of genetic material
◆ Most clinically significant aberrations arise during meiosis
◆ Potential contributing factors include maternal age, radiation, and use of some therapeutic or illicit drugs
◆ Translocation occurs when chromosomes split apart and rejoin in an abnormal arrangement; however, cells still have a normal amount of genetic material; often no visible abnormalities

Key facts about errors in chromosome number

◆ During meiosis and mitosis, failure to separate (*nondisjunction*) causes an unequal distribution of chromosomes
◆ Incidence increases with parental age
◆ Presence of one chromosome less than normal is monosomy
◆ Presence of an extra chromosome is trisomy
◆ Combination of trisomic and normal cells called mosaicism— two or more cell lines in the same person
◆ Effect of mosaicism depends on the proportion and anatomic location of abnormal cells

Teratogens and associated disorders (continued)

TERATOGENS	ASSOCIATED DISORDERS
Drugs, chemicals, and physical agents (continued)	
Methotrexate	◆ Intrauterine growth retardation ◆ Decreased ossification of skull ◆ Prominent eyes ◆ Limb abnormalities ◆ Mild developmental delay
Radiation	◆ Microcephaly ◆ Mental retardation
Tetracycline	◆ Brown staining of decidual teeth ◆ Dental caries ◆ Enamel hypoplasia
Vitamin A derivatives	◆ Facial defects ◆ Cardiac defects ◆ CNS defects ◆ Incomplete development of thymus
Warfarin (Coumadin)	◆ Intrauterine growth retardation ◆ Mental retardation ◆ Seizures ◆ Nasal hypoplasia ◆ Abnormal calcification of axial skeleton

Adapted with permission. Hansen, M. *Pathophysiology: Foundations of Disease and Clinical Intervention.* Philadephia: W.B. Saunders Co., 1998.

CHROMOSOME DEFECTS

Aberrations in chromosome structure or number cause a class of disorders called *congenital anomalies,* or *birth defects.* The aberration may be loss, addition, or rearrangement of genetic material. If the remaining genetic material is sufficient to maintain life, an endless variety of clinical manifestations may occur. Most clinically significant chromosome aberrations arise during meiosis. Meiosis is an incredibly complex process that can go wrong in many ways. Potential contributing factors include maternal age, radiation, and use of some therapeutic or illicit drugs.

Translocation, the shifting of chromosomal material, occurs when chromosomes split apart and rejoin in an abnormal arrangement. The cells still have a normal amount of genetic material; however, the children of parents with translocated chromosomes may have serious genetic defects, such as monosomies or trisomies. Parental age doesn't seem to be a factor in translocation.

Errors in chromosome number

During meiosis and mitosis, chromosomes normally separate in a process called *disjunction.* Failure to separate, called *nondisjunction,* causes an unequal distribution of chromosomes between the two resulting cells. If nondisjunction occurs during mitosis soon after fertilization, it may affect all the resulting cells. Gain or loss of chromosomes is usually caused by nondisjunction of autosomes or sex chromo-

CLOSER LOOK

Chromosomal disjunction and nondisjunction

This illustration shows normal chromosomal disjunction and nondisjunction of an ovum. When disjunction proceeds normally, fertilization with a normal sperm results in a zygote with the correct number of chromosomes. In nondisjunction, the sister chromatids fail to separate; the result is one trisomic cell and one monosomic cell.

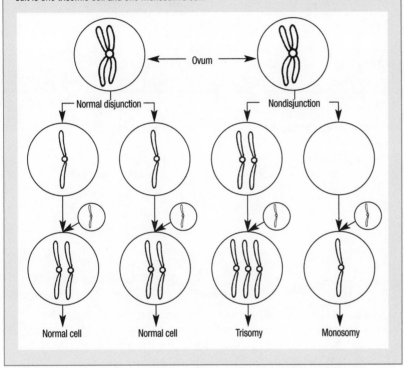

somes during meiosis. The incidence of nondisjunction increases with parental age. (See *Chromosomal disjunction and nondisjunction.*)

The presence of one chromosome less than the normal number is called *monosomy;* an autosomal monosomy is nonviable. The presence of an extra chromosome is called a *trisomy.* A mixture of both trisomic and normal cells results in mosaicism, which is the presence of two or more cell lines in the same person. The effect of mosaicism depends on the proportion and anatomic location of abnormal cells.

CLEFT LIP AND CLEFT PALATE

Cleft lip and cleft palate, polygenic multifactorial disorders, may occur separately or in combination. They originate in the second month of pregnancy if the front and sides of the face and the palatine shelves fuse imperfectly. Cleft lip with or without cleft palate occurs twice as often in males than females. Cleft palate without cleft lip is more common in females.

Cleft lip deformities can occur unilaterally, bilaterally or, rarely, in the midline. Only the lip may be involved, or the defect may extend into the upper jaw or nasal cavity. (See *Types of cleft deformities,* page 122.)

Characteristics of cleft lip and cleft palate

✦ Originate in the second month of pregnancy if the front and sides of the face and the palatine shelves fuse imperfectly
✦ Cleft lip with or without cleft palate occurs twice as often in males as in females
✦ Cleft palate without cleft lip is more common in females
✦ Cleft lip deformities can occur unilaterally, bilaterally or, rarely, in the midline
✦ Defect may extend into the upper jaw or nasal cavity
✦ Incidence is highest in children with a family history of cleft defects
✦ Cleft lip with or without cleft palate occurs in about 1 in 1,000 births

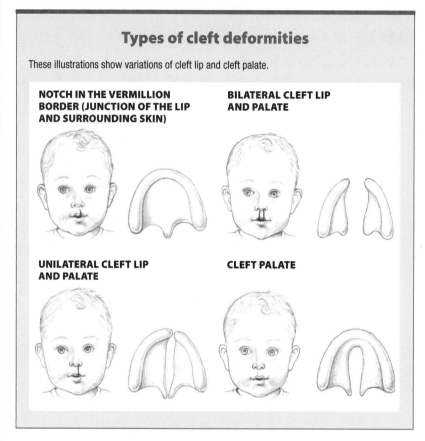

Types of cleft deformities

These illustrations show variations of cleft lip and cleft palate.

NOTCH IN THE VERMILLION BORDER (JUNCTION OF THE LIP AND SURROUNDING SKIN)

BILATERAL CLEFT LIP AND PALATE

UNILATERAL CLEFT LIP AND PALATE

CLEFT PALATE

Causes

♦ Chromosomal or Mendelian syndrome

♦ Exposure to teratogens during fetal development

♦ Combined genetic and environmental factors

How it happens

♦ During second month of pregnancy lip or palate fuses imperfectly

♦ Result of chromosomal abnormality, exposure to teratogens, genetic abnormality, environmental factors

Incidence is highest in children with a family history of cleft defects. Cleft lip with or without cleft palate occurs in about 1 in 1,000 births among Whites; the incidence is higher in Asians (1.7 in 1,000) and Native Americans (more than 3.6 in 1,000) but lower in Blacks (1 in 2,500).

CAUSES

Possible causes of cleft lip or cleft palate include chromosomal or Mendelian syndrome (cleft defects are associated with more than 300 syndromes), exposure to teratogens during fetal development, and combined genetic and environmental factors.

PATHOPHYSIOLOGY

During the second month of pregnancy, the front and sides of the face and the palatine shelves develop. Because of a chromosomal abnormality, exposure to teratogens, genetic abnormality, or environmental factors, the lip or palate fuses imperfectly.

The deformity may range from a simple notch to a complete cleft. A cleft palate may be partial or complete. A complete cleft includes the soft palate, the bones of the maxilla, and the alveolus on one or both sides of the premaxilla.

A double cleft is the most severe of the deformities. The cleft runs from the soft palate forward to either side of the nose. A double cleft separates the maxilla and premaxilla into freely moving segments. The tongue and other muscles can displace the segments, enlarging the cleft.

CLINICAL ALERT Isolated cleft palate is more commonly associated with other congenital defects than isolated cleft lip with or without cleft palate. The constellation of U-shaped cleft palate, mandibular hypoplasia, and glossoptosis is known as *Pierre Robin sequence,* or *Robin sequence.* Robin sequence can occur as an isolated defect or one feature of many different syndromes; therefore, a comprehensive genetic evaluation is suggested for infants with Robin sequence. Because of the mandibular hypoplasia and glossoptosis, careful evaluation and management of the airway are mandatory for infants with Robin sequence.

SIGNS AND SYMPTOMS

Signs and symptoms may include obvious cleft lip or cleft palate and feeding difficulties due to incomplete fusion of the palate.

COMPLICATIONS

Complications may include malnutrition, because the abnormal lip and palate affect nutritional intake; hearing impairment, often due to middle-ear damage or recurrent infections; and permanent speech impediment, even after surgical repair.

DIAGNOSIS

A typical clinical picture confirms the diagnosis. Cleft lip with or without cleft palate is obvious at birth; occasionally, more severe defects may be seen with diagnostic prenatal ultrasonography. Cleft palate without cleft lip may not be detected until a mouth examination is performed or until feeding difficulties develop.

TREATMENT

Treatment consists of surgical correction, but the timing of surgery varies. Some plastic surgeons repair cleft lips within the first few days of life to make feeding the baby easier. However, many surgeons delay lip repairs for 8 to 10 weeks (sometimes as long as 6 to 8 months) to allow the infant to grow and mature, thereby minimizing surgical and anesthesia risks, ruling out associated congenital anomalies, and allowing time for parental bonding. Cleft palate repair is usually completed by the 12th to 18th month. Some surgeons repair cleft palates in two steps, repairing the soft palate between ages 6 and 18 months and the hard palate as late as age 5. In all cases, surgery is performed only after the infant is gaining weight and infection-free.

Surgery must be coupled with speech therapy. Because the palate is essential to speech formation, structural changes, even in a repaired cleft, can permanently affect speech patterns. To compound the problem, children with cleft palates often have hearing difficulties because of middle ear damage or infections.

Use of a contoured speech bulb attached to the posterior of a denture to occlude the nasopharynx helps the child develop intelligible speech when a wide horseshoe defect makes surgery impossible. Special nipples and other feeding devices are available to improve feeding patterns and promote nutrition in infants with a cleft lip or palate.

 CLINICAL ALERT Daily use of folic acid before conception decreases the risk for isolated (not associated with another genetic or congenital malformation) cleft lip or palate by up to 25%. Women of childbearing age should be encouraged to take a daily multivitamin containing folic acid until menopause or until they're no longer fertile.

Alert!
+ Careful evaluation and management of the airway are mandatory for infants with Pierre Robin sequence.

Key signs and symptoms
+ Obvious cleft lip or cleft palate
+ Feeding difficulties due to incomplete fusion of the palate

Complications
+ Malnutrition
+ Hearing impairment
+ Permanent speech impediment, even after surgical repair

Diagnosis
+ Typical clinical picture confirms the diagnosis
+ More severe defects may be seen with diagnostic prenatal ultrasonography
+ Cleft palate without cleft lip may not be detected until a mouth examination is performed or until feeding difficulties develop

Treatment
+ Surgical correction
+ Speech therapy
+ Contoured speech bulb attached to the posterior of a denture helps the child develop intelligible speech
+ Special nipples improve feeding

Alert!
+ Daily use of folic acid before conception decreases the risk for isolated cleft lip or palate by up to 25%.

Alert!

✦ Never place a child with Pierre Robin sequence on his back because his tongue could fall back and obstruct his airway.

Key nursing actions

✦ Encourage taking 0.4 mg of folic acid twice daily before conception

✦ Maintain adequate nutrition to ensure normal growth and development.

✦ Teach the parents how best to feed the infant.

✦ Encourage the mother of an infant with cleft lip to breast-feed if the cleft doesn't prevent effective sucking.

✦ After surgery, record intake and output and maintain good nutrition.

✦ Provide care to curved metal bow (if used) over a repaired cleft lip to minimize tension on the suture line. Remove the gauze before feedings, and replace it frequently.

✦ Help the parents cope with their feelings about the child's deformity.

NURSING CONSIDERATIONS

✦ Recent research has indicated that ingestion of 0.4 mg of folic acid twice daily before conception may decrease the risk of isolated cleft defects.

 CLINICAL ALERT Never place a child with Pierre Robin sequence on his back because his tongue could fall back and obstruct his airway. Place the infant on his side for sleeping. Most other infants with a cleft palate can sleep on their backs without difficulty.

✦ Maintain adequate nutrition to ensure normal growth and development. Experiment with feeding devices. An infant with a cleft palate has an excellent appetite but commonly has difficulty feeding because of air leaks around the cleft and nasal regurgitation. He usually feeds better from a bottle and nipple designed specifically for feeding infants with cleft defects. These bottles come with special nipples or regular nipples with enlarged holes. Both types of nipples may be used with cleft palate bottles.

✦ Teach the parents how best to feed the infant. Advise them to hold the infant in a near-sitting position, with the flow directed to the side or back of the infant's tongue. Tell them to burp the infant frequently because he tends to swallow a lot of air. If the underside of the nasal septum becomes ulcerated and the child refuses to suck because of the pain, instruct the parents to direct the nipple to the side of the mouth to give the mucosa time to heal. Tell them to gently clean the palatal cleft with a cotton-tipped applicator dipped in half-strength hydrogen peroxide or water after each feeding.

✦ Encourage the mother of an infant with cleft lip to breast-feed if the cleft doesn't prevent effective sucking. Breast-feeding an infant with a cleft palate or one who has just had corrective surgery isn't usually possible. (Postoperatively, the infant can't suck for 6 to 10 weeks.) However, if the mother desires, suggest that she use a breast pump to express breast milk and then feed it to her infant from a bottle.

✦ After surgery, record intake and output and maintain good nutrition. To prevent atelectasis and pneumonia, the physician may gently suction the nasopharynx (this may be necessary before surgery, too). Restrain the infant to prevent him from hurting himself. Elbow restraints allow the infant to move his hands while keeping them away from his mouth. When necessary, use an infant seat to keep the child in a comfortable sitting position. Hang toys within reach of his restrained hands.

✦ Surgeons sometimes place a curved metal bow over a repaired cleft lip to minimize tension on the suture line. Remove the gauze before feedings, and replace it frequently. Moisten it with normal saline solution until the sutures are removed. Check your facility's policy to confirm this procedure.

✦ Help the parents cope with their feelings about the child's deformity. Start by telling them about it and showing them their infant as soon as possible. Because society places undue importance on physical appearance, many parents feel shock, disappointment, and guilt when they see the child. Help them by being calm and providing positive information.

✦ Direct the parents' attention to their child's assets. Stress the fact that surgical repairs can be made. Include the parents in the care and feeding of the child right from the start to encourage normal bonding. Provide the instructions, emotional support, and reassurance that the parents will need to take proper care of their child at home.

✦ Refer them to a social worker who can guide them to community resources, if needed, and to a genetic counselor to determine the recurrence risk.

CYSTIC FIBROSIS

In cystic fibrosis, dysfunction of the exocrine glands affects multiple organ systems. The disease affects males as well as females and is the most common fatal genetic disease in white children.

Cystic fibrosis, transmitted as an autosomal recessive trait, is accompanied by many complications and now carries an average life expectancy of 32 years. The disorder is characterized by chronic airway infection leading to bronchiectasis, bronchiolectasis, exocrine pancreatic insufficiency, intestinal dysfunction, abnormal sweat gland function, and reproductive dysfunction.

The incidence of cystic fibrosis varies with ethnic origin. It occurs in 1 of 2,000 births in Whites of North America and northern European descent, 1 in 17,000 births in Blacks, and 1 in 90,000 births in the Asian population in Hawaii.

CAUSES

The gene responsible for cystic fibrosis is on chromosome 7q; it encodes a membrane-associated protein called the *cystic fibrosis transmembrane regulator* (CFTR). The exact function of CFTR remains unknown, but it appears to help regulate chloride and sodium transport across epithelial membranes.

Causes of cystic fibrosis include abnormal coding found on as many as 350 CFTR alleles and autosomal recessive inheritance.

PATHOPHYSIOLOGY

Most cases of cystic fibrosis arise from a mutation that affects the genetic coding for a single amino acid, resulting in a protein (CFTR) that doesn't function properly. The CFTR resembles other transmembrane transport proteins, but lacks the phenylalanine in the protein produced by normal genes. This regulator interferes with cAMP-regulated chloride channels and transport of other ions by preventing adenosine triphosphate from binding to the protein or by interfering with activation by protein kinase.

The mutation affects volume-absorbing epithelia (in the airways and intestines), salt-absorbing epithelia (in sweat ducts), and volume-secretory epithelia (in the pancreas). Lack of phenylalanine leads to dehydration, increasing the viscosity of mucous-gland secretions, leading to obstruction of glandular ducts. Cystic fibrosis has a varying effect on electrolyte and water transport.

SIGNS AND SYMPTOMS

Respiratory symptoms may include thick secretions and dehydration due to ionic imbalance; chronic airway infections caused by *Staphylococcus aureus, Pseudomonas aeruginosa,* and *Pseudomonas cepacea,* possibly due to abnormal airway surface fluids and failure of lung defenses; and dyspnea from an accumulation of thick secretions in the bronchioles and alveoli.

Other respiratory signs include paroxysmal cough due to stimulation of the secretion-removal reflex; barrel chest, cyanosis, and clubbing of the fingers and toes from chronic hypoxia; crackles on auscultation due to thick, airway-occluding secretions; and wheezes heard on auscultation from constricted airways.

Retention of bicarbonate and water due to the absence of the CFTR chloride channel in the pancreatic ductile epithelia limits membrane function and leads to retention of pancreatic enzymes, chronic cholecystitis and cholelithiasis, and ultimate destruction of the pancreas.

Key signs and symptoms

- ✦ Thick secretions and dehydration
- ✦ Chronic airway infections
- ✦ Dyspnea
- ✦ Paroxysmal cough
- ✦ Barrel chest
- ✦ Cyanosis
- ✦ Clubbing of the fingers and toes
- ✦ Crackles and wheezes
- ✦ Retention of bicarbonate, water, and pancreatic enzymes
- ✦ Rectal prolapse in infants and children

Complications

- ✦ Obstructed glandular ducts
- ✦ Diabetes
- ✦ Pancreatitis
- ✦ Hepatic failure
- ✦ Malnutrition and malabsorption

Alert!

- ✦ The sweat test may be inaccurate in very young infants because they may not produce enough sweat for a valid test.

Diagnosis

- ✦ Sweat tests to detect elevated sodium chloride levels
- ✦ Presence of an obstructive pulmonary disease
- ✦ Confirmed pancreatic insufficiency or failure to thrive
- ✦ DNA testing

The GI effects of cystic fibrosis include obstruction of the small and large intestines because of the inhibited secretion of chloride and water and the excessive absorption of liquid, biliary cirrhosis from retention of biliary secretions, and esophageal varices due to cirrhosis and portal hypertension. Fatal shock and arrhythmias caused by hyponatremia and hypochloremia from sodium lost in sweat may result in death.

Poor weight gain, poor growth, distended abdomen, thin extremities, and sallow skin with poor turgor due to malabsorption result in failure to thrive. Clotting problems, retarded bone growth, and delayed sexual development are caused by a deficiency of fat-soluble vitamins. Rectal prolapse in infants and children results from malnutrition and wasting of perirectal supporting tissues.

COMPLICATIONS

One possible complication of cystic fibrosis is obstructed glandular ducts (leading to peribronchial thickening), which is caused by the increased viscosity of bronchial, pancreatic, and other mucous-gland secretions. Atelectasis or emphysema are due to respiratory effects of cystic fibrosis. Diabetes, pancreatitis, and hepatic failure result from effects on the intestines, pancreas, and liver.

Other complications include malnutrition and malabsorption of fat-soluble vitamins (A, D, E, and K), which are caused by deficiencies of trypsin, amylase, and lipase from obstructed pancreatic ducts, preventing the conversion and absorption of fat and protein in the intestinal tract.

In addition, lack of sperm in the semen (azoospermia) leaves many males infertile; secondary amenorrhea and increased mucus in the reproductive tract often blocks the passage of ova.

DIAGNOSIS

The Cystic Fibrosis Foundation has developed certain criteria for a definitive diagnosis. Two sweat tests detect elevated sodium chloride levels using a pilocarpine solution (a sweat inducer). The presence of an obstructive pulmonary disease, confirmed pancreatic insufficiency or failure to thrive, or a family history of cystic fibrosis must also be present.

 CLINICAL ALERT The sweat test may be inaccurate in very young infants because they may not produce enough sweat for a valid test. The test may need to be repeated.

Chest X-rays indicate early signs of obstructive lung disease. Stool specimen analysis indicates the absence of trypsin, suggesting pancreatic insufficiency.

Additional test results may support the diagnosis. DNA testing can locate the presence of the Delta F 508 deletion (found in about 70% of patients with cystic fibrosis, although the disease can cause more than 100 other mutations). It allows prenatal diagnosis in families with a previously affected child. Pulmonary function tests indicate decreased vital capacity, elevated residual volume due to air entrapments, and decreased forced expiratory volume in 1 second. This test is used if pulmonary exacerbation already exists. Liver enzyme tests may identify hepatic insufficiency. Sputum culture reveals organisms that cystic fibrosis patients typically and chronically colonize, such as *Staphylococcus* and *Pseudomonas.* Serum albumin measurement helps assess nutritional status and electrolyte analysis assesses hydration status.

TREATMENT

The aim of treatment is to help the child lead as normal a life as possible. The type of treatment depends on the organ system involved.

Hypertonic radiocontrast materials are delivered by enema to treat acute intestinal obstructions due to meconium ileus. Breathing exercises, postural drainage, and chest percussion clear pulmonary secretions. Antibiotics treat lung infection and are guided by sputum culture results.

Drugs are administered to increase mucus clearance. Inhaled beta-adrenergic agonists control airway constriction while pancreatic enzyme replacement maintains adequate nutrition. A sodium-channel blocker decreases sodium reabsorption from secretions and improves viscosity. Uridine triphosphate stimulates chloride secretion by a non-CFTR and salt supplements replace electrolytes lost through sweat. Dornase alfa (Pulmozyme), a genetically engineered pulmonary enzyme, helps liquefy mucus; recombinant alpha-antitrypsin counteracts excessive proteolytic activity produced during airway inflammation.

Gene therapy introduces normal CFTR into affected epithelial cells and the transplantation of the heart or lungs is performed in severe organ failure.

NURSING CONSIDERATIONS

✦ Throughout the illness, teach the patient and his family about the disease and its treatment. The Cystic Fibrosis Foundation can provide educational and support services.
✦ Although many males with cystic fibrosis are infertile, females with the illness may become pregnant (due to increased life expectancies). As a result, more cystic fibrosis patients are now facing difficult reproductive decisions. Refer such patients (or the parents of an affected child) for genetic counseling so they can discuss family planning issues or prenatal diagnosis options if they're considering having more children.
✦ Be aware that some patients have recently undergone lung transplants to reduce the effects of the disease. Also, clinical trials of aerosol gene therapy show promise in reducing pulmonary symptoms.
✦ Recent research indicates that the genetic defect responsible for cystic fibrosis has also been identified in individuals experiencing some forms of unexplained pancreatitis.

DOWN SYNDROME

Down syndrome, or *trisomy 21,* is a spontaneous chromosome abnormality that causes characteristic facial features, other distinctive physical abnormalities, and mental retardation; 60% of affected persons also have cardiac defects. It occurs in 1 of 650 to 700 live births. Improved treatment for heart defects, respiratory and other infections, and acute leukemia has significantly increased life expectancy. Fetal and neonatal mortality remain high, usually resulting from complications of associated heart defects.

CAUSES

Causes of Down syndrome include advanced parental age (when the mother is age 35 or older at delivery or the father is age 42 or older) and cumulative effects of environmental factors, such as radiation and viruses.

Treatment
✦ Hypertonic radiocontrast materials
✦ Breathing exercises
✦ Postural drainage
✦ Chest percussion
✦ Antibiotics and mucus clearance drugs
✦ Inhaled beta-adrenergic agonists
✦ Pancreatic enzyme replacement
✦ Sodium-channel blockers
✦ Transplantation of the heart or lungs

Key nursing actions
✦ Throughout the illness, teach the patient and his family about the disease and its treatment.
✦ Refer patients who become pregnant for genetic counseling.

Characteristics of Down syndrome
✦ A spontaneous chromosome abnormality
✦ Causes characteristic facial features, other distinctive physical abnormalities, and mental retardation
✦ 60% of affected persons also have cardiac defects
✦ Also called *trisomy 21*
✦ Improved treatment for physical defects has significantly increased life expectancy

Causes
✦ Advanced parental age
✦ Cumulative effects of environmental factors, such as radiation and viruses

How it happens

Alert!

Key signs and symptoms

Complications

Diagnosis

PATHOPHYSIOLOGY

Nearly all cases of Down syndrome result from trisomy 21 (three copies of chromosome 21). The result is a karyotype of 47 chromosomes instead of the usual 46. (See *Karyotype of Down syndrome.*) In 4% of patients, Down syndrome results from an unbalanced translocation or chromosomal rearrangement in which the long arm of chromosome 21 breaks off and attaches to another chromosome.

Some affected persons and some asymptomatic parents may have chromosomal mosaicism, a mixture of two cell types, some with the normal 46 and some with 47 (an extra chromosome 21).

SIGNS AND SYMPTOMS

CLINICAL ALERT The physical signs of Down syndrome are apparent at birth. The infant is lethargic and has distinctive craniofacial features.

Other signs and symptoms include distinctive facial features (low nasal bridge, epicanthic folds, protruding tongue, and low-set ears); small open mouth and disproportionately large tongue; single transverse crease on the palm (Simian crease); small white spots on the iris (Brushfield's spots); mental retardation (estimated IQ of 30 to 70); developmental delay due to hypotonia and decreased cognitive processing; congenital heart disease, mainly septal defects and especially of the endocardial cushion; and impaired reflexes due to decreased muscle tone in limbs.

COMPLICATIONS

Possible complications include early death due to cardiac defects; increased susceptibility to leukemia; premature senile dementia, usually in the 4th decade if the patient survives; increased susceptibility to acute and chronic infections; and strabismus and cataracts as the child grows. Females may menstruate and be fertile. Males may be infertile with low serum testosterone levels and often with undescended testes.

DIAGNOSIS

A karyotype showing the chromosomal abnormality confirms the diagnosis of Down syndrome. Other tests can reveal Down syndrome before birth. For example, prenatal ultrasonography can suggest Down syndrome if a duodenal obstruction or an atrioventricular canal defect is present. Reduced levels of alpha-fetoprotein (AFP) may indicate Down syndrome; a simple blood test for AFP is routinely offered to most pregnant women.

Amniocentesis also allows prenatal diagnosis; 80% of all amniocenteses are done for this purpose and are recommended for pregnant women older than age 35. Amniocentesis is also indicated for a pregnant woman of any age when either she or the father carries a translocated chromosome.

Additional medical tests confirm the presence of associated conditions. Developmental screening tests, such as the Denver Developmental Screening Test, determine the severity of retardation and chart the patient's progress in response to intervention or education programs.

TREATMENT

Surgery to correct cardiac defects and other related congenital abnormalities, antibiotic therapy for recurrent infections, and thyroid hormone replacement for hy-

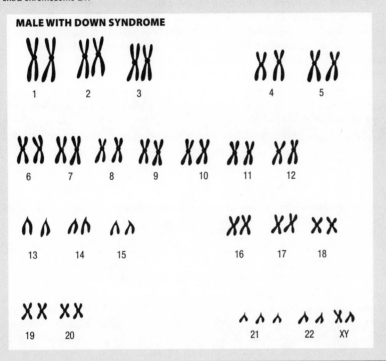

Karyotype of Down syndrome

Each autosome is normally one of a pair. A patient with Down syndrome, or trisomy 21, has an extra chromosome 21.

MALE WITH DOWN SYNDROME

pothyroidism have improved life expectancy considerably for patients with Down syndrome. Plastic surgery may correct the characteristic facial traits, especially the protruding tongue, cleft lip, and cleft palate. Benefits beyond improved appearance may include improved speech, reduced susceptibility to dental caries, and fewer orthodontic problems later in life.

When possible, parents of Down syndrome children are encouraged to keep their children at home rather than in an institution. Early intervention (such as infant stimulation programs) increases sensory awareness and has proved helpful with some patients. Special education programs, mandated in most communities, permit the child to maximize his potential and promote self-esteem. His physical condition and self-image can also benefit from special athletic programs. As adults, many Down syndrome patients become productive workers at jobs that match their intellectual abilities.

NURSING CONSIDERATIONS

Support for the parents of a child with Down syndrome is vital. By following the guidelines listed here, you can help them meet their child's physical and emotional needs.

✦ Establish a trusting relationship with the parents and encourage communication during the difficult period soon after diagnosis. Recognize signs of grieving.

Treatment

✦ Surgery to correct cardiac defects and other related congenital abnormalities
✦ Antibiotic therapy for recurrent infections
✦ Thyroid hormone replacement for hypothyroidism
✦ Plastic surgery
✦ Special education
✦ Special athletic programs

Key nursing actions

+ Encourage communication with parents during the difficult period soon after diagnosis.
+ Teach parents the importance of exercise and a balanced diet for the child.
+ Encourage the parents to hold and nurture their child.
+ Refer the parents to Down syndrome organizations.

Characteristics of hemophilia

+ X-linked recessive bleeding in 20 of 100,000 male births
+ Severity and prognosis vary
+ Results from a deficiency of specific clotting factors

Causes

+ Defect in a specific gene on the X chromosome that codes for factor VIII synthesis (hemophilia A)
+ One of more than 300 different base-pair substitutions involving the factor IX gene on the X chromosome (hemophilia B)

How it happens

+ Deficiency or nonfunction of factor VIII causes hemophilia A; deficiency or nonfunction of factor IX causes hemophilia B
+ Platelet plug forms, but clotting factor deficiency impairs formation of a stable fibrin clot

---

✦ Teach parents the importance of a balanced diet for the child. Stress the need for patience while feeding the infant, who may have difficulty sucking and may be less demanding and seem less eager to eat than other infants.

✦ Encourage the parents to hold and nurture their child.

✦ Emphasize the importance of adequate exercise and maximal environmental stimulation; refer the parents for infant stimulation classes, which may begin in the early months of life.

✦ Help the parents set realistic goals for their child. Explain that, although the child's mental development may seem normal at first, they shouldn't view this early development as a sign of future progress. By the time he's age 1, the child's development may begin to lag behind that of other children.

✦ Refer the parents and older siblings for genetic and psychological counseling, as appropriate, to help them evaluate future reproductive risks. Discuss options for prenatal testing.

✦ Encourage the parents to remember the emotional needs of the other children in the family.

✦ Refer the parents to national or local Down syndrome organizations and support groups.

HEMOPHILIA

Hemophilia is an X-linked recessive bleeding disorder; the severity and prognosis of bleeding vary with the degree of deficiency, or nonfunction, and the site of bleeding. Hemophilia occurs in 20 of 100,000 male births and results from a deficiency of specific clotting factors.

Hemophilia A, or classic hemophilia, is a deficiency of clotting factor VIII; it's more common than type B, affecting more than 80% of all hemophiliacs. Hemophilia B, or Christmas disease, affects 15% of all hemophiliacs and results from a deficiency of factor IX. There's no relationship between factor VIII and factor IX inherited defects.

CAUSES

Causes of hemophilia may include a defect in a specific gene on the X chromosome that codes for factor VIII synthesis (hemophilia A) or more than 300 different base-pair substitutions involving the factor IX gene on the X chromosome (hemophilia B).

PATHOPHYSIOLOGY

Hemophilia is an X-linked recessive genetic disease that causes abnormal bleeding because of a specific clotting factor malfunction. Factors VIII and IX are components of the intrinsic clotting pathway; factor IX is an essential factor and factor VIII is a critical cofactor. Factor VIII accelerates the activation of factor X by several thousandfold. Excessive bleeding occurs when these clotting factors are reduced by more than 75%. A deficiency or nonfunction of factor VIII causes hemophilia A; a deficiency or nonfunction of factor IX causes hemophilia B.

Hemophilia may be severe, moderate, or mild, depending on the degree of activation of clotting factors. Patients with severe disease have no detectable factor VIII or factor IX activity or less than 1% of normal. Moderately afflicted patients have 1% to 4% of normal clotting activity, and mildly afflicted patients have 5% to 25% of normal clotting activity.

A person with hemophilia forms a platelet plug at a bleeding site, but clotting factor deficiency impairs the ability to form a stable fibrin clot. Delayed bleeding is more common than immediate hemorrhage.

SIGNS AND SYMPTOMS

Hemophilia produces abnormal bleeding, which may be mild, moderate, or severe, depending on the degree of factor deficiency.

Mild hemophilia commonly goes undiagnosed until adulthood because the patient doesn't bleed spontaneously or after minor trauma but has prolonged bleeding if challenged by major surgery or trauma. Postoperative bleeding continues as a slow ooze, or ceases and starts up again, up to 8 days after surgery.

Moderate hemophilia causes symptoms similar to severe hemophilia but produces only occasional spontaneous bleeding episodes.

Severe hemophilia causes spontaneous bleeding. In many cases, the first sign of severe hemophilia is excessive bleeding after circumcision. Later, spontaneous bleeding or severe bleeding after minor trauma may produce large subcutaneous and deep intramuscular hematomas. Bleeding into joints and muscles causes pain, swelling, extreme tenderness and, possibly, permanent deformity.

COMPLICATIONS

Complications may include peripheral neuropathy, pain, paresthesia, and muscle atrophy due to bleeding near peripheral nerves; ischemia and gangrene due to impaired blood flow through a major vessel distal to the bleeding site; and decreased tissue perfusion and hypovolemic shock (exhibited as restlessness, anxiety, confusion, pallor, cool and clammy skin, chest pain, decreased urine output, hypotension, and tachycardia).

DIAGNOSIS

Development of a large cephalohematoma or intracranial hemorrhage after prolonged labor or delivery by forceps or vacuum extraction may be the first indication of a bleeding problem. After the neonatal period, a history of prolonged bleeding after surgery (including dental extractions) or trauma or episodes of spontaneous bleeding into muscles or joints usually indicates some defect in the hemostatic mechanism.

Hemophilia A and B may be clinically indistinguishable, but specific coagulation factor assays can diagnose the type and severity of the disease. A positive family history, prenatal diagnosis, and carrier testing can also help diagnose hemophilia; however, nearly one-third of all patients have no family history.

Characteristic findings in hemophilia A include factor VIII-C assay of 0% to 30% of normal and a prolonged partial thromboplastin time (PTT). Patients have a normal platelet count and function, bleeding time, and prothrombin time.

Characteristics of hemophilia B include a deficient factor IX-C and baseline coagulation results similar to hemophilia A, except for a normal factor VIII level.

TREATMENT

Hemophilia isn't curable, but treatment can prevent crippling deformities and prolong life expectancy. Treatment of hemophilia includes cryoprecipitate (for hemophilia A) or lyophilized factor VIII or IX to increase clotting factor levels and to permit normal hemostasis levels.

Treatment

+ Cryoprecipitate; lyophilized factor VIII or IX
+ Factor IX concentrate during bleeding
+ Aminocaproic acid for oral bleeding
+ DDAVP before dental procedures or minor surgery

Alert!

+ To help prevent injury, young children should wear padding on knees and elbows.

Key nursing actions

During bleeding episodes

+ Give clotting agents, as ordered. Repeat infusions as ordered until bleeding stops.
+ Restrict activity for 48 hours after bleeding is under control.
+ Control pain with an analgesic.

If the patient has bled into a joint

+ Immediately elevate the joint.
+ Begin ROM exercises, if ordered.

After bleeding episodes and surgery

+ Watch closely for signs of further bleeding and monitor PTT.
+ Refer new patients to hemophilia treatment centers for evaluation.

Characteristics of Marfan syndrome

+ Rare degenerative, generalized disease of the connective tissue
+ Results from elastin and collagen defects and causes ocular, skeletal, and cardiovascular anomalies

In hemophilia B, administration of factor IX concentrate during bleeding episodes increases factor IX levels. Aminocaproic acid (Amicar) administered for oral bleeding inhibits plasminogen activator substances.

Prophylactic desmopressin (DDAVP) administered before dental procedures or minor surgery releases stored von Willebrand's factor and factor VIII to reduce bleeding.

 CLINICAL ALERT To help prevent injury, young children should wear clothing with padded patches on the knees and elbows. Older children should avoid contact sports.

NURSING CONSIDERATIONS

During bleeding episodes

+ Give clotting agents, as ordered. The body uses up antihemophilic factor in 48 to 72 hours, so repeat infusions as ordered until bleeding stops.
+ Apply cold compresses or ice bags and raise the injured part.
+ To prevent recurrence of bleeding, restrict activity for 48 hours after bleeding is under control.
+ Control pain with an analgesic, such as acetaminophen, propoxyphene, codeine, or meperidine, as ordered. Avoid I.M. injections because of possible hematoma formation at the injection site. Aspirin and aspirin-containing medications are contraindicated because they decrease platelet adherence and may increase the bleeding. Caution should be used when trying other nonsteroidal anti-inflammatory drugs—for example, ibuprofen or ketoprofen.

If the patient has bled into a joint

+ Immediately elevate the joint.
+ To restore joint mobility, begin range-of-motion exercises, if ordered, at least 48 hours after the bleeding is controlled. Tell the patient to avoid weight bearing until bleeding stops and swelling subsides.

After bleeding episodes and surgery

+ Watch closely for signs of further bleeding, such as increased pain and swelling, fever, or symptoms of shock.
+ Closely monitor PTT.
+ Teach the parents special precautions to prevent bleeding episodes.
+ Refer a new patient to a hemophilia treatment center for evaluation. The center will devise a treatment plan for the patient's primary physician and is a resource for other medical and school personnel, dentist, and others involved in care.
+ Persons who have been exposed to human immunodeficiency virus through contaminated blood products need special support.
+ Refer patients and carriers for genetic counseling.

MARFAN SYNDROME

Marfan syndrome is a rare degenerative, generalized disease of the connective tissue. It results from elastin and collagen defects and causes ocular, skeletal, and cardiovascular anomalies. Death occurs from cardiovascular complications from early infancy to adulthood. The syndrome occurs in 1 of 20,000 individuals, affecting males and females equally.

CAUSES

Causes of Marfan syndrome in patients with a negative family history (15% of all patients) may include autosomal dominant mutation and, possibly, advanced paternal age.

PATHOPHYSIOLOGY

Marfan syndrome is caused by a mutation in a single allele of a gene located on chromosome 15; the gene codes for fibrillin, a glycoprotein component of connective tissue. These small fibers are abundant in large blood vessels and the suspensory ligaments of the ocular lenses. The effect on connective tissue is varied and includes excessive bone growth, ocular disorders, and cardiac defects.

SIGNS AND SYMPTOMS

The most common signs and symptoms of Marfan syndrome are skeletal abnormalities, particularly excessively long tubular bones and an arm span that exceeds the patient's height. The patient is usually taller than average for his family (in the 95th percentile for his age), with the upper half of his body shorter than average and the lower half, longer. His fingers are long and slender (arachnodactyly). Weakness of ligaments, tendons, and joint capsules results in joints that are loose, hyperextensible, and habitually dislocated. Excessive growth of the rib bones gives rise to chest deformities such as pectus excavatum (funnel chest).

Eye problems are also common; 75% of patients have crystalline lens displacement (ectopia lentis), the ocular hallmark of Marfan syndrome. Quivering of the iris with eye movement (iridodonesis) typically suggests this disorder. Most patients are severely myopic, many have retinal detachment, and some have glaucoma.

The most serious complications occur in the cardiovascular system and include weakness of the aortic media, which leads to progressive dilation or dissecting aneurysm of the ascending aorta. Such dilation appears first in the coronary sinuses and is often preceded by aortic insufficiency. Less-common cardiovascular complications include mitral valve prolapse and endocarditis.

COMPLICATIONS

Possible complications include weak joints and ligaments, predisposing to injury; cataracts due to lens displacement; retinal detachments and retinal tears; severe mitral valve insufficiency due to mitral valve prolapse; spontaneous pneumothorax due to chest wall instability; inguinal and incisional hernias; and dilation of the dural sac (portion of the dura mater beyond caudal end of the spinal cord).

DIAGNOSIS

Because no specific test confirms Marfan syndrome, diagnosis is based on a positive family history in one parent (85% of patients) and typical clinical features. These features include the presence of lens displacement and aneurysm of the ascending aorta without other symptoms or familial tendency.

Useful supplementary procedures, although not definitive, include X-rays confirming skeletal abnormalities, echocardiogram showing dilation of the aortic root, and DNA analysis.

Causes
+ Autosomal dominant mutation
+ Advanced paternal age

How it happens
+ Mutation in a single allele of a gene on chromosome 15
+ Effect on connective tissue varies; includes excessive bone growth and ocular disorders

Key signs and symptoms
+ Long tubular bones and an arm span exceeding the patient's height
+ Upper half of body shorter than average and lower half longer
+ Fingers are long and slender
+ Loose and dislocated joints
+ Severe myopia, retinal detachment, and glaucoma
+ Weakness of the aortic media

Complications
+ Weak joints and ligaments
+ Cataracts and retinal detachments
+ Severe mitral valve insufficiency
+ Spontaneous pneumothorax
+ Inguinal and incisional hernias
+ Dilation of the dural sac

Diagnosis
+ Positive family history in one parent and typical clinical features
+ Presence of lens displacement
+ X-rays confirming skeletal abnormalities

Treatment

+ Relief of symptoms
+ Surgical repair of aneurysms and ocular deformities
+ Steroid and sex hormone therapy
+ Surgical replacement of the aortic and mitral valves
+ Mechanical bracing

Key nursing actions

+ High school and college athletes who fit the criteria should undergo a careful clinical and cardiac examination before being allowed to play.
+ Provide supportive care.
+ Educate the patient and his family about the course of the disease and its potential complications.
+ Stress the need for frequent checkups to detect and treat degenerative changes early.

Characteristics of NTDs

+ Serious birth defects that involve the spine or skull
+ Result from failure of the neural tube to close at approximately 28 days after conception
+ Common forms are spina bifida, anencephaly, and encephalocele

Causes

+ Exposure to a teratogen
+ Isolated birth defects
+ Combination of genetic and environmental factors

TREATMENT

Treatment for Marfan syndrome is aimed at relieving symptoms. It may involve surgical repair of aneurysms to prevent rupture, surgical correction of ocular deformities to improve vision, and steroid and sex hormone therapy to induce early epiphyseal closure and limit adult height. In young patients, prompt treatment with beta-adrenergic blockers may delay or prevent aortic dilation.

Extreme dilation of the aorta requires surgical replacement of the aortic and mitral valves. Mechanical bracing and physical therapy are prescribed for mild scoliosis if the curvature is greater than 20 degrees; surgery is performed if the curvature is greater than 45 degrees.

NURSING CONSIDERATIONS

+ High school and college athletes (particularly basketball players) who fit the criteria for Marfan syndrome should undergo a careful clinical and cardiac examination before being allowed to play to reduce the risk of sudden death from a dissecting aortic aneurysm or other cardiac complications.
+ Provide the patient with supportive care, as appropriate for his clinical status.
+ Educate the patient and his family about the course of the disease and its potential complications.
+ Stress the need for frequent checkups to detect and treat degenerative changes early.
+ Emphasize the importance of taking prescribed medications as ordered and avoiding contact sports and isometric exercise.
+ If recommended by the physician, encourage hormonal therapy to induce early epiphyseal closure, thus preventing abnormal adult height.
+ To encourage normal adolescent development, advise the parents to avoid unrealistic expectations for their child simply because he's tall and looks older than his years.
+ Refer the patient and his family to the National Marfan Foundation for additional information.

NEURAL TUBE DEFECTS

Neural tube defects (NTDs) are serious birth defects that involve the spine or skull; they result from failure of the neural tube to close at approximately 28 days after conception. The most common forms of NTD are spina bifida (50% of cases), anencephaly (40%), and encephalocele (10%). Spina bifida occulta is the most common and least severe spinal cord defect.

The incidence of NTDs varies greatly among countries and by region in the United States. For example, the incidence is significantly higher in the British Isles and low in southern China and Japan. In the United States, North and South Carolina have at least twice the incidence of NTDs as most other parts of the country. These birth defects are also less common in Blacks than in Whites.

CAUSES

Causes of NTDs may include exposure to a teratogen, part of a multiple malformation syndrome (for example, chromosomal abnormalities such as trisomy 18 or 13 syndrome) or, in isolated birth defects, a combination of genetic and environmental factors (mostly unknown, although possibly a lack of folic acid in the mother's diet).

PATHOPHYSIOLOGY

Neural tube closure normally occurs at 24 days' gestation in the cranial region and continues distally, with closure of the lumbar regions by 28 days. Spina bifida occulta is characterized by incomplete closure of one or more vertebrae without protrusion of the spinal cord or meninges.

In more severe forms of spina bifida, however, incomplete closure of one or more vertebrae causes protrusion of the spinal contents in an external sac or cystic lesion (spina bifida cystica). Spina bifida cystica has two classifications: myelomeningocele (meningomyelocele) and meningocele. In myelomeningocele, the external sac contains meninges, cerebrospinal fluid (CSF), and a portion of the spinal cord or nerve roots distal to the conus medullaris. When the spinal nerve roots end at the sac, motor and sensory functions below the sac are terminated. In meningocele, less severe than myelomeningocele, the sac contains only meninges and CSF. Meningocele may produce no neurologic symptoms.

In encephalocele, a saclike portion of the meninges and brain protrudes through a defective opening in the skull. Typically, it occurs in the occipital area, but it may also occur in the parietal, nasopharyngeal, or frontal area.

In anencephaly, the most severe form of NTD, the closure defect occurs at the cranial end of the neuroaxis and, as a result, the entire top of the skull or part of it is missing, severely damaging the brain. Portions of the brain stem and spinal cord may also be missing. No diagnostic or therapeutic efforts are helpful; this condition is invariably fatal.

SIGNS AND SYMPTOMS

Signs and symptoms depend on the type and severity of the NTD. Spina bifida occulta is often accompanied by a depression or dimple, tuft of hair, soft fatty deposits, port wine nevi, or a combination of these abnormalities on the skin over the spinal defect.

Spina bifida occulta doesn't usually cause neurologic dysfunction but occasionally is associated with foot weakness or bowel and bladder disturbances, especially likely during rapid growth phases. In both myelomeningocele and meningocele, a saclike structure protrudes over the spine.

Depending on the level of the defect, myelomeningocele causes permanent neurologic dysfunction, such as flaccid or spastic paralysis and bowel and bladder incontinence.

Associated disorders include trophic skin disturbances (ulcerations, cyanosis), clubfoot, knee contractures, hydrocephalus (in about 90% of patients), mental retardation, Arnold-Chiari syndrome (part of the brain protrudes into the spinal canal), and curvature of the spine.

Clinical effects of encephalocele vary with the degree of tissue involvement and location of the defect. Paralysis and hydrocephalus are common. Infants with this defect have a better chance of survival than anencephalic infants and usually suffer less paralysis; however, surviving infants are usually severely mentally retarded.

COMPLICATIONS

Complications may include paralysis below the level of the defect and infection such as meningitis.

How it happens

Spina bifida
- Incomplete closure of one or more vertebrae without protrusion of the spinal cord or meninges
- Myelomeningocele: the external sac contains meninges, CSF, and a portion of the spinal cord or nerve roots distal to the conus medullaris
- Meningocele: the sac contains only meninges and CSF

Encephalocele
- Saclike portion of the meninges and brain protrudes through a defective opening in the skull.
- Occurs in the occipital, parietal, nasopharyngeal, or frontal area

Anencephaly
- Closure defect occurs at the cranial end of the neuroaxis
- This condition is invariably fatal

Key signs and symptoms

- Depression or dimple, tuft of hair, soft fatty deposits, or port wine nevi on the skin on spinal defect
- Curvature of the spine
- Encephalocele
- Paralysis
- Hydrocephalus

Complications

- Paralysis below the level of the defect
- Infection

Diagnosis

Prenatal

+ Amniocentesis to detect elevated AFP levels in amniotic fluid
+ Measuring acetylcholinesterase levels
+ Fetal karyotype
+ Biochemical tests to detect chromosomal abnormalities
+ Maternal serum AFP screening

Neonatal

+ Palpation and spinal X-ray
+ Myelography
+ Pinprick examination of the legs and trunk
+ Skull X-rays
+ Cephalic measurements
+ Urine cultures

Treatment

Spina bifida occulta

+ Surgery doesn't reverse neurologic deficits and serious and permanent handicaps are likely
+ Fetal surgery to repair some open defects

Meningocele

+ Surgical closure of the protruding sac
+ Continual assessment of growth and development

Myelomeningocele

+ Repair of the sac and supportive measures to promote independence
+ Shunt to relieve associated hydrocephalus

Encephalocele

+ Surgery during infancy to place protruding tissues back in the skull, excise the sac, and correct associated craniofacial abnormalities

DIAGNOSIS

Amniocentesis can detect elevated AFP levels in amniotic fluid, which indicates the presence of an open NTD. Measuring acetylcholinesterase levels (not usually effective for closed NTDs) can confirm the diagnosis. Fetal karyotype should be performed in addition to biochemical tests to detect chromosomal abnormalities (present in 5% to 7% of NTDs).

Ultrasound may be used when the fetus has increased risk of open NTD, based on family history or abnormal serum screening results (not conclusive for open NTDs or ventral wall defects).

If the NTD isn't diagnosed before birth, other tests are used to make the diagnosis. Palpation and spinal X-ray can show the bone defect for spina bifida occulta. Myelography can differentiate spina bifida occulta from other spinal abnormalities, especially spinal cord tumors. Transillumination of the protruding sac can sometimes distinguish between myelomeningocele (typically doesn't transilluminate) and meningocele (typically does transilluminate). A pinprick examination of the legs and trunk shows the level of sensory and motor involvement in myelomeningocele. Skull X-rays, cephalic measurements, and computed tomography (CT) scan demonstrate associated hydrocephalus.

Appropriate laboratory tests in patients with myelomeningocele include urinalysis, urine cultures, and tests for renal function starting in the neonatal period and continuing at regular intervals. Additionally, encephalocele can be used; X-rays show a basilar bony skull defect. CT scan and ultrasonography further define the defect.

TREATMENT

Spina bifida occulta usually requires no treatment. Prompt neurosurgical repair and aggressive management may improve the condition of children with some NTDs. However, surgery doesn't reverse neurologic deficits and serious and permanent handicaps are likely. Fetal surgery has been successful at repairing some open defects, thereby reducing damage.

Treatment of meningocele consists of surgical closure of the protruding sac and continual assessment of growth and development. Treatment of myelomeningocele requires repair of the sac and supportive measures to promote independence and prevent further complications. A shunt may be needed to relieve associated hydrocephalus. Treatment of encephalocele includes surgery during infancy to place protruding tissues back in the skull, excise the sac, and correct associated craniofacial abnormalities.

NURSING CONSIDERATIONS

+ When an NTD has been diagnosed prenatally, refer the prospective parents to a genetic counselor, who can provide information and support the couple's decisions on how to manage the pregnancy.
+ Recent research sponsored by the March of Dimes and others has indicated that the risk of an open NTD may be reduced 50% to 70% in pregnant women who take a daily multivitamin with folic acid. Urge all women of childbearing age to take such a vitamin supplement until menopause or the end of childbearing potential. (See *Folic acid supplement recommendations.*)
+ The parents of a child with an NTD will need assistance from physicians, nurses, surgeons, rehabilitation providers, and social workers. Help to coordinate such assistance as needed. Obviously, care is most complex when the neurologic deficit is

Folic acid supplement recommendations

These recommendations for folic acid supplement dosages have been endorsed by the Centers for Disease Control and Prevention, the U.S. Public Health Service, the March of Dimes Birth Defects Foundation, and the Spina Bifida Association of America, among other groups.

ALL WOMEN OF CHILDBEARING AGE
All women who are capable of becoming pregnant should:
+ consume 0.4 mg of folic acid daily to reduce their risk of having a child with spina bifida or another neural tube defect (NTD)
+ continue to consume 0.4 mg of folic acid daily when pregnant until their health care provider prescribes other prenatal vitamins.

WOMEN AT HIGH RISK
Women with a previous pregnancy affected by an NTD should:
+ receive genetic counseling before their next pregnancy
+ consume 0.4 mg of folic acid daily
+ when actively trying to become pregnant (at least 1 month before conception), increase their dosage of folic acid to 4 mg daily (by taking a separate folic acid supplement, not by increasing their intake of multivitamins)
+ continue to take 4 mg of folic acid daily through the first 3 months of pregnancy.

severe. Immediate goals include psychological support to help the parents accept the diagnosis and preoperative and postoperative care. Long-term goals include patient and family teaching and measures to prevent contractures, pressure ulcers, urinary tract infections (UTIs), and other complications.

Before surgery
+ Prevent local infection by cleaning the defect gently with sterile saline solution or other solutions as ordered. Inspect the defect often for signs of infection and cover it with sterile dressings moistened with sterile saline solution. Prevent skin breakdown by placing sheepskin or a foam pad under the infant. Keep the infant's skin clean and apply lotion to his knees, elbows, chin, and other pressure areas. Give antibiotics as ordered.
+ Handle the infant carefully, and don't apply pressure to the defect. Typically, the infant can't wear a diaper or a shirt until after surgical correction because it will irritate the sac, so keep him warm in an infant Isolette. Hold and cuddle the infant. Place him on his abdomen on your lap; teach his parents to do the same.
+ Provide adequate time for parent-child bonding, if possible.
+ Measure the infant's head circumference daily and watch for signs of hydrocephalus and meningeal irritation, such as fever or nuchal rigidity. Be sure to mark the spot so you get accurate readings.
+ Contractures can be minimized by passive range-of-motion exercises and casting. To prevent hip dislocation, moderately abduct hips with a pad between the knees or with sandbags and ankle rolls.
+ Monitor intake and output. Watch for decreased skin turgor, dryness, or other signs of dehydration. Provide meticulous skin care to genitals and buttocks to prevent infection.
+ Ensure adequate nutrition.

Folic acid supplements
+ Women of childbearing age should take 0.4 mg of folic acid daily when pregnant
+ Women at high risk should consume 0.4 mg of folic acid daily and 4 mg of folic acid daily during the first three months of pregnancy

Key nursing actions

Before surgery
+ Inspect defect for signs of infection; cover it with sterile dressings moistened with sterile saline solution.
+ Prevent skin breakdown.
+ Keep the infant's skin clean and apply lotion to knees, elbows, chin, and other pressure areas.
+ Provide adequate time for parent-child bonding, if possible.
+ Measure the infant's head circumference daily.
+ Contractures can be minimized by passive ROM exercises and casting.
+ Ensure adequate nutrition.

Key nursing actions

After surgery

+ Watch for hydrocephalus, which often follows surgery.
+ Monitor vital signs often and check for bulging fontanels (the most telling sign of infant increased ICP).
+ Place infant prone to protect and assess the site.
+ Emphasize to the parents the need for increased fluid intake to prevent UTIs.
+ Stress the need for a high-bulk diet, exercise, and a stool softener as ordered.
+ Refer the parents to the Spina Bifida Association of America.

Characteristics of sickle cell anemia

+ A congenital hemolytic anemia resulting from defective hemoglobin molecules
+ One-half of the patients with sickle cell anemia die by their early 20s
+ Occurs primarily in persons of African and Mediterranean descent

Causes

+ Homozygous inheritance of gene that produces hemoglobin S
+ Heterozygous inheritance of this gene results in sickle cell trait, generally asymptomatic

After surgery

+ Watch for hydrocephalus, which often follows surgery. Measure the infant's head circumference as ordered.
+ Monitor vital signs often. Watch for signs of shock, infection, and increased intracranial pressure (ICP), such as projectile vomiting. Frequently assess the infant's fontanels. Remember that before age 2, infants don't show typical signs of increased ICP because suture lines aren't fully closed. In infants, the most telling sign is bulging fontanels.
+ Change the dressing regularly as ordered, and check and report signs of drainage, wound rupture, and infection.
+ Place the infant in the prone position to protect and assess the site.
+ If leg casts have been applied to treat deformities, watch for signs that the child is outgrowing the casts. Regularly check distal pulses to ensure adequate circulation.

To help the parents cope with their infant's physical problems and successfully meet long-term treatment goals:

+ Teach them to recognize early signs of complications, such as hydrocephalus, decubitus ulcers, and UTIs.
+ Provide psychological support and encourage a positive attitude. Help the parents work through their feelings of guilt, anger, and helplessness.
+ Encourage the parents to begin training their child in a bladder routine by age 3. Emphasize the need for increased fluid intake to prevent UTIs. Teach intermittent catheterization and conduit hygiene as ordered.
+ To prevent constipation and bowel obstruction, stress the need for increased fluid intake, a high-bulk diet, exercise, and a stool softener as ordered. If possible, teach the parents to help empty their child's bowel by telling him to bear down, and giving a glycerin suppository as needed.
+ Urge early recognition of developmental lags (a possible result of hydrocephalus). If present, stress the importance of follow-up IQ assessment to help plan realistic educational goals. The child may need to attend a school with special facilities. Also stress the need for stimulation to ensure maximum mental development. Help the parents plan activities appropriate to their child's age and abilities.
+ Refer the parents for genetic counseling and suggest that amniocentesis be performed in future pregnancies. Also refer the parents to the Spina Bifida Association of America.

SICKLE CELL ANEMIA

Sickle cell anemia is a congenital hemolytic anemia resulting from defective hemoglobin molecules. One-half of the patients with sickle cell anemia die by their early 20s; few live to middle age.

Sickle cell anemia occurs primarily in persons of African and Mediterranean descent, but it also affects populations in Puerto Rico, Turkey, India, and the Middle East.

CAUSE

Sickle cell anemia results from homozygous inheritance of the gene that produces hemoglobin S. Heterozygous inheritance of this gene results in sickle cell trait, generally an asymptomatic condition.

PATHOPHYSIOLOGY

Sickle cell anemia results from substitution of the amino acid valine for glutamic acid in the hemoglobin S gene encoding the beta chain of hemoglobin. Abnormal hemoglobin S, found in the red blood cells (RBCs) of patients, becomes insoluble during hypoxia. As a result, these cells become rigid, rough, and elongated, forming a crescent or sickle shape. (See *Characteristics of sickled cells,* page 140.) The sickling produces hemolysis. The altered cells also pile up in the capillaries and smaller blood vessels, making the blood more viscous. Normal circulation is impaired, causing pain, tissue infarctions, and swelling.

Each patient with sickle cell anemia has a different hypoxic threshold and different factors that trigger a sickle cell crisis. Illness, exposure to cold, stress, acidotic states, or a pathophysiologic process that pulls water out of the sickle cells precipitates a crisis in most patients. (See *Sickle cell crisis,* page 141.) The blockages then cause anoxic changes that lead to further sickling and obstruction.

SIGNS AND SYMPTOMS

 CLINICAL ALERT **Symptoms of sickle cell anemia don't develop until after age 6 months because fetal hemoglobin protects infants for the first few months after birth.**

Signs and symptoms may include tachycardia, cardiomegaly, chronic fatigue, unexplained dyspnea, hepatomegaly, joint swelling, aching bones, or chest pain. Severe pain in the abdomen, thorax, muscle, or bones characterizes a painful crisis (vasoocclusive crisis). Symptoms include jaundice, dark urine, and low-grade fever due to blood vessel obstruction by rigid, tangled, sickled cells leads to tissue anoxia and possibly necrosis. An increased susceptibility to *Streptococcus pneumoniae* sepsis due to autosplenectomy (splenic damage and scarring in patients with long-term disease) can be fatal without prompt treatment.

Suspect crisis in a patient with sickle cell anemia who exhibits pale lips, tongue, palms, or nail beds; lethargy; listlessness; sleepiness; irritability; severe pain; and fever. An aplastic (megaloblastic) crisis results from bone marrow depression and is associated with infection (usually viral) and is characterized by pallor, lethargy, sleepiness, dyspnea, possible coma, markedly decreased bone marrow activity, and RBC hemolysis.

In infants ages 8 months to 2 years, an acute sequestration crisis may cause lethargy, pallor, and hypovolemic shock due to the sudden massive entrapment of cells in the spleen and liver. A hemolytic crisis is quite rare and usually affects patients who also have glucose-6-phosphate dehydrogenase deficiency. Degenerative changes cause liver congestion and enlargement and chronic jaundice worsens.

COMPLICATIONS

Complications may include retinopathy, nephropathy, and cerebral vessel occlusion due to organ infarction; hypovolemic shock and death due to massive entrapment of cells, necrosis; infection; and gangrene.

How it happens

◆ Substitution of the amino acid valine for glutamic acid in the hemoglobin S gene encoding the beta chain of hemoglobin
◆ Abnormal hemoglobin S becomes insoluble during hypoxia.
◆ Cells become rigid and elongated
◆ Altered cells pile up in the capillaries and smaller blood vessels
◆ Triggers of a sickle cell crisis include illness, exposure to cold, stress, and acidotic states

Alert!

◆ Symptoms don't develop until after age 6 months.

Key signs and symptoms

◆ Tachycardia
◆ Cardiomegaly
◆ Chronic fatigue
◆ Joint swelling
◆ Jaundice
◆ Low-grade fever

Complications

◆ Retinopathy
◆ Nephropathy
◆ Cerebral vessel occlusion

Sickled cells

✦ 30- to 40-day life span
✦ Hb has decreased oxygen-carrying capacity
✦ 6 to 9 g/ml of Hb
✦ RBCs destroyed at accelerated rate

Diagnosis

✦ Positive family history and typical clinical features
✦ Hemoglobin electrophoresis showing hemoglobin S
✦ Stained blood smear shows sickle cells
✦ A lateral chest X-ray shows "Lincoln log" deformity in the vertebrae

Treatment

✦ Begins before age 4 months with prophylactic penicillin
✦ Hospitalization for a transfusion of packed RBCs if hemoglobin drops suddenly
✦ In a sequestration crisis: sedation, blood transfusion, and oxygen administration

Alert!

✦ Vaccines to prevent illness and anti-infectives should be considered to prevent complications in patients with sickle cell anemia.

Characteristics of sickled cells

Normal red blood cells (RBCs) and sickled cells vary in shape, life span, oxygen-carrying capacity, and the rate at which they're destroyed. These illustrations show normal and sickled cells; major differences between them are also listed.

NORMAL RBCs
✦ 120-day life span
✦ Hemoglobin (Hb) has normal oxygen-carrying capacity
✦ 12 to 14 g/ml of Hb
✦ RBCs destroyed at normal rate

SICKLED CELLS
✦ 30- to 40-day life span
✦ Hb has decreased oxygen-carrying capacity
✦ 6 to 9 g/ml of Hb
✦ RBCs destroyed at accelerated rate

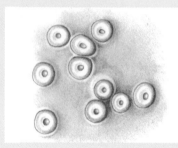
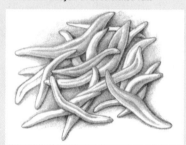

DIAGNOSIS

A positive family history and typical clinical features suggest sickle cell anemia. Hemoglobin electrophoresis showing hemoglobin S can also confirm it. Electrophoresis should be performed on umbilical cord blood to provide screening for all neonates at risk. A stained blood smear shows sickle cells. Additional laboratory studies may show low RBC counts, elevated white blood cell and platelet counts, decreased erythrocyte sedimentation rate, increased serum iron levels, decreased RBC survival, and reticulocytosis. Hemoglobin levels may be low or normal.

A lateral chest X-ray shows "Lincoln log" deformity in the vertebrae of many adults and some adolescents with sickle cell anemia. Some states mandate neonatal screening for hemoglobin abnormalities, including sickle cell anemia. Prenatal and preimplantation diagnosis is available, especially if the mutation in the family is known.

TREATMENT

Treatment begins before age 4 months with prophylactic penicillin. If the patient's hemoglobin drops suddenly or if his condition deteriorates rapidly, he'll need to be hospitalized for a transfusion of packed RBCs. In a sequestration crisis, treatment may include sedation, analgesics administration, blood transfusions, oxygen administration, and large amounts of oral and intravenous fluids.

A good antisickling agent isn't yet available; the most commonly used drug, sodium cyanate, has many adverse effects. Additional drugs administered include hydroxyurea to reduce painful episodes by increasing the production of fetal hemoglobin, which seems to alleviate symptoms, as well as iron and folic acid supplements to prevent anemia.

 CLINICAL ALERT Vaccines to prevent illness and anti-infectives, such as low-dose penicillin, should be considered to prevent complications in patients with sickle cell anemia.

Sickle cell crisis

Infection, exposure to cold, high altitudes, overexertion, or other situations that cause cellular oxygen deprivation may trigger a sickle cell crisis. The deoxygenated, sickle-shaped red blood cells stick to the capillary wall and each other, blocking blood flow and causing cellular hypoxia. The crisis worsens as tissue hypoxia and acidic waste products cause more sickling and cell damage. With each new crisis, organs and tissues are slowly destroyed, especially the spleen and kidneys.

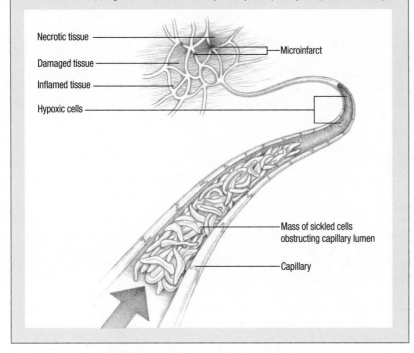

NURSING CONSIDERATIONS

Supportive measures during crises and precautions to avoid them are important.
✦ Apply warm compresses to painful areas, and cover the child with a blanket. (Never use cold compresses because they aggravate the condition.)
✦ Administer an analgesic-antipyretic, such as aspirin or acetaminophen. (Additional pain relief may be required during an acute crisis.)
✦ Encourage bed rest, and place the patient in a sitting position. If dehydration or severe pain occurs, hospitalization may be necessary.
✦ When cultures indicate, give antibiotics as ordered.

During remissions

✦ Advise the patient to avoid tight clothing that restricts circulation.
✦ Warn against strenuous exercise, vasoconstricting medications, cold temperatures (including drinking large amounts of ice water and swimming), unpressurized aircraft, high altitude, and other conditions that provoke hypoxia.

Key nursing actions

✦ Supportive measures during crises and precautions to avoid them are important.
✦ Apply warm compresses to painful areas, and cover the child with a blanket.
✦ Administer an analgesic-antipyretic.

During remissions

✦ Advise the patient to avoid tight clothing that restricts circulation.
✦ Warn against strenuous exercise, vasoconstricting medications, cold temperatures, unpressurized aircraft, high altitude, and other conditions that provoke hypoxia.
✦ Emphasize the need for prompt treatment of infection.
✦ Inform the patient of the need to increase fluid intake to prevent dehydration due to impaired ability to concentrate urine properly.

Key nursing actions

During pregnancy or surgery

✦ Warn women with sickle cell anemia that they may have increased obstetrical risks.

✦ If a woman with sickle cell anemia does become pregnant, encourage her to maintain a balanced diet and to take a folic acid supplement.

General tips

✦ Warn parents against being overprotective; the child can enjoy most everyday activities.

✦ Refer parents of children with sickle cell anemia for genetic counseling.

✦ Adolescents or adult males with sickle cell anemia may develop sudden, painful episodes of priapism.

✦ Stress the importance of normal childhood immunizations, meticulous wound care, good oral hygiene, regular dental checkups, and a balanced diet as safeguards against infection.

✦ Emphasize the need for prompt treatment of infection.

✦ Inform the patient of the need to increase fluid intake to prevent dehydration due to impaired ability to concentrate urine properly. Tell the parents to encourage their child to drink more fluids, especially in the summer, by offering fluids in such forms as milkshakes, ice pops, and eggnog.

During pregnancy or surgery

✦ Warn women with sickle cell anemia that they may have increased obstetrical risks. However, use of oral contraceptives may also be risky; refer them for birth control counseling to a qualified obstetric-gynecologic health care provider.

✦ If a woman with sickle cell anemia does become pregnant, encourage her to maintain a balanced diet and to take a folic acid supplement.

✦ During general anesthesia, a sickle cell anemia patient requires optimal ventilation to prevent hypoxic crisis. Make sure the surgeon and the anesthesiologist know that the patient has sickle cell anemia. Provide a preoperative transfusion of packed RBCs, as needed.

General tips

✦ To encourage normal mental and social development, warn the parents against being overprotective. Although the child must avoid strenuous exercise, he can enjoy most everyday activities.

✦ Refer parents of children with sickle cell anemia for genetic counseling to answer their questions about the risk to future offspring. Recommend screening of other family members to determine if they're heterozygote carriers. These parents may also need psychological counseling to cope with guilt feelings. In addition, suggest they join an appropriate community support group.

✦ Adolescents or adult males with sickle cell anemia may develop sudden, painful episodes of priapism. Such episodes are common and, if prolonged, can have serious reproductive consequences. Advise the patient to contact his physician when these episodes occur.

Cardiovascular system

The cardiovascular system begins its activity when the fetus is barely 4 weeks old and is the last system to cease activity at the end of life. This body system is so vital that it helps define the presence of life.

The heart, arteries, veins, and lymphatics form the cardiovascular network that serves as the body's transport system. This system brings life-supporting oxygen and nutrients to cells, removes metabolic waste products, and carries hormones from one part of the body to another.

The cardiovascular system, commonly called the *circulatory system,* is divided into two branches: pulmonary and systemic circulations. In *pulmonary circulation,* blood picks up oxygen and liberates the waste product carbon dioxide. In *systemic circulation* (which includes coronary circulation), blood carries oxygen and nutrients to all active cells and transports waste products to the kidneys, liver, and skin for excretion.

Circulation requires normal heart function, which propels blood through the system by continuous rhythmic contractions. Blood circulates through three types of vessels: arteries, veins, and capillaries. The sturdy, pliable walls of the arteries adjust to the volume of blood leaving the heart. The aorta is the major artery arching out of the left ventricle; its segments and branches ultimately divide into minute, thin-walled (one cell thick) capillaries. Capillaries pass the blood to the veins, which return it to the heart. In the veins, valves prevent blood backflow.

PATHOPHYSIOLOGIC CHANGES

Pathophysiologic manifestations of cardiovascular disease may stem from aneurysm, cardiac shunts, embolus, release of cardiac enzymes and proteins, stenosis, thrombus, and valve incompetence.

The cardiovascular system

+ Begins when the fetus is barely 4 weeks old; last system to cease activity
+ Helps define presence of life
+ Comprises the heart, arteries, veins, and lymphatics
+ Serves as the body's transport system
+ Brings oxygen and nutrients to cells, removes metabolic waste products, and carries hormones
+ Commonly called the *circulatory system*
+ Pulmonary circulation: blood picks up oxygen and eliminates carbon dioxide
+ Systemic circulation: blood carries oxygen and nutrients to active cells and transports waste for excretion
+ Blood circulates through arteries, veins, and capillaries

143

Aneurysm

+ Localized outpouching or dilation of a weakened arterial wall
+ Can be the result of atherosclerotic plaque formation or the loss of elastin and collagen in the vessel wall
+ May result from abnormalities in media of arterial wall, trauma, and infections
+ Ruptured aneurysm may cause massive hemorrhage and death
+ Four types: saccular, fusiform, dissecting, and false

Cardiac shunts

+ Provide communication between pulmonary and systemic circulations
+ Blood flows through a shunt from area of high pressure to area of low pressure or from area of high resistance to area of low resistance

Left-to-right shunts

+ Blood flows from left side of heart to right side through defect
+ Can flow from aorta to pulmonary artery through a patent ductus arteriosus
+ Blood in left side of heart is rich in oxygen
+ Blood flow increases as blood is continually recirculated to the lungs, leading to hypertrophy of pulmonary vessels
+ Right- or left-sided heart failure may occur

ANEURYSM

An aneurysm is a localized outpouching or dilation of a weakened arterial wall. This weakness can be the result of atherosclerotic plaque formation that erodes the vessel wall or the loss of elastin and collagen in the vessel wall. Congenital abnormalities in the media of the arterial wall, trauma, and infections, such as syphilis, may also lead to aneurysm formation. A ruptured aneurysm may cause massive hemorrhage and death.

Several types of aneurysms can occur. A *saccular aneurysm* occurs when increased pressure in the artery pushes out a pouch on one side of the artery, creating a bulge. (See *Types of aortic aneurysms.*)

When the arterial wall weakens around its circumference, a spindle-shaped aneurysm called a *fusiform aneurysm* is created.

A third type of aneurysm, a *dissecting aneurysm,* occurs when blood is forced between the layers of the arterial wall, causing them to separate and creating a false lumen.

Lastly, a *false aneurysm* develops when there's a break in all layers of the arterial wall. Blood leaks out but it's contained by surrounding structures, creating a pulsatile hematoma.

An aneurysm most commonly occurs in one of four locations. An abdominal aortic aneurysm — an abnormal dilation of the arterial wall — generally occurs in the aorta between the renal artery and the iliac branches. A thoracic aortic aneurysm is an abnormal widening of the ascending, transverse, or descending part of the aorta. A localized dilation of a cerebral artery that may arise at an arterial junction in the circle of Willis — the circular anastomosis forming the major cerebral arteries at the base of the brain — is called a cerebral aneurysm. Lastly, femoral and popliteal aneurysms (sometimes called peripheral arterial aneurysms) are the end result of progressive atherosclerotic changes occurring in the walls (medial layer) of the femoral and popliteal arteries.

CARDIAC SHUNTS

A cardiac shunt provides communication between the pulmonary and systemic circulations. Before birth, shunts between the right and left sides of the heart and between the aorta and pulmonary artery are a normal part of fetal circulation. Following birth, however, the mixing of pulmonary and systemic blood or the movement of blood between the left and right sides of the heart is abnormal. Blood flows through a shunt from an area of high pressure to an area of low pressure or from an area of high resistance to an area of low resistance.

Left-to-right shunts

In a left-to-right shunt, blood flows from the left side of the heart to the right side through an atrial or ventricular septal defect or from the aorta to the pulmonary artery through a patent ductus arteriosus. Because the blood in the left side of the heart is rich in oxygen, a left-to-right shunt delivers oxygenated blood back to the right side of the heart or to the lungs. Consequently, a left-to-right shunt that occurs as a result of a congenital heart defect is called an *acyanotic defect.*

In a left-to-right shunt, pulmonary blood flow increases as blood is continually recirculated to the lungs, leading to hypertrophy of the pulmonary vessels. The increased amount of blood circulated from the left side of the heart to the right side can result in right-sided heart failure. Eventually, left-sided heart failure may also occur.

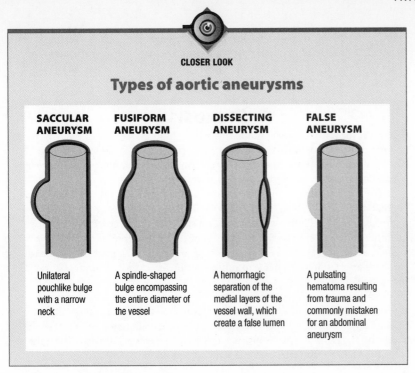

Types of aortic aneurysms

SACCULAR ANEURYSM

Unilateral pouchlike bulge with a narrow neck

FUSIFORM ANEURYSM

A spindle-shaped bulge encompassing the entire diameter of the vessel

DISSECTING ANEURYSM

A hemorrhagic separation of the medial layers of the vessel wall, which create a false lumen

FALSE ANEURYSM

A pulsating hematoma resulting from trauma and commonly mistaken for an abdominal aneurysm

Right-to-left shunts

♦ Occur when blood flows from right to left side of heart
♦ Blood returning to the right side of heart and the pulmonary artery is low in oxygen
♦ Add deoxygenated blood to systemic circulation, causing hypoxia and cyanosis
♦ Related to poor tissue and organ perfusion

Right-to-left shunts

A right-to-left shunt occurs when blood flows from the right side of the heart to the left side, as in tetralogy of Fallot. Because blood returning to the right side of the heart and the pulmonary artery is low in oxygen, a right-to-left shunt adds deoxygenated blood to the systemic circulation, causing hypoxia and cyanosis. Congenital defects that involve right-to-left shunts are therefore called *cyanotic defects*. Common manifestations of a right-to-left shunt that are related to poor tissue and organ perfusion include fatigue, increased respiratory rate, and clubbing of the fingers.

Embolus

♦ Substance that circulates from one location in the body to another through bloodstream
♦ Most are blood clots from thrombus
♦ May consist of pieces of tissue, an air bubble, amniotic fluid, fat, bacteria, or tumor cells
♦ May cause pulmonary infarction and possibly death
♦ May lodge in organs causing ischemia or infarction

EMBOLUS

An embolus is a substance that circulates from one location in the body to another through the bloodstream. Although most emboli are blood clots from a thrombus, they may also consist of pieces of tissue, an air bubble, amniotic fluid, fat, bacteria, tumor cells, or a foreign substance.

Emboli that originate in the venous circulation (such as those from deep vein thrombosis) travel to the right side of the heart to the pulmonary circulation and eventually lodge in a capillary, causing pulmonary infarction and, possibly, death. Most emboli in the arterial system originate from the left side of the heart from such conditions as arrhythmias, valvular heart disease, myocardial infarction, heart failure, or endocarditis. Arterial emboli may lodge in organs, such as the brain, kidneys, or extremities, causing ischemia or infarction.

Release of cardiac enzymes and proteins

♦ Cardiac enzymes and proteins released; measured in bloodstream when heart is damaged
♦ Released enzymes: creatine kinase and lactate dehydrogenase
♦ Proteins released include troponin T, troponin I, and myoglobin

RELEASE OF CARDIAC ENZYMES AND PROTEINS

When the heart muscle is damaged, the cell membrane's integrity is impaired and intracellular contents—including cardiac enzymes and proteins—are released and can be measured in the bloodstream. The release follows a characteristic rising and falling of enzyme and protein values. The released enzymes include creatine kinase, lactate dehydrogenase, and aspartate aminotransferase; the proteins released include troponin T, troponin I, and myoglobin. (See *Release of cardiac enzymes and proteins.*)

STENOSIS

Stenosis
+ Narrowing of a tubular structure
+ Tissues and organs perfused by the blood vessel may become ischemic, function abnormally, or die
+ Blood flow through valve is reduced
+ Pressure in the chamber increases, heart has to work harder, resulting in hypertrophy; increased need for oxygen
+ Diseased coronary arteries may be unable to sufficiently increase oxygen supply to meet demand

Stenosis is the narrowing of a tubular structure (blood vessel or heart valve). When an artery is stenosed, the tissues and organs perfused by that blood vessel may become ischemic, function abnormally, or die. An occluded vein may result in venous congestion and chronic venous insufficiency.

When a heart valve is stenosed, blood flow through that valve is reduced, causing blood to accumulate in the chamber behind the valve; pressure in the chamber increases, to enable pumping against the resistance of the stenosed valve. Consequently, the heart has to work harder, resulting in hypertrophy. Hypertrophy and an increase in workload raise the heart's oxygen demands. A heart with diseased coronary arteries may be unable to sufficiently increase oxygen supply to meet the increased demand.

When stenosis occurs in a valve on the left side of the heart, the increased pressure leads to greater pulmonary venous pressure and pulmonary congestion. As pulmonary vascular resistance rises, right-sided heart failure may occur. Stenosis in a valve on the right side of the heart causes an increase in pressures on the right side of the heart, leading to systemic venous congestion.

THROMBUS

Thrombus
+ Blood clot that forms anywhere within the vascular system
+ Virchow's triad: endothelial injury, sluggish blood flow, and increased coagulability
+ Consequences include occlusion of blood vessel or formation of an embolus

A thrombus is a blood clot, consisting of platelets, fibrin, and red and white blood cells, that forms anywhere within the vascular system, such as the arteries, veins, heart chambers, or heart valves.

Three conditions, known as Virchow's triad, promote thrombus formation: endothelial injury, sluggish blood flow, and increased coagulability. When a blood vessel wall is injured, the endothelial lining attracts platelets and other inflammatory mediators, which may stimulate clot formation. Sluggish or abnormal blood flow also promotes thrombus formation by allowing platelets and clotting factors to accumulate and adhere to the blood vessel walls. Conditions that increase the coagulability of blood also promote clot formation.

The consequences of thrombus formation include occlusion of the blood vessel or the formation of an embolus (if a portion of a thrombus breaks loose and travels through the circulatory system until it lodges in a smaller vessel).

VALVE INCOMPETENCE

Valve incompetence
+ Insufficiency or regurgitation
+ May affect valves of veins or heart
+ Valve leaflets close improperly, blood flows backward and pools, causing valve to weaken
+ Incompetent valves allow blood to flow in both directions through heart valve; cause involved heart chambers to dilate

Valve incompetence, also called insufficiency or regurgitation, occurs when valve leaflets don't completely close. Incompetence may affect valves of the veins or heart.

In the veins, valves keep the blood flowing in one direction, toward the heart. When valve leaflets close improperly, blood flows backward and pools above the valve, causing that valve to weaken and become incompetent. Eventually, the veins become distended, which may result in varicose veins, chronic venous insufficiency, and venous stasis ulcers. Blood clots may form as blood flow becomes sluggish.

In the heart, incompetent valves allow blood to flow in both directions through the valve, increasing the volume of blood that must be pumped (as well as the heart's workload) and resulting in hypertrophy. As blood volume in the heart in-

Release of cardiac enzymes and proteins

Because they're released by damaged tissue, serum proteins and isoenzymes (catalytic proteins that vary in concentration in specific organs) can help identify the compromised organ and assess the extent of damage. After acute myocardial infarction, cardiac enzymes and proteins rise and fall in a characteristic pattern, as shown in this graph.

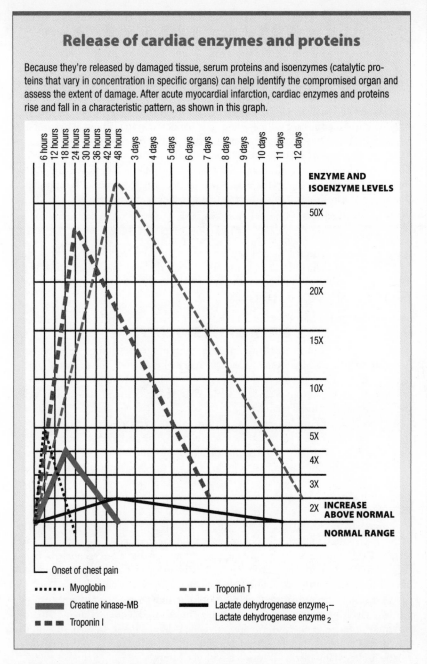

creases, the involved heart chambers dilate to accommodate the increased volume. Although incompetence may occur in any heart valve, it's more common in the mitral and aortic valves.

Characteristics of ACS
+ Involve the rupture or erosion of plaque as initiating event
+ Rupture results in platelet adhesions, fibrin clot formation, and activation of thrombin
+ Acute MI and unstable angina now part of this group
+ Death commonly results

Causes
+ Family history
+ Obesity
+ Smoking
+ High-fat/high-carbohydrate diet
+ Sedentary lifestyle

How it happens
+ Thrombus progresses and occludes blood flow
+ Degree of blockage and time affected vessel determines type of infarct that occurs
+ Imbalance in myocardial oxygen supply and demand
+ Distal microthrombi cause necrosis in some myocytes
+ Smaller vessels infarct, placing patient at risk for non–Q-wave MI
+ When infarct occurs myocardial cells have died
+ Infarcted muscle becomes edematous and cyanotic; leukocytes infiltrate necrotic area and begin to remove necrotic cells, thinning ventricular wall; scar formation begins

ACUTE CORONARY SYNDROMES

Acute coronary syndromes (ACS) are clinical conditions that involve the rupture or erosion of plaque—an unstable and lipid-rich substance—as the initiating event. The rupture results in platelet adhesions, fibrin clot formation, and activation of thrombin. Acute myocardial infarction (MI), (Q-wave and non–Q-wave) and unstable angina are now recognized as part of this group.

Cardiovascular disease is the leading cause of death in the United States and Western Europe. Death commonly results from cardiac damage or complications of MI. Each year, approximately 900,000 people in the United States experience MI. Mortality is high when treatment is delayed, and almost one-half of sudden deaths due to MI occur before hospitalization (within 1 hour of the onset of symptoms). The prognosis improves if vigorous treatment begins immediately.

CAUSES

A patient with certain risk factors appears to face a greater likelihood of developing ACS. These factors include a family history of heart disease, obesity, smoking, high-fat and high-carbohydrate diet, sedentary lifestyle, menopause, stress, diabetes, hypertension, and hyperlipoproteinemia.

PATHOPHYSIOLOGY

An ACS most commonly results when a thrombus progresses and occludes blood flow (an early thrombus doesn't necessarily block blood flow). The degree of blockage and the time that the affected vessel remains occluded are major determinants for the type of infarct that occurs. The underlying effect is an imbalance in myocardial oxygen supply and demand.

In a patient with unstable angina, a thrombus full of platelets partially occludes a coronary vessel. (See *Viewing the coronary vessels.*) The partially occluded vessel may have distal microthrombi that cause necrosis in some myocytes. The smaller vessels infarct, placing the patient at higher risk for progression to a non–Q-wave MI. A Q-wave MI occurs when a thrombus fully occludes the vessel for a prolonged time. In this type of MI, a greater concentration of thrombin and fibrin is noted. (See *Understanding thrombus formation,* page 150.)

Progressive occlusion of a vessel results in muscle and tissue damage. Ischemia, which occurs first, indicates that blood flow and oxygen demand are out of balance. Ischemia can be resolved by improving blood flow or reducing oxygen needs. Injury occurs next. It's the result of prolonged ischemia, which causes damage to an area of the heart. Lastly, when infarct occurs, myocardial cells have died.

All MIs have a central area of necrosis or infarction surrounded by a zone of potentially viable hypoxic injury. This zone may be salvaged if circulation is restored, or it may progress to necrosis. An area of viable ischemic tissue, in turn, surrounds the zone of injury. Although ischemia begins immediately, the size of the infarct can be limited if circulation is restored within 6 hours.

As the heart muscle is damaged, cardiac enzyme levels (creatine kinase [CK], lactate dehydrogenase, and aspartate aminotransferase) and serum cardiac protein levels (troponin T, troponin I, and myoglobin) become elevated.

Within 24 hours, the infarcted muscle becomes edematous and cyanotic. During the next several days, leukocytes infiltrate the necrotic area and begin to remove necrotic cells, thinning the ventricular wall. Scar formation begins by the third week after MI, and by the sixth week, scar tissue is well established.

Viewing the coronary vessels

If an occlusion in a coronary artery causes a myocardial infarction (MI), the amount of damage to the myocardium depends on several factors. The area of the heart supplied by the affected vessel is a concern as well as the demand for oxygen in the affected area of the heart. In addition, the collateral circulation in the affected area of the heart affects the outcome. Collateral circulation is an alternate circulation that develops when blood flow to a tissue is blocked. This illustration shows the major coronary vessels that may be involved in an MI.

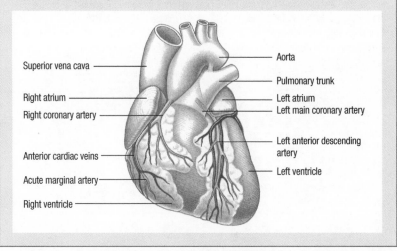

Coronary vessels concerns

✦ Area of the heart supplied by the affected vessel
✦ Demand for oxygen in the affected area of the heart
✦ Collateral circulation in the affected area

The scar tissue that forms on the necrotic area inhibits contractility. When this occurs, the compensatory mechanisms (vascular constriction, increased heart rate, and renal retention of sodium and water) try to maintain cardiac output. Ventricular dilation may also occur in a process called remodeling. Functionally, an MI may cause reduced contractility with abnormal wall motion, altered left ventricular compliance, reduced stroke volume, reduced ejection fraction, and elevated left ventricular end-diastolic pressure.

SIGNS AND SYMPTOMS

A patient with angina typically experiences burning, squeezing, and a crushing tightness in the substernal or precordial chest that may radiate to the left arm, neck, jaw, or shoulder blade.

Angina usually follows physical exertion, but may also follow emotional excitement, exposure to cold, or a large meal. Angina is commonly relieved by nitroglycerin. It's less severe and of shorter duration than the pain of acute MI.

Angina has four major forms. In the stable form, pain is predictable in frequency and duration, and it can be relieved with nitrates and rest. Unstable angina is marked by increased pain that's easily induced. Prinzmetal's (or variant) angina is pain from unpredictable coronary artery spasm. Microvascular angina is angina-like chest pain due to impairment of vasodilator reserve in a patient with normal coronary arteries.

A patient with MI experiences severe, persistent chest pain that isn't relieved by rest or nitroglycerin. He may describe the pain as crushing or squeezing; it's usually substernal, but may radiate to the left arm, jaw, neck, or shoulder blades.

Key signs and symptoms

✦ Angina as burning, squeezing, and a crushing tightness in chest
✦ Usually follows physical exertion, emotional excitement, exposure to cold, or a large meal
✦ Four major forms: stable, unstable, Prinzmetal's (or variant), and microvascular
✦ Patient experiences severe, persistent chest pain not relieved by rest in MI
✦ Patient may have feeling of impending doom

Thrombus formation

- Area of plaque ruptures or erodes
- Platelets adhere to the damaged area and are exposed to activating factors
- Activation causes expression of glycoprotein IIb/IIa receptors
- Platelet aggregation and adhesion occurs
- Thrombus is enlarged

Understanding thrombus formation

Acute coronary syndrome most commonly results when plaque erodes or ruptures, leading to thrombus formation and subsequent coronary artery occlusion. Here's how it happens.

1. An area of plaque may rupture or erode because of weakening due to inflammation in the subendothelial layer of the blood vessel, blood flow velocity and turbulence, or vessel anatomy.

3. Platelet activation causes expression of glycoprotein IIb/IIIa receptors that bind fibrinogen.

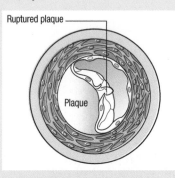

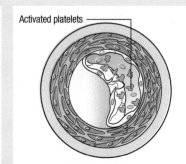

2. The ruptured surface is thombogenic. Platelets adhere to the damaged area and are exposed to activating factors, including collagen, thrombin, and von Willebrand (VW) factor.

4. This leads to further platelet aggregation and adhesion, and enlarges the thrombus.

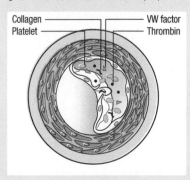

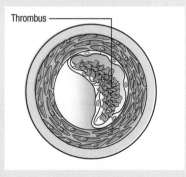

Complications

- Arrhythmias
- Cardiogenic shock
- Heart failure
- Pericarditis
- Rupture of atrial or ventricular septum, ventricular wall, or valves
- Death

Other signs and symptoms of MI include a feeling of impending doom, fatigue, nausea and vomiting, shortness of breath, cool extremities, perspiration, anxiety, hypotension or hypertension, palpable precordial pulse, and muffled heart sounds.

COMPLICATIONS

Complications may include arrhythmias; cardiogenic shock; heart failure, causing pulmonary edema; pericarditis; rupture of the atrial or ventricular septum, ventricular wall, or valves; mural thrombi causing cerebral or pulmonary emboli; ventricular aneurysms; myocardial rupture; extensions of the original infarction; and death.

A patient with ACS is at risk for complications for up to 12 weeks following the acute episode. In addition, for approximately the next 6 months, the patient is at risk for additional episodes until the area of the initiating plaque heals.

DIAGNOSIS

The following tests help diagnose ACS:

✦ Electrocardiogram (ECG) during an anginal episode shows ischemia. Serial 12-lead ECGs may be normal or inconclusive during the first few hours after an MI. Abnormalities include serial ST-segment depression in non–Q-wave MI and ST-segment elevation and Q waves, representing scarring and necrosis, in a Q-`wave MI. (See *Pinpointing myocardial infarction,* page 152.)

✦ Coronary angiography reveals coronary artery stenosis or obstruction and collateral circulation and shows the condition of the arteries beyond the narrowing.

✦ Myocardial perfusion imaging with thallium-201 during treadmill exercise discloses ischemic areas of the myocardium, visualized as "cold spots."

✦ With MI, serial serum cardiac marker measurements show elevated CK, especially the CK-MB isoenzyme (the cardiac muscle fraction of CK), troponins T and I, and myoglobin.

✦ With a Q-wave MI, echocardiography shows decreased ventricular wall movement.

TREATMENT

For patients with angina, the goal of treatment is to reduce myocardial oxygen demand or increase oxygen supply. Nitrates are administered to reduce myocardial oxygen consumption. Beta-adrenergic blockers may be administered to reduce the workload and oxygen demands of the heart. If angina is caused by coronary artery spasm, calcium channel blockers may be given. Antiplatelet drugs minimize platelet aggregation and the danger of coronary occlusion. Antilipemic drugs can reduce elevated serum cholesterol or triglyceride levels. Obstructive lesions may necessitate coronary artery bypass grafting or percutaneous transluminal coronary angioplasty (PTCA). Other alternatives include laser angioplasty, minimally invasive surgery, rotational atherectomy, or stent placement.

Enhanced external counterpulsation (EECP) is another treatment for angina. Used to reduce the symptoms of angina, this noninvasive procedure is believed to work by increasing coronary blood flow to ischemic areas of the heart. EECP involves the use of a series of compressive cuffs that are sequentially inflated and deflated and placed around the patient's calves, lower thighs, and upper thighs. Inflation and deflation of the cuffs are controlled by events in the cardiac cycle. During diastole, the cuffs are inflated to increase venous return and cardiac output, thereby increasing coronary perfusion. During systole, the cuffs are deflated to reduce resistance and decrease the heart's workload. Treatment sessions last for 1 hour and are well tolerated; there are no reported complications and the patient shouldn't experience pain during the procedure.

The goals of treatment for MI are to relieve pain, stabilize heart rhythm, revascularize the coronary artery, preserve myocardial tissue, and reduce cardiac workload. (See *Treating myocardial infarction,* pages 154 and 155.) Thrombolytic therapy should be started within 3 hours of the onset of symptoms (unless contraindications exist). Thrombolytic therapy involves the administration of streptokinase

Diagnosis

✦ ECG during an anginal episode shows ischemia
✦ Coronary angiography
✦ Myocardial perfusion imaging with thallium-201 during treadmill exercise
✦ With MI, serial serum cardiac marker measurements show elevated CK, especially CK-MB isoenzyme, troponins T and I, and myoglobin
✦ With a Q-wave MI, echocardiography shows decreased ventricular wall movement

Treatment

Angina
✦ Nitrates to reduce myocardial oxygen consumption
✦ Beta-adrenergic blockers to reduce workload and oxygen demands
✦ Antiplatelet drugs
✦ Coronary artery bypass grafting or PTCA
✦ Laser angioplasty
✦ Stent placement
✦ EECP

Types of MI

+ Inferior
+ Anterior
+ Septal
+ Lateral
+ Anterolateral
+ Posterior
+ Right ventricular

Treatment

MI

+ Thrombolytic therapy should be started within 3 hours of onset of symptoms
+ PTCA
+ Oxygen and nitroglycerin, unless contraindicated
+ Lidocaine
+ Transcutaneous pacing patches (or a transvenous pacemaker)
+ Defibrillation
+ Epinephrine
+ I.V. beta-adrenergic blocker followed by oral therapy
+ ACE inhibitors
+ Stent placement
+ Transmyocardial revascularization
+ Lipid-lowering drugs

Pinpointing myocardial infarction

Depending on its location, ischemia or infarction causes changes in these electrocardiographic leads.

TYPE OF MYOCARDIAL INFARCTION	LEADS
Inferior	II, III, aV_F
Anterior	V_3, V_4
Septal	V_1, V_2
Lateral	I, aV_L, V_5, V_6
Anterolateral	I, aV_L, V_3 to V_6
Posterior	V_1, V_2, V_7, V_8, V_9
Right ventricular	II, III, aV_F, V_{4R} to V_{6R}

(Streptase), alteplase (Activase), anistreplase (Eminase), or reteplase (Retavase). PTCA is an option for opening blocked or narrowed arteries.

Oxygen is administered to increase oxygenation of the blood. Nitroglycerin is administered sublingually to relieve chest pain, unless systolic blood pressure is less than 90 mm Hg or heart rate is less than 50 or greater than 100 beats/minute. Morphine is administered as analgesia because pain stimulates the sympathetic nervous system, leading to an increase in heart rate and vasoconstriction. Aspirin is administered to inhibit platelet aggregation. I.V. heparin is given to patients who have received tissue plasminogen activator to increase the chances of patency in the affected coronary artery. Physical activity is limited for the first 12 hours to reduce cardiac workload, thereby limiting the area of necrosis.

Lidocaine, transcutaneous pacing patches (or a transvenous pacemaker), defibrillation, or epinephrine may be used if arrhythmias are present. I.V. nitroglycerin is administered for 24 to 48 hours to patients without hypotension, bradycardia, or excessive tachycardia, to reduce afterload and preload and relieve chest pain. Glycoprotein IIb/IIIa inhibitors (such as abciximab [ReoPro]) are administered to patients with continued unstable angina or acute chest pain or following invasive cardiac procedures to reduce platelet aggregation. An I.V. beta-adrenergic blocker is administered early to patients with evolving acute MI; it's followed by oral therapy to reduce heart rate and contractibility and reduce myocardial oxygen requirements. Angiotensin-converting enzyme (ACE) inhibitors are administered to those with evolving MI with ST-segment elevation or left bundle-branch block, to reduce afterload and preload and prevent remodeling. Laser angioplasty, atherectomy, stent placement, or transmyocardial revascularization may be initiated. Lipid-lowering drugs are administered to patients with elevated low-density lipoprotein and cholesterol levels.

NURSING CONSIDERATIONS

✦ On admission to a monitored setting, monitor and record the patient's ECG, blood pressure, temperature, and heart and breath sounds. Also, assess and record the pain's severity, location, type, and duration. Obtain a 12-lead ECG and assess heart rate and blood pressure when the patient is experiencing acute chest pain.

✦ Monitor the patient's hemodynamic status closely, and be alert for indicators suggesting decreased cardiac output, such as decreased blood pressure, increased heart rate, increased pulmonary artery pressure, increased pulmonary artery wedge pressure, decreased cardiac output measurements, and decreased right atrial pressure.

✦ During episodes of chest pain, monitor the ECG, blood pressure and pulmonary catheter measurements (if applicable) to determine changes.

✦ Assess urine output hourly for at least the first 4 hours; continue assessments according to your facility's policy.

✦ Monitor the patient's oxygen saturation levels and continue oxygen administration as ordered. Notify the physician if oxygen saturation falls below 90%.

✦ Check the patient's blood pressure after giving nitroglycerin (especially after the first dose).

✦ Frequently monitor ECG rhythm strips to detect heart rate changes and arrhythmias.

✦ Obtain serial measurements of cardiac enzyme levels as ordered.

✦ Assess for crackles, cough, tachypnea, and edema, which may indicate impending left-sided heart failure. Carefully monitor daily weight, intake and output, respiratory rate, and periodically auscultate for adventitious breath sounds as well as for S_3 or S_4 gallops.

✦ Prepare the patient for reperfusion therapy as indicated.

✦ Administer and titrate medications as ordered. Avoid giving I.M. injections because absorption from muscles is unpredictable; I.V. administration provides more rapid symptomatic relief.

✦ Organize patient care and activities to allow periods of uninterrupted rest. Assist with range-of-motion exercises. If the patient is immobilized, turn him often and use antiembolism stockings or intermittent compression devices. Gradually increase the patient's activity level as tolerated and as indicated by acceptable monitoring parameters.

✦ Provide a clear-liquid diet until nausea subsides. Anticipate the possibility for a low-cholesterol, low-sodium, caffeine-free diet.

✦ Provide a stool softener to prevent straining during defecation. Allow the patient to use a bedside commode if appropriate, and provide as much privacy as possible.

✦ Provide emotional support and help reduce stress and anxiety; administer antianxiety agents as needed.

✦ Advise the patient to report typical or atypical chest pain. Post-MI syndrome may develop, producing chest pain that must be differentiated from recurrent MI, pulmonary infarction, and heart failure.

✦ Encourage the patient to participate in a cardiac rehabilitation exercise program that includes progressive activities.

✦ Stress the need to stop smoking. If necessary, refer the patient to a support group.

(Text continues on page 156.)

Key nursing actions

✦ Assess and record the pain's severity, location, type, and duration.

✦ Obtain a 12-lead ECG and assess heart rate and blood pressure when the patient is experiencing acute chest pain.

✦ During chest pain, monitor the ECG, blood pressure and pulmonary catheter measurements.

✦ Assess urine output hourly for at least the first 4 hours.

✦ Monitor the patient's oxygen saturation levels and continue oxygen administration as ordered. Notify the physician if oxygen saturation falls below 90%.

✦ Check the patient's blood pressure after giving nitroglycerin.

✦ Advise the patient to report typical or atypical chest pain.

Treating myocardial infarction

This chart shows how treatments can be applied to myocardial infarction at various stages of its development. Without such treatment, various complications can result.

Treatments	Pathophysiology
✦ ASPIRIN ✦ ANTIPLATELET AGGREGATES	Change in the condition of plaque in the coronary artery
	Activation of platelets
✦ GLYCOPROTEIN IIB/IIIA RECEPTOR BLOCKING AGENTS	Formation of thrombus
✦ THROMBOLYTIC THERAPY ✦ PERCUTANEOUS TRANSLUMINAL CORONARY ANGIOPLASTY	Coronary blood supply less than demand
✦ NITRATES	Ischemia of tissue in the region supplied by the artery
✦ BETA-ADRENERGIC BLOCKERS	Myocardial cell death
✦ OXYGEN ✦ BED REST	
✦ VASODILATORS	
✦ MORPHINE	Stimulation of the sympathetic nervous system
✦ BETA-ADRENERGIC BLOCKERS	
	Increased heart rate Increased afterload Increased O_2 needs
✦ NITRATES ✦ VASODILATORS	Vasoconstriction

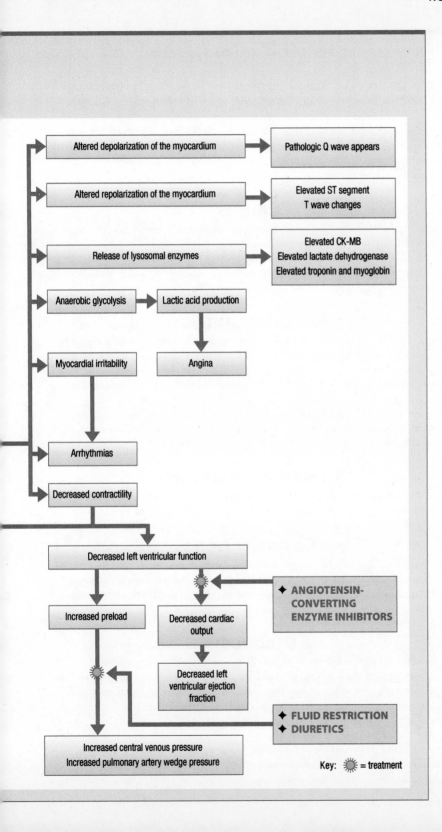

ARTERIAL OCCLUSIVE DISEASE

Arterial occlusive disease is the obstruction or narrowing of the lumen of the aorta and its major branches, causing an interruption of blood flow, usually to the legs and feet. This disorder may affect the carotid, vertebral, innominate, subclavian, mesenteric, and celiac arteries. (See *Possible sites of major artery occlusion.*)

Arterial occlusive disease is more common in males than in females. The prognosis depends on the occlusion's location, the development of collateral circulation to counteract reduced blood flow and, in acute disease, the time elapsed between occlusion and its removal.

CAUSES

Arterial occlusive disease is a common complication of atherosclerosis. The occlusive mechanism may be endogenous, due to emboli formation or thrombosis, or exogenous, due to trauma or fracture. Predisposing factors include smoking; aging; conditions such as hypertension, hyperlipidemia, and diabetes; and a family history of vascular disorders, myocardial infarction, or stroke.

PATHOPHYSIOLOGY

Arterial occlusive disease is almost always the result of atherosclerosis, in which fatty, fibrous plaques narrow the lumen of blood vessels. This occlusion can occur acutely or progressively over 20 to 40 years, with areas of vessel branching, or bifurcation, being the most common sites. The narrowing of the lumens reduces the blood volume that can flow through them, causing arterial insufficiency to the affected area. Ischemia usually occurs after the vessel lumens have narrowed by at least 50%, reducing blood flow to a level at which it no longer meets the needs of tissue and nerves.

SIGNS AND SYMPTOMS

Signs and symptoms of arterial occlusive disease depend on the site of the occlusion. (See *Signs and symptoms of arterial occlusive disease,* page 158.)

COMPLICATIONS

Complications of arterial occlusive disease may include severe ischemia and necrosis; skin ulceration; gangrene, which can lead to limb amputation; impaired nail and hair growth; stroke or transient ischemic attack; and peripheral or systemic embolism.

DIAGNOSIS

Diagnosis is usually indicated by patient history and physical examination. Pertinent tests support the diagnosis of arterial occlusive disease. Arteriography demonstrates the type (thrombus or embolus), location, and degree of obstruction and the collateral circulation. Arteriography is particularly useful in chronic disease or for evaluating candidates for reconstructive surgery.

Also useful are Doppler ultrasonography and plethysmography—noninvasive tests that show decreased blood flow distal to the occlusion in acute disease. To help determine the degree of obstruction in the internal carotid artery by comparing ophthalmic artery pressure to brachial artery pressure on the affected side, use an

Possible sites of major artery occlusion

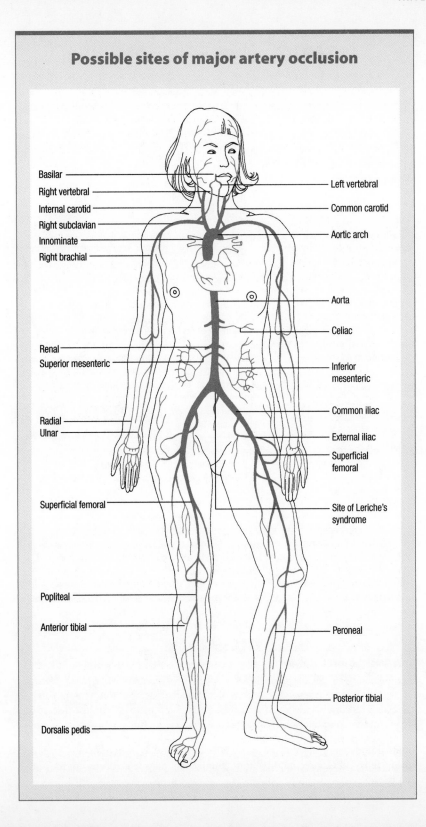

Basilar
Right vertebral
Internal carotid
Right subclavian
Innominate
Right brachial

Left vertebral
Common carotid
Aortic arch

Aorta
Celiac

Renal
Superior mesenteric

Inferior mesenteric

Radial
Ulnar

Common iliac
External iliac
Superficial femoral

Superficial femoral

Site of Leriche's syndrome

Popliteal

Anterior tibial

Peroneal

Posterior tibial

Dorsalis pedis

Sites of major artery occulsion

♦ Basilar
♦ Right vertebral
♦ Left vertebral
♦ Internal or common carotid
♦ Right subclavian
♦ Innominate
♦ Aortic arch
♦ Right brachial
♦ Aorta
♦ Celiac
♦ Renal
♦ Radial
♦ Superior or inferior mesenteric
♦ Ulnar
♦ Common or external iliac
♦ Superficial femoral
♦ Site of Leriche's syndrome
♦ Popliteal
♦ Peroneal
♦ Anterior or posterior tibial
♦ Dorsalis pedis

Signs and symptoms of arterial occlusive disease

SITE OF OCCLUSION	SIGNS AND SYMPTOMS
Carotid arterial system ✦ Internal carotids ✦ External carotids	Neurologic dysfunction: transient ischemic attacks (TIAs) due to reduced cerebral circulation produce unilateral sensory or motor dysfunction (transient monocular blindness, hemiparesis), possible aphasia or dysarthria, confusion, decreased mentation, and headache. These recurrent clinical features usually last 5 to 10 minutes, but may persist up to 24 hours and may herald a stroke. Absent or decreased pulsation with an auscultatory bruit over the affected vessels.
Vertebrobasilar system ✦ Vertebral arteries ✦ Basilar arteries	Neurologic dysfunction: TIAs of brain stem and cerebellum produce binocular visual disturbances, vertigo, dysarthria, and "drop attacks" (falling down without loss of consciousness). Less common than carotid TIA.
Innominate ✦ Brachiocephalic artery	Neurologic dysfunction: signs and symptoms of vertebrobasilar occlusion. Indications of ischemia (claudication) of right arm; possible bruit over right side of neck.
Subclavian artery	Subclavian steal syndrome (characterized by blood backflow from the brain through the vertebral artery on the same side as the occlusion, into the subclavian artery distal to the occlusion); clinical effects of vertebrobasilar occlusion and exercise-induced arm claudication. Possible gangrene, usually limited to the digits.
Mesenteric artery ✦ Superior (most commonly affected) ✦ Celiac axis ✦ Inferior	Bowel ischemia, infarct necrosis, and gangrene; sudden, acute abdominal pain; nausea and vomiting; diarrhea; leukocytosis; and shock due to massive intraluminal fluid and plasma loss.
Aortic bifurcation (saddle block occlusion, a medical emergency associated with cardiac embolization)	Sensory and motor deficits (muscle weakness, numbness, paresthesias, paralysis) and signs of ischemia (sudden pain and cold, pale legs with decreased or absent peripheral pulses) in both legs.
Iliac artery (Leriche's syndrome)	Intermittent claudication of lower back, buttocks, and thighs, relieved by rest; absent or reduced femoral or distal pulses; possible bruit over femoral arteries; impotence in males.
Femoral and popliteal artery (associated with aneurysm formation)	Intermittent claudication of the calves on exertion; ischemic pain in feet; pretrophic pain (heralds necrosis and ulceration); leg pallor and coolness; blanching of feet on elevation; gangrene; no palpable pulses in ankles and feet.

Key signs and symptoms of arterial occlusive disease

✦ Neurologic dysfunction
✦ Subclavian steal syndrome
✦ Bowel ischemia
✦ Sensory and motor deficits
✦ Intermittent claudication of lower back, buttocks, and thighs
✦ Intermittent claudication of calves

ophthalmodynamometer. More than a 20% difference between pressures suggests insufficiency. EEG and computed tomography scan may be necessary to rule out brain lesions.

TREATMENT

Treatment of arterial occlusive disease depends on the cause, location, and size of the obstruction. For mild chronic disease, supportive measures include smoking cessation, hypertension control, and mild exercise such as walking. For carotid artery occlusion, antiplatelet therapy may begin with ticlopidine (Ticlid) or clopidogrel (Plavix) and aspirin. For intermittent claudication of chronic occlusive disease, pentoxifylline (Trental) and cilostazol may improve blood flow through the capillaries, particularly for patients who are poor candidates for surgery.

If a patient has acute arterial occlusive disease, his condition will usually require surgery to restore circulation to the affected area. Several different surgical options are available. For example:

✦ *Embolectomy:* a balloon-tipped Fogarty catheter is used to remove thrombotic material from the artery. Embolectomy is commonly used for mesenteric, femoral, or popliteal artery occlusive disease.

✦ *Thromboendarterectomy:* opening of the occluded artery and direct removal of the obstructing thrombus and the medial layer of the arterial wall; usually performed after angiography and commonly used with autogenous vein or Dacron bypass surgery (femoral-popliteal or aortofemoral).

✦ *Patch grafting:* the thrombosed arterial segment is removed and replaced with an autogenous vein or Dacron graft.

✦ *Bypass graft:* blood flow is diverted through an anastomosed autogenous or Dacron graft past the thrombosed segment.

✦ *Thrombolytic therapy:* urokinase, streptokinase, or alteplase causes lysis of the clot around or in the plaque.

✦ *Atherectomy:* plaque is excised using a drill or slicing mechanism.

✦ *Balloon angioplasty:* balloon inflation compresses the obstruction.

✦ *Laser angioplasty:* the obstruction is excised and vaporized using hot-tip lasers.

✦ *Stents:* meshes of wires that stretch and mold to the arterial wall are inserted to prevent reocclusion. This adjunct therapy follows laser angioplasty or atherectomy.

Combined therapy, which is simply the concomitant use of any of these surgical treatments, may be appropriate. Also, lumbar sympathectomy is a possible adjunct to surgery, depending on the condition of the sympathetic nervous system.

Amputation becomes necessary if arterial reconstructive surgery fails or if gangrene, persistent infection, or intractable pain develops.

Other therapy includes heparin to prevent emboli (for embolic occlusion) and bowel resection after restoration of blood flow (for mesenteric artery occlusion).

NURSING CONSIDERATIONS

✦ Provide comprehensive patient teaching such as proper foot care.
✦ Explain all diagnostic tests and procedures.
✦ Advise the patient to stop smoking and to follow the prescribed medical regimen.

Before surgery, during an acute episode

✦ Assess the patient's circulatory status by checking for the most distal pulses and by inspecting his skin color and temperature.
✦ Provide pain relief as needed.
✦ Administer heparin by continuous I.V. drip, as ordered, using an infusion pump to ensure the proper flow rate.
✦ Wrap the patient's affected foot in soft cotton batting, and reposition it frequently to prevent pressure on any one area.
✦ Strictly avoid elevating or applying heat to the affected leg.

Treatment

Mild chronic disease
✦ Smoking cessation
✦ Hypertension control
✦ Mild exercise

Carotid artery occlusion
✦ Antiplatelet therapy with ticlopidine or clopidogrel and aspirin

Chronic occlusive disease
✦ Pentoxifylline and cilostazol

Acute arterial occlusive disease
✦ Embolectomy
✦ Thromboendarterectomy
✦ Patch grafting
✦ Bypass graft
✦ Thrombolytic therapy
✦ Atherectomy
✦ Balloon angioplasty
✦ Laser angioplasty
✦ Stents

Key nursing actions

✦ Provide comprehensive patient teaching such as proper foot care.
✦ Advise the patient to stop smoking and to follow the prescribed medical regimen.

Before surgery, during an acute episode

✦ Assess the patient's circulatory status by checking for the most distal pulses and by inspecting his skin color and temperature.
✦ Wrap the patient's affected foot in soft cotton batting, and reposition it frequently to prevent pressure on any one area.
✦ Strictly avoid elevating or applying heat to the affected leg.

Key nursing actions

After surgery to restore circulation

- In carotid, innominate, vertebral, or subclavian artery occlusion, assess neurologic status.
- In mesenteric artery occlusion: connect an NG tube to low intermittent suction.
- In saddle block occlusion: check distal pulses for adequate circulation.
- In iliac artery occlusion: monitor urine output for renal failure.
- In femoral and popliteal artery occlusions: assist the patient with early ambulation.
- After amputation, check the patient's stump carefully for drainage.

Characteristics of cardiac arrhythmias

- Abnormal electrical conduction or automaticity changes heart's rate and rhythm
- Mild to catastrophic
- Classified by origin
- Effect on cardiac output and blood pressure determines clinical significance

Causes

- Congenital defects
- Myocardial ischemia
- Drug toxicity
- Degeneration of conductive tissue
- Hypertrophy of heart muscle
- Acid-base imbalances

✦ Watch for signs of fluid and electrolyte imbalance, and monitor intake and output for signs of renal failure (urine output less than 30 ml/hour).
✦ If the patient has carotid, innominate, vertebral, or subclavian artery occlusion, monitor him for signs of stroke, such as numbness in his arm or leg and intermittent blindness.

After surgery to restore circulation

✦ Monitor the patient's vital signs. Continuously assess his circulatory function by inspecting skin color and temperature and by checking for distal pulses. When charting, compare earlier assessments and observations. Watch closely for signs of hemorrhage (tachycardia and hypotension), and check dressings for excessive bleeding.
✦ In carotid, innominate, vertebral, or subclavian artery occlusion, assess the patient's neurologic status frequently for changes in level of consciousness, muscle strength, and pupil size.
✦ In mesenteric artery occlusion, connect a nasogastric tube to low intermittent suction. Monitor the patient's intake and output (low urine output may indicate damage to renal arteries during surgery). Check bowel sounds for return of peristalsis. Increased abdominal distention and tenderness may indicate extension of bowel ischemia with resulting gangrene, necessitating further excision, or it may indicate peritonitis.
✦ In saddle block occlusion, check distal pulses for adequate circulation. Watch for signs of renal failure and mesenteric artery occlusion (severe abdominal pain) as well as cardiac arrhythmias, which may precipitate embolus formation.
✦ In iliac artery occlusion, monitor urine output for signs of renal failure from decreased perfusion to the kidneys as a result of surgery. Provide meticulous catheter care.
✦ In femoral and popliteal artery occlusions, assist the patient with early ambulation; discourage prolonged sitting.
✦ After amputation, check the patient's stump carefully for drainage and record its color and amount and the time. Elevate the stump, as ordered, and administer adequate analgesic medication. Because phantom limb pain is common, explain this phenomenon to the patient, and administer analgesics as ordered.
✦ When preparing the patient for discharge, instruct him to watch for signs of recurrence (pain, pallor, numbness, paralysis, and absence of pulse) that can result from graft occlusion or occlusion at another site. Warn him against wearing constrictive clothing.

CARDIAC ARRHYTHMIAS

In arrhythmias, abnormal electrical conduction or automaticity changes the heart's rate and rhythm. Arrhythmias vary in severity, from those that are mild, asymptomatic, and require no treatment (such as sinus arrhythmia, in which heart rate increases and decreases with respiration) to catastrophic ventricular fibrillation, which requires immediate resuscitation. Arrhythmias are generally classified according to their origin (ventricular or supraventricular). Their effect on cardiac output and blood pressure, partially influenced by the site of origin, determines their clinical significance.

CAUSES

Common causes of arrhythmias include congenital defects, myocardial ischemia, myocardial infarction (MI), organic heart disease, drug toxicity, degeneration of the conductive tissue, connective tissue disorders, electrolyte imbalances, cellular hypoxia, hypertrophy of the heart muscle, acid-base imbalances, and emotional stress.

However, each arrhythmia may have its own specific causes. (See *Types of cardiac arrhythmias*, pages 162 to 169.)

PATHOPHYSIOLOGY

Arrhythmias may result from enhanced automaticity, reentry, escape beats, or abnormal electrical conduction. (See *Comparing normal and abnormal conduction*, pages 170 and 171.)

SIGNS AND SYMPTOMS

Signs and symptoms of arrhythmias result from reduced cardiac output and altered perfusion to the organs. These signs and symptoms may include dyspnea; hypotension; dizziness, syncope, and weakness; chest pain; cool, clammy skin; altered level of consciousness; and reduced urinary output.

COMPLICATIONS

Complications of arrhythmias may include sudden cardiac death, MI, heart failure, and thromboembolism.

DIAGNOSIS

Various tests help identify arrhythmias. Electrocardiography (ECG) detects arrhythmias as well as ischemia and infarction that may result in arrhythmias. Laboratory testing may reveal serum electrolyte abnormalities, acid-base abnormalities, or toxic drug levels that may cause arrhythmias. Holter monitoring, event monitoring, and loop recording can detect arrhythmias and the effectiveness of drug therapy during a patient's daily activities. Exercise testing may detect exercise-induced arrhythmias. Electrophysiologic testing, an invasive procedure, identifies the mechanism of an arrhythmia and the location of accessory pathways. This test also assesses the effectiveness of antiarrhythmic drugs, radiofrequency ablation, and implanted cardioverter-defibrillators.

TREATMENT

Follow the specific treatment guidelines for each arrhythmia. (See *Types of cardiac arrhythmias*, pages 162 to 169.)

NURSING CONSIDERATIONS

✦ Take the patient's pulse.
✦ If the patient's pulse is abnormally rapid, slow, or irregular, watch for signs of hypoperfusion, such as hypotension, decreased level of consciousness, and diminished urine output.
✦ Document arrhythmias in a monitored patient, and assess for possible causes and effects.
✦ When life-threatening arrhythmias develop, rapidly assess respirations, pulse rate, and level of consciousness.
✦ Initiate cardiopulmonary resuscitation, if indicated.
✦ Evaluate the patient for altered cardiac output resulting from arrhythmias.

(Text continues on page 168.)

How it happens
✦ Enhanced automaticity
✦ Reentry
✦ Escape beats
✦ Abnormal electrical conduction

Key signs and symptoms
✦ Dyspnea
✦ Hypotension
✦ Dizziness
✦ Syncope
✦ Chest pain
✦ Cool, clammy skin
✦ Reduced urinary output

Complications
✦ Sudden cardiac death
✦ MI
✦ Heart failure
✦ Thromboembolism

Diagnosis
✦ ECG
✦ Laboratory testing
✦ Holter and event monitoring
✦ Loop recording

Key nursing actions
✦ Assess the patient for rhythm disturbances.
✦ Watch for hypoperfusion.
✦ When life-threatening arrhythmias develop, rapidly assess respirations, pulse rate, and consciousness.
✦ Monitor for predisposing factors and signs of drug toxicity.
✦ If the patient has a permanent pacemaker, warn him about environmental hazards.

Types of cardiac arrhythmias

This chart reviews many common cardiac arrhythmias and outlines their features, causes, and treatments. Use a normal electrocardiogram strip, if available, to compare normal cardiac rhythm configurations with the rhythm strips here. Characteristics of normal sinus rhythm include:
- ✦ ventricular and atrial rates of 60 to 100 beats/minute
- ✦ regular and uniform QRS complexes and P waves
- ✦ PR interval of 0.12 to 0.20 second
- ✦ QRS duration < 0.12 second
- ✦ identical atrial and ventricular rates, with constant PR intervals.

ARRHYTHMIA AND FEATURES

Sinus tachycardia

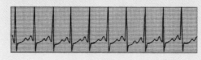

- ✦ Atrial and ventricular rhythms regular
- ✦ Rate > 100 beats/minute; rarely, > 160 beats/minute
- ✦ Normal P wave preceding each QRS complex

Sinus bradycardia

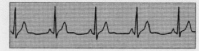

- ✦ Atrial and ventricular rhythms regular
- ✦ Rate < 60 beats/minute
- ✦ Normal P waves preceding each QRS complex

Paroxysmal supraventricular tachycardia

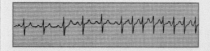

- ✦ Atrial and ventricular rhythms regular
- ✦ Rate > 160 beats/minute; rarely exceeds 250 beats/minute
- ✦ P waves regular but aberrant; difficult to differentiate from preceding T wave
- ✦ P wave preceding each QRS complex
- ✦ Sudden onset and termination of arrhythmia

ECG characteristics: Sinus tachycardia

- ✦ Atrial and ventricular rhythms regular
- ✦ Rate > 100 beats/minute; rarely > 160 beats/minute
- ✦ Normal P wave preceding each QRS complex

ECG characteristics: Sinus bradycardia

- ✦ Atrial and ventricular rhythms regular
- ✦ Rate < 60 beats/minute
- ✦ Normal P waves preceding each QRS complex

CAUSES	TREATMENT
✦ Normal physiologic response to fever, exercise, anxiety, pain, dehydration; may also accompany shock, left-sided heart failure, cardiac tamponade, hyperthyroidism, anemia, hypovolemia, pulmonary embolism, and anterior wall myocardial infarction (MI) ✦ May also occur with atropine, epinephrine, isoproterenol (Isuprel), quinidine (Quinaglute), caffeine, alcohol, cocaine, amphetamine, and nicotine use	✦ Correction of underlying cause ✦ Beta-adrenergic blockers or calcium channel blockers for symptomatic patients
✦ Normal, in well-conditioned heart, as in an athlete ✦ Increased intracranial pressure; increased vagal tone due to straining during defecation, vomiting, intubation, or mechanical ventilation; sick sinus syndrome; hypothyroidism; and inferior wall MI ✦ May also occur with anticholinesterase, beta-adrenergic blocker, digoxin (Lanoxin), and morphine use	✦ Correction of underlying cause ✦ For low cardiac output, dizziness, weakness, altered level of consciousness, or low blood pressure; advanced cardiac life support (ACLS) protocol for administration of atropine ✦ Temporary or permanent pacemaker ✦ Dopamine or epinephrine infusion
✦ Intrinsic abnormality of atrioventricular (AV) conduction system ✦ Physical or psychological stress, hypoxia, hypokalemia, cardiomyopathy, congenital heart disease, MI, valvular disease, Wolff-Parkinson-White syndrome, cor pulmonale, hyperthyroidism, and systemic hypertension ✦ Digoxin toxicity; use of caffeine, marijuana, or central nervous system stimulants	✦ If the patient is unstable, immediate cardioversion ✦ If the patient is stable, vagal stimulation, Valsalva's maneuver, and carotid sinus massage ✦ If cardiac function is preserved, treatment priority: calcium channel blocker, beta-adrenergic blocker, digoxin, and cardioversion; then consider procainamide, amiodarone, or sotalol if each preceding treatment is ineffective in rhythm conversion ✦ If the ejection fraction is less than 40% or if the patient is in heart failure, treatment order: digoxin, amiodarone, then diltiazem

ECG characteristics: Paroxysmal supraventricular tachycardia

✦ Atrial and ventricular rhythms regular
✦ Rate > 160 beats/minute; rarely exceeds 250 beats/minute
✦ P waves regular but aberrant; difficult to differentiate from preceding T wave
✦ P wave preceding each QRS complex
✦ Sudden onset and termination of arrhythmia

(continued)

ECG characteristics: Atrial flutter

- ✦ Atrial rhythm regular, rate 250 to 400 beats/minute
- ✦ Ventricular rate variable, depending on degree of AV block (usually 60 to 100 beats/minute)
- ✦ Sawtooth P-wave configuration possible (F waves)
- ✦ QRS complexes uniform in shape but often irregular in rate

ECG characteristics: Atrial fibrillation

- ✦ Atrial rhythm grossly irregular; rate > 400 beats/minute
- ✦ Ventricular rhythm irregular
- ✦ QRS complexes of uniform configuration and duration
- ✦ PR interval indiscernible
- ✦ No P waves or P waves that appear as erratic, irregular, baseline fibrillatory waves

Types of cardiac arrhythmias *(continued)*

ARRHYTHMIA AND FEATURES

Atrial flutter

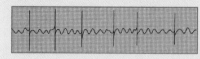

- ✦ Atrial rhythm regular; rate 250 to 400 beats/minute
- ✦ Ventricular rate variable, depending on degree of AV block (usually 60 to 100 beats/minute)
- ✦ Sawtooth P-wave configuration possible (F waves)
- ✦ QRS complexes uniform in shape, but often irregular in rate

Atrial fibrillation

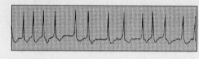

- ✦ Atrial rhythm grossly irregular; rate > 400 beats/minute
- ✦ Ventricular rhythm irregular
- ✦ QRS complexes of uniform configuration and duration
- ✦ PR interval indiscernible
- ✦ No P waves or P waves that appear as erratic, irregular, baseline fibrillatory waves (F waves)

Junctional rhythm

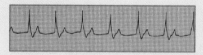

- ✦ Atrial and ventricular rhythms regular; atrial rate 40 to 60 beats/minute; ventricular rate usually 40 to 60 beats/minute (60 to 100 beats/minute is accelerated junctional rhythm)
- ✦ P waves preceding, hidden within (absent), or after QRS complex; usually inverted if visible
- ✦ PR interval (when present) < 0.12 second
- ✦ QRS complex configuration and duration normal, except in aberrant conduction

First-degree AV block

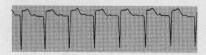

- ✦ Atrial and ventricular rhythms regular
- ✦ PR interval > 0.20 second
- ✦ P wave precedes QRS complex
- ✦ QRS complex normal

CAUSES	TREATMENT
✦ Heart failure, tricuspid or mitral valve disease, pulmonary embolism, cor pulmonale, inferior wall MI, and pericarditis ✦ Digoxin toxicity	✦ If the patient is unstable with a ventricular rate > 150 beats/minute, immediate cardioversion ✦ If the patient is stable drug therapy may include calcium channel blockers, beta-adrenergic blockers, or antiarrhythmics ✦ Anticoagulation therapy (heparin, enoxaparin [Lovenox]) or warfarin (Coumadin) may also be necessary ✦ Radiofrequency ablation to control rhythm
✦ Heart failure, chronic obstructive pulmonary disease, thyrotoxicosis, constrictive pericarditis, ischemic heart disease, sepsis, pulmonary embolus, rheumatic heart disease, hypertension, mitral stenosis, atrial irritation, or complication of coronary bypass or valve replacement surgery ✦ Nifedipine (Procardia or Adalat) and digoxin use	✦ If the patient is unstable with a ventricular rate > 150 beats/minute, immediate cardioversion ✦ If the patient is stable, follow ACLS protocol for cardioversion and drug therapy, which may include calcium channel blockers, beta-adrenergic blockers, or antiarrhythmics ✦ Anticoagulants, such as heparin, enoxaparin, or warfarin. ✦ Class III antiarrhythmic, dofetilide (Tikosyn) for conversion of atrial fibrillation and atrial flutter to normal sinus rhythm ✦ Radiofrequency catheter ablation to the bundle of His to interrupt all conduction between atria and the ventricles (in resistant patients with recurring symptomatic atrial fibrillation) ✦ Maze procedure, in which sutures are placed in strategic places in the atrial myocardium to prevent electrical circuits from developing perpetuating atrial fibrillation
✦ Inferior wall MI or ischemia, hypoxia, vagal stimulation, and sick sinus syndrome ✦ Acute rheumatic fever ✦ Valve surgery ✦ Digoxin toxicity, response to calcium channel blocker	✦ Correction of underlying cause ✦ Atropine for symptomatic slow rate ✦ Pacemaker insertion if the patient doesn't respond to drugs ✦ Discontinuation of digoxin if appropriate
✦ May be seen in healthy people ✦ Inferior wall MI or ischemia, hypothyroidism, hypokalemia, and hyperkalemia ✦ Digoxin toxicity; use of quinidine, procainamide (Pronestyl), beta-adrenergic blockers, calcium channel blockers, or amiodarone (Cordarone)	✦ Correction of underlying cause ✦ Possibly atropine if severe symptomatic bradycardia develops ✦ Cautious use of digoxin, calcium channel blockers, and beta-adrenergic blockers *(continued)*

ECG characteristics: Junctional rhythm

✦ Atrial and ventricular rhythms regular; atrial rate 40 to 60 beats/minute; ventricular rate usually 40 to 60 beats/minute (60 to 100 beats/minute is accelerated junctional rhythm)
✦ P waves preceding, hidden within (absent), or after QRS complex; inverted if visible
✦ PR interval (when present) < 0.12 second
✦ QRS complex configuration and duration normal, except in aberrant conduction

ECG characteristics: First-degree AV block

✦ Atrial and ventricular rhythms regular
✦ PR interval > 0.20 second
✦ P wave precedes QRS complex
✦ QRS complex normal

ECG characteristics: Second-degree AV block (Mobitz I)

✦ Atrial rhythm regular
✦ Ventricular rhythm irregular
✦ Atrial rate exceeds ventricular rate
✦ PR interval progressively longer with each cycle until QRS complex disappears; PR interval shorter after dropped beat

ECG characteristics: Second-degree AV block (Mobitz II)

✦ Atrial rhythm regular
✦ Ventricular rhythm regular or irregular with varying degree of block
✦ PR interval constant
✦ QRS complexes periodically absent

Types of cardiac arrhythmias *(continued)*

ARRHYTHMIA AND FEATURES

Second-degree AV block
Mobitz I (Wenckebach)

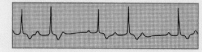

✦ Atrial rhythm regular
✦ Ventricular rhythm irregular
✦ Atrial rate exceeds ventricular rate
✦ PR interval progressively, but only slightly, longer with each cycle until QRS complex disappears (dropped beat); PR interval shorter after dropped beat

Second-degree AV block
Mobitz II

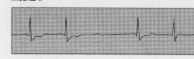

✦ Atrial rhythm regular
✦ Ventricular rhythm regular or irregular, with varying degree of block
✦ PR interval constant
✦ QRS complexes periodically absent

Third-degree AV block
(complete heart block)

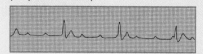

✦ Atrial rhythm regular
✦ Ventricular rhythm regular and rate slower than atrial rate
✦ No relation between P waves and QRS complexes
✦ No constant PR interval
✦ QRS interval normal (nodal pacemaker) or wide and bizarre (ventricular pacemaker)
✦ P wave may be buried in QRS complexes or T wave
✦ QRS complex normal

Premature ventricular contraction (PVC)

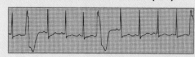

✦ Atrial rhythm regular
✦ Ventricular rhythm irregular
✦ QRS complex premature, usually followed by a complete compensatory pause
✦ QRS complex wide and distorted, usually > 0.14 second
✦ Premature QRS complexes occurring alone, in pairs, or in threes, alternating with normal beats; focus from one or more sites
✦ Ominous when clustered, multifocal, with R wave on T pattern

CAUSES	TREATMENT
✦ Inferior wall MI, cardiac surgery, acute rheumatic fever, and vagal stimulation ✦ Digoxin toxicity; use of propranolol (Inderal), quinidine, or procainamide	✦ Treatment of underlying cause ✦ Atropine or temporary pacemaker for symptomatic bradycardia ✦ Discontinuation of digoxin if appropriate
✦ Severe coronary artery disease, anterior wall MI, and acute myocarditis ✦ Digoxin toxicity	✦ Temporary or permanent pacemaker ✦ Atropine, dopamine, or epinephrine for symptomatic bradycardia ✦ Discontinuation of digoxin if appropriate
✦ Inferior or anterior wall MI, congenital abnormality, rheumatic fever, hypoxia, postoperative complication of mitral valve replacement, postprocedure complication of radiofrequency ablation in or near AV nodal tissue, Lev's disease (fibrosis and calcification that spreads from cardiac structures to the conductive tissue), and Lenègre's disease (conductive tissue fibrosis) ✦ Digoxin toxicity	✦ Atropine, dopamine, or epinephrine for symptomatic bradycardia ✦ Temporary or permanent pacemaker
✦ Heart failure; old or acute MI, ischemia, or contusion; myocardial irritation by ventricular catheter or a pacemaker; hypercapnia; hypokalemia; hypocalcemia; and hypomagnesemia ✦ Drug toxicity (digoxin, aminophylline, tricyclic antidepressants, beta-adrenergic blockers, isoproterenol, or dopamine [Intropin]) ✦ Caffeine, tobacco, or alcohol use ✦ Psychological stress, anxiety, pain, or exercise	✦ If warranted, procainamide, amiodarone, or lidocaine I.V. ✦ Treatment of underlying cause ✦ Discontinuation of drug causing toxicity ✦ Potassium chloride I.V., if PVC induced by hypokalemia ✦ Magnesium sulfate I.V., if PVC induced by hypomagnesemia

(continued)

ECG characteristics: Third-degree AV block

✦ Atrial rhythm regular
✦ Ventricular rate slower than atrial rate and rhythm regular
✦ No relation between P waves and QRS complexes
✦ No constant PR interval
✦ QRS interval normal (nodal pacemaker) or wide and bizarre (ventricular pacemaker)
✦ P wave may be buried in QRS complexes or T wave
✦ QRS complex normal

ECG characteristics: PVC

✦ Atrial rhythm regular
✦ Ventricular rhythm irregular
✦ QRS complex premature, usually followed by a complete compensatory pause
✦ QRS complex wide and distorted, usually > 0.14 second
✦ Premature QRS complexes occurring singly, in pairs, or in threes, alternating with normal beats; focus from one or more sites
✦ Ominous when clustered, multifocal, with R wave on T pattern

ECG characteristics: Ventricular tachycardia

✦ Ventricular rate 140 to 220 beats/minute, rhythm regular or irregular
✦ QRS complexes wide, bizarre, and independent of P waves
✦ P waves not discernible
✦ May start and stop suddenly

ECG characteristics: Ventricular fibrillation

✦ Ventricular rhythm chaotic; rate rapid
✦ QRS complexes wide and irregular; no visible P waves

Types of cardiac arrhythmias *(continued)*

ARRHYTHMIA AND FEATURES

Ventricular tachycardia (VT)

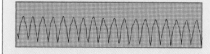

✦ Ventricular rate 140 to 220 beats/minute, rhythm regular or irregular
✦ QRS complexes wide, bizarre, and independent of P waves
✦ P waves not discernible
✦ May start and stop suddenly

Ventricular fibrillation

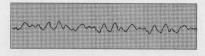

✦ Ventricular rhythm chaotic; rate rapid
✦ QRS complexes wide and irregular; no visible P waves

Asystole

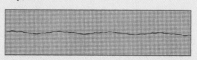

✦ No atrial or ventricular rate or rhythm
✦ No discernible P waves, QRS complexes, or T waves

✦ Administer medications as ordered, and prepare to assist with medical procedures, if indicated (for example, cardioversion).
✦ Monitor for predisposing factors — such as fluid and electrolyte imbalances — and signs of drug toxicity, especially with digoxin (Lanoxin). If you suspect drug toxicity, report such signs to the physician immediately and withhold the next dose.
✦ To prevent arrhythmias in a postoperative cardiac patient, provide adequate oxygen and reduce the heart's workload while carefully maintaining metabolic, neurologic, respiratory, and hemodynamic status.
✦ To avoid temporary pacemaker malfunction, install a fresh battery before each insertion. Carefully secure the external catheter wires and the pacemaker box. As-

CAUSES	TREATMENT
✦ Myocardial ischemia, MI, or aneurysm; coronary artery disease; rheumatic heart disease; mitral valve prolapse; heart failure; cardiomyopathy; ventricular catheters; hypokalemia; hypercalcemia; hypomagnesemia; and pulmonary embolism ✦ Digoxin, procainamide, epinephrine, or quinidine toxicity ✦ Anxiety	✦ Pulseless: Initiate CPR; follow ACLS protocol for defibrillation, endotracheal (ET) intubation, and administration of epinephrine or vasopressin (Pitressin), followed by amiodarone or lidocaine and, if ineffective, magnesium sulfate or procainamide ✦ With pulse: If hemodynamically stable, monomorphic VT administration of procainamide, sotalol, amiodarone or lidocaine (follow ACLS protocol); if drugs are ineffective, initiate synchronized cardioversion ✦ If polymorphic VT, administer beta-adrenergic blockers, lidocaine, amiodarone, procainamide, or sotalol (follow ACLS protocol); if drug is unsuccessful, initiate synchronized cardioversion ✦ If torsades, magnesium I.V., then overdrive pacing if rhythm persists; may also administer isoproterenol, phenytoin (Dilantin), or lidocaine ✦ Implanted cardioverter defibrillator if recurrent VT
✦ Myocardial ischemia, MI, untreated ventricular tachycardia, R-on-T phenomenon, hypokalemia, hyperkalemia, hypercalcemia, hypoxemia, alkalosis, electric shock, and hypothermia ✦ Digoxin, epinephrine, or quinidine toxicity	✦ Pulseless CPR: follow ACLS defibrillation protocol for ET intubation, and administration of epinephrine or vasopressin, amiodarone, or lidocaine, and if ineffective, magnesium sulfate or procainamide and atropine. ✦ Implanted cardioverter defibrillator if risk for recurrent ventricular fibrillation.
✦ Myocardial ischemia, MI, aortic valve disease, heart failure, hypoxia, hypokalemia, severe acidosis, electric shock, ventricular arrhythmia, AV block, pulmonary embolism, heart rupture, cardiac tamponade, hyperkalemia, and electromechanical dissociation ✦ Cocaine overdose	✦ Continue CPR, follow ACLS protocol for ET intubation, transcutaneous or transvenous pacing, and administration of epinephrine and atropine.

ECG characteristics: Asystole

✦ No atrial or ventricular rate or rhythm
✦ No discernible P waves, QRS complexes, or T waves

sess the threshold daily. Watch closely for premature contractions, a sign of myocardial irritation.
✦ To avert permanent pacemaker malfunction, restrict the patient's activity after insertion, as ordered. Monitor the pulse rate regularly, and watch for signs of decreased cardiac output.
✦ If the patient has a permanent pacemaker, warn him about environmental hazards, as indicated by the pacemaker's manufacturer. Although hazards may not present a problem, 24-hour Holter monitoring may be helpful. Tell the patient to report light-headedness or syncope, and stress the importance of regular checkups.

Cardiac conduction

Normal
+ Begins at SA node
+ Impulse travels through atria along Bachmann's bundle to the AV node
+ Ends up at Purkinje fibers to the ventricles

Abnormal
+ Altered automacity increases the intrinsic rate of the SA node
+ Ischemia or a deformity causes abnormal circuit within conductive fibers
+ Alternative reentry mechanism depends on presence of congenial accessory pathway linking the atria and ventricles
+ Conduction disturbances occur when impulses are conducted too quickly or slowly

Characteristics of cardiomyopathy
+ Life-threatening
+ Disease of heart muscle fibers
+ Occurs in three main forms: dilated, hypertrophic, and restrictive
+ Second most common direct cause of sudden death
+ Approximately 5 to 8 per 100,000 U.S. residents have dilated cardiomyopathy; prognosis is poor
+ Two types of hypertrophic cardiomyopathy: obstructive and nonobstructive
+ Restrictive cardiomyopathy results from fibrosis of cardiac muscle

---

CLOSER LOOK

Comparing normal and abnormal conduction

NORMAL CARDIAC CONDUCTION
The heart's conduction system, shown here, begins at the sinoatrial (SA) node — the heart's pacemaker. When an impulse leaves the SA node, it travels through the atria along Bachmann's bundle and the internodal pathways to the atrioventricular (AV) node, and then down the bundle of His, along the bundle branches and, finally, down the Purkinje fibers to the ventricles.

ABNORMAL CARDIAC CONDUCTION
Altered automaticity, reentry, or conduction disturbances may cause cardiac arrhythmias.

Altered automaticity
Altered automaticity is the result of partial depolarization, which may increase the intrinsic rate of the SA node or latent pacemakers, or may induce ectopic pacemakers to reach threshold and depolarize.

Automaticity may be altered by drugs, such as epinephrine (Adrenalin), atropine, and digoxin (Lanoxin), and such conditions as acidosis, alkalosis, hypoxia, myocardial infarc-tion (MI), hypokalemia, and hypocalcemia. Examples of arrhythmias caused by altered automaticity include atrial fibrillation and flutter; supraventricular tachycardia; premature atrial, junctional, and ventricular complexes; ventricular tachycardia (VT) and fibrillation; and accelerated idioventricular and junctional rhythms.

Reentry
Ischemia or a deformity causes an abnormal circuit to develop within conductive fibers. Although current flow is blocked in one direction within the circuit, the descending impulse can travel in the other direction. By the time the impulse completes the circuit, the previously depolarized tissue within the circuit is no longer refractory to stimulation, allowing reentry of the impulse and repetition of this cycle.

Conditions that increase the likelihood of reentry include hyperkalemia, myocardial ischemia, and the use of certain antiarrhythmic drugs. Reentry may be responsible for such arrhythmias as paroxysmal supraventricular

---

▼ LIFE-THREATENING DISORDER

CARDIOMYOPATHY

Cardiomyopathy generally applies to disease of the heart muscle fibers, and it occurs in three main forms: dilated, hypertrophic, and restrictive (extremely rare). Cardiomyopathy is the second most common direct cause of sudden death; coronary artery disease (CAD) is first. Approximately 5 to 8 per 100,000 U.S. residents have *dilated cardiomyopathy,* the most common type. At greatest risk for dilated cardiomyopathy are males and blacks; other risk factors include CAD, hypertension, pregnancy, viral infections, and alcohol or illegal drug use. Because dilated cardiomyopathy usually isn't diagnosed until its advanced stages, the prognosis is generally poor.

Hypertrophic cardiomyopathy can occur in very young and aged patients. However, it's most common in young adults and athletic patients and puts them at risk for sudden death. There are two types of hypertrophic cardiomyopathy: obstructive hypertrophic cardiomyopathy and nonobstructive hypertrophic cardiomyopathy.

Restrictive cardiomyopathy occurs as a result of fibrosis of the cardiac muscle due to a process of infiltration.

tachycardia; premature atrial, junctional, and ventricular complexes; and VT.

An alternative reentry mechanism depends on the presence of a congenital accessory pathway linking the atria and the ventricles outside the AV junction; for example, Wolff-Parkinson-White syndrome.

Conduction disturbances
Conduction disturbances occur when impulses are conducted too quickly or too slowly. Possible causes include trauma, drug toxicity, myocardial ischemia, MI, and electrolyte abnormalities. The AV blocks occur as a result of conduction disturbances.

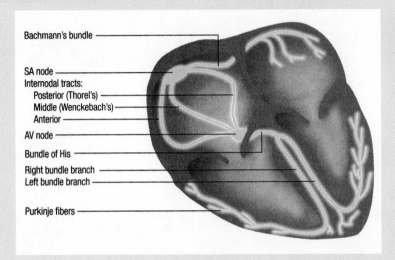

Bachmann's bundle
SA node
Internodal tracts:
Posterior (Thorel's)
Middle (Wenckebach's)
Anterior
AV node
Bundle of His
Right bundle branch
Left bundle branch
Purkinje fibers

CAUSES

Most patients with dilated cardiomyopathy have idiopathic, or primary, disease; however, some are secondary to identifiable causes. (See *Comparing the cardiomyopathies,* pages 172 and 173.)

Hypertrophic cardiomyopathy can be transmitted as an autosomal genetic disorder or may have no genetic component at all. Restrictive cardiomyopathy can be caused by amyloidosis, sarcoidosis, hemochromatosis, or may be the result of a parasitic infection.

PATHOPHYSIOLOGY

Dilated cardiomyopathy results from extensively damaged myocardial muscle fibers. Consequently, there's reduced contractility in the left ventricle. As systolic function declines, stroke volume, ejection fraction, and cardiac output fall. As end-diastolic volumes rise, pulmonary congestion may occur. The elevated end-diastolic volume is a compensatory response to preserve stroke volume despite a reduced ejection fraction. The sympathetic nervous system is also stimulated to increase heart rate and contractility. The kidneys are stimulated to retain sodium and water to maintain cardiac output, and vasoconstriction also occurs as the renin-angiotensin system is stimulated. When these compensatory mechanisms can no longer maintain cardiac output, the heart begins to fail. Left ventricular dilation oc-

Causes
+ Idiopathic disease
+ Secondary to identifiable causes
+ Hypertrophic cardiomyopathy can be transmitted as an autosomal genetic disorder or may have no genetic component
+ Restrictive cardiomyopathy can be caused by amyloidosis, sarcoidosis, hemochromatosis, or may be result of a parasitic infection

How it happens
Dilated cardiomyopathy
+ Extensively damaged myocardial muscle fibers
+ Left ventricle contractility reduced
+ Systolic function declines; stroke volume, ejection fraction, and cardiac output fall
+ End-diastolic volumes rise; pulmonary congestion may occur
+ Vasoconstriction occurs as renin-angiotensin system is stimulated
+ Heart begins to fail when compensatory systems fail
+ Left ventricular dilation occurs as venous return and systemic vascular resistance rise
+ Atria dilate as more work is needed to pump blood into full ventricles
+ Cardiomegaly occurs as a consequence of dilation of atria and ventricles

Key signs of dilated cardiomyopathy

✦ Increased chamber size
✦ Increased myocardial mass
✦ Decreased contractility

Comparing the cardiomyopathies

Cardiomyopathies include a variety of structural or functional abnormalities of the ventricles. They're grouped into three main pathophysiologic types—dilated, hypertrophic, and restrictive. These conditions may lead to heart failure by impairing myocardial structure and function.

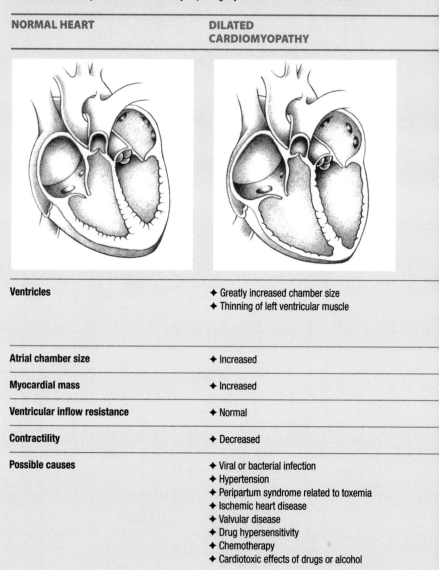

	NORMAL HEART	DILATED CARDIOMYOPATHY
Ventricles		✦ Greatly increased chamber size ✦ Thinning of left ventricular muscle
Atrial chamber size		✦ Increased
Myocardial mass		✦ Increased
Ventricular inflow resistance		✦ Normal
Contractility		✦ Decreased
Possible causes		✦ Viral or bacterial infection ✦ Hypertension ✦ Peripartum syndrome related to toxemia ✦ Ischemic heart disease ✦ Valvular disease ✦ Drug hypersensitivity ✦ Chemotherapy ✦ Cardiotoxic effects of drugs or alcohol

curs as venous return and systemic vascular resistance rise. Eventually, the atria also dilate, as more work is required to pump blood into the full ventricles. Cardiomegaly occurs as a consequence of dilation of the atria and ventricles. Blood pooling in the ventricles increases the risk of emboli.

HYPERTROPHIC CARDIOMYOPATHY

RESTRICTIVE CARDIOMYOPATHY

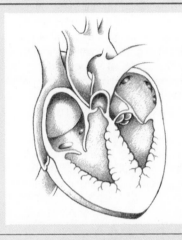

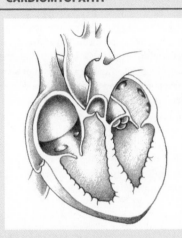

Hypertrophic cardiomyopathy	Restrictive cardiomyopathy
✦ Normal right and decreased left chamber size ✦ Left ventricular hypertrophy ✦ Thickened interventricular septum (obstructive hypertrophic cardiomyopathy)	✦ Decreased ventricular chamber size ✦ Left ventricular hypertrophy
✦ Increased on left	✦ Increased
✦ Increased	✦ Normal
✦ Increased	✦ Increased
✦ Increased or decreased	✦ Decreased
✦ Autosomal dominant trait (obstructive hypertrophic cardiomyopathy) ✦ Hypertension ✦ Obstructive valvular disease ✦ Thyroid disease	✦ Amyloidosis ✦ Sarcoidosis ✦ Hemochromatosis ✦ Infiltrative neoplastic disease

CLINICAL ALERT Barth syndrome is a rare genetic disorder that can cause dilated cardiomyopathy in boys. This syndrome may be associated with skeletal muscle changes, short stature, neutropenia, and increased susceptibility to bacterial infections. Evidence of dilated cardiomyopathy may appear as early as the first few days or months of life.

Key signs of hypertrophic cardiomyopathy

✦ Increased atrial chamber size (on left)
✦ Increased myocardial mass
✦ Increased or decreased contractility

Key signs of restrictive cardiomyopathy

✦ Increased atrial chamber size
✦ Normal myocardial mass
✦ Decreased contractility

Alert!

✦ Barth syndrome is a rare genetic disorder that can cause dilated cardiomyopathy in boys.
✦ Evidence of dilated cardiomyopathy may appear as early as the first few days or months of life.

How it happens

Nonobstructive hypertrophic cardiomyopathy

✦ Affects diastolic function
✦ Hypertrophied ventricle becomes stiff, noncompliant, and unable to relax during ventricular filling
✦ Ventricular filling reduced; left ventricular filling pressure rises
✦ Compensatory response leads to low cardiac output

Obstructive hypertrophic cardiomyopathy

✦ Asymmetrical left ventricular or intraventricular septum hypertrophy
✦ Rapid contractions of left ventricle
✦ Forceful ejection of blood draws anterior leaflet of mitral valve to intraventricular septum
✦ Early closure of outflow tract, decreasing ejection fraction results

Restrictive cardiomyopathy

✦ Stiffness of ventricle due to left ventricular hypertrophy and endocardial fibrosis and thickening
✦ Ability of ventricle to relax and fill during diastole reduced

Key signs and symptoms

Dilated cardiomyopathy

✦ Shortness of breath
✦ Orthopnea
✦ Hepatomegaly
✦ Jugular vein distention

Hypertrophic cardiomyopathy

✦ Dyspnea
✦ Fatigue
✦ Angina
✦ Pulsus biferiens

Restrictive cardiomyopathy

✦ Fatigue
✦ Liver engorgement
✦ S_3 or S_4 gallop rhythms

Unlike dilated cardiomyopathy, which affects systolic function, nonobstructive hypertrophic cardiomyopathy primarily affects diastolic function. The hypertrophied ventricle becomes stiff, noncompliant, and unable to relax during ventricular filling. Consequently, ventricular filling is reduced and left ventricular filling pressure rises, causing a rise in left atrial and pulmonary venous pressures and leading to venous congestion and dyspnea. Ventricular filling time is further reduced as a compensatory response to tachycardia leading to low cardiac output. If papillary muscles become hypertrophied and don't close completely during contraction, mitral insufficiency occurs.

The features of obstructive hypertrophic cardiomyopathy include asymmetrical left ventricular hypertrophy; hypertrophy of the intraventricular septum; rapid, forceful contractions of the left ventricle; impaired relaxation; and obstruction to left ventricular outflow. The forceful ejection of blood draws the anterior leaflet of the mitral valve to the intraventricular septum. This causes early closure of the outflow tract, decreasing ejection fraction. Moreover, intramural coronary arteries are abnormally small and may not be sufficient to supply the hypertrophied muscle with enough blood and oxygen to meet the increased needs of the hyperdynamic muscle.

Restrictive cardiomyopathy is characterized by stiffness of the ventricle caused by left ventricular hypertrophy and endocardial fibrosis and thickening, thus reducing the ability of the ventricle to relax and fill during diastole. Moreover, the rigid myocardium fails to contract completely during systole. As a result, cardiac output falls.

SIGNS AND SYMPTOMS

A patient with dilated cardiomyopathy may present with respiratory symptoms, such as shortness of breath, orthopnea, dyspnea on exertion, paroxysmal nocturnal dyspnea, and a dry cough at night, due to left-sided heart failure. He may have peripheral edema, hepatomegaly, jugular vein distention, and may have experienced weight gain due to right-sided heart failure.

A decrease in cardiac output results in decreased renal perfusion and worsening renal function, peripheral cyanosis, and tachycardia (a compensatory response). A pansystolic murmur may be present. This murmur is associated with mitral and tricuspid insufficiency and is secondary to cardiomegaly and weak papillary muscles. S_3 and S_4 gallop rhythms may also be heard and are associated with heart failure. The patient may have an irregular pulse if atrial fibrillation exists.

In hypertrophic cardiomyopathy, dyspnea is due to elevated left ventricular filling pressure and fatigue is due to reduced cardiac output. In this condition the intramural coronary arteries can't supply enough oxygen to meet the demands of the hypertrophied heart. This causes the patient to experience angina. Vigorous left ventricular contractions cause an abrupt arterial pulse and powerful left ventricular contractions. The rapid ejection of blood during systole causes a peripheral pulse with a characteristic double impulse, which is called *pulsus biferiens*. If the enlarged atrium causes atrial fibrillation, the patient will have an irregular pulse.

A systolic ejection murmur along the left sternal border at the apex is caused by mitral insufficiency. Syncope results from arrhythmias or reduced ventricular filling leading to reduced cardiac output. Activity intolerance is a result of worsening outflow tract obstruction from exercise induced catecholamine release. In patients with obstructive hypertrophic cardiomyopathy symptoms occur at rest. Patients with latent hypertrophic cardiomyopathy are symptomatic when standing or while exercising. Those with nonobstructive hypertrophic cardiomyopathy exhibit no signs or symptoms.

Clinical manifestations of restrictive cardiomyopathy may include fatigue, dyspnea, orthopnea, chest pain, edema, liver engorgement, peripheral cyanosis, pallor, and S_3 or S_4 gallop rhythms due to heart failure. Systolic murmurs are caused by mitral and tricuspid insufficiency.

COMPLICATIONS

Cardiomyopathy may result in such complications as heart failure, arrhythmias, systemic or pulmonary embolization, or sudden death.

DIAGNOSIS

Along with a physical examination, tests are available to help diagnose cardiomyopathy. Echocardiography can confirm a diagnosis of dilated cardiomyopathy, while a chest X-ray may reveal cardiomegaly associated with any of the cardiomyopathies. A cardiac catheterization is a diagnostic test that allows for possible heart biopsy, which can be definitive with obstructive hypertrophic cardiomyopathy. A diagnosis of cardiomyopathy requires elimination of other possible causes of heart failure and arrhythmias. (*See Comparing diagnostic tests in cardiomyopathy,* pages 176 and 177.)

TREATMENT

Dilated cardiomyopathy

Treatment of dilated cardiomyopathy seeks to correct the underlying causes and to improve the heart's pumping ability. Angiotensin-converting enzyme (ACE) inhibitors reduce afterload through vasodilation, thereby reducing heart failure. Diuretics are commonly given with an ACE inhibitor to reduce fluid retention. For the patient without improvement of symptoms on an ACE inhibitor and diuretic, digoxin (Lanoxin) may improve myocardial contractility.

Hydralazine (Apresoline) and isosorbide (Isordil), in combination, produce vasodilation. Antiarrhythmics, cardioversion, and pacemakers may be used to control arrhythmias. Although controversial, anticoagulants may be prescribed to reduce the risk of emboli. Treatment may also include oxygen, a sodium-restricted diet, and bed rest.

Surgical interventions in carefully selected patients may include revascularization such as coronary artery bypass grafting if ischemia is the cause of dilated cardiomyopathy; valvular repair or replacement, if dilated cardiomyopathy is due to valve dysfunction; cardiomyoplasty, in which the latissimus dorsi muscle is wrapped around the ventricles to assist the ventricles to pump more efficiently, may be considered when medical treatment fails; or a cardiomyostimulator delivering bursts of electrical impulses during systole to help the myocardium contract. Heart transplantation may be considered for patients who fail to respond to other treatments.

Lifestyle modifications, such as smoking cessation, a restricted diet (low-fat, low-sodium), physical activity, and abstinence from alcohol, are also important.

Hypertrophic cardiomyopathy

Treatment of hypertrophic cardiomyopathy seeks to relax the ventricle and to relieve outflow tract obstruction. Propranolol (Inderal), a beta-adrenergic blocker, slows heart rate and increases ventricular filling by relaxing the obstructing muscle, thereby reducing angina, syncope, dyspnea, and arrhythmias. However, propranolol

Complications
+ Heart failure
+ Arrhythmias
+ Systemic or pulmonary embolization
+ Sudden death

Diagnosis
+ Physical examination
+ Echocardiography
+ Chest X-ray
+ Cardiac catheterization

Treatment
Dilated cardiomyopathy
+ ACE inhibitors
+ Diuretics with an ACE inhibitor
+ Digoxin, hydralazine, and isosorbide
+ Antiarrhythmics
+ Cardioversion
+ Pacemakers
+ Heart transplantation
+ Smoking cessation
+ Restricted diet
+ Physical activity
+ Abstinence from alcohol

Hypertrophic cardiomyopathy
+ Propranolol
+ Calcium channel blockers
+ Antiarrhythmic drugs
+ Cardioversion
+ Anticoagulant therapy
+ Ventricular myotomy
+ Mitral valve replacement

Test results in dilated cardiomyopathy

Electrocardiography
+ Biventricular hypertrophy
+ Sinus tachycardia
+ Bundle branch block

Echocardiography
+ Left ventricular thrombi
+ Global hypokinesia

Chest X-ray
+ Cardiomegaly
+ Pulmonary hypertension

Cardiac catheterization
+ Elevated left atrial and left ventricular end-diastolic pressure
+ Left ventricular enlargement

Radionuclide studies
+ Left ventricular dilation
+ Reduced ejection fraction

Test results in nonobstructive hypertrophic cardiomyopathy

Electrocardiography
+ Left ventricular hypertrophy
+ ST-segment and T-wave abnormalities
+ Ventricular arrhythmias

Echocardiography
+ Symmetrical thickening of left ventricular wall
+ Left atrial dilation

Chest X-ray
+ Cardiomegaly

Cardiac catheterization
+ Elevated ventricular end-diastolic pressure
+ Mitral insufficiency

Radionuclide studies
+ Reduced left ventricular volume
+ Ischemia

Comparing diagnostic tests in cardiomyopathy

Cardiomyopathies include a variety of structural or functional abnormalities of the ventricles. They're grouped into four main pathophysiologic types: dilated, nonobstructive and obstructive hypertrophic, and restrictive. These conditions may lead to heart failure by impairing myocardial structure and function.

DILATED CARDIOMYOPATHY	NONOBSTRUCTIVE HYPERTROPHIC CARDIOMYOPATHY
Electrocardiography	
Biventricular hypertrophy, sinus tachycardia, atrial enlargement, atrial and ventricular arrhythmias, bundle branch block, and ST-segment and T-wave abnormalities	Left ventricular hypertrophy, ST-segment and T-wave abnormalities, left anterior hemiblock, Q waves in precordial and inferior leads, ventricular arrhythmias and, possibly, atrial fibrillation
Echocardiography	
Left ventricular thrombi, global hypokinesia, enlarged atria, left ventricular dilation and, possibly, valvular abnormalities	Symmetrical thickening of the left ventricular wall and intraventricular septum and left atrial dilation
Chest X-ray	
Cardiomegaly, pulmonary congestion, pulmonary venous hypertension, and pleural or pericardial effusions	Cardiomegaly
Cardiac catheterization	
Elevated left atrial and left ventricular end-diastolic pressures, left ventricular enlargement, and mitral and tricuspid incompetence; may identify coronary artery disease as a cause	Elevated ventricular end-diastolic pressure and, possibly, mitral insufficiency, hyperdynamic systolic function, and aortic valve pressure gradient if aortic valve is stenotic
Radionuclide studies	
Left ventricular dilation and hypokinesis, reduced ejection fraction	Reduced left ventricular volume, increased muscle mass, and ischemia

may aggravate symptoms of cardiac decompensation. Calcium channel blockers may be prescribed to relax the heart muscle and improve ventricular filling. Antiarrhythmic drugs may be prescribed to treat arrhythmias. Atrial fibrillation necessitates cardioversion to treat the arrhythmia and, because of the high risk of systemic embolism, anticoagulant therapy until fibrillation subsides.

If drug therapy fails, the patient may undergo surgery. Ventricular myotomy (resection of the hypertrophied septum) alone or combined with mitral valve replacement may ease outflow tract obstruction and relieve symptoms. This experimental procedure can cause complications, such as complete heart block and ventricular

OBSTRUCTIVE HYPERTROPHIC CARDIOMYOPATHY	RESTRICTIVE CARDIOMYOPATHY
Left ventricular hypertrophy with QRS complexes tallest across mid-precordium, ST-segment and T-wave abnormalities, left axis deviation, left atrial abnormality, supraventricular tachycardia, and ventricular tachycardia	Low voltage, hypertrophy, atrioventricular conduction defects, and arrhythmias
Asymmetrical septal hypertrophy; anterior movement of the anterior mitral leaflet during systole, early termination of left ventricular ejection that worsens with dobutamine (Dobutrex) or nitrate provocation, mitral insufficiency, and atrial dilation	Increased left ventricular muscle mass, normal or reduced left ventricular cavity size, and decreased systolic function; rules out constrictive pericarditis
Normal or mild cardiomegaly	Cardiomegaly, pericardial effusion, and pulmonary congestion
Asymmetrical septal hypertrophy, early termination of systole with decreased ejection fraction, outflow tract pressure gradient increasing from the apex to just below the aortic valve, and mitral insufficiency	Reduced systolic function and myocardial infiltration; increased left ventricular end-diastolic pressure; rules out constrictive pericarditis
Reduced left ventricular volume, increased septal muscle mass, septal ischemia	Left ventricular hypertrophy with restricted ventricular filling and reduced ejection fraction

Test results in obstructive hypertrophic cardiomyopathy

Electrocardiography
+ Left ventricular hypertrophy
+ ST-segment abnormalities

Echocardiography
+ Atrial dilation

Chest X-ray
+ Normal or mild cardiomegaly

Cardiac catheterization
+ Asymetrical septal hypertrophy
+ Mitral insufficiency

Radionuclide studies
+ Reduced left ventricular volume
+ Increased septal muscle mass

Test results in restrictive cardiomyopathy

Electrocardiography
+ Low voltage and hypertrophy

Echocardiography
+ Increased left ventricular muscle mass
+ Decreased systolic function

Chest X-ray
+ Cardiomegaly
+ Pulmonary congestion

Cardiac catheterization
+ Reduced systolic function
+ Increased left ventricular end-diastolic pressure

Radionuclide studies
+ Left ventricular hypertrophy

septal defect. Dual-chamber pacing can prevent progression of hypertrophy and obstruction. Implantable defibrillators may be used in patients with ventricular arrhythmias.

Restrictive cardiomyopathy

Although no therapy currently exists for restricted ventricular filling, digoxin, diuretics, and a sodium-restricted diet can ease symptoms. Anticoagulant therapy may prevent thrombophlebitis in the patient on prolonged bed rest.

Treatment

Restrictive cardiomyopathy
+ No therapy currently exists for restricted ventricular filling
+ Digoxin, diuretics, sodium-restricted diet can ease symptoms

NURSING CONSIDERATIONS

For the patient with dilated cardiomyopathy in acute failure

✦ Monitor the patient for signs of progressive failure (increasing crackles and dyspnea and increased jugular vein distention) and compromised renal perfusion (oliguria, elevated blood urea nitrogen and creatinine levels, and electrolyte imbalances). Weigh the patient daily.

✦ If the patient is receiving vasodilators, check blood pressure and heart rate. If he becomes hypotensive, stop the infusion and place him in a supine position with his legs elevated to increase venous return and to ensure cerebral blood flow.

✦ If the patient is receiving diuretics, monitor for signs of resolving congestion (decreased crackles and dyspnea) or too vigorous diuresis. Check serum potassium level for hypokalemia, especially if therapy includes digoxin. Monitor intake and output closely.

✦ Therapeutic restrictions and an uncertain prognosis usually cause profound anxiety and depression, so offer emotional support and let the patient express his feelings. Be flexible with visiting hours but emphasize to the patient and his family members that adequate rest is imperative.

✦ Before discharge, teach the patient about his illness and its treatment. Emphasize the need to avoid alcohol, to restrict sodium intake, to watch for weight gain, and to take digoxin as prescribed and watch for its adverse effects (anorexia, nausea, vomiting, and yellow vision).

✦ Encourage family members to learn cardiopulmonary resuscitation (CPR).

For the patient with hypertrophic cardiomyopathy

✦ Warn the patient against strenuous physical activity such as running because syncope or sudden death may follow well-tolerated exercise.

✦ Administer medications as prescribed. Avoid nitroglycerin, digoxin, and diuretics because they can worsen obstruction. Warn the patient not to stop taking propranolol abruptly because doing so may increase myocardial demands. To determine the patient's tolerance for an increased dosage of propranolol, take his pulse to check for bradycardia. Also take his blood pressure while he's in a supine position and standing (a drop in blood pressure [greater than 10 mm Hg] when standing may indicate orthostatic hypotension).

✦ Administer prophylaxis for subacute infective endocarditis before dental work or surgery.

✦ Provide psychological support. If the patient is hospitalized for a long time, be flexible with visiting hours, and encourage occasional weekends away from the hospital, if possible. Refer the patient for psychosocial counseling to help him and his family accept his restricted lifestyle and poor prognosis.

✦ If the patient is a child, have his parents arrange for him to continue his studies in the health care facility.

✦ Urge the patient's family to learn CPR because sudden cardiac arrest is possible.

For the patient with restrictive cardiomyopathy

✦ In the acute phase, monitor heart rate and rhythm, blood pressure, urine output, and pulmonary artery pressure readings to help guide treatment.

✦ Give psychological support. Provide appropriate diversionary activities for the patient restricted to prolonged bed rest. Because a poor prognosis may cause profound anxiety and depression, be especially supportive and understanding, and encourage the patient to express his fears. Refer him for psychosocial counseling, as necessary, for assistance in coping with his restricted lifestyle. Be flexible with visiting hours whenever possible.

Key nursing actions

Dilated cardiomyopathy in acute failure

✦ Monitor for signs of progressive failure and compromised renal perfusion.

✦ If the patient is receiving vasodilators, check blood pressure and heart rate; if he's receiving diuretics, monitor for signs of resolving congestion or too vigorous diuresis.

✦ Emphasize the need to avoid alcohol, to maintain a prescribed diet, and to take digoxin as prescribed.

✦ Urge family members to learn CPR.

Hypertrophic cardiomyopathy

✦ Warn the patient against strenuous physical activity.

✦ Administer prophylaxis for subacute infective endocarditis before dental work or surgery.

✦ Provide psychological support.

✦ Urge family members to learn CPR.

Restrictive cardiomyopathy

✦ Monitor heart rate and rhythm, blood pressure, urine output, and pulmonary artery pressure readings to help guide treatment.

✦ Give psychological support.

✦ Before discharge, teach the patient to watch for and report signs of digoxin toxicity.

✦ Before discharge, teach the patient to watch for and report signs of digoxin toxicity (anorexia, nausea, vomiting, and yellow vision); to record and report weight gain; and, if sodium restriction is ordered, to avoid canned foods, pickles, smoked meats, and use of table salt.

COARCTATION OF THE AORTA

Coarctation is a narrowing of the aorta, usually just below the left subclavian artery, near the site where the ligamentum arteriosum (the remnant of the ductus arteriosus, a fetal blood vessel) joins the pulmonary artery to the aorta. Coarctation may occur with aortic valve stenosis (usually of a bicuspid aortic valve) and with severe cases of hypoplasia of the aortic arch, patent ductus arteriosus (PDA), and ventricular septal defect (VSD). The obstruction to blood flow results in ineffective pumping of the heart and increases the risk for heart failure.

This acyanotic condition accounts for about 7% of all congenital heart defects in children and is twice as common in males as in females. When coarctation of the aorta occurs in females, it's commonly associated with Turner's syndrome, a chromosomal disorder that causes ovarian dysgenesis.

The prognosis depends on the severity of associated cardiac anomalies. If corrective surgery is performed before isolated coarctation induces severe systemic hypertension or degenerative changes in the aorta, the prognosis is good.

CAUSES

Although the cause of this defect is unknown in females, it may be associated with Turner's syndrome.

PATHOPHYSIOLOGY

Coarctation of the aorta may develop as a result of spasm and constriction of the smooth muscle in the ductus arteriosus as it closes. Possibly, this contractile tissue extends into the aortic wall, causing narrowing. The obstructive process causes hypertension in the aortic branches above the constriction (arteries that supply the arms, neck, and head) and diminished pressure in the vessel below the constriction.

Restricted blood flow through the narrowed aorta increases the pressure load on the left ventricle and causes ventricular hypertrophy and dilation of the proximal aorta.

As oxygenated blood leaves the left ventricle, a portion travels through the arteries that branch off the aorta proximal to the coarctation. If PDA is present, the rest of the blood travels through the coarctation, mixes with deoxygenated blood from the PDA, and travels to the legs. If the ductus arteriosus is closed, the legs and lower portion of the body must rely solely on the blood that gets through the coarctation.

Untreated, coarctation of the aorta leads to left ventricular hypertrophy and may eventually lead to left-sided heart failure and, rarely, to cerebral hemorrhage and aortic rupture. If VSD accompanies coarctation, blood shunts from left to right, straining the right side of the heart. This leads to pulmonary hypertension and, eventually, right-sided heart hypertrophy and failure.

If coarctation is asymptomatic in infancy, it usually remains so throughout adolescence as collateral circulation develops to bypass the narrowed segment.

SIGNS AND SYMPTOMS

The patient with coarctation of the aorta may present with such signs and symptoms as tachypnea, dyspnea, pulmonary edema, pallor, tachycardia, failure to

---

Characteristics of coarctation of the aorta

✦ Acyanotic condition; narrowing of aorta, usually just below left subclavian artery
✦ May occur with aortic valve stenosis, and severe cases of hypoplasia of aortic arch, PDA, and VSD
✦ Obstruction results in ineffective pumping of heart
✦ Accounts for 7% of all congenital heart defects in children
✦ Prognosis depends on severity of associated cardiac anomalies
✦ Prognosis is good if surgery is performed in time

Causes

✦ Associated with Turner's syndrome in females

How it happens

✦ Develops as a result of spasm and constriction of smooth muscle in ductus arteriosus as it closes
✦ Contractile tissue may extend into aortic wall
✦ Causes hypertension in aortic branches above constriction, diminished pressure in vessel below
✦ Restricted blood flow increases pressure load on left ventricle
✦ Oxygenated blood leaves left ventricle, travels through arteries that branch off aorta proximal to coarctation

Key signs and symptoms

+ Tachypnea
+ Dyspnea
+ Pulmonary edema
+ Pallor
+ Tachycardia
+ Failure to thrive
+ Cardiomegaly
+ Pink upper extremities
+ Cyanotic lower extremities

Complications

+ Heart failure
+ Severe hypertension
+ Cerebral aneurysm and hemorrhage
+ Rupture of aorta
+ Aortic aneurysm
+ Infective endocarditis

Diagnosis

+ Infective endocarditis
+ Wide pulse pressure
+ Chest X-rays
+ Left ventricular hypertrophy
+ Electrocardiography

Treatment

+ Digoxin
+ Diuretics
+ Sedatives
+ Prostaglandin infusion
+ Antibiotics
+ Surgery in preschool years
+ Reconstruct aorta
+ Balloon angioplasty or resection with end-to-end anastomosis or use of a tubular graft

thrive, cardiomegaly, and hepatomegaly due to heart failure during an infant's first year of life. He may also experience claudication due to reduced blood flow to the legs.

The patient may be hypertensive in the upper body due to increased pressure in the arteries proximal to the coarctation and may have headache, vertigo, and epistaxis secondary to hypertension.

He may present with pink upper extremities and cyanotic lower extremities due to reduced oxygenated blood reaching the legs and absent or diminished femoral pulses due to restricted blood flow to the lower extremities through the constricted aorta.

In most cases, normal heart sounds are heard unless a coexisting cardiac defect is present. The patient's chest and arms may be more developed than his legs because circulation to the legs is restricted.

COMPLICATIONS

Coarctation of the aorta may result in serious complications. These include heart failure, severe hypertension, cerebral aneurysms and hemorrhage, rupture of the aorta, aortic aneurysm, and infective endocarditis.

DIAGNOSIS

A diagnosis of coarctation of the aorta may be made with the help of various tests. A physical examination will reveal the cardinal signs — resting systolic hypertension in the upper body, absent or diminished femoral pulses, and a wide pulse pressure. In addition, chest X-rays may be used. These may demonstrate left ventricular hypertrophy, heart failure, a wide ascending and descending aorta, and notching of the undersurfaces of the ribs due to erosion by collateral circulation.

Electrocardiography may reveal left ventricular hypertrophy and echocardiography may show increased left ventricular muscle thickness, coexisting aortic valve abnormalities, and the coarctation site. To evaluate collateral circulation and measure pressure in the right and left ventricles and in the ascending and descending aortas (on both sides of the obstruction), a cardiac catheterization should be used. In addition, aortography locates the site and extent of coarctation.

TREATMENT

Treatment of coarctation of the aorta may involve the use of medications, such as digoxin (Lanoxin), diuretics, and sedatives for infants with heart failure.

Prostaglandin infusion is used to keep the ductus open. Antibiotics provide prophylaxis against infective endocarditis before and after surgery. For children with previously undetected coarctation, antihypertensive therapy is employed until surgery is performed.

The family of the infant with heart failure or hypertension is generally prepared for early corrective surgery; however, surgery is sometimes delayed until the preschool years. A flap of the left subclavian artery may be used to reconstruct the aorta. Alternatively, balloon angioplasty or resection with end-to-end anastomosis or the use of a tubular graft may also be performed.

NURSING CONSIDERATIONS

+ When coarctation in an infant requires a rapid loading dose of digoxin (Lanoxin), monitor vital signs closely and watch for digoxin toxicity (poor feeding and vomiting).

✦ Balance intake and output carefully, especially if the infant is receiving diuretics with fluid restriction.
✦ Because the infant may be unable to maintain proper body temperature, regulate environmental temperature with an overbed warmer, if needed.
✦ Monitor blood glucose levels to detect possible hypoglycemia, which may occur as glycogen stores become depleted.
✦ Offer the parents emotional support and an explanation of the disorder. Also explain diagnostic procedures, surgery, and drug therapy. Tell the parents what to expect postoperatively.
✦ For an older child, assess the blood pressure in his extremities regularly, explain exercise restrictions, stress the need to take medications properly and to watch for adverse effects, and teach him about tests and other procedures.

After corrective surgery
✦ Monitor the patient's blood pressure closely, using an intra-arterial line. Take his blood pressure in all extremities. Monitor intake and output.
✦ If the patient develops hypertension and requires nitroprusside (Nipriate) or trimethaphan (Arfonad), administer it as ordered by continuous I.V. infusion, using an infusion pump. Watch for severe hypotension, and regulate the dosage according to parameters.
✦ Provide pain relief, and encourage a gradual increase in activity.
✦ Promote adequate respiratory functioning through turning, coughing, and deep breathing.
✦ Watch for abdominal pain or rigidity and signs of GI or urinary bleeding.
✦ Teach an older child and his parents about antihypertensives if he needs to continue them after surgery.
✦ Stress the importance of continued endocarditis prophylaxis.

HEART FAILURE

Heart failure occurs when the heart can't pump enough blood to meet the body's metabolic needs. Heart failure results in intravascular and interstitial volume overload and poor tissue perfusion. An individual with heart failure experiences reduced exercise tolerance, a reduced quality of life, and a shortened life span.

Although the most common cause of heart failure is coronary artery disease, it also occurs in infants, children, and adults with congenital and acquired heart defects. The incidence of heart failure increases with age. Approximately 1% of people older than age 50 experience heart failure; it occurs in 10% of people older than age 80. About 700,000 Americans die of heart failure each year. Mortality from heart failure is greater for males, blacks, and elderly people.

Although advances in diagnostic and therapeutic techniques have greatly improved the outlook for patients with heart failure, the prognosis still depends on the underlying cause and its response to treatment.

CAUSES

Cardiovascular disorders that lead to heart failure include atherosclerotic heart disease, myocardial infarction (MI), hypertension, rheumatic heart disease, congenital heart disease, ischemic heart disease, cardiomyopathy, valvular diseases, and arrhythmias.

Noncardiovascular causes of heart failure include pregnancy and childbirth, increased environmental temperature or humidity, severe physical or mental stress,

Causes

+ Atherosclerotic, rheumatic, congenital, or ischemic heart disease
+ MI
+ Hypertension
+ Cardiomyopathy
+ Valvular diseases
+ Arrhythmias
+ COPD

How it happens

Left-sided heart failure
+ Ineffective left ventricular contractile function
+ Pumping ability of left ventricle fails, cardiac output falls
+ Blood backs up into left atrium and then into lungs

Right-sided heart failure
+ Ineffective right ventricular contractile function
+ Blood backs up into right atrium and peripheral circulation
+ Patient gains weight and develops peripheral edema

Systolic dysfunction
+ Left ventricle can't pump enough blood out to systemic circulation
+ Blood backs up into pulmonary circulation and pressure increases in pulmonary venous system
+ Cardiac output falls; weakness and fatigue occur

Diastolic dysfunction
+ Ability of left ventricle to relax and fill during diastole is reduced and stroke volume falls
+ Higher volumes needed in ventricles to maintain cardiac output

thyrotoxicosis, acute blood loss, pulmonary embolism, severe infection, and chronic obstructive pulmonary disease.

PATHOPHYSIOLOGY

Heart failure may be classified according to the side of the heart affected (left- or right-sided heart failure) or by the cardiac cycle involved (systolic or diastolic dysfunction).

Left-sided heart failure

Left-sided heart failure occurs as a result of ineffective left ventricular contractile function. As the pumping ability of the left ventricle fails, cardiac output falls. Blood is no longer effectively pumped out into the body; it backs up into the left atrium and then into the lungs, causing pulmonary congestion, dyspnea, and activity intolerance. If the condition persists, pulmonary edema and right-sided heart failure may result. Common causes include left ventricular infarction, hypertension, and aortic and mitral valve stenosis.

Right-sided heart failure

Right-sided heart failure results from ineffective right ventricular contractile function. Consequently, blood isn't pumped effectively through the right ventricle to the lungs, causing blood to back up into the right atrium and the peripheral circulation. The patient gains weight and develops peripheral edema and engorgement of the kidney and other organs. It may be due to an acute right ventricular infarction, pulmonary hypertension, or a pulmonary embolus. However, the most common cause is profound backward blood flow due to left-sided heart failure. (See *Understanding left- and right-sided heart failure*.)

Systolic dysfunction

Systolic dysfunction occurs when the left ventricle can't pump enough blood out to the systemic circulation during systole and the ejection fraction falls. Consequently, blood backs up into the pulmonary circulation and pressure increases in the pulmonary venous system. Cardiac output falls; weakness, fatigue, and shortness of breath may occur. Causes of systolic dysfunction include MI and dilated cardiomyopathy.

Diastolic dysfunction

Diastolic dysfunction occurs when the ability of the left ventricle to relax and fill during diastole is reduced and the stroke volume falls. Therefore, higher volumes are needed in the ventricles to maintain cardiac output. Consequently, pulmonary congestion and peripheral edema develop. Diastolic dysfunction may occur as a result of left ventricular hypertrophy, hypertension, or restrictive cardiomyopathy. This type of heart failure is less common than systolic dysfunction, and its treatment isn't as clear.

All causes of heart failure eventually lead to reduced cardiac output, which triggers compensatory mechanisms, such as increased sympathetic activity, activation of the renin-angiotensin-aldosterone system, ventricular dilation, and hypertrophy. These mechanisms improve cardiac output at the expense of increased ventricular work.

Increased sympathetic activity—a response to decreased cardiac output and blood pressure—enhances peripheral vascular resistance, contractility, heart rate,

Understanding left- and right-sided heart failure

These illustrations show how myocardial damage leads to heart failure.

LEFT-SIDED HEART FAILURE

1. Increased workload and end-diastolic volume enlarge the left ventricle (see illustration at right). Because of lack of oxygen, the ventricle enlarges with stretched tissue rather than functional tissue. The patient may experience increased heart rate, pale and cool skin, tingling in the extremities, decreased cardiac output, and arrhythmias.

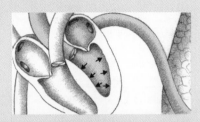

2. Diminished left ventricular function allows blood to pool in the ventricle and the atrium and eventually back up into the pulmonary veins and capillaries, as shown at right. At this stage, the patient may experience dyspnea on exertion, confusion, dizziness, orthostatic hypotension, decreased peripheral pulses and pulse pressure, cyanosis, and an S_3 gallop.

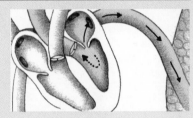

3. As the pulmonary circulation becomes engorged, rising capillary pressure pushes sodium (Na) and water (H_2O) into the interstitial space (as shown at right), causing pulmonary edema. You'll note coughing, subclavian retractions, crackles, tachypnea, elevated pulmonary artery pressure, diminished pulmonary compliance, and increased partial pressure of carbon dioxide.

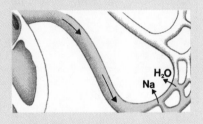

H_2O

Na

4. When the patient lies down, fluid in the extremities moves into the systemic circulation. Because the left ventricle can't handle the increased venous return, fluid pools in the pulmonary circulation, worsening pulmonary edema. You may note decreased breath sounds, dullness on percussion, crackles, and orthopnea.

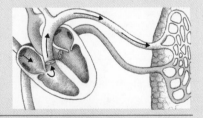

5. The right ventricle may now become stressed because it's pumping against greater pulmonary vascular resistance and left ventricular pressure (see illustration at right). When this occurs, the patient's symptoms worsen.

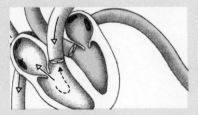

Left-sided heart failure

✦ Increased workload and end-diastolic volume enlarge the left ventricle

✦ Diminished function allows blood to pool in the ventricle and atrium and back up into the pulmonary veins and capillaries

✦ Rising capillary pressure pushes sodium and water into interstitial space

✦ Fluid in the extremities moves into the systemic circulation

✦ Right ventricle becomes stressed because it's pumping against greater pulmonary vascular resistance and left ventricle pressure

(continued)

Right-sided heart failure

- ✦ Stressed right ventricle enlarges with the formation of stretched tissue
- ✦ Blood pools in the right ventricle and right atrium
- ✦ Backed-up blood also distends the visceral veins
- ✦ Rising capillary pressure forces excess fluid from the capillaries into the interstitial space

Understanding left- and right-sided heart failure *(continued)*

RIGHT-SIDED HEART FAILURE

6. The stressed right ventricle enlarges with the formation of stretched tissue (see illustration at right). Increasing conduction time and deviation of the heart from its normal axis can cause arrhythmias. If the patient doesn't already have left-sided heart failure, he may experience increased heart rate, cool skin, cyanosis, decreased cardiac output, palpitations, and dyspnea.

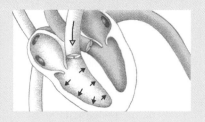

7. Blood pools in the right ventricle and right atrium. The backed-up blood causes pressure and congestion in the vena cava and systemic circulation (as shown at right). The patient will have elevated central venous pressure, jugular vein distention, and hepatojugular reflux.

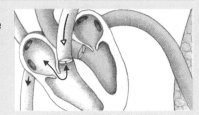

8. Backed-up blood also distends the visceral veins, especially the hepatic vein. As the liver and spleen become engorged (see illustration at right), their function is impaired. The patient may develop anorexia, nausea, abdominal pain, palpable liver and spleen, weakness, and dyspnea secondary to abdominal distention.

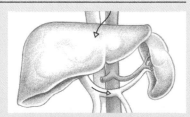

9. Rising capillary pressure forces excess fluid from the capillaries into the interstitial space (as shown at right). This causes tissue edema, especially in the lower extremities and abdomen. The patient may experience weight gain, pitting edema, and nocturia.

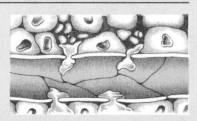

and venous return. Signs of increased sympathetic activity, such as cool extremities and clamminess, may indicate impending heart failure.

Increased sympathetic activity also restricts blood flow to the kidneys, causing them to secrete renin which, in turn, converts angiotensinogen to angiotensin I, which then becomes angiotensin II — a potent vasoconstrictor. Angiotensin causes the adrenal cortex to release aldosterone, leading to sodium and water retention and an increase in circulating blood volume. This renal mechanism is initially helpful; however, if it persists unchecked, it can aggravate heart failure as the heart struggles to pump against the increased volume.

In ventricular dilation, an increase in end-diastolic ventricular volume (preload) causes increased stroke work and stroke volume during contraction, stretching cardiac muscle fibers so that the ventricle can accept the increased intravascular volume. Eventually, the muscle becomes stretched beyond optimum limits and contractility declines.

In ventricular hypertrophy, an increase in ventricular muscle mass allows the heart to pump against increased resistance to the outflow of blood, improving cardiac output. However, this increased muscle mass also increases myocardial oxygen requirements. An increase in the ventricular diastolic pressure necessary to fill the enlarged ventricle may compromise diastolic coronary blood flow, limiting the oxygen supply to the ventricle and causing ischemia and impaired muscle contractility.

In heart failure, counterregulatory substances—prostaglandins and atrial natriuretic factor—are produced in an attempt to reduce the negative effects of volume overload and vasoconstriction caused by the compensatory mechanisms.

The kidneys release the prostaglandins, prostacyclin and prostaglandin E_2, which are potent vasodilators. These vasodilators also act to reduce volume overload produced by the renin-angiotensin-aldosterone system by inhibiting sodium and water reabsorption by the kidneys.

Atrial natriuretic factor is a hormone secreted mainly by the atria in response to stimulation of the stretch receptors in the atria caused by excess fluid volume. B-type natriuretic factor is secreted by the ventricles because of fluid volume overload. These natriuretic factors work to counteract the negative effects of sympathetic nervous system stimulation and the renin-angiotensin-aldosterone system by producing vasodilation and diuresis.

SIGNS AND SYMPTOMS

The early clinical manifestations of left-sided heart failure are generally respiratory in nature. The patient may experience dyspnea, which is caused by pulmonary congestion. He may report orthopnea as blood is redistributed from the legs to the central circulation when the patient lies down at night, paroxysmal nocturnal dyspnea due to the reabsorption of interstitial fluid when lying down, and reduced sympathetic stimulation while sleeping. In addition, pulmonary congestion can cause a nonproductive cough.

Another early manifestation of left-sided heart failure is fatigue—the result of reduced oxygenation and an inability to increase cardiac output in response to physical activity.

Later respiratory clinical manifestations of left-sided heart failure include crackles due to pulmonary congestion and hemoptysis resulting from bleeding veins in the bronchial system caused by venous distention.

One of the later cardiac clinical manifestations is displacement of the point of maximal impulse toward the left anterior axillary line caused by left ventricular hypertrophy. Other findings include tachycardia due to sympathetic stimulation, S_3 caused by rapid ventricular filling, and S_4 resulting from atrial contraction against a noncompliant ventricle.

On physical exam, the patient may have cool, pale skin resulting from peripheral vasoconstriction, and he may be restless and confused due to reduced cardiac output.

Clinical manifestations of right-sided heart failure include jugular vein distention, positive hepatojugular reflux, and hepatomegaly—all secondary to venous congestion. The patient may report right upper quadrant pain caused by liver engorgement, and anorexia, fullness, and nausea, which may be due to congestion of the liver and intestines.

Nocturia may be present as fluid is redistributed and reabsorbed at night. The patient may experience weight gain, edema, ascites, and anasarca due to sodium and water retention and fluid volume excess.

Key signs and symptoms

Left-sided heart failure
+ Dyspnea
+ Orthopnea
+ Paroxysmal nocturnal dyspnea
+ Reduced sympathetic stimulation while sleeping
+ Pulmonary congestion
+ Tachycardia
+ S_3
+ S_4
+ Cool, pale skin
+ Restlessness

Right-sided heart failure
+ Jugular vein distention
+ Positive hepatojugular reflux
+ Hepatomegaly

Complications

+ Pulmonary edema
+ Acute renal failure
+ Arrhythmias
+ Activity intolerance
+ Renal impairment
+ Cardiac cachexia

Diagnosis

+ Increased pulmonary vascular markings
+ Interstitial edema
+ Pleural effusion
+ Tachycardia
+ Extrasystoles
+ Abnormal liver function tests
+ Elevated BUN and creatinine
+ Prothrombin time may be prolonged
+ Elevated pulmonary artery and pulmonary artery wedge pressures
+ Radionuclide ventriculography, diastolic dysfunction, ejection fraction may be normal

Treatment

+ Diuretics
+ ACE inhibitors
+ Vasodilators
+ Digoxin
+ Beta-adrenergic blockers
+ Sodium-restricted diet
+ Antiembolism stockings
+ Surgical valve replacement
+ Coronary artery bypass grafting
+ PTCA
+ Stenting
+ Mechanical VAD

COMPLICATIONS

Acute complications of heart failure include pulmonary edema, acute renal failure, and arrhythmias. Activity intolerance, renal impairment, cardiac cachexia, metabolic impairment, and thromboembolism are chronic complications of the disease.

DIAGNOSIS

These tests help diagnose heart failure:
+ Chest X-rays show increased pulmonary vascular markings, interstitial edema, or pleural effusion and cardiomegaly.
+ Electrocardiography may indicate hypertrophy, ischemic changes, or infarction and may also reveal tachycardia and extrasystoles.
+ Laboratory testing may reveal abnormal liver function tests and elevated blood urea nitrogen (BUN) and creatinine levels. Prothrombin time may be prolonged as congestion impairs the liver's ability to synthesize procoagulants.
+ Brain natriuretic peptide (BNP) assay, a blood test, may show elevated levels. Along with such clinical signs as edematous ankles, elevated BNP levels strongly indicate heart failure.
+ Echocardiography may reveal left ventricular hypertrophy, dilation, and abnormal contractility.
+ Pulmonary artery monitoring typically demonstrates elevated pulmonary artery and pulmonary artery wedge pressures, left ventricular end-diastolic pressure in left-sided heart failure, and elevated right atrial pressure or central venous pressure in right-sided heart failure.
+ Radionuclide ventriculography may reveal an ejection fraction less than 40%; in diastolic dysfunction, the ejection fraction may be normal.

TREATMENT

Treatment for heart failure can be determined by using the New York Heart Association classification system and the American College of Cardiology/American Heart Association (ACC/AHA) guidelines. (See *Classifying signs and symptoms to determine treatment.*)

Treatment measures include diuretics that reduce preload by decreasing total blood volume and circulatory congestion. Angiotensin-converting enzyme (ACE) inhibitors dilate blood vessels and decrease systemic vascular resistance, thereby reducing the workload of the heart. Vasodilators may be given to the patient who can't tolerate ACE inhibitors. Vasodilators increase cardiac output by reducing impedance to ventricular outflow, thereby decreasing afterload. Digoxin (Lanoxin) may help strengthen myocardial contractility. Beta-adrenergic blockers may prevent cardiac remodeling (left ventricular dilation and hypertrophy). Nesiritide (Natrecor), a human B-type natriuretic peptide, may be administered to augment diuresis and to decrease afterload. Positive inotropic agents, such as I.V. dopamine (Intropin) or dobutamine (Dobutrex), are reserved for those with end-stage heart failure or those awaiting heart transplantation.

The patient must alternate periods of rest with periods of activity and follow a sodium-restricted diet with smaller, more frequent meals. He may have to wear antiembolism stockings to prevent venostasis and possible thromboembolism formation. The doctor may also order oxygen therapy.

Although controversial, surgery may be performed if the patient's heart failure doesn't improve after therapy and lifestyle modifications. If the patient with valve dysfunction has recurrent acute heart failure, he may undergo surgical valve replacement. Coronary artery bypass grafting, percutaneous transluminal coronary

Classifying signs and symptoms to determine treatment

Two sets of guidelines are available to help direct treatment of the patient with heart failure. The New York Heart Association (NYHA) classification is based on functional capacity. The American College of Cardiology/American Heart Association (ACC/AHA) guidelines are based on objective assessment. These guidelines are compared side-by-side below.

NYHA CLASSIFICATION	ACC/AHA GUIDELINES	RECOMMENDATIONS
	Stage A. Patient at high risk for developing heart failure but without structural heart disease or signs and symptoms of heart failure	✦ Treatment of hypertension, lipid disorders, and diabetes ✦ Encouraging patient to stop smoking and to exercise regularly ✦ Discouraging use of alcohol and illicit drugs ✦ Angiotensin-converting enzyme (ACE) inhibitor if indicated
Class I. Ordinary physical activity doesn't cause undue fatigue, palpitations, dyspnea, or angina.	*Stage B.* Structural heart disease, but without signs and symptoms of heart failure	✦ All stage A therapies ✦ ACE inhibitor (unless contraindicated) ✦ Beta-adrenergic blocker (unless contraindicated)
Class II. Slight limitation of physical activity but asymptomatic at rest. Ordinary physical activity causes fatigue, palpitations, dyspnea, or anginal pain. *Class III.* Marked limitation of physical activity, but typically asymptomatic at rest. Less than ordinary physical activity causes fatigue, palpitations, dyspnea, or angina.	*Stage C.* Structural heart disease with prior or current signs and symptoms of heart failure	✦ All stage A and B therapies ✦ Sodium-restricted diet ✦ Diuretics ✦ Digoxin (Lanoxin) ✦ Avoiding or withdrawing antiarrhythmic agents, most calcium channel blockers, and nonsteroidal anti-inflammatory drugs ✦ Drug therapy, including aldosterone antagonists, angiotensin receptor blockers, hydralazine (Apresoline), and nitrates
Class IV. Unable to perform any physical activity without discomfort; symptoms may be present at rest. Discomfort increases with physical activity.	*Stage D.* End-stage disease requiring specialized treatment strategies, such as mechanical circulatory support, continuous inotropic infusion, or heart transplant	✦ All therapies for stages A, B, and C ✦ Mechanical assist device, such as biventricular pacemaker or left ventricular assist device ✦ Continuous inotropic therapy ✦ Hospice care

Used with permission from Davis, S.L. "How the Heart Failure Picture has Changed," *Nursing2002* (32)11:36-44, November 2002.

ACC/AHA treatment guidelines

Stage A
✦ Treat underlying disorder
✦ Encourage smoking cessation
✦ ACE inhibitors

Stage B
✦ Stage A therapies
✦ Beta-adrenergic blocker

Stage C
✦ Stage A and B therapies
✦ Diuretics
✦ Digoxin
✦ Drug therapy

Stage D
✦ Stage A, B, and C therapies
✦ Mechanical assist device
✦ Hospice care

angioplasty, or stenting may be performed in a patient with heart failure caused by ischemia.

The Dor procedure, also called partial left ventriculectomy or ventricular remodeling, involves the removal of nonviable heart muscle to reduce the size of the hypertrophied ventricle, thereby allowing the heart to pump more efficiently. Patients with severe heart failure may benefit from a mechanical ventricular assist device (VAD) or from cardiac transplantation. An internal cardioverter-defibrillator may be implanted to treat life-threatening arrhythmias. A biventricular pacemaker may be placed to control ventricular dyssynchrony.

Other surgery or invasive procedures may be recommended in the patient with severe limitations or repeated hospitalizations, despite maximal medical therapy. Some procedures are controversial and may include cardiomyoplasty, insertion of an intra-aortic balloon pump, use of a mechanical VAD, and implanting an internal cardioverter-defibrillator.

 CLINICAL ALERT Heart failure in children occurs mainly as a result of congenital heart defects. Therefore, treatment guidelines are directed toward the specific cause.

NURSING CONSIDERATIONS

During the acute phase of heart failure
✦ Place the patient in Fowler's position and give him supplemental oxygen to help him breathe more easily.
✦ Weigh the patient daily, and check for peripheral edema. Carefully monitor intake and output, vital signs, and mental status. Auscultate the heart for abnormal sounds (S_3 gallop) and the lungs for crackles or rhonchi. Report changes immediately.
✦ Frequently monitor BUN, creatinine, and serum potassium, sodium, chloride, and magnesium levels.
✦ Make sure the patient has continuous cardiac monitoring during acute and advanced stages to identify and treat arrhythmias promptly.
✦ To prevent deep vein thrombosis due to vascular congestion, assist the patient with range-of-motion exercises. Enforce bed rest, and apply antiembolism stockings. Check the patient regularly for calf pain and tenderness.
✦ Allow adequate rest periods.

To prepare the patient for discharge
✦ Advise the patient to avoid foods high in sodium, such as canned or commercially prepared foods and dairy products, to curb fluid overload.
✦ Encourage the patient to participate in an outpatient cardiac rehabilitation program.
✦ Explain to the patient that the potassium he loses through diuretic therapy may need to be replaced by taking a prescribed potassium supplement and eating high-potassium foods, such as bananas and apricots.
✦ Stress the need for regular checkups.
✦ Stress the importance of taking digoxin exactly as prescribed. Tell the patient to watch for and immediately report signs of toxicity, such as anorexia, vomiting, and yellow vision.
✦ Tell the patient to notify the physician promptly if his pulse is unusually irregular or measures less than 60 beats/minute; if he experiences dizziness, syncope, blurred vision, shortness of breath, a persistent dry cough, palpitations, increased fatigue, paroxysmal nocturnal dyspnea, swollen ankles, or decreased urine output; or if he notices rapid weight gain (3 to 5 lb [1.5 to 2.5 kg] in 1 week).

HYPERTENSION

Hypertension, an elevation in diastolic or systolic blood pressure, occurs as two major types: essential (primary) hypertension, the most common, and secondary hypertension, which results from renal disease or another identifiable cause. Malignant hypertension is a severe, fulminant form of hypertension common to both types. Hypertension is a major cause of stroke, cardiac disease, and renal failure.

Hypertension affects 15% to 20% of adults in the United States. The risk of hypertension increases with age and is higher for blacks than whites and in those with less education and lower income. Men have a higher incidence of hypertension in young and early middle adulthood; thereafter, women have a higher incidence.

Essential hypertension usually begins insidiously as a benign disease, slowly progressing to a malignant state. If untreated, even mild cases can cause major complications and death. Carefully managed treatment, which may include lifestyle modifications and drug therapy, improves the prognosis. Untreated, it carries a high mortality rate. Severely elevated blood pressure (hypertensive crisis) may be fatal.

CAUSES

Those with a family history and those of advanced age are at risk for primary hypertension.

 CLINICAL ALERT Elderly people may have isolated systolic hypertension, in which just the systolic blood pressure is elevated, as atherosclerosis causes a loss of elasticity in large arteries. Previously, it was believed that isolated systolic hypertension was a normal part of the aging process and shouldn't be treated. Results of the Systolic Hypertension in the Elderly Program, however, found that treating isolated systolic hypertension with antihypertensive drugs lowered the incidence of stroke, coronary artery disease (CAD), and left-sided heart failure.

Also at risk for primary hypertension are those with sleep apnea, diabetes mellitus, excess renin, and mineral deficiencies (calcium, potassium, and magnesium). Primary hypertension is most common in blacks, making race a factor as well.

 CLINICAL ALERT Blacks are at an increased risk for primary hypertension when predisposition to low plasma renin levels diminishes the ability to excrete excess sodium. Hypertension develops at an earlier age and is more severe than in Whites.

Lifestyle factors that increase someone's risk for primary hypertension include tobacco use, excessive alcohol consumption, a sedentary lifestyle, and high stress levels. Obesity heightens the risk of primary hypertension as does the influences of a high dietary intake of sodium and saturated fat.

Causes of secondary hypertension include coarctation of the aorta, renal artery stenosis, renal parenchymal disease, brain tumor, quadriplegia, head injury, pheochromocytoma, Cushing's syndrome, hyperaldosteronism, and thyroid, pituitary, or parathyroid dysfunction. Secondary hypertension may also be induced by pregnancy.

The use of hormonal contraceptives, cocaine, epoetin alfa, sympathetic stimulants, monoamine oxidase inhibitors (taken with tyramine,) estrogen replacement therapy, nonsteroidal anti-inflammatory drugs, and excessive alcohol consumption are all causes of secondary hypertension.

Characteristics of hypertension

- ✦ Elevation in diastolic or systolic blood pressure
- ✦ Two types: essential or secondary
- ✦ Major cause of stroke, cardiac disease, and renal failure
- ✦ Risk increases with age; higher for blacks than whites

Alert!

- ✦ Elderly people may have isolated systolic hypertension, in which just the systolic blood pressure is elevated.
- ✦ Blacks are at an increased risk for primary hypertension when predisposition to low plasma renin levels diminishes the ability to excrete excess sodium.

Causes

Primary hypertension
- ✦ Sleep apnea
- ✦ Diabetes mellitus
- ✦ Race
- ✦ Tobacco use
- ✦ Excessive alcohol consumption
- ✦ Obesity

Secondary hypertension
- ✦ Coarctation of aorta
- ✦ Renal artery stenosis
- ✦ Renal parenchymal disease
- ✦ Head injury
- ✦ Pregnancy
- ✦ Hormonal contraceptives

Intrinsic blood pressure regulators

+ Renin-angiotensin system
+ Autoregulation
+ Sympathetic nervous system
+ Antidiuretic hormone

How it happens

Primary hypertension
+ Peripheral resistance is increased by factors that increase blood viscosity or reduce lumen size of vessels
+ Changes in arteriolar bed cause increased peripheral vascular resistance
+ Increased blood volume results from renal or hormonal dysfunction
+ Increase in arteriolar thickening caused by genetic factors
+ Abnormal renin release, resulting in formation of angiotensin II
+ Increases heart's workload as resistance to left ventricular ejection increases
+ Left ventricle hypertrophies, raising heart's oxygen demands and workload
+ Causes vascular damage, leading to accelerated atherosclerosis and target organ damage

---

Understanding blood pressure regulation

Hypertension may result from a disturbance in one of these intrinsic mechanisms.

RENIN-ANGIOTENSIN SYSTEM
The renin-angiotensin system acts to increase blood pressure through these mechanisms:
+ sodium depletion, reduced blood pressure, and dehydration stimulate renin release
+ renin reacts with angiotensin, a liver enzyme, and converts it to angiotensin I, which increases preload and afterload
+ angiotensin I converts to angiotensin II in the lungs; angiotensin II is a potent vasoconstrictor that targets the arterioles
+ angiotensin II works to increase preload and afterload by stimulating the adrenal cortex to secrete aldosterone; this increases blood volume by conserving sodium and water.

AUTOREGULATION
Several intrinsic mechanisms work to change an artery's diameter to maintain tissue and organ perfusion despite fluctuations in systemic blood pressure. These mechanisms include stress relaxation and capillary fluid shifts:

+ in stress relaxation, blood vessels gradually dilate when blood pressure increases to reduce peripheral resistance
+ in capillary fluid shift, plasma moves between vessels and extravascular spaces to maintain intravascular volume.

SYMPATHETIC NERVOUS SYSTEM
When blood pressure drops, baroreceptors in the aortic arch and carotid sinuses decrease their inhibition of the medulla's vasomotor center. The consequent increases in sympathetic stimulation of the heart by norepinephrine increases cardiac output by strengthening the contractile force, raising the heart rate, and augmenting peripheral resistance by vasoconstriction. Stress can also stimulate the sympathetic nervous system to increase cardiac output and peripheral vascular resistance.

ANTIDIURETIC HORMONE
The release of antidiuretic hormone can regulate hypotension by increasing reabsorption of water by the kidney. With reabsorption, blood plasma volume increases, thus raising blood pressure.

PATHOPHYSIOLOGY

Arterial blood pressure is a product of total peripheral resistance and cardiac output. Cardiac output is increased by conditions that increase heart rate, stroke volume, or both. Peripheral resistance is increased by factors that increase blood viscosity or reduce the lumen size of vessels, especially the arterioles.

Several theories help to explain the development of hypertension, including:
+ changes in the arteriolar bed, causing increased peripheral vascular resistance
+ abnormally increased tone in the sympathetic nervous system that originates in the vasomotor system centers, causing increased peripheral vascular resistance
+ increased blood volume resulting from renal or hormonal dysfunction
+ an increase in arteriolar thickening caused by genetic factors, leading to increased peripheral vascular resistance
+ abnormal renin release, resulting in the formation of angiotensin II, which constricts the arteriole and increases blood volume. (See *Understanding blood pressure regulation*.)

Prolonged hypertension increases the heart's workload as resistance to left ventricular ejection increases. To increase contractile force, the left ventricle hypertrophies, raising the heart's oxygen demands and workload. Cardiac dilation and failure may occur when hypertrophy can no longer maintain sufficient cardiac output. Because hypertension promotes coronary atherosclerosis, the heart may be further compromised by reduced blood flow to the myocardium, resulting in angina or myocardial infarction (MI). Hypertension also causes vascular damage, leading to accelerated atherosclerosis and target organ damage, such as retinal injury, renal failure, stroke, and aortic aneurysm and dissection.

The pathophysiology of secondary hypertension is related to the underlying disease. For example:

✦ The most common cause of secondary hypertension is chronic renal disease. Insult to the kidney from chronic glomerulonephritis or renal artery stenosis interferes with sodium excretion, the renin-angiotensin-aldosterone system, or renal perfusion, causing blood pressure to increase.

✦ In Cushing's syndrome, increased cortisol levels raise blood pressure by increasing renal sodium retention, angiotensin II levels, and vascular response to norepinephrine.

✦ In primary aldosteronism, increased intravascular volume, altered sodium concentrations in vessel walls, or very high aldosterone levels cause vasoconstriction and increased resistance.

✦ Pheochromocytoma is a chromaffin cell tumor of the adrenal medulla that secretes epinephrine and norepinephrine. Epinephrine increases cardiac contractility and rate, whereas norepinephrine increases peripheral vascular resistance.

SIGNS AND SYMPTOMS

Hypertension is frequently asymptomatic but there are signs and symptoms that may occur. Examination findings may include elevated blood pressure readings on at least two consecutive occasions after the initial screening.

 CLINICAL ALERT Because many older adults have a wide auscultatory gap — the hiatus between the first Korotkoff sound and the next sound — failure to pump the blood pressure cuff up high enough can lead to missing the first beat and underestimating systolic blood pressure. To avoid missing the first Korotkoff sound, palpate the radial artery and inflate the cuff to a point approximately 20 mm beyond which the pulse beat disappears.

The patient may describe an occipital headache that may worsen on rising in the morning as a result of increased intracranial pressure, and may report associated nausea and vomiting.

He may experience epistaxis due to vascular involvement. Dizziness, confusion, and fatigue are caused by decreased tissue perfusion due to vasoconstriction of blood vessels, and blurry vision is a result of retinal damage.

Nocturia is caused by an increase in blood flow to the kidneys and an increase in glomerular filtration. Edema is caused by increased capillary pressure. Bruits may be heard over the abdominal aorta or carotid, renal, and femoral arteries. They're caused by stenosis or aneurysm.

If secondary hypertension exists, other signs and symptoms may be related to the cause. For example, Cushing's syndrome may cause truncal obesity and purple striae, whereas patients with pheochromocytoma may develop headache, nausea, vomiting, palpitations, pallor, and profuse perspiration.

COMPLICATIONS

Complications of hypertension include hypertensive crisis, peripheral artery disease, dissecting aortic aneurysm, CAD, angina, MI, heart failure, arrhythmias, and sudden death. (See *What happens in hypertensive crisis,* page 192.) Transient ischemic attacks, stroke, retinopathy, hypertensive encephalopathy, and renal failure may also occur.

How it happens
Secondary hypertension
✦ Insult to kidney from chronic renal disease interferes with systems causing blood pressure to increase
✦ Primary aldosteronism
✦ Pheochromocytoma increasing blood pressure

Alert!
✦ Because many older adults have a wide auscultatory gap, failure to pump the blood pressure cuff up high enough can lead to missing the first beat and underestimating systolic blood pressure.
✦ Palpate the radial artery and inflate the cuff to a point approximately 20 mm beyond which the pulse beat disappears.

Key signs and symptoms
✦ Frequently asymptomatic
✦ Occipital headache
✦ Associated nausea and vomiting
✦ Epistaxis
✦ Dizziness
✦ Bruits
✦ Cushing's syndrome
✦ Pheochromocytoma

Complications
✦ Hypertensive crisis
✦ Peripheral artery disease
✦ Dissecting aortic aneurysm
✦ MI
✦ Heart failure

What happens in hypertensive crisis

Hypertensive crisis is a severe increase in arterial blood pressure caused by a disturbance in one or more of the regulating mechanisms. If untreated, hypertensive crisis may result in renal, cardiac, or cerebral complications and possibly, death.

Hypertensive crisis

- Disturbance occurs
- Prolonged hypertension
- Inflammation and necrosis of arterioles
- Narrowing of blood vessels
- Restriction of blood flow to major organs
- Organ damage
- Renal, cardiac, or cerebral complications occur

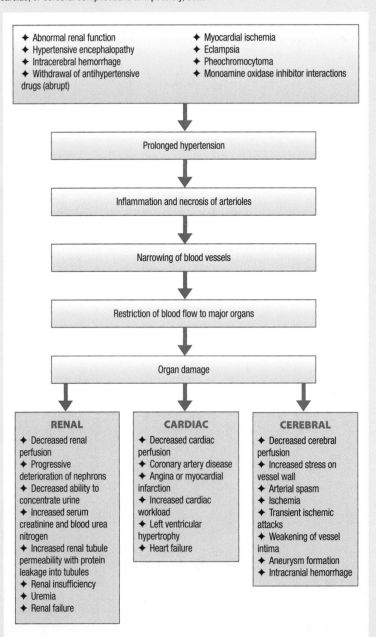

- Abnormal renal function
- Hypertensive encephalopathy
- Intracerebral hemorrhage
- Withdrawal of antihypertensive drugs (abrupt)
- Myocardial ischemia
- Eclampsia
- Pheochromocytoma
- Monoamine oxidase inhibitor interactions

Prolonged hypertension

Inflammation and necrosis of arterioles

Narrowing of blood vessels

Restriction of blood flow to major organs

Organ damage

RENAL
- Decreased renal perfusion
- Progressive deterioration of nephrons
- Decreased ability to concentrate urine
- Increased serum creatinine and blood urea nitrogen
- Increased renal tubule permeability with protein leakage into tubules
- Renal insufficiency
- Uremia
- Renal failure

CARDIAC
- Decreased cardiac perfusion
- Coronary artery disease
- Angina or myocardial infarction
- Increased cardiac workload
- Left ventricular hypertrophy
- Heart failure

CEREBRAL
- Decreased cerebral perfusion
- Increased stress on vessel wall
- Arterial spasm
- Ischemia
- Transient ischemic attacks
- Weakening of vessel intima
- Aneurysm formation
- Intracranial hemorrhage

DIAGNOSIS

These tests help diagnose hypertension:

♦ Serial blood pressure measurements reveal patterns and trends.

♦ Urinalysis may show protein, casts, red blood cells, or white blood cells, suggesting renal disease; presence of catecholamines associated with pheochromocytoma; or glucose, suggesting diabetes.

♦ Laboratory testing may reveal elevated blood urea nitrogen and serum creatinine levels suggestive of renal disease, or hypokalemia indicating adrenal dysfunction (primary hyperaldosteronism).

♦ Complete blood count may reveal other causes of hypertension, such as polycythemia or anemia.

♦ Lipid profile (including high- and low-density lipoprotein cholesterol levels as well as triglycerides) help determine the patient's risk of CAD.

♦ Chest X-rays may show cardiomegaly.

♦ Echocardiography may reveal left ventricular hypertrophy.

TREATMENT

Goals for treating hypertension include reducing further disease or death related to cardiovascular and renal complications. Target blood pressures are less than 140/90 mm Hg to decrease cardiovascular complications, and less than 130/80 mm Hg for patients with hypertension and diabetes or renal disease. The National Institutes of Health recommend the following approach to treating hypertension. (See *Classifying and managing blood pressure,* pages 194 and 195.)

One treatment option centers around lifestyle modifications, including weight loss, adopting the Dietary Approaches to Stop Hypertension (DASH) eating plan, dietary sodium restrictions, physical activity, and moderation of alcohol consumption. The DASH eating plan involves a diet that is potassium- and calcium-rich and low in saturated fat.

Drug therapy based on the patient's blood pressure classification is also a treatment option. Thiazide diuretics (such as chlorothiazide [Diuril]) should be used as initial therapy for most patients with hypertension and may be used either alone or in combination with other recommended classes of drugs.

Other recommended antihypertensives include angiotensin-converting enzyme inhibitors, angiotensin receptor blockers, beta-adrenergic blockers, calcium channel blockers, and other diuretics. When the use of a single drug fails to achieve target blood pressure, a second drug in a different class should be added.

Treatment of secondary hypertension focuses on correcting the underlying cause and controlling hypertensive effects.

Typically, hypertensive emergencies require parenteral administration of a vasodilator or an adrenergic inhibitor or oral administration of a selected drug, such as nifedipine (Procardia or Adalat), captopril (Capoten), clonidine (Catapres), or labetalol (Normodyne), to rapidly reduce blood pressure. The initial goal is to reduce mean arterial blood pressure by no more than 25% (within minutes to hours) then to 160/110 mm Hg within 2 hours while avoiding excessive decreases in blood pressure that can precipitate renal, cerebral, or myocardial ischemia.

Examples of hypertensive emergencies include hypertensive encephalopathy, intracranial hemorrhage, acute left-sided heart failure with pulmonary edema, and dissecting aortic aneurysm. Hypertensive emergencies are also associated with eclampsia or severe pregnancy-induced hypertension, unstable angina, and acute MI.

Hypertension without accompanying symptoms or target-organ disease seldom requires emergency drug therapy.

Diagnosis

♦ Serial blood pressure measurements
♦ Urinalysis laboratory testing
♦ Elevated blood urea nitrogen
♦ Elevated creatinine levels
♦ Hypokalemia
♦ Polycythemia
♦ Anemia

Treatment

Primary hypertension
♦ Weight loss
♦ Dietary sodium restrictions
♦ Physical activity
♦ Moderation of alcohol consumption
♦ DASH eating plan
♦ Thiazide diuretics
♦ Antihypertensives
♦ Beta-adrenergic blockers
♦ Calcium channel blockers

Secondary hypertension
♦ Parenteral administration of a vasodilator or an adrenergic inhibitor

Classifying blood pressure

✦ Normal = systolic blood pressure < 120
✦ Hypertension = systolic blood pressure 120 to 139
✦ Stage 1 hypertension = systolic blood pressure 140 to 159
✦ Stage 2 hypertension = systolic blood pressure ≥ 160

Classifying and managing blood pressure

In 2003, the National Institutes of Health issued a revised method of classifying blood pressure. This new system adds a prehypertension category, which will help to identify those at increased risk for hypertension. Patients with prehypertension have twice the risk for developing hypertension as those with normal blood pressures.

The revised categories are based on the average of two or more readings, properly measured and taken while seated, and obtained on separate visits after an initial screening. They apply to adults age 18 and older.

BLOOD PRESSURE CLASSIFICATION	SYSTOLIC BLOOD PRESSURE* (MM HG)	DIASTOLIC BLOOD PRESSURE* (MM HG)	LIFESTYLE MODIFICATION
Normal	< 120	AND < 80	Encourage
Prehypertension	120 to 139	OR 80 to 89	Yes
Stage 1 hypertension	140 to 159	OR 90 to 99	Yes
Stage 2 hypertension	≥ 160	OR > 100	Yes

*　Treatment determined by highest blood pressure category.

**　Initial combined therapy should be used cautiously in those at risk for orthostatic hypotension.

***　Compelling indications include heart failure, postmyocardial infarction, high risk for coronary artery disease, diabetes, chronic kidney disease, and risk for recurrent stroke.

****　Treat patients with chronic kidney disease or diabetes to blood pressure goal of < 130/80 mm Hg.

Key nursing actions

✦ Suggest that the patient establish a daily routine for taking his medication.
✦ Encourage a change in dietary habits. Help the obese patient plan a weight-reduction diet.
✦ Help the patient examine and modify his lifestyle.
✦ If a patient is hospitalized with hypertension, find out if he was taking his prescribed medication.

NURSING CONSIDERATIONS

✦ To encourage adherence to antihypertensive therapy, suggest that the patient establish a daily routine for taking his medication. Warn that uncontrolled hypertension may cause stroke and heart attack. Tell him to report adverse drug effects. Also, advise him to avoid high-sodium antacids and over-the-counter cold and sinus medications, which contain harmful vasoconstrictors.

✦ Encourage a change in dietary habits. Help the obese patient plan a weight-reduction diet; tell him to avoid high-sodium foods (pickles, potato chips, canned soups, and cold cuts) and table salt.

✦ Help the patient examine and modify his lifestyle (for example, by reducing stress and exercising regularly).

✦ If a patient is hospitalized with hypertension, find out if he was taking his prescribed medication. If he wasn't, ask why. If the patient can't afford the medication, refer him to an appropriate social service agency. Tell the patient and his family to keep a record of drugs used in the past, noting especially which ones were or weren't effective. Suggest recording this information on a card so that the patient can show it to his physician.

INITIAL DRUG THERAPY		
	WITHOUT COMPELLING INDICATION	**WITH COMPELLING INDICATIONS***
	No antihypertensive drug indicated	Drugs for the compelling indications****
	Thiazide-type diuretics for most; may consider angiotensin-converting enzyme (ACE) inhibitors, angiotensin receptor blockers, beta-adrenergic blockers, calcium channel blockers, or combination	Drugs for the compelling indications****; other antihypertensive drugs (diuretics, ACE inhibitors, angiotensin receptor blockers, beta-adrenergic blockers, or calcium channel blockers as needed)
	Two-drug combination for most** (usually thiazide diuretic and ACE inhibitor or angiotensin receptor blocker, beta-adrenergic blocker, or calcium channel blocker)	Same as stage 1

Initial drug therapy for managing blood pressure
+ Normal and prehypertension: no antihypertensive drug indicated
+ Stage 1 hypertension: Thiazide-type diuretics
+ Stage 2 hypertension: Two-drug combination for most patients

✦ When routine blood pressure screening reveals elevated pressure, make sure the cuff size is appropriate for the patient's upper arm circumference. Take the pressure measurement at least twice, after the patient has been sitting quietly in a chair (with feet on the floor and arm supported at heart level) for at least 5 minutes. Blood pressure measurement taken in the standing position is indicated periodically, especially if the patient is at risk for postural hypotension. Ask the patient if he smoked, drank a beverage containing caffeine, or was emotionally upset before the test. Advise the patient to return for blood pressure testing at frequent, regular intervals.

✦ To help identify hypertension and prevent untreated hypertension, participate in public education programs dealing with hypertension and ways to reduce risk factors. Encourage public participation in blood pressure screening programs. Routinely screen all patients, especially those at risk (blacks and people with family histories of hypertension, stroke, or heart attack).

Key nursing actions
(continued)
✦ When routine blood pressure screening reveals elevated pressure, make sure the cuff size is appropriate for the patient's upper arm circumference. Take the pressure measurement at least twice.
✦ To help identify hypertension and prevent untreated hypertension, participate in public education programs dealing with hypertension and ways to reduce risk factors.

Characteristics of metabolic syndrome

+ Also called *syndrome X, insulin resistance syndrome, dysmetabolic syndrome,* and *multiple metabolic syndrome*
+ Cluster of conditions characterized by abdominal obesity, high blood sugar, insulin resistance, high blood cholesterol and triglycerides, and high blood pressure
+ Increased risk of heart disease, stroke, dying of myocardial infarction
+ First defined in May 15, 2001; commonly goes unrecognized

Causes

+ May be a genetic predisposition
+ Abdominal obesity
+ Type 2 diabetes mellitus
+ Insulin resistance
+ Dyslipidemia
+ Hypertension

How it happens

+ Glucose is insulin resistant
+ Excess insulin required to overcome resistance
+ Excess quantity/force of insulin causes damage to lining of arteries, promotes fat storage deposits, prevents fat breakdown
+ Can lead to diabetes, blood clots, and coronary events

METABOLIC SYNDROME

Metabolic syndrome — also called *syndrome X, insulin resistance syndrome, dysmetabolic syndrome,* and *multiple metabolic syndrome* — is a cluster of conditions characterized by abdominal obesity, high blood sugar (type II diabetes mellitus), insulin resistance, high blood cholesterol and triglycerides, and high blood pressure. More than 22% of people in the United States meet three or more of these criteria for metabolic syndrome, raising their risk of heart disease and stroke and placing them at high risk for dying of myocardial infarction. Metabolic syndrome was first defined in the Third Report of the National Cholesterol Education Program Expert Panel on Detection, Evaluation, and Treatment of High Blood Cholesterol in Adults on May 15, 2001, and commonly goes unrecognized.

CAUSES

There may be a genetic predisposition for metabolic syndrome. Risk factors for acquired metabolic syndrome include abdominal obesity, type 2 diabetes mellitus, insulin resistance, dyslipidemia, and hypertension.

Abdominal obesity is a strong predictor of metabolic syndrome; excess weight around the waist increases the risk more than in people who are just as overweight but with the weight distributed around the hips. Intra-abdominal fat tends to be more resistant to insulin than fat in other areas of the body. This increases the release of free fatty acid into the portal system, leading to increased apolipoprotein B, increased low-density lipoprotein (LDL), decreased high-density lipoprotein (HDL), and increased triglycerides. As a result, the risk of cardiovascular disease is increased.

Type 2 diabetes mellitus is a risk factor because a hallmark for metabolic syndrome is a fasting glucose level greater than 110 mg/dL. People with diabetes have atherosclerotic heart disease at a younger age, affecting more women than men. Diabetes also increases the risk of macrovascular disease (ischemic heart disease, stroke, and peripheral vascular disease) and is a coronary heart disease risk equivalent.

Another risk factor is insulin resistance. In insulin resistance, cells have an abnormal response to insulin. For people who are genetically inclined to insulin resistance and abdominal obesity and those with a sedentary lifestyle, metabolic syndrome becomes a greater risk. Insulin resistance leads to hyperinsulinemia, hyperglycemia, abnormal glucose and lipid metabolism, damaged endothelium, and cardiovascular disease.

Dyslipidemia can also be a risk factor for metabolic syndrome. Normally, insulin reduces the amount of free fatty acids in the liver. However, in people with insulin resistance, there's an increase in the amount of free fatty acids reaching the liver. As a result, triglycerides and LDL levels rise, producing an abnormal endothelium and atherosclerosis.

High blood pressure is another risk factor. The combination of insulin resistance, hyperinsulinemia, and abdominal obesity leads to hypertension and its harmful cardiovascular effects. Moreover, insulin resistance promotes salt sensitivity in people with high blood pressure.

PATHOPHYSIOLOGY

In the normal digestion process, food is broken down in the intestines into basic components, one of which is glucose. Glucose provides energy for cellular activity, and excess glucose is stored in cells for future use. Insulin, a hormone secreted in the pancreas, guides glucose into storage cells.

In people with metabolic syndrome, glucose is insulin resistant. It doesn't respond to insulin's attempt to guide it into storage cells. Excess insulin is then required to overcome this resistance. This excess in quantity and force of insulin causes damage to the lining of the arteries, promotes fat storage deposits, and prevents fat breakdown. This series of events can lead to diabetes, blood clots, and coronary events.

SIGNS AND SYMPTOMS

Assessment commonly reveals a history of hypertension, abdominal obesity, sedentary lifestyle, poor diet, and a family member with metabolic syndrome. Physical findings include abdominal obesity: a waist more than 40″ (101.6 cm) around in men and 35″ (88.9 cm) in women. Commonly, blood pressure is found to be 130/85 mm Hg or more; fasting blood glucose is found to be 100 or more. The patient may feel tired, especially after eating, and may have difficulty losing weight.

COMPLICATIONS

Complications may include coronary artery disease, diabetes, hyperlipidemia, and premature death.

DIAGNOSIS

Blood studies commonly indicate elevated blood glucose levels, hyperinsulinemia, and elevated serum uric acid. Use of lipid profile studies reveal elevated LDL levels, low HDL levels, and elevated triglycerides. Further diagnostic procedures are nonspecific and may be performed to detect hypertension, diabetes, hyperlipidemia, and hyperinsulinemia.

TREATMENT

Treatment may consist of lifestyle modifications, pharmacologic therapy, surgical intervention, or a combination of these therapies.

Lifestyle modifications

Therapeutic lifestyle change is a program of lifestyle modifications focused on weight reduction and exercise. Modest weight reduction through diet and exercise considerably improves hemoglobin A_{1c} levels, reduces insulin resistance, improves blood lipid levels, and decreases blood pressure—all elements of metabolic syndrome. Recent studies have shown that in patients with impaired glucose tolerance, losing an average of 7% of body weight reduced the risk of developing type 2 diabetes by 58%.

To improve cardiovascular health, a diet rich in vegetables, fruits, whole grains, fish, and low-fat dairy products combined with regular exercise is recommended. Moreover, nutrient-dense, low-energy foods should replace low-nutrient high-calorie foods. Meal replacements and shakes may also improve risk factors for metabolic syndrome and improve weight loss. (See *Therapeutic lifestyle change diet*, page 198.)

A regular exercise program of moderate physical activity, in addition to dietary modifications, promotes weight loss maintenance, improves insulin sensitivity, and reduces blood glucose levels. According to the Surgeon General's Report on Physical Activity and Health, a person should exercise moderately for a minimum of

Key signs and symptoms
- Family history of syndrome or contributing factors
- Abdominal obesity
- High blood pressure
- Fasting blood glucose is found to be 100 or more
- Fatigue after eating
- Difficulty losing weight

Complications
- Coronary artery disease
- Diabetes
- Hyperlipidemia
- Premature death

Diagnosis
- Elevated blood glucose levels
- Hyperinsulinemia
- Elevated serum uric acid
- Elevated LDL levels
- Low HDL levels
- Elevated triglycerides
- Hypertension
- Diabetes
- Hyperlipidemia
- Hyperinsulinemia

Treatment
Lifestyle modifications
- Modest weight reduction
- Nutrient-dense diet
- Regular exercise program of moderate physical activity

Key areas of a therapeutic lifestyle change diet

+ Total fat: 25% to 35% of total calories
+ Fiber: 20 to 30 g/day
+ Protein: approximately 15% of calories
+ Total calories: balance energy intake and expenditure to maintain desirable body weight

Therapeutic lifestyle change diet

This table shows the nutrient composition of the therapeutic lifestyle change diet.

NUTRIENT	RECOMMENDED INTAKE
Saturated fat*	< 7% of total calories
Polyunsaturated fat	Up to 10% of total calories
Monounsaturated fat	Up to 20% of total calories
Total fat	25% to 35% of total calories
Carbohydrate**	50% to 60% of total calories
Fiber	20 to 30 g/day
Protein	Approximately 15% of total calories
Cholesterol	< 200 mg/day
Total calories***	Balance energy intake and expenditure to maintain desirable body weight and prevent weight gain

* Trans fatty acids are another low-density lipoprotein-raising fat that should be kept at a low intake.

** Carbohydrates should be derived predominantly from foods rich in complex carbohydrates, including grains — especially whole grains, fruits, and vegetables.

*** Daily expenditure should include at least moderate physical activity (approximately 200 kcal/day.)

"Executive Summary of the Third Report of the National Cholesterol Education Program (NCEP) Expert Panel on Detection, Evaluation, and Treatment of High Blood Cholesterol in Adults (Adult Treatment Panel III)," *JAMA* 285:2486-97, 2001.

30 minutes on most (if not all) days of the week. Others have even recommended 60 minutes of daily physical activity. The selected exercise program should improve cardiovascular conditioning, increase strength through resistance training, and improve flexibility.

Treatment

Pharmacologic therapy
+ Phentermine
+ Orlistat
+ Sibutramine
+ Vitamin supplements

Pharmacologic therapy

Medications may be used in the treatment of metabolic syndrome for those who have a body mass index (BMI) of 27 kg/m^2 or greater in the presence of other risk factors (such as diabetes, hypertension, and hyperlipidemia) or for those with a BMI of 30 kg/m^2 or greater without other risk factors. Weight loss medications may also be added to lifestyle changes if the patient hasn't achieved weight loss after 12 weeks.

Phentermine (Adipex-P) is used for short-term treatment of obesity in conjunction with diet and exercise. Currently, the only two medications that have been approved for long-term weight loss are orlistat (Xenical) and sibutramine (Meridia).

Orlistat works by decreasing the absorption of dietary fat by inhibiting pancreatic lipase, which is needed for the breakdown and absorption of fat. Adverse effects of orlistat include steatorrhea, increased defecation, fecal urgency, and flatus. Because absorption of fat-soluble vitamins is reduced, the patient may require vitamin supplements. Studies show that when obese patients took orlistat in conjunction with dieting, they achieved greater weight loss and serum glucose control than diet alone.

Sibutramine promotes weight loss by inhibiting the reuptake of serotonin, norepinephrine, and dopamine and increases the satiety-producing effects of serotonin. Further, it reduces the drop in metabolic rate that often occurs with weight loss. The most frequent adverse effects include diarrhea, dyspepsia, and vomiting.

Surgical interventions

Surgical treatment of obesity produces a greater degree and duration of weight loss than other therapies and improves or resolves most of the factors of metabolic syndrome. Candidates for surgical intervention include patients with a BMI greater than 40 kg/m^2 or those with a BMI greater than 35 kg/m^2 with obesity-related medical conditions.

Gastric bypass procedures such as Roux-en-Y produce permanent weight loss in the majority of patients. This type of surgery requires a multidisciplinary approach for safe and effective weight loss.

NURSING CONSIDERATIONS

✦ Monitor the patient's blood pressure, blood glucose levels, blood cholesterol levels, and insulin levels.
✦ Because research indicates that longer lifestyle modification programs are associated with improved weight loss maintenance, encourage patients with metabolic syndrome to begin an exercise and weight loss program with a friend or family member. Assist him in exploring options and support his efforts.
✦ To improve compliance, schedule frequent follow-up appointments with the patient. At that time, review his food diaries and exercise logs. Be positive and promote his active participation and partnership in his treatment plan.

PATENT DUCTUS ARTERIOSUS

The ductus arteriosus is a fetal blood vessel that connects the pulmonary artery to the descending aorta, just distal to the left subclavian artery. Normally, the ductus closes within days to weeks after birth. In patent ductus arteriosus (PDA), the lumen of the ductus remains open after birth. This creates a left-to-right shunt of blood from the aorta to the pulmonary artery and results in recirculation of arterial blood through the lungs. Initially, PDA may produce no clinical effects, but over time it can precipitate pulmonary vascular disease, causing symptoms to appear by age 40. PDA affects twice as many females as males and is the most common acyanotic congenital heart defect found in adults.

The prognosis is good if the shunt is small or surgical repair is effective. Otherwise, PDA may advance to intractable heart failure, which may be fatal.

CAUSES

PDA has been linked to premature birth, probably as a result of abnormalities in oxygenation or the relaxant action of prostaglandin E, which prevents ductal spasm and contracture necessary for closure. It has also been associated with rubella syndrome, coarctation of the aorta, ventricular septal defect, pulmonary and aortic stenosis, and living at high altitudes.

Treatment

Surgical intervention
✦ Candidates for surgery must have a BMI greater than 40 kg/m^2 or greater than 35 kg/m^2 with obesity-related medical conditions
✦ Gastric bypass

Key nursing actions
✦ Monitor the patient's blood pressure and blood glucose, blood cholesterol, and insulin levels.
✦ Encourage patients to begin an exercise and weight loss program with a friend.
✦ To improve compliance, schedule frequent follow-up appointments with the patient.

Characteristics of PDA
✦ Lumen of ductus remains open after birth
✦ Creates a left-to-right shunt of blood from aorta to pulmonary artery
✦ Results in recirculation of arterial blood through lungs
✦ Can precipitate pulmonary vascular disease
✦ Most common acyanotic congenital heart defect found in adults
✦ Prognosis is good if shunt is small or surgery is effective

Causes
✦ Premature birth
✦ Rubella syndrome
✦ Coarctation of the aorta

How it happens

+ Relative resistances in vasculature and size of ductus determine quantity of blood shunted
+ Oxygenated blood is shunted from aorta through ductus arteriosus to pulmonary artery
+ Blood returns to left side of heart and is pumped back to aorta
+ Left atrium and left ventricle must accommodate
+ Causes left ventricular hypertrophy, possibly heart failure
+ Shunt can cause chronic pulmonary artery hypertension

Key signs and symptoms

+ Respiratory distress with signs of heart failure in infants
+ Gibson murmur — may be absent
+ Thrill may be palpated at left sternal border
+ Prominent left ventricular impulse

Complications

+ Infective endocarditis
+ Heart failure
+ Recurrent pneumonia

Diagnosis

+ Increased pulmonary vascular markings
+ Prominent pulmonary arteries
+ Enlargement of left ventricle and aorta
+ ECG normal or indicate left atrial or ventricular hypertrophy
+ Echocardiography detects and estimates size of a PDA

PATHOPHYSIOLOGY

The ductus arteriosus normally closes as prostaglandin levels from the placenta fall and oxygen levels rise. This process should begin as soon as the neonate takes its first breath, but may take as long as 3 months in some children.

In PDA, relative resistances in pulmonary and systemic vasculature and the size of the ductus determine the quantity of blood that's shunted from left to right. Because of increased aortic pressure, oxygenated blood is shunted from the aorta through the ductus arteriosus to the pulmonary artery. The blood returns to the left side of the heart and is pumped out to the aorta once more.

The left atrium and left ventricle must accommodate the increased pulmonary venous return, which increases filling pressure and workload on the left side of the heart, causes left ventricular hypertrophy and, possibly, heart failure. In the final stages of untreated PDA, the left-to-right shunt leads to chronic pulmonary artery hypertension that becomes fixed and unreactive. This causes the shunt to reverse so that unoxygenated blood enters systemic circulation, causing cyanosis.

SIGNS AND SYMPTOMS

One sign of PDA is respiratory distress with signs of heart failure in infants, especially those who are premature. This is due to the tremendous volume of blood shunted to the lungs through a PDA and the increased workload on the left side of the heart.

Another sign is a classic machinery, or Gibson, murmur. This murmur is continuous and is heard throughout systole and diastole in older children and adults due to shunting of blood from the aorta to the pulmonary artery throughout systole and diastole. It's best heard at the base of the heart, at the second intercostal space under the left clavicle. The murmur may obscure S_2. However, in a right-to-left shunt, this murmur may be absent.

Upon physical examination, a thrill may be palpated at the left sternal border caused by the shunting of blood from the aorta to the pulmonary artery. The patient may have a prominent left ventricular impulse due to left ventricular hypertrophy and bounding peripheral pulses (Corrigan's pulse) due to the high-flow state.

A widened pulse pressure may be evident because of an elevated systolic blood pressure and, primarily, a drop in diastolic blood pressure as blood is shunted through the PDA, thus reducing peripheral resistance.

The patient may exhibit slow motor development, heart failure, and failure to thrive as a result of fatigue and dyspnea on exertion, which may develop in adults with undetected PDA.

COMPLICATIONS

Possible complications of PDA may include infective endocarditis, heart failure, and recurrent pneumonia.

DIAGNOSIS

Certain tests help diagnose PDA. Chest X-rays may show increased pulmonary vascular markings, prominent pulmonary arteries, and enlargement of the left ventricle and aorta. An electrocardiography (ECG) may be normal or may indicate left atrial or ventricular hypertrophy and, in pulmonary vascular disease, biventricular hypertrophy.

Use of an echocardiography detects and estimates the size of a PDA, while also revealing an enlarged left atrium and left ventricle, or right ventricular hypertrophy from pulmonary vascular disease.

Because of the influx of aortic blood, higher pulmonary arterial oxygen content than right ventricular content is seen in a cardiac catheterization. Increased pulmonary artery pressure indicates a large shunt or, if it exceeds systemic arterial pressure, severe pulmonary vascular disease. In addition, cardiac catheterization allows for the calculation of blood volume crossing the ductus, and can rule out associated cardiac defects. Injection of a contrast agent can conclusively demonstrate PDA.

TREATMENT

Correction of PDA may require surgery to ligate the ductus if medical management can't control heart failure. Asymptomatic infants with PDA don't require immediate treatment and, if symptoms are mild, surgical ligation of the PDA is usually delayed until age 1.

PDA may be treated with indomethacin (Indocin) (a prostaglandin inhibitor) that will induce ductus spasm and closure in premature infants.

Prophylactic antibiotics protect patients against infective endocarditis.

Treatment of PDA may also include management of heart failure with fluid restriction, diuretics, and digoxin.

Cardiac catheterization may be performed in order to deposit a plug or umbrella in the ductus to stop shunting.

NURSING CONSIDERATIONS

✦ PDA necessitates careful monitoring, patient and family teaching, and emotional support.

✦ Watch carefully for signs of PDA in all premature infants.

✦ Be alert for respiratory distress symptoms resulting from heart failure, which may develop rapidly in a premature infant. Frequently assess vital signs, ECG, electrolyte levels, and intake and output. Record responses to diuretics and other therapies.

✦ If the infant receives indomethacin for ductus closure, watch for possible adverse effects, such as diarrhea, jaundice, bleeding, and renal dysfunction.

✦ Before surgery, carefully explain all treatments and tests to the parents. Include the child in your explanations. Arrange for the child and his parents to meet the intensive care unit staff. Tell them about expected I.V. lines, monitoring equipment, and postoperative procedures.

✦ Immediately after surgery, the child may have a central venous pressure catheter and an arterial line in place. Carefully assess vital signs, intake and output, and arterial and venous pressures. Provide pain relief, as needed.

✦ Before discharge, review instructions with the parents about activity restrictions based on the child's tolerance and energy levels. Advise parents not to become overprotective as their child's tolerance for physical activity increases.

✦ Stress the need for regular medical follow-up examinations. Advise parents to inform any physician who treats their child about his history of surgery for PDA — even if the child is being treated for an unrelated medical problem.

Treatment

✦ Surgery
✦ Indomethacin
✦ Prophylactic antibiotics
✦ Management of heart failure
✦ Cardiac catheterization

Key nursing actions

✦ PDA necessitates careful monitoring, patient and family teaching, and emotional support.
✦ Watch carefully for signs of PDA in all premature infants.
✦ Be alert for respiratory distress symptoms from heart failure.
✦ Before surgery, carefully explain all treatments and tests to the parents.
✦ Immediately after surgery, the child may have a central venous pressure catheter and an arterial line in place.
✦ Before discharge, review instructions with the parents about activity restrictions based on the child's tolerance and energy levels.

PERICARDITIS

Pericarditis is an inflammation of the pericardium — the fibroserous sac that envelops, supports, and protects the heart. It occurs in acute and chronic forms. Acute pericarditis can be fibrinous or effusive, with purulent, serous, or hemorrhagic exudate. Chronic constrictive pericarditis is characterized by dense fibrous pericardial thickening. The prognosis depends on the underlying cause, but is generally good in acute pericarditis, unless constriction occurs.

CAUSES

Common causes of pericarditis include neoplasms (primary or metastases from lungs, breasts, or other organs), high-dose radiation to the chest, uremia, hypersensitivity reactions, or autoimmune diseases, such as acute rheumatic fever (most common cause of pericarditis in children), systemic lupus erythematosus, and rheumatoid arthritis. Other causes include previous cardiac injury, such as myocardial infarction (Dressler's syndrome), trauma, or surgery (postcardiotomy syndrome), that leaves the pericardium intact but causes blood to leak into the pericardial cavity, and drugs, such as hydralazine (Apresoline) or procainamide (Pronestyl).

Idiopathic factors most commonly cause acute pericarditis, whereas bacterial, fungal, or viral infections cause infectious pericarditis. Two of the less common causes of pericarditis are aortic aneurysm with pericardial leakage and myxedema with cholesterol deposits in the pericardium.

PATHOPHYSIOLOGY

Pericardial tissue damaged by bacteria or other substances results in the release of chemical mediators of inflammation (prostaglandins, histamines, bradykinins, and serotonin) into the surrounding tissue, thereby initiating the inflammatory process. Friction occurs as the inflamed pericardial layers rub against each other. Histamines and other chemical mediators dilate vessels and increase vessel permeability. Vessel walls then leak fluids and protein (including fibrinogen) into tissues, causing extracellular edema. Macrophages already present in the tissue begin to phagocytize the invading bacteria and are joined by neutrophils and monocytes. After several days, the area fills with an exudate composed of necrotic tissue and dead and dying bacteria, neutrophils, and macrophages. Eventually, the contents of the cavity autolyze and are gradually reabsorbed into healthy tissue.

A pericardial effusion develops if fluid accumulates in the pericardial cavity. Cardiac tamponade results when there's a rapid accumulation of fluid in the pericardial space, compressing the heart and preventing it from filling during diastole and resulting in a drop in cardiac output.

Chronic constrictive pericarditis develops if the pericardium becomes thick and stiff from chronic or recurrent pericarditis, encasing the heart in a stiff shell and preventing it from properly filling during diastole. This causes an increase in left- and right-sided filling pressures, leading to a drop in stroke volume and cardiac output.

SIGNS AND SYMPTOMS

Signs and symptoms of pericarditis may include a pericardial friction rub caused by the roughened pericardial membranes rubbing against one another. Although the rub may be heard intermittently, it's best heard when the patient leans forward and exhales.

The patient may report a sharp and typically sudden pain, usually starting over the sternum and radiating to the neck (especially the left trapezius ridge), shoulders, back, and arms due to inflammation and irritation of the pericardial membranes. The pain is often pleuritic, increasing when the patient sits up and leans forward, pulling the heart away from the diaphragmatic pleurae of the lungs. The patient's respirations may be shallow and rapid in an attempt to reduce pleuritic pain.

Upon auscultation, the patient may have muffled and distant heart sounds due to fluid build up. He may also have a pericardial knock in early diastole that's produced by restricted ventricular filling and heard best along the left sternal border.

The patient may experience dyspnea, orthopnea, and tachycardia as well as other signs of heart failure as fluid builds up in the pericardial space and causes pericardial effusion, a major complication of acute pericarditis.

Pallor, clammy skin, hypotension, pulsus paradoxus, jugular vein distention and, eventually, cardiovascular collapse may occur with the rapid fluid accumulation of cardiac tamponade.

Fluid retention, ascites, hepatomegaly, jugular vein distention, and other signs of chronic right-sided heart failure may occur with chronic constrictive pericarditis as the systemic venous pressure gradually increases. The patient may exhibit a positive Kussmaul's sign—increased jugular vein distention on inspiration, due to restricted right-sided filling—and may experience a mild fever caused by the inflammatory process.

DIAGNOSIS

These tests help diagnose pericarditis:

✦ Electrocardiography may reveal diffuse ST-segment elevation in the limb leads and most precordial leads that reflects the inflammatory process. Downsloping PR segments and upright T waves are present in most leads. QRS segments may be diminished when pericardial effusion exists. Arrhythmias, such as atrial fibrillation and sinus arrhythmias, may occur. In chronic constrictive pericarditis, there may be low-voltage QRS complexes, T-wave inversion or flattening, and P mitrale (wide P waves) in leads I, II, and V_6.

✦ Laboratory testing may reveal an elevated erythrocyte sedimentation rate as a result of the inflammatory process or a normal or elevated white blood cell count, especially in infectious pericarditis; blood urea nitrogen may detect uremia as a cause of pericarditis.

✦ Blood cultures may identify an infectious cause.

✦ Antistreptolysin-O titers may be positive if pericarditis is due to rheumatic fever.

✦ Purified protein derivative skin test may be positive if pericarditis is due to tuberculosis.

✦ Echocardiography may show an echo-free space between the ventricular wall and the pericardium and reduced pumping action of the heart.

✦ Chest X-rays may be normal with acute pericarditis. The cardiac silhouette may be enlarged with a water bottle shape caused by fluid accumulation if pleural effusion is present.

TREATMENT

Correcting pericarditis typically involves bed rest while fever and pain persist, to reduce metabolic needs. It also involves treatment of the underlying cause—if it can be identified. For example, antibacterial, antifungal, or antiviral therapy will be administered if an infectious cause is suspected.

Key signs and symptoms

✦ Pericardial friction rub
✦ Sharp sudden pain over sternum and radiating to neck, shoulders, back, and arms
✦ Shallow, rapid respirations
✦ Muffled and distant heart sounds
✦ Pericardial knock in early diastole
✦ Dyspnea
✦ Orthopnea
✦ Tachycardia
✦ Other signs of heart failure

Diagnosis

✦ Downsloping PR segments and upright T waves
✦ QRS segments may be diminished
✦ Arrhythmias
✦ Low-voltage QRS complexes, T-wave inversion or flattening, and P mitrale in leads I, II, and V_6
✦ Elevated erythrocyte
✦ Elevated WBC count
✦ Cardiac silhouette may be enlarged with a water bottle shape in chest X-ray

Treatment

+ Bed rest
+ Treatment of underlying cause
+ Antibacterials
+ Antifungals
+ Antiviral therapy
+ NSAIDs
+ Pericardiocentesis
+ Partial or total pericardectomy

Key nursing actions

+ A patient with pericarditis needs complete bed rest.
+ The patient should be placed in an upright position to relieve dyspnea and chest pain.
+ Provide analgesics and oxygen.
+ Monitor the patient for decreased blood pressure, increased central venous pressure, and pulsus paradoxus.

Characteristics of pulmonary hypertension

+ Life-threatening disorder
+ When PAP is above normal
+ No definitive set of values used to diagnose; NIH requires a mean PAP of 25 mm Hg or more

Primary

+ Increased PAP and pulmonary vascular resistance
+ Most common in women ages 20 to 40

Secondary

+ Prognosis depends on underlying disorder
+ Patient may have no symptoms until lung damage is severe

Alert!

+ Mortality is highest in pregnant women.

Nonsteroidal anti-inflammatory drugs (NSAIDs), such as aspirin and indomethacin, are prescribed to relieve pain and reduce inflammation. Corticosteroids may be employed if NSAIDs are ineffective and no infection exists. (Corticosteroids must be administered cautiously because episodes may recur when therapy is discontinued.)

Procedures such as a pericardiocentesis may be performed to remove excess fluid from the pericardial space. A partial pericardectomy, which allows for the creation of a window that fosters drainage of fluid into the pleural space, may be performed in order to treat recurrent pericarditis. A total pericardectomy permits adequate filling and contraction of the heart; it's used to treat constrictive pericarditis.

Idiopathic pericarditis may be benign and self-limiting and may not require aggressive treatment.

NURSING CONSIDERATIONS

A patient with pericarditis needs complete bed rest. In addition, the patient's pain level should be assessed in relation to respiration and body position to distinguish pericardial pain from myocardial ischemic pain.

+ The patient should be placed in an upright position to relieve dyspnea and chest pain.

+ Analgesics and oxygen should be administered and the patient with acute pericarditis should be reassured that his condition is temporary and treatable.

+ The patient should be monitored for decreased blood pressure, increased central venous pressure, and pulsus paradoxus. These are signs of cardiac compression and cardiac tamponade, which are both complications of pericardial effusion. Because cardiac tamponade requires immediate treatment, keep a pericardiocentesis set handy whenever pericardial effusion is suspected.

+ As always, tests and treatments must be explained to the patient. If surgery is necessary, he should learn deep-breathing and coughing exercises before the procedure. Postoperative care includes monitoring the patient for arrhythmias and hypotension. Vital signs, arterial blood gas analysis, intake and output, daily weight, blood chemistries, chest X-rays, and pulmonary artery catheter readings should be monitored closely.

▼ *LIFE-THREATENING DISORDER*

PULMONARY HYPERTENSION

Pulmonary hypertension occurs when pulmonary artery pressure (PAP) rises above normal for reasons other than aging or altitude. No definitive set of values is used to diagnose pulmonary hypertension, but the National Institutes of Health requires a mean PAP of 25 mm Hg or more. Primary or idiopathic pulmonary hypertension is characterized by increased PAP and increased pulmonary vascular resistance. This form is most common in women ages 20 to 40 and is usually fatal within 3 to 4 years.

 CLINICAL ALERT Mortality is highest in pregnant women.

Secondary pulmonary hypertension results from existing cardiac or pulmonary disease or both. The prognosis in secondary pulmonary hypertension depends on the severity of the underlying disorder.

The patient may have no signs or symptoms of the disorder until lung damage becomes severe. In fact, it may not be diagnosed until an autopsy is performed.

CAUSES

Causes of primary pulmonary hypertension are unknown, but may include hereditary factors or altered immune mechanisms.

Secondary pulmonary hypertension results from hypoxemia caused by various conditions, including:

✦ alveolar hypoventilation resulting from chronic obstructive pulmonary disease, sarcoidosis, diffuse interstitial pneumonia, malignant metastases, scleroderma, obesity, or kyphoscoliosis

✦ vascular obstruction resulting from pulmonary embolism, vasculitis, left atrial myxoma, idiopathic veno-occlusive disease, fibrosing mediastinitis, or mediastinal neoplasm

✦ primary cardiac disease resulting from patent ductus arteriosus (PDA), atrial septal defect, or ventricular septal defect (VSD).

Conditions causing acquired cardiac disease include rheumatic valvular disease and mitral stenosis.

PATHOPHYSIOLOGY

In primary pulmonary hypertension, the smooth muscle in the pulmonary artery wall hypertrophies, narrowing the small pulmonary artery (arterioles) or obliterating it completely. The reason the artery wall hypertrophies is unknown. Fibrous lesions form around the vessels, impairing distensibility and increasing vascular resistance. Pressures in the left ventricle, which receives blood from the lungs, remain normal. However, the increased pressures generated in the lungs are transmitted to the right ventricle, which supplies the pulmonary artery. Eventually, the right ventricle fails (cor pulmonale). Although oxygenation isn't severely affected initially, hypoxia and cyanosis eventually occur. Death results from cor pulmonale.

Alveolar hypoventilation can result from diseases caused by alveolar destruction or from disorders that prevent the chest wall from expanding sufficiently to allow air into the alveoli. The resulting decreased ventilation increases pulmonary vascular resistance. Hypoxemia resulting from this ventilation-perfusion mismatch also causes vasoconstriction, further increasing vascular resistance and resulting in pulmonary hypertension.

Coronary artery disease or mitral valvular disease causing increased left ventricular filling pressures may result in secondary pulmonary hypertension. VSD and PDA cause secondary pulmonary hypertension by increasing blood flow through the pulmonary circulation through left-to-right shunting. Pulmonary emboli and chronic destruction of alveolar walls (as in emphysema) cause secondary pulmonary hypertension by obliterating or obstructing the pulmonary vascular bed. Secondary pulmonary hypertension can also occur by vasoconstriction of the vascular bed, such as through hypoxemia, acidosis, or both. Conditions resulting in vascular obstruction can also cause pulmonary hypertension because blood isn't allowed to flow appropriately through the vessels.

Secondary pulmonary hypertension can be reversed if the disorder is resolved. If hypertension persists, hypertrophy occurs in the medial smooth muscle layer of the arterioles. The larger arteries stiffen, and hypertension progresses. Pulmonary pressures begin to equal systemic blood pressure, causing right ventricular hypertrophy and eventually cor pulmonale.

Primary cardiac diseases may be congenital or acquired. Congenital defects cause a left-to-right shunt, rerouting blood through the lungs twice and causing pulmonary hypertension. Acquired cardiac diseases, such as rheumatic valvular disease and mitral stenosis, result in left-sided heart failure that diminishes the flow of

Causes

Primary
✦ Hereditary factors
✦ Altered immune mechanisms

Secondary
✦ Hypoxemia, caused by alveolar hypoventilation, vascular obstruction, primary cardiac disease, and conditions causing acquired cardiac disease

How it happens

Primary
✦ Smooth muscle in pulmonary artery wall hypertrophies
✦ Small pulmonary artery narrowed or obliterated
✦ Fibrous lesions form around vessels
✦ Pressures in left ventricle remain normal
✦ Increased pressure generated in lungs transmitted to right ventricle
✦ Right ventricle fails
✦ Hypoxia and cyanosis occur
✦ Death results from cor pulmonale

Secondary
✦ Alveolar hypoventilation can result from diseases
✦ Decreased ventilation increases pulmonary vascular resistance
✦ Hypoxemia causes vasoconstriction
✦ Coronary artery disease or mitral valvular disease causes increased left ventricular filling pressures
✦ Vascular obstruction prevents appropriate blood flow through vessels

oxygenated blood from the lungs. This increases pulmonary vascular resistance and right ventricular pressure.

SIGNS AND SYMPTOMS

Most patients complain of increasing dyspnea on exertion from left-sided heart failure and weakness, syncope, and fatigability from diminished tissue oxygenation. Many also show signs of right-sided heart failure, including peripheral edema, ascites, jugular vein distention, and hepatomegaly.

Hypoxia may cause tachycardia, decreased level of consciousness, confusion, and memory loss. Possible displacement of the point of maximal impulse beyond the midclavicular line may occur due to fluid accumulation. Fluid accumulation in the lungs may result in decreased breath sounds. Other clinical effects vary with the underlying disorder.

COMPLICATIONS

Possible complications of pulmonary hypertension include cor pulmonale, cardiac failure, and cardiac arrest.

DIAGNOSIS

These tests help diagnose pulmonary hypertension:

+ Arterial blood gas (ABG) analysis reveals hypoxemia.
+ In right ventricular hypertrophy, electrocardiography shows right axis deviation and tall or peaked P waves in inferior leads.
+ Cardiac catheterization reveals pulmonary systolic pressure above 30 mm Hg. It may also show an increased pulmonary artery wedge pressure (PAWP) if the underlying cause is left atrial myxoma, mitral stenosis, or left-sided heart failure; otherwise, PAWP is normal.
+ Pulmonary angiography detects filling defects in pulmonary vasculature such as those that develop with pulmonary emboli.
+ Pulmonary function studies may show decreased flow rates and increased residual volume in underlying obstructive disease; in underlying restrictive disease, they may show reduced total lung capacity.
+ Radionuclide imaging detects abnormalities in right and left ventricular functioning.
+ Open lung biopsy may determine the type of disorder.
+ Echocardiography allows the assessment of ventricular wall motion and possible valvular dysfunction. It can also demonstrate right ventricular enlargement, abnormal septal configuration consistent with right ventricular pressure overload, and reduction in left ventricular cavity size.
+ Perfusion lung scanning may produce normal or abnormal results, with multiple patchy and diffuse filling defects that don't suggest pulmonary embolism.

TREATMENT

Managing pulmonary hypertension typically involves oxygen therapy to correct hypoxemia and the resulting increased pulmonary vascular resistance. It also involves fluid restriction in right-sided heart failure to decrease the heart's workload.

Drug therapy may include digoxin to increase cardiac output; diuretics to decrease intravascular volume and extravascular fluid accumulation; vasodilators to reduce myocardial workload and oxygen consumption; calcium channel blockers to reduce myocardial workload and oxygen consumption; bronchodilators to relax

Key signs and symptoms

+ Increasing dyspnea on exertion
+ Syncope
+ Fatigability
+ Tachycardia
+ Decreased level of consciousness
+ Confusion
+ Memory loss
+ Displacement of point of maximal impulse beyond midclavicular line

Complications

+ Cor pulmonale
+ Cardiac failure
+ Cardiac arrest

Diagnosis

+ ABG analysis reveals hypoxemia
+ Electrocardiography shows right axis deviation, tall/peaked P waves in inferior leads in right ventricular hypertrophy
+ Pulmonary systolic pressure above 30 mm Hg
+ Pulmonary angiography detects filling defects in pulmonary vasculature
+ Reduced total lung capacity
+ Radionuclide imaging detects abnormalities in right and left ventricular function
+ Echocardiography for assessment of ventricular wall motion and possible valvular dysfunction
+ Perfusion lung scanning may produce normal or abnormal results

smooth muscles and increase airway patency; and beta-adrenergic blockers to improve oxygenation.

Treatment of the underlying cause is necessary to correct pulmonary edema. In severe cases, a heart-lung transplant may be indicated.

NURSING CONSIDERATIONS

Pulmonary hypertension requires keen observation and careful monitoring as well as skilled supportive care.

✦ Administer oxygen therapy as ordered and observe the patient's response. Report signs of increasing dyspnea to the physician so he can adjust treatment accordingly.

✦ Monitor ABG levels for acidosis and hypoxemia. Report changes in level of consciousness at once.

✦ When caring for a patient with right-sided heart failure, especially one receiving diuretics, record her weight daily, carefully measure intake and output, and explain all medications and diet restrictions. Check for worsening jugular vein distention, which may indicate fluid overload.

✦ Monitor vital signs, especially blood pressure and heart rate. Watch for hypotension and tachycardia. If the patient has a pulmonary artery catheter, check PAP and PAWP as ordered. Report changes.

✦ Before discharge, help the patient adjust to the limitations imposed by this disorder. Advise against overexertion, and suggest frequent rest periods between activities. Refer the patient to the social services department if she needs special equipment, such as oxygen equipment, for home use. Make sure she understands the prescribed medications and diet and the need to weigh herself daily.

RAYNAUD'S DISEASE

Raynaud's disease is one of several primary arteriospastic disorders characterized by episodic vasospasm in the small peripheral arteries and arterioles, precipitated by exposure to cold or stress. This condition occurs bilaterally and usually affects the hands or, less commonly, the feet. Raynaud's disease is most prevalent in females, particularly between puberty and age 40. It's a benign condition, requiring no specific treatment and causing no serious sequelae.

Raynaud's phenomenon, however, a condition usually associated with several connective disorders—such as scleroderma, systemic lupus erythematosus (SLE), or polymyositis—has a progressive course, leading to ischemia, gangrene, and amputation. Distinguishing between the two disorders is difficult because some patients who experience mild symptoms of Raynaud's disease for several years may later develop overt connective tissue disease, especially scleroderma.

CAUSES

Although family history is a risk factor, the cause of this disorder is unknown.

Raynaud's phenomenon may develop secondary to connective tissue disorders, such as scleroderma, rheumatoid arthritis, SLE, or polymyositis; pulmonary hypertension; thoracic outlet syndrome; arterio-occlusive disease; myxedema; trauma; serum sickness; exposure to heavy metals; previous damage from cold exposure; and long-term exposure to cold, vibrating machinery (such as operating a jackhammer) or pressure to the fingertips (such as in typists and pianists).

Treatment
✦ Oxygen therapy
✦ Fluid restriction
✦ Digoxin
✦ Diuretics
✦ Vasodilators
✦ Calcium channel blockers
✦ Beta-adrenergic blockers

Key nursing actions
✦ Administer oxygen therapy and observe the patient's response.
✦ Monitor ABG levels for acidosis and hypoxemia.
✦ Monitor vital signs, especially blood pressure and heart rate.
✦ Before discharge, help the patient adjust to the limitations imposed by this disorder.

Characteristics of Raynaud's disease
✦ One of several primary arteriospastic disorders
✦ Episodic vasospasm in small peripheral arteries and arterioles, precipitated by exposure to cold or stress
✦ Usually affects hands or feet
✦ Most prevalent in females, particularly between puberty and age 40
✦ Benign condition
✦ Raynaud's phenomenon has a progressive course, leading to ischemia, gangrene, and amputation

Causes
✦ Family history is a risk factor
✦ Cause of disorder unknown
✦ May develop secondary to connective tissue disorders

How it happens

+ Hyperactive response of intrinsic vascular wall to exposure to cold to account for reduced digital blood flow
+ Increased vasomotor tone due to sympathetic stimulation
+ Antigen-antibody immune response

Key signs and symptoms

+ Blanching of fingers bilaterally after exposure to cold or stress
+ Fingers turn red as blood rushes back into arterioles
+ Cold and numb feeling
+ Aching pain

Complications

+ Cutaneous gangrene

Diagnosis

+ Skin color changes
+ Bilateral involvement
+ Absence of gangrene or minimal cutaneous gangrene
+ Normal arterial pulses
+ Patient history of symptoms for at least 2 years
+ ANA titer used to identify autoimmune disease as an underlying cause of Raynaud's phenomenon

Treatment

+ Avoid triggers
+ Keep fingers and toes warm
+ Calcium channel blockers
+ Biofeedback exercises
+ Amputation in cases of gangrene

PATHOPHYSIOLOGY

Although the cause is unknown, several theories to explain the cause exist. The first theory looks to the hyperactive response of the intrinsic vascular wall to exposure to cold to account for reduced digital blood flow. The second theory looks at increased vasomotor tone due to sympathetic stimulation as the cause. Lastly, the third theory is based on antigen-antibody immune response. It's the most likely theory because abnormal immunologic test results accompany Raynaud's phenomenon.

SIGNS AND SYMPTOMS

A patient with Raynaud's disease may present with blanching of the fingers bilaterally after exposure to cold or stress as vasoconstriction or vasospasm reduces blood flow. This blanching is followed by cyanosis due to increased oxygen extraction resulting from sluggish blood flow. As the spasm resolves, the fingers turn red as blood rushes back into the arterioles. The patient may report that his digits feel cold and numb. These sensations may occur during the vasoconstrictive phase because of ischemia. He may also complain of throbbing, aching pain, swelling, and tingling. These symptoms most likely occur during the hyperemic phase. Trophic changes, such as sclerodactyly, ulcerations, or chronic paronychia, occur as a result of ischemia in longstanding disease.

COMPLICATIONS

Cutaneous gangrene may occur as a result of prolonged ischemia, necessitating amputation of one or more digits (although extremely rare).

DIAGNOSIS

There are tests to help diagnose Raynaud's disease. Clinical criteria include skin color changes induced by cold or stress; bilateral involvement; absence of gangrene or, if present, minimal cutaneous gangrene; normal arterial pulses; and patient history of symptoms for at least 2 years.

Antinuclear antibody (ANA) titer is used to identify autoimmune disease as an underlying cause of Raynaud's phenomenon; further tests must be performed if ANA titer is positive. The results of an arteriography can rule out arterial occlusive disease; a Doppler ultrasonography may show reduced blood flow if symptoms result from arterial occlusive disease.

TREATMENT

The patient should be taught to avoid triggers, such as cold and mechanical or chemical injury. He should be encouraged to stop smoking, to avoid decongestants and caffeine, and to keep his fingers and toes warm to reduce vasoconstriction.

Calcium channel blockers, such as nifedipine (Procardia or Adalat), diltiazem (Cardizem), and nicardipine (Cardene) may be prescribed to produce vasodilation and prevent vasospasm and adrenergic blockers, such as phenoxybenzamine (Dibenzyline) or reserpine (Resa), may improve blood flow to fingers or toes.

Biofeedback and relaxation exercises have been found to help reduce stress and improve circulation. Sympathectomy may be performed to promote vasodilation and to prevent ischemic ulcers (necessary in less than 25% of patients). If ischemia causes ulceration and gangrene, amputation may be necessary.

NURSING CONSIDERATIONS

✦ Warn the patient against exposure to the cold. Tell him to wear mittens or gloves in cold weather or when handling cold items or defrosting the freezer.
✦ Advise the patient to avoid stressful situations and to stop smoking.
✦ Instruct the patient to inspect his skin frequently and to seek immediate care for signs of skin breakdown or infection.
✦ Teach the patient about prescribed medications and their adverse effects.
✦ Provide psychological support and reassurance to allay the patient's fear of amputation and disfigurement.

▼ *LIFE-THREATENING DISORDER*

SHOCK

Shock isn't a disease, but rather a clinical syndrome leading to reduced tissue and organ perfusion and, eventually, organ dysfunction and failure. Shock can be classified into three major categories based on the precipitating factors: distributive (neurogenic, septic, and anaphylactic), cardiogenic, and hypovolemic shock. Even with treatment, shock has a high mortality rate after the body's compensatory mechanisms fail. (See *Types of shock,* page 210.)

CAUSES

Causes of neurogenic shock may include spinal cord injury, spinal anesthesia, vasomotor center depression, severe pain, medications, and hypoglycemia.

Causes of septic shock may include gram-negative bacteria (most common cause), gram-positive bacteria, viruses, fungi, *Rickettsiae*, parasites, yeast, protozoa, or mycobacteria.

 CLINICAL ALERT The immature immune system of neonates and infants and the weakened immune system of older adults, commonly accompanied by chronic illness, make these populations more susceptible to septic shock.

Causes of anaphylactic shock may include medications, vaccines, venom, foods, contrast media, and ABO-incompatible blood.

Causes of cardiogenic shock may include myocardial infarction (MI) (most common cause), heart failure, cardiomyopathy, arrhythmias, obstruction, pericardial tamponade, tension pneumothorax, and pulmonary embolism.

Causes of hypovolemic shock may include blood loss (most common cause), GI fluid loss, burns, renal loss (diabetic ketoacidosis, diabetes insipidus, and adrenal insufficiency), fluid shifts, ascites, peritonitis, and hemothorax.

PATHOPHYSIOLOGY

There are three basic stages common to each type of shock: compensatory, progressive, and irreversible, or refractory.

Compensatory stage

When arterial pressure and tissue perfusion are reduced, compensatory mechanisms are activated to maintain perfusion to the heart and brain. As the baroreceptors in the carotid sinus and aortic arch sense a decrease in blood pressure, epinephrine and norepinephrine are secreted to increase peripheral resistance, blood

---

Key nursing actions
✦ Warn patient to avoid exposure to cold.
✦ Advise patient to avoid stressful situations and to stop smoking.
✦ Instruct patient to inspect his skin frequently.
✦ Allay patient's fear of amputation and disfigurement.

Characteristics of shock
✦ Life-threatening disorder
✦ Leads to reduced tissue and organ perfusion and eventual organ dysfunction and failure
✦ Three categories: distributive, cardiogenic, and hypovolemic
✦ High mortality rate after compensatory mechanisms fail

Alert!
✦ Neonates, infants, and older adults are more susceptible to septic shock.

Causes

Neurogenic shock
✦ Spinal cord injury
✦ Spinal anesthesia

Septic shock
✦ Gram-negative/positive bacteria
✦ Viruses

Anaphylactic shock
✦ Medications and vaccines
✦ Venom

Cardiogenic shock
✦ MI
✦ Heart failure

Hypovolemic shock
✦ Blood loss or GI fluid loss
✦ Renal loss

Types of shock

+ Distributive: neurogenic, septic, and anaphylactic; vasodilation causes a state of hypovolemia
+ Cardiogenic: left ventricle can't maintain an adequate cardiac output
+ Hypovolemic: preload decreases ventricular filling

How it happens

Compensatory stage

+ Arterial pressure and tissue perfusion are reduced
+ Compensatory mechanisms activated
+ Epinephrine and norepinephrine are secreted
+ Renin-angiotensin-aldosterone system activates
+ Cardiac output and tissue perfusion are maintained

Types of shock

DISTRIBUTIVE SHOCK
In this type of shock, vasodilation causes a state of hypovolemia.

+ *Neurogenic shock.* A loss of sympathetic vasoconstrictor tone in the vascular smooth muscle and reduced autonomic function lead to widespread arterial and venous vasodilation. Venous return is reduced as blood pools in the venous system, leading to a drop in cardiac output and hypotension.

+ *Septic shock.* An immune response is triggered when bacteria release endotoxins. In response, macrophages secrete tumor necrosis factor (TNF) and interleukins. These mediators are responsible for an increased release of platelet-activating factor (PAF), prostaglandins, leukotrienes, thromboxane A_2, kinins, and complement. The consequences are vasodilation and vasoconstriction, increased capillary permeability, reduced systemic vascular resistance, microemboli, and an elevated cardiac output. Endotoxins also stimulate the release of histamine, further increasing capillary permeability. Moreover, myocardial depressant factor, TNF, PAF, and other factors depress myocardial function. Cardiac output falls, resulting in multisystem organ failure.

+ *Anaphylactic shock.* Triggered by an allergic reaction, anaphylactic shock occurs when a person is exposed to an antigen to which he has already been sensitized. Exposure results in the production of specific immunoglobulin (Ig) E antibodies by plasma cells that bind to membrane receptors on mast cells and basophils. On reexposure, the antigen binds to IgE antibodies or cross-linked IgE receptors, triggering the release of powerful chemical mediators from mast cells. IgG or IgM enters into the reaction and activates the release of complement factors. At the same time, the chemical mediators bradykinin and leukotrienes induce vascular collapse by stimulating contraction of certain groups of smooth muscles and by increasing vascular permeability, leading to decreased peripheral resistance and plasma leakage into the extravascular tissues, thereby reducing blood volume and causing hypotension, hypovolemic shock, and cardiac dysfunction. Bronchospasm and laryngeal edema also occur.

CARDIOGENIC SHOCK
In cardiogenic shock, the left ventricle can't maintain an adequate cardiac output. Compensatory mechanisms increase heart rate, strengthen myocardial contractions, promote sodium and water retention, and cause selective vasoconstriction. However, these mechanisms increase myocardial workload and oxygen consumption, which reduces the heart's ability to pump blood, especially if the patient has myocardial ischemia. Consequently, blood backs up, resulting in pulmonary edema. Eventually, cardiac output falls and multisystem organ failure develops as the compensatory mechanisms fail to maintain perfusion.

HYPOVOLEMIC SHOCK
When fluid is lost from the intravascular space through external losses or the shift of fluid from the vessels to the interstitial or intracellular spaces, venous return to the heart is reduced. This reduction in preload decreases ventricular filling, leading to a drop in stroke volume. Then, cardiac output falls, causing reduced perfusion of the tissues and organs.

---

pressure, and myocardial contractility. Reduced blood flow to the kidney activates the renin-angiotensin-aldosterone system, causing vasoconstriction and sodium and water retention, leading to increased blood volume and venous return. As a result of these compensatory mechanisms, cardiac output and tissue perfusion are maintained.

Progressive stage

The progressive stage of shock begins as compensatory mechanisms fail to maintain cardiac output. Tissues become hypoxic because of poor perfusion. As cells switch to anaerobic metabolism, lactic acid builds up, producing metabolic acidosis. This acidotic state depresses myocardial function. Tissue hypoxia also promotes the release of endothelial mediators, which produce vasodilation and endothelial abnormalities, leading to venous pooling and increased capillary permeability. Sluggish blood flow increases the risk of disseminated intravascular coagulation (DIC).

Irreversible (refractory) stage

As the shock syndrome progresses, permanent organ damage occurs as compensatory mechanisms can no longer maintain cardiac output. Reduced perfusion damages cell membranes, lysosomal enzymes are released, and energy stores are depleted, possibly leading to cell death. As cells use anaerobic metabolism, lactic acid accumulates, increasing capillary permeability and the movement of fluid out of the vascular space. This loss of intravascular fluid further contributes to hypotension. Perfusion to the coronary arteries is reduced, causing myocardial depression and a further reduction in cardiac output. Eventually, circulatory and respiratory failures occur. Death is inevitable.

SIGNS AND SYMPTOMS

In the compensatory stage of shock, sympathetic stimulation results in tachycardia and a bounding pulse. The patient may become tachypneic in order to compensate for hypoxia and may be restless and irritable as a result of cerebral hypoxia. Vasoconstriction causes decreased urinary output and cool, pale skin. In septic shock, the skin will be warm and dry as a result of vasodilation.

In the progressive stage of shock, as compensatory mechanisms fail, hypotension occurs. The patient may have a narrowed pulse pressure with a reduced stroke volume; a weak, rapid, thready pulse caused by decreased cardiac output; shallow respirations as weakness progresses; and reduced urinary output as poor renal perfusion continues. Vasoconstriction results in cold, clammy skin and hypoxia causes cyanosis.

 CLINICAL ALERT Hypotension, an altered level of consciousness, and hyperventilation may be the only signs of septic shock in infants and elderly people.

In the irreversible stage, reduced cerebral perfusion, acid-base imbalance, or electrolyte abnormalities can lead to unconsciousness and absent reflexes. Hypotension worsens as decompensation occurs and a reduced cardiac output causes a weak pulse. Slow, shallow, or Cheyne-Stokes respirations occur secondary to respiratory center depression, and the patient may become anuric due to renal failure.

COMPLICATIONS

Possible complications of shock include acute respiratory distress syndrome, acute tubular necrosis, DIC, cerebral hypoxia, and death.

DIAGNOSIS

These tests help diagnose shock:
+ Hematocrit may be reduced in hemorrhage or elevated in other types of shock due to hypovolemia.
+ Blood, urine, and sputum cultures may identify the organism responsible for septic shock.

How it happens

Progressive stage
+ Compensatory mechanisms fail
+ Tissues become hypoxic
+ Cells switch to anaerobic metabolism; metabolic acidosis occurs
+ Acidotic state depresses myocardial function
+ Venous pooling and increased capillary permeability result

Irreversible stage
+ Reduced perfusion damages cell membranes
+ Lysosomal enzymes are released, energy stores depleted
+ Cells use anaerobic metabolism, lactic acid accumulates
+ Hypotension occurs
+ Perfusion to coronary arteries and cardiac output is reduced

Key signs and symptoms

Compensatory stage
+ Tachycardia and bounding pulse
+ Tachypneic state
+ Restlessness

Progressive stage
+ Hypotension
+ Narrowed pulse pressure
+ Reduced stroke volume

Irreversible stage
+ Unconsciousness reflexes
+ Hypotension worsens
+ Slow, Cheyne-Stokes respirations

Alert!

+ Hypotension and hyperventilation may be the only signs of septic shock in infants and elderly people.

Diagnosis

+ Hematocrit may be reduced in hemorrhage or elevated in other types of shock
+ Blood, urine, and sputum cultures may identify organism responsible for septic shock
+ Increased WBC count
+ Increased serum lactate
+ Elevated serum glucose
+ ABG may reveal respiratory alkalosis or acidosis, respiratory depression, metabolic acidosis
+ Urine specific gravity may be high
+ Echocardiography determines left ventricular function, reveals valvular abnormalities

Treatment

+ Identify and treat underlying cause if possible
+ Intubation and mechanical ventilation
+ Supplemental oxygen
+ Continuous cardiac monitoring
+ Antiarrhythmics
+ Two I.V. lines for fluid and drug administration
+ I.V. fluids, crystalloids, or blood products to increase or maintain intravascular volume

Hypovolemic shock
+ Pneumatic antishock garment
+ Packed RBCs

Cardiogenic shock
+ Inotropic drugs
+ Vasodilators
+ Thrombolytic therapy

+ Coagulation studies may detect coagulopathy from DIC.
+ Laboratory testing may reveal increased white blood cell count and erythrocyte sedimentation rate due to injury and inflammation; elevated blood urea nitrogen and creatinine levels due to reduced renal perfusion; serum lactate may be increased secondary to anaerobic metabolism; and serum glucose may be elevated in the early stages of shock as the liver releases glycogen stores in response to sympathetic stimulation.
+ Cardiac enzymes and proteins may be elevated, indicating MI as a cause of cardiogenic shock.
+ Arterial blood gas (ABG) analysis may reveal respiratory alkalosis in early shock associated with tachypnea, respiratory acidosis in later stages associated with respiratory depression, and metabolic acidosis in later stages secondary to anaerobic metabolism.
+ Urine specific gravity may be high in response to effects of antidiuretic hormone.
+ Chest X-rays may be normal in early stages; pulmonary congestion may be seen in later stages.
+ Hemodynamic monitoring may reveal characteristic patterns of intracardiac pressures and cardiac output, which are used to guide fluid and drug management. (See *Putting hemodynamic monitoring to use.*)
+ Electrocardiography (ECG) determines the heart rate and detects arrhythmias, ischemic changes, and MI.
+ Echocardiography determines left ventricular function and reveals valvular abnormalities.

TREATMENT

To correct shock, the underlying cause must be identified and treated, if possible. If the patient develops respiratory distress, intubation and mechanical ventilation may be necessary to maintain a patent airway. Supplemental oxygen by way of a face mask or mechanical ventilator may be necessary to increase oxygenation.

Detection of changes in heart rate and rhythm is accomplished through continuous cardiac monitoring, and antiarrhythmics are administered as necessary.

At least two I.V. lines with large-gauge needles should be initiated and maintained for fluid and drug administration. I.V. fluids, crystalloids, or blood products may be given to increase or maintain intravascular volume.

Additional therapies for hypovolemic shock include the use of a pneumatic antishock garment, which may be applied to control internal and external hemorrhage by direct pressure. Initially, fluids, such as normal saline solution or lactated Ringer's solution, are administered to restore filling pressures, and packed red blood cells are given to restore blood loss and improve the blood's oxygen-carrying capacity.

Additional measures for cardiogenic shock may include inotropic drugs, such as dopamine (Intropin), dobutamine (Dobutrex), inamrinone (Inocor), and epinephrine (Adrenalin), which increase heart contractility and cardiac output. Vasodilators, such as nitroglycerin (Triaul) or nitroprusside (Nipride), are given with a vasopressor to reduce the left ventricle's workload. If the patient has fluid volume overload, preload may be reduced through the use of diuretics. Intra-aortic balloon pump (IABP) therapy is used to reduce the work of the left ventricle by decreasing systemic vascular resistance. (Diastolic pressure is increased, resulting in improved coronary artery perfusion.) Thrombolytic therapy or coronary artery revascularization restores coronary artery blood flow, if cardiogenic shock is due to an acute MI; and emergency surgery repairs papillary muscle rupture or ventricular septal de-

Putting hemodynamic monitoring to use

Hemodynamic monitoring provides information on intracardiac pressures and cardiac output. To understand intracardiac pressures, picture the cardiovascular system as a continuous loop with constantly changing pressure gradients that keep the blood moving.

RIGHT ATRIAL PRESSURE (RAP), OR CENTRAL VENOUS PRESSURE (CVP)

The RAP reflects right atrial, or right side of the heart, function and end-diastolic pressure.
+ Normal: 1 to 6 mm Hg (1.34 to 8 cm H_2O). (To convert mm Hg to cm H_2O, multiply mm Hg by 1.34.)
+ Elevated value suggests: right ventricular (RV) failure, volume overload, tricuspid valve stenosis or insufficiency, constrictive pericarditis, pulmonary hypertension, cardiac tamponade, or RV infarction.
+ Low value suggests: reduced circulating blood volume.

RV PRESSURE

RV systolic pressure normally equals pulmonary artery systolic pressure, RV end-diastolic pressure, which equals RAP, reflects RV function.
+ Normal: systolic, 15 to 25 mm Hg; diastolic, 0 to 8 mm Hg.
+ Elevated value suggests: mitral stenosis or insufficiency, pulmonary disease, hypoxemia, constrictive pericarditis, chronic heart failure, atrial and ventricular septal defects, and patent ductus arteriosus.

PULMONARY ARTERY PRESSURE

Pulmonary artery systolic pressure reflects RV function and pulmonary circulation pressures. Pulmonary artery diastolic pressure reflects left ventricular (LV) pressures, specifically LV end-diastolic pressure.
+ Normal: systolic, 15 to 25 mm Hg; diastolic, 8 to 15 mm Hg; mean, 10 to 20 mm Hg.

+ Elevated value suggests: LV failure, increased pulmonary blood flow (left or right shunting, as in atrial or ventricular septal defects), mitral stenosis or insufficiency, and any condition causing increased pulmonary arteriolar resistance.

PULMONARY ARTERY WEDGE PRESSURE (PAWP)

PAWP reflects left atrial and LV pressures unless the patient has mitral stenosis. Changes in PAWP reflect changes in LV filling pressure. The heart momentarily relaxes during diastole as it fills with blood from the pulmonary veins; this permits the pulmonary vasculature, left atrium, and left ventricle to act as a single chamber.
+ Normal: mean pressure, 6 to 12 mm Hg.
+ Elevated value suggests: LV failure, mitral stenosis or insufficiency, and pericardial tamponade.
+ Low value suggests: hypovolemia.

LEFT ATRIAL PRESSURE

This value reflects LV end-diastolic pressure in patients without mitral valve disease.
+ Normal: 6 to 12 mm Hg.

CARDIAC OUTPUT

Cardiac output is the amount of blood ejected by the heart each minute.
+ Normal: 4 to 8 L; varies with a patient's weight, height, and body surface area. Adjusting the cardiac output to the patient's size yields a measurement called the cardiac index.

What hemodynamic monitoring measures

+ RAP or CVP
+ RV pressure
+ Pulmonary artery pressure
+ PAWP
+ Left atrial pressure
+ Cardiac output

Normal values in hemodynamic monitoring

+ RAP or CVP — 1 to 6 mm Hg (1.34 to 8 cm H_2O)
+ RV pressure — systolic: 15 to 25 mm Hg; diastolic: 0 to 8 mm Hg
+ Pulmonary artery pressure — systolic: 15 to 25 mm Hg; diastolic: 8 to 15 mm Hg; mean: 10 to 20 mm Hg
+ PAWP — mean pressure: 6 to 12 mm Hg
+ Left atrial pressure — 6 to 12 mm Hg
+ Cardiac output — 4 to 8 L

fect, if either is the cause of cardiogenic shock. A ventricular assist device can assist the pumping action of the heart when IABP and drug therapy fail. Heart transplantation may be considered when other medical and surgical therapeutic measures fail.

Antibiotic therapy may be used to eradicate the causative organism in septic shock. Inotropic and vasopressor drugs, such as dopamine (Intropin), dobutamine (Dobutrex), and norepinephrine (Levophed), improve perfusion and maintain blood pressure. Although still investigational, monoclonal antibodies to tumor

Treatment

Septic shock
✦ Antibiotic therapy

Neurogenic shock
✦ Vasopressor drugs
✦ Fluid replacement

Key nursing actions

✦ Record vital signs and peripheral pulses every 15 minutes and ECG continuously.
✦ Start I.V. lines with normal saline solution or lactated Ringer's solution, using a large-bore catheter (14G).
✦ If output is less than 30 ml/hour in adults, increase the fluid infusion rate.
✦ Draw a sample to measure ABG levels.
✦ Draw venous blood for complete blood count, electrolyte levels, type and crossmatch, and coagulation studies.
✦ During therapy, assess skin color and temperature, and note changes.
✦ Watch for signs of impending coagulopathy.

Alert!

✦ Don't start I.V. administration in the legs of a patient in shock who has suffered abdominal trauma.
✦ Infused fluid may escape through the ruptured vessel into the abdomen.

necrosis factor, endotoxin, and interleukin-1, may be used to counteract septic shock mediators.

Therapy for neurogenic shock may include vasopressor drugs to raise blood pressure by vasoconstriction and fluid replacement to maintain blood pressure and cardiac output.

NURSING CONSIDERATIONS

Management of shock necessitates prompt, aggressive supportive measures and careful assessment and monitoring of vital signs. Follow these priorities:
✦ Check for a patent airway and adequate circulation. If blood pressure and heart rate are absent, start cardiopulmonary resuscitation.
✦ Record blood pressure, pulse rate, peripheral pulses, respiratory rate, and other vital signs every 15 minutes and the ECG continuously. Systolic blood pressure lower than 80 mm Hg usually results in inadequate coronary artery blood flow, cardiac ischemia, arrhythmias, and further complications of low cardiac output. When blood pressure drops below 80 mm Hg, increase the oxygen flow rate, and notify the physician immediately. A progressive decrease in blood pressure accompanied by a thready pulse generally signals inadequate cardiac output from reduced intravascular volume. Notify the physician and increase the infusion rate.
✦ Start I.V. lines with normal saline solution or lactated Ringer's solution, using a large-bore catheter (14G), which allows easier administration of blood transfusions, if required later.

 CLINICAL ALERT Don't start I.V. administration in the legs of a patient in shock who has suffered abdominal trauma because the infused fluid may escape through the ruptured vessel into the abdomen.

✦ An indwelling urinary catheter may be inserted to measure hourly urine output. If output is less than 30 ml/hour in adults, increase the fluid infusion rate, but watch for signs of fluid overload such as an increase in pulmonary artery wedge pressure (PAWP). Notify the physician if urine output doesn't improve. An osmotic diuretic such as mannitol (Osmitrol) may be ordered to increase renal blood flow and urine output. Determine how much fluid to give by checking blood pressure, urine output, central venous pressure (CVP), or PAWP. (To increase accuracy, CVP should be measured at the level of the right atrium, using the same reference point on the chest each time.)
✦ Draw an arterial blood sample to measure ABG levels. Administer oxygen by face mask or airway to ensure adequate tissue oxygenation. Adjust the oxygen flow rate to a higher or lower level, as determined by ABG measurements.
✦ Draw venous blood for complete blood count, electrolyte levels, type and crossmatch, and coagulation studies.
✦ During therapy, assess skin color and temperature, and note changes. Cold, clammy skin may be a sign of continuing peripheral vascular constriction, indicating progressive shock.
✦ Watch for signs of impending coagulopathy (petechiae, bruising, and bleeding or oozing from gums or venipuncture sites).
✦ Explain all procedures and their purpose to the patient. Throughout these emergency measures, provide emotional support to the patient and his family.

Myocardial infarction

If coronary artery occlusion causes prolonged ischemia, lasting longer than 30 to 45 minutes, irreversible myocardial cell damage and muscle death occur.

The site of the myocardial infarction (MI) depends on the vessels involved. Occlusion of the circumflex branch of the left coronary artery causes a lateral wall infarction; occlusion of the anterior descending branch of the left coronary artery causes an anterior wall infarction.

True posterior or inferior wall infarctions generally result from occlusion of the right coronary artery or one of its branches.

All infarcts have a central area of necrosis (infarction) surrounded by an area of potentially viable hypoxic injury, which may be salvaged if circulation is restored, or may progress to necrosis. The zone of injury, in turn, is surrounded by viable ischemic tissue.

TISSUE DESTRUCTION IN MI

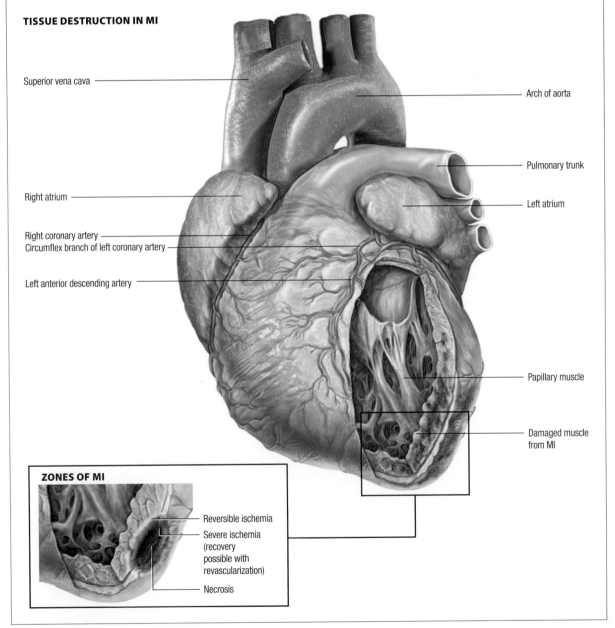

Superior vena cava

Arch of aorta

Pulmonary trunk

Right atrium

Left atrium

Right coronary artery
Circumflex branch of left coronary artery

Left anterior descending artery

Papillary muscle

Damaged muscle from MI

ZONES OF MI

Reversible ischemia

Severe ischemia (recovery possible with revascularization)

Necrosis

Coronary artery disease

Coronary artery disease (CAD) results as atherosclerotic plaque fills the lumens of the coronary arteries and obstructs blood flow. The primary effect of CAD is a diminished supply of oxygen and nutrients to myocardial tissue.

PROGRESSION OF CAD IN ATHEROSCLEROSIS

NORMAL HEART

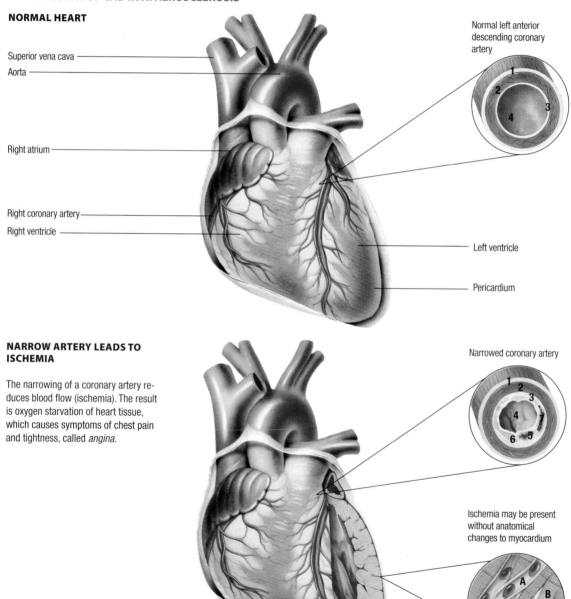

Superior vena cava

Aorta

Right atrium

Right coronary artery

Right ventricle

Normal left anterior descending coronary artery

Left ventricle

Pericardium

NARROW ARTERY LEADS TO ISCHEMIA

The narrowing of a coronary artery reduces blood flow (ischemia). The result is oxygen starvation of heart tissue, which causes symptoms of chest pain and tightness, called *angina*.

Narrowed coronary artery

Ischemia may be present without anatomical changes to myocardium

BLOCKED ARTERY LEADS TO MYOCARDIAL INFARCTION (MI)

Sudden insufficient blood supply (ischemia) is commonly caused by ruptured plaque and thrombus formation that occludes the artery lumen. This produces an area of necrosis in heart muscle, which results in an MI.

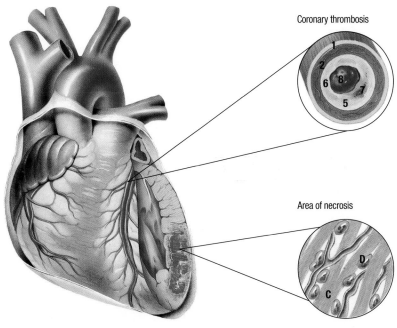

Coronary thrombosis

Area of necrosis

RECOVERY THROUGH COLLATERAL BLOOD SUPPLY

Collateral (accessory) blood supply from adjacent vessels travels to the region affected by the MI to provide fresh blood.

Collateral blood supply

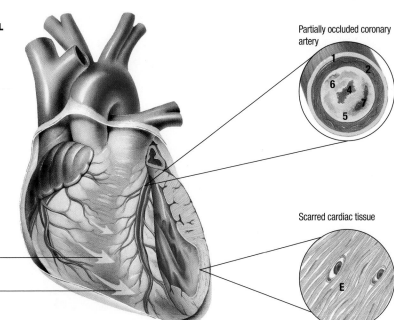

Partially occluded coronary artery

Scarred cardiac tissue

KEY TO CIRCULAR INSETS

Coronary artery
1 Adventitia
2 Media
3 Intima
4 Lumen
5 Advanced plaque
6 Fatty deposits
7 Hemorrhage
8 Thrombus

Myocardium
A Capillaries
B Muscle fibers
C Dead muscle fibers
D Leukocytes
E Scar tissue

Heart failure

Heart failure occurs when the heart can't pump enough blood to meet the metabolic needs of the body. It may be classified according to the side of the heart affected.

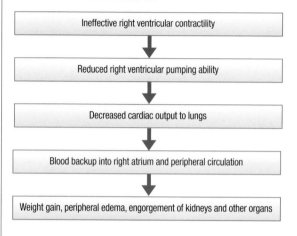

RIGHT-SIDED HEART FAILURE

Ineffective right ventricular contractility

⬇

Reduced right ventricular pumping ability

⬇

Decreased cardiac output to lungs

⬇

Blood backup into right atrium and peripheral circulation

⬇

Weight gain, peripheral edema, engorgement of kidneys and other organs

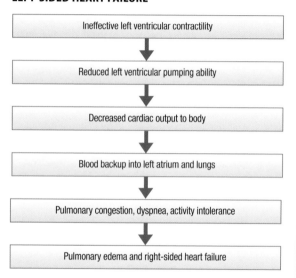

LEFT-SIDED HEART FAILURE

Ineffective left ventricular contractility

⬇

Reduced left ventricular pumping ability

⬇

Decreased cardiac output to body

⬇

Blood backup into left atrium and lungs

⬇

Pulmonary congestion, dyspnea, activity intolerance

⬇

Pulmonary edema and right-sided heart failure

NORMAL CARDIAC CIRCULATION

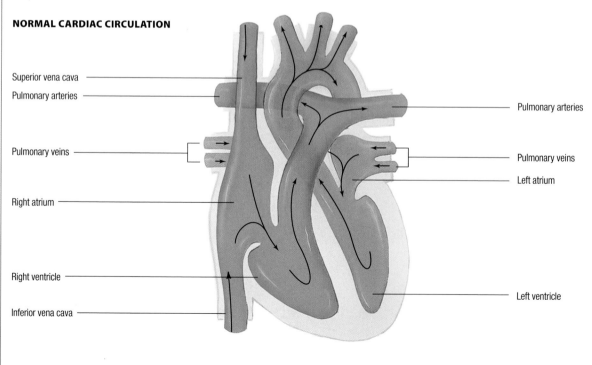

Superior vena cava
Pulmonary arteries
Pulmonary veins
Right atrium
Right ventricle
Inferior vena cava

Pulmonary arteries
Pulmonary veins
Left atrium
Left ventricle

Chronic bronchitis

Chronic bronchitis, a form of chronic obstructive pulmonary disease, is characterized by hypersecretion of mucus and a chronic productive cough. It develops when irritants are inhaled for a prolonged period.

The irritants inflame the tracheobronchial tree, leading to increased mucus production and a narrowed or blocked airway. As the inflamma-tion continues, changes in the cells lining the respiratory tract increase resistance in the small airways, and severe imbalance in the ventilation-perfusion ratio decreases arterial oxygenation.

MUCUS BUILDUP IN CHRONIC BRONCHITIS

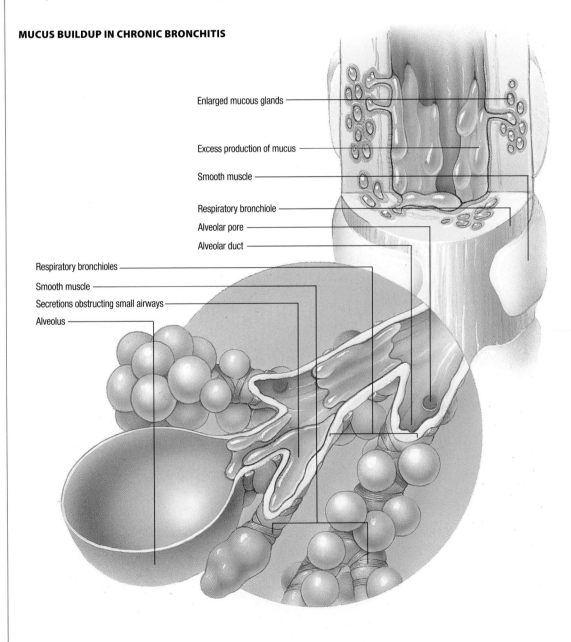

Enlarged mucous glands

Excess production of mucus

Smooth muscle

Respiratory bronchiole

Alveolar pore

Alveolar duct

Respiratory bronchioles

Smooth muscle

Secretions obstructing small airways

Alveolus

Asthma

In asthma, bronchial linings overreact to various stimuli, causing smooth muscle spasms that severely constrict the airways. When the hypersensitive patient inhales a triggering substance, abnormal antibodies stimulate mast cells in the lung interstitium to release both histamine and leukotrienes. Histamine attaches to receptor sites in the larger bronchi, where it causes swelling in smooth muscles.

Leukotrienes attach to receptor sites in the smaller bronchi and cause swelling of smooth muscle there. Leukotrienes also cause fatty acids called *prostaglandins* to travel through the bloodstream to the lungs, where they enhance histamine's effects. Histamine stimulates the mucous membranes to secrete excessive mucus, further narrowing the bronchial lumen.

On inhalation, the narrowed bronchial lumen can still expand slightly, allowing air to reach the alveoli. On exhalation, increased intrathoracic pressure closes the bronchial lumen completely. Mucus fills the lung bases, inhibiting alveolar ventilation. Blood, shunted to alveoli in other lung parts, can't compensate for diminished ventilation.

ASTHMATIC BRONCHUS

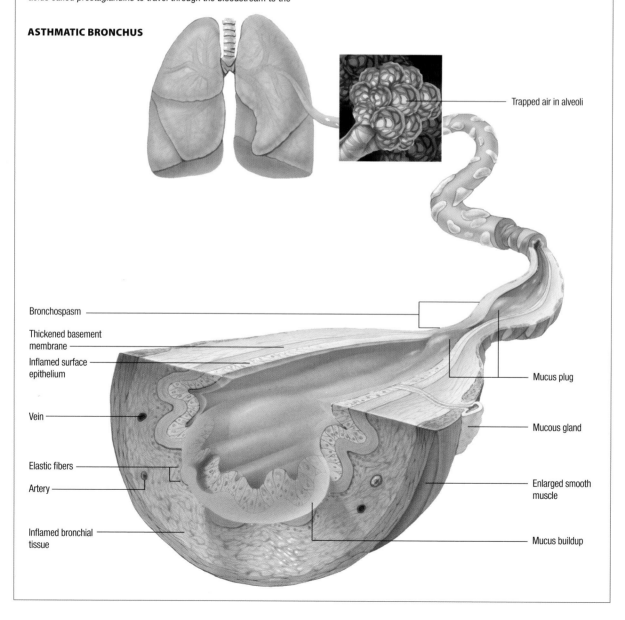

Trapped air in alveoli

Bronchospasm

Thickened basement membrane

Inflamed surface epithelium

Mucus plug

Vein

Mucous gland

Elastic fibers

Artery

Enlarged smooth muscle

Inflamed bronchial tissue

Mucus buildup

Emphysema

In emphysema, obstruction results from tissue changes rather than mucus production, which occurs in asthma and chronic bronchitis. The distinguishing characteristic of emphysema is airflow limitation caused by lack of elastic recoil in the lungs.

The recurrent inflammation in emphysema is associated with the release of proteolytic enzymes from lung cells. This causes irreversible enlargement of the air spaces distal to the terminal bronchioles. Enlargement of air spaces destroys the alveolar walls, which results in a breakdown of elasticity and loss of fibrous and muscle tissue, making the lungs less compliant.

The alveoli are left unable to recoil normally after expanding, resulting in bronchiolar collapse on expiration. The damaged or destroyed alveolar walls can't support the airways to keep them open. The amount of air that can be exhaled passively is diminished, trapping air in the lungs and leading to overdistention. Hyperinflation of the alveoli produces bullae and air spaces adjacent to the pleura.

LUNG CHANGES IN EMPHYSEMA

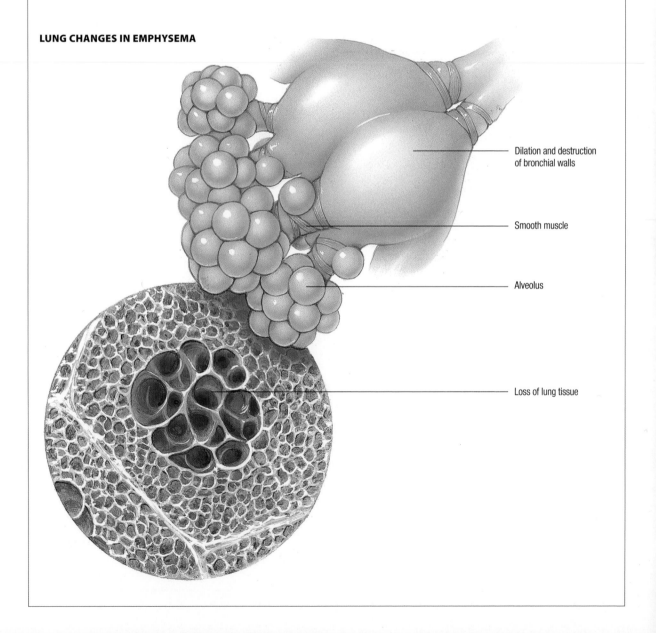

Dilation and destruction of bronchial walls

Smooth muscle

Alveolus

Loss of lung tissue

Pulmonary edema

Pulmonary edema is an accumulation of fluid in the extravascular spaces of the lungs. It's a common complication of cardiac disorders and may occur as a chronic condition or may develop quickly and rapidly become fatal.

NORMAL ALVEOLI

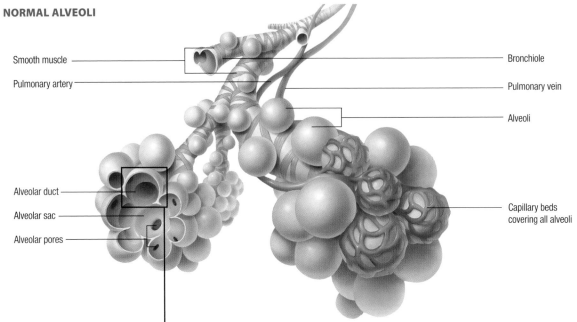

Smooth muscle

Pulmonary artery

Alveolar duct

Alveolar sac

Alveolar pores

Bronchiole

Pulmonary vein

Alveoli

Capillary beds covering all alveoli

HOW PULMONARY EDEMA DEVELOPS

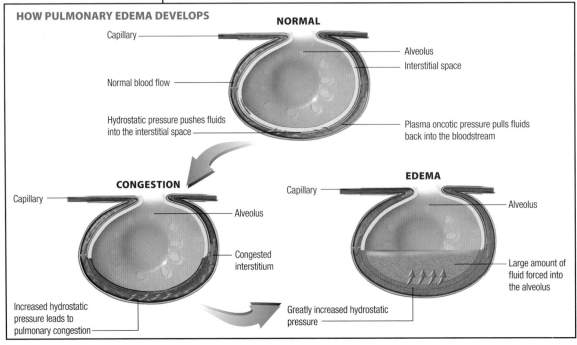

NORMAL

Capillary

Normal blood flow

Hydrostatic pressure pushes fluids into the interstitial space

Alveolus

Interstitial space

Plasma oncotic pressure pulls fluids back into the bloodstream

CONGESTION

Capillary

Alveolus

Congested interstitium

Increased hydrostatic pressure leads to pulmonary congestion

EDEMA

Capillary

Alveolus

Large amount of fluid forced into the alveolus

Greatly increased hydrostatic pressure

TETRALOGY OF FALLOT

Tetralogy of Fallot is a combination of four cardiac defects: ventricular septal defect (VSD), right ventricular outflow tract obstruction (pulmonic stenosis), right ventricular hypertrophy, and dextroposition of the aorta, with overriding of the VSD. Blood shunts from right to left through the VSD, allowing unoxygenated blood to mix with oxygenated blood and resulting in cyanosis. This cyanotic heart defect sometimes coexists with other congenital acyanotic heart defects, such as patent ductus arteriosus or atrial septal defect. It accounts for about 10% of all congenital defects and occurs equally in males and females. Before surgical advances made correction possible, about one-third of these children died in infancy.

CAUSES

The cause of tetralogy of Fallot is unknown, but may be associated with fetal alcohol syndrome and thalidomide use during pregnancy.

PATHOPHYSIOLOGY

In tetralogy of Fallot, unoxygenated venous blood returning to the right side of the heart may pass through the VSD to the left ventricle, bypassing the lungs, or it may enter the pulmonary artery, depending on the extent of the pulmonic stenosis. Rather than originating from the left ventricle, the aorta overrides both ventricles.

The VSD usually lies in the outflow tract of the right ventricle and is generally large enough to permit equalization of right and left ventricular pressures. However, the ratio of systemic vascular resistance to pulmonic stenosis affects the direction and magnitude of shunt flow across the VSD. Severe obstruction of right ventricular outflow produces a right-to-left shunt, causing decreased systemic arterial oxygen saturation, cyanosis, reduced pulmonary blood flow, and hypoplasia of the entire pulmonary vasculature. Right ventricular hypertrophy develops in response to the extra force needed to push blood into the stenotic pulmonary artery. Milder forms of pulmonic stenosis result in a left-to-right shunt or no shunt at all.

SIGNS AND SYMPTOMS

Cyanosis, the hallmark sign of tetralogy of Fallot, is caused by a right-to-left shunt. Cyanotic or "blue" spells (Tet spells) are another sign of the disorder. They are characterized by dyspnea; deep, sighing respirations; bradycardia; fainting; seizures; and loss of consciousness following exercise, crying, straining, infection, or fever. It may result from reduced oxygen to the brain because of increased right-to-left shunting, possibly caused by spasm of the right ventricular outflow tract, increased systemic venous return, or decreased systemic arterial resistance.

As a result of poor oxygenation, clubbing, diminished exercise tolerance, increasing dyspnea on exertion, growth retardation, and eating difficulties occur. To reduce venous return of unoxygenated blood from the legs and to increase systemic arterial resistance, the patient may squat with shortness of breath.

A loud systolic murmur is best heard along the left sternal border. This murmur may diminish or obscure the pulmonic component of S_2. In a patient with a large patent ductus, a continuous ductus murmur may obscure systolic murmur. Abnormal blood flow through the heart may result in a thrill at the left sternal order. An obvious right ventricular impulse and prominent inferior sternum are associated with right ventricular hypertrophy.

Characteristics of tetralogy of Fallot

+ Combination of four cardiac defects: VSD, pulmonic stenosis, right ventricular hypertrophy, and dextroposition of aorta, with overriding of VSD
+ Blood shunts from right to left
+ Unoxygenated blood mixes with oxygenated blood; cyanosis occurs
+ Accounts for about 10% of all congenital defects

Causes

+ Fetal alcohol syndrome
+ Thalidomide use

How it happens

+ Unoxygenated venous blood returns to right side of heart, passes through VSD to left ventricle; may enter pulmonary artery
+ Aorta overrides both ventricles
+ Ratio of systemic vascular resistance to pulmonic stenosis affects direction and magnitude of shunt flow across VSD
+ Right ventricular hypertrophy develops in response to extra force

Key signs and symptoms

+ Cyanosis
+ Clubbing
+ Loud systolic murmur best heard along left sternal border
+ Obvious right ventricular impulse and prominent inferior sternum

Complications
+ Pulmonary or venous thrombosis
+ Cerebral embolism
+ Infective endocarditis
+ Risk of spontaneous abortion

Diagnosis
+ Chest X-rays show pulmonary vascular marking and enlarged right ventricle
+ Electrocardiography shows right ventricular hypertrophy
+ Echocardiography shows septal overriding of aorta, VSD, and pulmonic stenosis
+ Laboratory testing shows diminished oxygen saturation and polycythemia
+ Cardiac catheterization confirms diagnosis, measures degree of oxygen saturation in aortic blood

Treatment
+ Child should assume a knee-chest position and be given oxygen and morphine during cyanotic spells
+ Palliative surgery with Blalock-Taussig procedure
+ Prophylactic antibiotics
+ Phlebotomy

Key nursing actions
+ Explain tetralogy of Fallot to the parents.
+ Teach parents to recognize serious hypoxic spells.
+ Warn parents to keep their child away from people with infections.

COMPLICATIONS

Possible complications of tetralogy of Fallot include pulmonary thrombosis, venous thrombosis, cerebral embolism, infective endocarditis, risk of spontaneous abortion, premature birth, and low-birth-weight infants born to women with tetralogy of Fallot.

DIAGNOSIS

Certain tests help diagnose tetralogy of Fallot. Chest X-rays may demonstrate decreased pulmonary vascular marking (depending on the severity of the pulmonary obstruction), an enlarged right ventricle, and a boot-shaped cardiac silhouette. An electrocardiography shows right ventricular hypertrophy, right axis deviation and, possibly, right atrial hypertrophy.

To identify septal overriding of the aorta, the VSD, and pulmonic stenosis, and to detect the hypertrophied walls of the right ventricle, an echocardiography should be used. In addition, laboratory testing reveals diminished oxygen saturation and polycythemia (hematocrit may be more than 60%) if the cyanosis is severe and longstanding, predisposing the patient to thrombosis.

Cardiac catheterization confirms the diagnosis by providing visualization of pulmonic stenosis, the VSD, and the overriding aorta and ruling out other cyanotic heart defects. This test also measures the degree of oxygen saturation in aortic blood.

TREATMENT

In tetralogy of Fallot, the child should assume a knee-chest position and should be given oxygen and morphine to improve oxygenation during cyanotic spells.

Palliative surgery with a Blalock-Taussig procedure, which enhances blood flow to the lungs and reduces hypoxia, may be performed to join the subclavian artery to the pulmonary artery.

Prophylactic antibiotics may be administered to prevent infective endocarditis or cerebral abscesses.

Polycythemia may be reduced by phlebotomy, and corrective surgery may be done to relieve pulmonic stenosis and close the VSD, directing left ventricular outflow to the aorta.

NURSING CONSIDERATIONS

+ Explain tetralogy of Fallot to the parents. Inform them that their child will set his own exercise limits and will know when to rest. Make sure they understand that their child can engage in physical activity, and advise them not to be overprotective.
+ Teach parents to recognize serious hypoxic spells, which can cause dramatically increased cyanosis; deep, sighing respirations; and loss of consciousness. Tell them to place their child in the knee-chest position and to report such spells immediately. Emergency treatment may be necessary.
+ To prevent infective endocarditis and other infections, warn parents to keep their child away from people with infections. Urge them to encourage good dental hygiene, and tell them to watch for ear, nose, and throat infections and dental caries, all of which necessitate immediate treatment. When dental care, infections, or surgery requires prophylactic antibiotics, tell the parents to make sure the child completes the prescribed regimen.

✦ If the child requires medical attention for an unrelated problem, advise the parents to inform the physician immediately of the child's history of tetralogy of Fallot because any treatment must take this serious heart defect into consideration.

✦ During hospitalization, alert the staff to the child's condition. Because of the right-to-left shunt through the VSD, treat I.V. lines like arterial lines. Remember, a clot dislodged from a catheter tip in a vein can cross the VSD and cause cerebral embolism. The same thing can happen if air enters the venous lines.

After palliative surgery

✦ Monitor oxygenation and arterial blood gas (ABG) values closely in the intensive care unit.

✦ If the child has undergone the Blalock-Taussig procedure, don't use the arm on the operative side for measuring blood pressure, inserting I.V. lines, or drawing blood samples because blood perfusion on this side diminishes greatly until collateral circulation develops. Note this on the child's chart and at his bedside.

After corrective surgery

✦ Watch for right bundle-branch block or more serious disturbances of atrioventricular conduction and for ventricular ectopic beats.

✦ Be alert for other postoperative complications, such as bleeding, right-sided heart failure, and respiratory failure. After surgery, transient heart failure is common and may require treatment with digoxin (Lanoxin) and diuretics.

✦ Monitor left atrial pressure directly. A pulmonary artery catheter may also be used to check central venous and pulmonary artery pressures.

✦ Frequently check color and vital signs. Obtain ABG measurements regularly to assess oxygenation. As needed, suction to prevent atelectasis and pneumonia. Monitor mechanical ventilation.

✦ Monitor and record intake and output accurately.

✦ If atrioventricular block develops with a low heart rate, a temporary external pacemaker may be necessary.

✦ If blood pressure or cardiac output is inadequate, catecholamines may be ordered by continuous I.V. infusion. To decrease left ventricular workload, administer nitroprusside (Nipride), if ordered. Provide analgesics, as needed.

✦ Keep the parents informed about their child's progress. After discharge, the child may require digoxin (Lanoxin), diuretics, and other drugs. Stress the importance of complying with the prescribed regimen, and make sure the parents know how and when to administer these medications. Teach parents to watch for signs of digoxin toxicity (anorexia, nausea, and vomiting). Prophylactic antibiotics to prevent infective endocarditis will still be required. Advise the parents to avoid becoming overprotective as the child's tolerance for physical activity increases.

TRANSPOSITION OF THE GREAT ARTERIES

Transposition of the great arteries is a cyanotic congenital heart defect in which the great arteries are reversed such that the aorta arises from the right ventricle and the pulmonary artery from the left ventricle, producing two noncommunicating circulatory systems (pulmonic and systemic).

The right-to-left shunting of blood leads to an increased risk of heart failure and anoxia. Transposition accounts for about 5% of all congenital heart defects and commonly coexists with other congenital heart defects, such as ventricular septal

Key nursing actions
(continued)

✦ During hospitalization, alert the staff to the child's condition. Because of the right-to-left shunt through the VSD, treat I.V. lines like arterial lines.

After palliative surgery

✦ Monitor oxygenation and ABG values closely in the ICU.

✦ If the child has undergone Blalock-Taussig procedure, don't use the arm on the operative side for measuring blood pressure, inserting I.V. lines, or drawing blood samples.

After corrective surgery

✦ Watch for right bundle-branch block or more serious disturbances of atrioventricular conduction and for ventricular ectopic beats.

✦ Be alert for other postoperative complications.

✦ Monitor left atrial pressure directly.

✦ Keep the parents informed about their child's progress.

Characteristics of transposition of the great arteries

✦ Cyanotic congenital heart defect
✦ Great arteries are reversed
✦ Produces two noncommunicating circulatory systems
✦ Right-to-left shunting of blood leads to increased risk of heart failure and anoxia
✦ Commonly coexists with other congenital heart defects
✦ Affects two to three times more males than females
✦ Cause is unknown

How it happens
+ Results from faulty embryonic development
+ Oxygenated blood returning to left side of heart is carried back to lungs
+ Unoxygenated blood returning to right side of heart is carried to systemic circulation
+ In infants, blood mixes only at patent foramen ovale and at PDA, resulting in slight mixing of systemic and pulmonary blood

Key signs and symptoms
+ Cyanosis and tachypnea worsen with crying hours after birth
+ Within days to weeks: gallop rhythm, tachycardia, dyspnea, hepatomegaly, and cardiomegaly
+ Murmurs of ASD, VSD, or PDA
+ Diminished exercise tolerance, fatigability, and clubbing

Complications
+ Heart failure
+ Infective endocarditis

Diagnosis
+ Chest X-rays show oblong heart
+ Electrocardiography shows right axis deviation and right ventricular hypertrophy
+ Echocardiography shows reversed position of aorta and pulmonary artery
+ Cardiac catheterization reveals decreased oxygen saturation in left ventricular blood and aortic blood

defect (VSD), VSD with pulmonic stenosis, atrial septal defect (ASD), and patent ductus arteriosus (PDA). It affects two to three times more males than females.

CAUSES
The cause of this disorder is unknown.

PATHOPHYSIOLOGY
Transposition of the great arteries results from faulty embryonic development. Oxygenated blood returning to the left side of the heart is carried back to the lungs by a transposed pulmonary artery. Unoxygenated blood returning to the right side of the heart is carried to the systemic circulation by a transposed aorta.

Communication between the pulmonary and systemic circulations is necessary for survival. In infants with isolated transposition, blood mixes only at the patent foramen ovale and at the PDA, resulting in slight mixing of unoxygenated systemic blood and oxygenated pulmonary blood. In infants with concurrent cardiac defects, greater mixing of blood occurs.

SIGNS AND SYMPTOMS
When no other heart defects exist that allow mixing of systemic and pulmonary blood, cyanosis and tachypnea that worsen with crying occur within the first few hours after birth. Cyanosis may be minimized with associated defects, such as ASD, VSD, or PDA.

Within days to weeks gallop rhythm, tachycardia, dyspnea, hepatomegaly, and cardiomegaly occur as a result of heart failure. A loud S_2 can be auscultated because the anteriorly transposed aorta is directly behind the sternum. Murmurs of ASD, VSD, or PDA may also be heard. Reduced oxygenation causes diminished exercise tolerance, fatigability, and clubbing.

COMPLICATIONS
Transposition of the great arteries may be complicated by heart failure or infective endocarditis.

DIAGNOSIS
Certain tests help diagnose transposition of the great arteries. Chest X-rays are normal in the first days after birth. Within days to weeks, right atrial and right ventricular enlargements characteristically cause the heart to appear oblong. X-ray may also show increased pulmonary vascular markings, except when pulmonic stenosis exists. A right axis deviation and right ventricular hypertrophy can be revealed in an electrocardiography; however, an electrocardiography may be normal in a neonate.

An echocardiography demonstrates the reversed position of the aorta and pulmonary artery and records echoes from both semilunar valves simultaneously because of aortic valve displacement. It also detects other cardiac defects.

To reveal decreased oxygen saturation in left ventricular blood and aortic blood use cardiac catheterization. This test also shows increased right atrial, right ventricular, and pulmonary artery oxygen saturation; and right ventricular systolic pressure equal to systemic pressure. Dye injection reveals the transposed vessels and the presence of other cardiac defects.

In addition, an arterial blood gas (ABG) analysis indicates hypoxia and secondary metabolic acidosis.

TREATMENT

Treatment of this disorder may involve prostaglandin infusion to keep the ductus arteriosus patent until surgical correction. Atrial balloon septostomy (Rashkind procedure) may be performed during cardiac catheterization, if needed, as a palliative measure until surgery can be performed. It enlarges the patent foramen ovale and thereby improves oxygenation and alleviates hypoxia by allowing greater mixing of blood from the pulmonary and systemic circulations.

After atrial balloon septostomy, diuretics and digoxin (Lanoxin) may be administered to lessen heart failure until the infant is ready to withstand corrective surgery (usually between birth and age 1). Depending on the physiology of the defect, surgery may be performed to correct the transposition.

NURSING CONSIDERATIONS

✦ Explain cardiac catheterization and all necessary procedures to the parents. Offer emotional support.
✦ Monitor vital signs, ABG values, urine output, and central venous pressure, watching for signs of heart failure. Give digoxin and I.V. fluids, being careful to avoid fluid overload.
✦ Teach the parents to recognize signs of heart failure and digoxin toxicity (poor feeding and vomiting). Stress the importance of regular checkups to monitor cardiovascular status.
✦ Teach the parents to protect their infant from infection and to give antibiotics.
✦ Tell the parents to let their child develop normally. They don't need to restrict activities; he'll set his own limits.
✦ If the patient is scheduled for surgery, explain the procedure to the parents and child, if old enough. Teach them about the intensive care unit, and introduce them to the staff. Also explain postoperative care.
✦ Preoperatively, monitor ABG values, acid-base balance, intake and output, and vital signs.

After corrective surgery
✦ Monitor cardiac output by checking blood pressure, skin color, heart rate, urine output, central venous and left atrial pressures, and level of consciousness; report abnormalities or changes.
✦ Carefully measure ABG levels.
✦ To detect supraventricular conduction blocks and arrhythmias, monitor the patient closely. Watch for signs of atrioventricular block, atrial arrhythmia, and faulty sinoatrial function.
✦ After Mustard or Senning procedures, watch for signs of baffle obstruction such as marked facial edema.
✦ Encourage the parents to help their child assume new activity levels and independence. Teach them about postoperative antibiotic prophylaxis for endocarditis.

VALVULAR HEART DISEASE

In valvular heart disease, three types of mechanical disruption can occur: stenosis, or narrowing, of the valve opening; incomplete closure of the valve; or valve pro-

Treatment
✦ Prostaglandin infusion
✦ Rashkind procedure during cardiac catheterization until surgery can be performed
✦ Diuretics and digoxin until infant can withstand corrective surgery
✦ Surgery to correct transposition

Key nursing actions
✦ Monitor vital signs, ABG values, urine output, and central venous pressure.
✦ Teach the parents to recognize signs of heart failure and digoxin toxicity.
✦ Teach the parents to protect their infant from infection and to give antibiotics.

After corrective surgery
✦ Monitor cardiac output by checking blood pressure, skin color, heart rate, urine output, central venous and left atrial pressures, and level of consciousness; report abnormalities or changes.
✦ Carefully measure ABG levels.
✦ To detect supraventricular conduction blocks and arrhythmias, monitor the patient closely.
✦ After Mustard or Senning procedures, watch for signs of baffle obstruction.

Characteristics of valvular heart disease
✦ Three types: stenosis, incomplete closure of valve, valve prolapse
✦ Occurs most commonly in children due to a congenital heart defect
✦ Rheumatic heart disease is a common cause in adults

How it happens

Mitral insufficiency

+ Abnormality of mitral leaflets, mitral annulus, chordae tendineae, papillary muscles, left atrium, left ventricle can lead to mitral insufficiency
+ Blood from left ventricle flows into left atrium during systole
+ Atrium enlarges to accommodate backflow
+ Left- and right-sided heart failure result

Mitral stenosis

+ Valve narrowing obstructs blood flow from left atrium to left ventricle; left atrial volume and pressure rise, chamber dilates
+ Greater resistance to blood flow causes pulmonary hypertension, right ventricular hypertrophy, right-sided heart failure

Aortic insufficiency

+ Blood flows back into left ventricle during diastole
+ Excess volume causes fluid overload in left atrium and pulmonary system
+ Left-sided heart failure and pulmonary edema result

Aortic stenosis

+ Increased left ventricular pressure tries to overcome resistance of narrowed valvular opening
+ Diminished cardiac output causes poor coronary artery perfusion and left-sided heart failure

Pulmonic stenosis

+ Obstructed right ventricular outflow causes right ventricular hypertrophy
+ Right-sided heart failure results

lapse. Valvular disorders in children and adolescents most commonly occur as a result of congenital heart defects. In adults, rheumatic heart disease is a common cause.

CAUSES

The causes of valvular heart disease are varied and are different for each type of valve disorder. (See *Types of valvular heart disease,* pages 222 to 225.)

PATHOPHYSIOLOGY

Pathophysiology of valvular heart disease varies according to the valve and the disorder.

Mitral insufficiency

An abnormality of the mitral leaflets, mitral annulus, chordae tendineae, papillary muscles, left atrium, or left ventricle can lead to mitral insufficiency. Blood from the left ventricle flows back into the left atrium during systole, causing the atrium to enlarge to accommodate the backflow. As a result, the left ventricle also dilates to accommodate the increased blood volume from the atrium and to compensate for diminishing cardiac output. Ventricular hypertrophy and increased end-diastolic pressure result in increased pulmonary artery pressure, eventually leading to left-sided and right-sided heart failure.

Mitral stenosis

Narrowing of the valve by valvular abnormalities, fibrosis, or calcification obstructs blood flow from the left atrium to the left ventricle. Consequently, left atrial volume and pressure rise and the chamber dilates. Greater resistance to blood flow causes pulmonary hypertension, right ventricular hypertrophy, and right-sided heart failure. Also, inadequate filling of the left ventricle produces low cardiac output.

Aortic insufficiency

Blood flows back into the left ventricle during diastole, causing fluid overload in the ventricle, which dilates and hypertrophies. The excess volume causes fluid overload in the left atrium and, finally, the pulmonary system. Left-sided heart failure and pulmonary edema eventually result.

Aortic stenosis

Increased left ventricular pressure tries to overcome the resistance of the narrowed valvular opening. The added workload increases the demand for oxygen, and diminished cardiac output causes poor coronary artery perfusion, ischemia of the left ventricle, and left-sided heart failure.

Pulmonic stenosis

Obstructed right ventricular outflow causes right ventricular hypertrophy, eventually resulting in right-sided heart failure.

SIGNS AND SYMPTOMS

The clinical manifestations vary according to the type of valvular defect. (See *Types of valvular heart disease,* pages 222 to 225, for specific clinical features of each valve disorder.)

COMPLICATIONS

Possible complications of valvular heart disease include heart failure, pulmonary edema, thromboembolism, endocarditis, and arrhythmias.

DIAGNOSIS

The diagnosis of valvular heart disease can be made through cardiac catheterization, chest X-rays, echocardiography, or electrocardiography. (See *Types of valvular heart disease,* pages 222 to 225.)

TREATMENT

Correcting this disorder typically involves digoxin (Lanoxin), a low-sodium diet, diuretics, vasodilators, and especially angiotensin-converting enzyme inhibitors to treat left-sided heart failure. In acute situations, oxygen is administered to increase oxygenation. Anticoagulants prevent thrombus formation around diseased or replaced valves and prophylactic antibiotics before and after surgery or dental care prevent endocarditis.

Nitroglycerin can relieve angina in conditions such as aortic stenosis. Beta-adrenergic blockers or digoxin slow the ventricular rate in atrial fibrillation or atrial flutter. Cardioversion converts atrial fibrillation to sinus rhythm.

To separate thick or adherent mitral valve leaflets, an open or closed commissurotomy may be performed or balloon valvuloplasty may be used to enlarge the orifice of a stenotic mitral, aortic, or pulmonic valve.

Anuloplasty or valvuloplasty may be used to reconstruct or repair the valve in mitral insufficiency and valve replacement with a prosthetic valve may be used for mitral and aortic valve disease.

NURSING CONSIDERATIONS

✦ Watch closely for signs of heart failure or pulmonary edema and for adverse effects of drug therapy.
✦ Teach the patient about diet restrictions, medications, and the importance of consistent follow-up care.
✦ If the patient has had surgery, watch for hypotension, arrhythmias, and thrombus formation. Monitor vital signs, arterial blood gas values, intake, output, daily weight, blood chemistries, chest X-rays, and pulmonary artery catheter readings.

Complications
✦ Heart failure
✦ Pulmonary edema
✦ Thromboembolism

Diagnosis
✦ Cardiac catheterization
✦ Chest X-rays
✦ Echocardiography
✦ Electrocardiography

Treatment
✦ Digoxin
✦ Diuretics
✦ ACE inhibitors
✦ Prophylactic antibiotics before and after surgery or dental care
✦ Nitroglycerin
✦ Beta-adrenergic blockers
✦ Valvuloplasty

Key nursing actions
✦ Watch closely for signs of heart failure or pulmonary edema.
✦ Teach the patient about diet restrictions and medications.
✦ If the patient has had surgery, watch for hypotension, arrhythmias, and thrombus formation.

(Text continues on page 224.)

Key causes of mitral stenosis
+ Rheumatic fever
+ Congenital abnormalities

Key causes of mitral insufficiency
+ Rheumatic fever
+ MI
+ Ruptured chordae tendineae
+ Congenital abnormalities

Key causes of aortic insufficiency
+ Rheumatic fever
+ Marfan syndrome
+ Ventricular septal defect

Key causes of aortic stenosis
+ Congenital aortic bicuspid valve
+ Rheumatic fever
+ Atherosclerosis

Types of valvular heart disease

CAUSES AND INCIDENCE	CLINICAL FINDINGS
Mitral stenosis	
+ Results from rheumatic fever (most common cause) or endocarditis + Most common in females + May be associated with other congenital anomalies	+ Dyspnea on exertion, paroxysmal nocturnal dyspnea, orthopnea, weakness, fatigue, and palpitations + Peripheral edema, jugular vein distention, ascites, and hepatomegaly (right ventricular failure) + Crackles, atrial fibrillation, and signs of systemic emboli + Auscultation revealing a loud S_1 or opening snap and a diastolic murmur at the apex
Mitral insufficiency	
+ Results from rheumatic fever, hypertrophic obstructive cardiomyopathy, mitral valve prolapse, myocardial infarction, severe left ventricular dilation or failure, or ruptured chordae tendineae + Associated with other congenital anomalies such as transposition of the great arteries + Rare in children without other congenital anomalies	+ Orthopnea, dyspnea, fatigue, angina, and palpitations + Peripheral edema, jugular vein distention, and hepatomegaly (right-sided heart failure) + Tachycardia, crackles, and pulmonary edema + Auscultation revealing a holosystolic murmur at apex, a possible split S_2, and an S_3
Aortic insufficiency	
+ Results from rheumatic fever, syphilis, hypertension, or endocarditis or may be idiopathic + Associated with Marfan syndrome + Most common in males + Associated with ventricular septal defect, even after surgical closure	+ Dyspnea, cough, fatigue, palpitations, angina, and syncope + Pulmonary congestion, left-sided heart failure, and "pulsating" nail beds (Quincke's sign) + Rapidly rising and collapsing pulses (pulsus biferiens), cardiac arrhythmias, and widened pulse pressure + Auscultation revealing an S_3 and a diastolic blowing murmur at left sternal border + Palpation and visualization of apical impulse in chronic disease
Aortic stenosis	
+ Results from congenital aortic bicuspid valve (associated with coarctation of the aorta), congenital stenosis of valve cusps, rheumatic fever, or atherosclerosis in the elderly + Most common in males	+ Dyspnea on exertion, paroxysmal nocturnal dyspnea, fatigue, syncope, angina, and palpitations + Pulmonary congestion and left-sided heart failure + Diminished carotid pulses, decreased cardiac output, and cardiac arrhythmias; may have pulsus alternans + Auscultation revealing systolic murmur heard at base or in carotids and, possibly, an S_4

DIAGNOSTIC MEASURES

♦ *Cardiac catheterization:* diastolic pressure gradient across valve, elevated left atrial pressure and pulmonary artery wedge pressure (PAWP) > 15 mm Hg with severe pulmonary hypertension, elevated right-sided heart pressure with decreased cardiac output, and abnormal contraction of the left ventricle
♦ *Chest X-rays:* left atrial and ventricular enlargement, enlarged pulmonary arteries, and mitral valve calcification
♦ *Echocardiography:* thickened mitral valve leaflets and left atrial enlargement
♦ *Electrocardiography (ECG):* left atrial hypertrophy, atrial fibrillation, right ventricular hypertrophy, and right axis deviation

♦ *Cardiac catheterization:* mitral insufficiency with increased left ventricular end-diastolic volume and pressure, increased atrial pressure and PAWP, and decreased cardiac output
♦ *Chest X-rays:* left atrial and ventricular enlargement and pulmonary venous congestion
♦ *Echocardiography:* abnormal valve leaflet motion and left atrial enlargement
♦ *ECG:* may show left atrial and ventricular hypertrophy, sinus tachycardia, and atrial fibrillation

♦ *Cardiac catheterization:* reduction in arterial diastolic pressures, aortic insufficiency, other valvular abnormalities, and increased left ventricular end-diastolic pressure
♦ *Chest X-rays:* left ventricular enlargement and pulmonary venous congestion
♦ *Echocardiography:* left ventricular enlargement, alterations in mitral valve movement (indirect indication of aortic valve disease), and mitral thickening
♦ *ECG:* sinus tachycardia, left ventricular hypertrophy, and left atrial hypertrophy in severe disease

♦ *Cardiac catheterization:* pressure gradient across valve (indicating obstruction) and increased left ventricular end-diastolic pressures
♦ *Chest X-rays:* valvular calcification, left ventricular enlargement, and pulmonary venous congestion
♦ *Echocardiography:* thickened aortic valve and left ventricular wall, possibly coexistent with mitral valve stenosis
♦ *ECG:* left ventricular hypertrophy

(continued)

Diagnosing mitral stenosis

♦ Cardiac catheterization: diastolic pressure gradient across valve
♦ Chest X-ray: left atrial and ventricular enlargement
♦ Echocardiography: thickened mitral valve leaflets
♦ ECG: left atrial hypertrophy

Diagnosing mitral insufficiency

♦ Cardiac catheterization: mitral insufficiency
♦ Chest X-ray: left atrial and ventricular enlargement
♦ Echocardiography: abnormal valve leaflet motion
♦ ECG: left atrial and ventricular hypertrophy

Diagnosing aortic insufficiency

♦ Cardiac catheterization: reduced arterial diastolic pressure
♦ Chest X-ray: left ventricular enlargement and pulmonary venous congestion
♦ Echocardiography: left ventricular enlargement
♦ ECG: sinus tachycardia

Diagnosing aortic stenosis

♦ Cardiac catheterization: pressure gradient across valve
♦ Chest X-ray: valvular calcification
♦ Echocardiography: thickened aortic valve
♦ ECG: left ventricular hypertrophy

Key causes of pulmonic stenosis

✦ Congenital stenosis
✦ Tetralogy of Fallot

Diagnosing pulmonic stenosis

✦ Cardiac catheterization: increased right ventricular pressure
✦ ECG: right ventricular hypertrophy

Characteristics of varicose veins

✦ Veins are dilated, tortuous veins, engorged with blood
✦ Result from improper venous valve function
✦ Primary: originate in superficial veins; secondary: originate in deep veins

Causes

Primary
✦ Congenital weakness of valves or venous wall
✦ Pregnancy
✦ Obesity

Secondary
✦ Deep vein thrombosis
✦ Venous malformation

How it happens

✦ Valves become incompetent
✦ Pressure increases and vein becomes distended
✦ Vein walls weaken, lose elasticity
✦ Veins enlarge, become lumpy and tortuous
✦ Hydrostatic pressure increases; plasma forced out of veins; edema results

Types of valvular heart disease *(continued)*	
CAUSES AND INCIDENCE	**CLINICAL FINDINGS**
Pulmonic stenosis	
✦ Results from congenital stenosis of valve cusp or rheumatic heart disease (uncommon) ✦ Associated with tetralogy of Fallot	✦ Asymptomatic or symptomatic with dyspnea on exertion, fatigue, chest pain, and syncope ✦ May cause jugular vein distention or right-sided heart failure ✦ Auscultation revealing a systolic murmur at the left sternal border and a split S_2 with a delayed or absent pulmonic component

VARICOSE VEINS

Varicose veins are dilated, tortuous veins, engorged with blood and resulting from improper venous valve function. They can be primary, originating in the superficial veins, or secondary, occurring in the deep veins.

Primary varicose veins tend to be familial; they affect both legs and are twice as common in females as in males. They account for approximately 90% of varicose veins; about 10% to 20% of Americans have primary varicose veins. Usually, secondary varicose veins occur in one leg. Both types are more common in middle adulthood.

Without treatment, varicose veins continue to enlarge. Although there's no cure, certain measures, such as walking and using compression stockings, can reduce symptoms. Surgery may remove varicose veins, but the condition can occur in other veins.

CAUSES

Primary varicose veins can result from congenital weakness of the valves or venous wall or from conditions that produce prolonged venous stasis or increased intra-abdominal pressure, such as pregnancy, obesity, constipation, or wearing tight clothes.

Also at an increased risk for developing primary varicose veins are those with occupations that necessitate standing for extended periods and those with a family history of varicose veins.

Secondary varicose veins can result from deep vein thrombosis, venous malformation, arteriovenous fistulas, trauma to the venous system, and occlusion.

PATHOPHYSIOLOGY

Veins are thin-walled, distensible vessels with valves that keep blood flowing in one direction. Any condition that weakens, destroys, or distends these valves allows blood backflow to the previous valve. If a valve can't hold the pooling blood, it can become incompetent, allowing even more blood to flow backward. As the volume of venous blood builds, pressure in the vein increases and the vein becomes distended. As the veins are stretched, their walls weaken and they lose their elasticity. As the veins enlarge, they become lumpy and tortuous. As hydrostatic pressure in-

DIAGNOSTIC MEASURES

◆ *Cardiac catheterization:* increased right ventricular pressure, decreased pulmonary artery pressure, and abnormal valve orifice
◆ *ECG:* may show right ventricular hypertrophy, right axis deviation, right atrial hypertrophy, and atrial fibrillation

creases, plasma is forced out of the veins and into the surrounding tissues, resulting in edema.

People who stand for prolonged periods may also develop venous pooling because there's no muscular contraction in the legs, forcing blood back up to the heart. If the valves in the veins are too weak to hold the pooling blood, they begin to leak, allowing blood to flow backward.

SIGNS AND SYMPTOMS

Varicose veins generally appear dilated, tortuous, purplish, and ropelike, particularly in the calves, due to venous pooling. Venous pooling also causes leg heaviness that worsens in the evening and in warm weather.

Deep vein incompetence causes edema of the calves and ankles. After prolonged standing or walking, tissue breakdown may cause a dull aching in the leg and increased fluid retention may cause an aching during menses.

COMPLICATIONS

Possible complications of varicose veins include blood clots secondary to venous stasis, venous stasis ulcers, and chronic venous insufficiency.

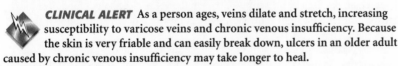 **CLINICAL ALERT** As a person ages, veins dilate and stretch, increasing susceptibility to varicose veins and chronic venous insufficiency. Because the skin is very friable and can easily break down, ulcers in an older adult caused by chronic venous insufficiency may take longer to heal.

DIAGNOSIS

Certain tests help diagnose varicose veins. A manual compression test detects a palpable impulse when the vein is firmly occluded at least 8″ (20.3 cm) above the point of palpation, indicating incompetent valves in the vein.

Performing a Trendelenburg's test (retrograde filling test) will help detect incompetent deep and superficial vein valves. In addition, a photoplethysmography characterizes venous blood flow by noting changes in the skin's circulation.

To detect the presence or absence of venous backflow in a patient's deep or superficial veins a Doppler ultrasonography should be performed. While venous outflow and reflux plethysmography detect deep venous occlusion, it's an invasive (therefore, not routinely used) test. Another test, ascending and descending venography, demonstrates venous occlusion and patterns of collateral flow.

Key signs and symptoms
◆ Veins appear dilated, purplish, and ropelike
◆ Leg heaviness that worsens in evening, warm weather
◆ Edema of calves and ankles
◆ Dull aching in legs after prolonged standing or walking

Complications
◆ Blood clots
◆ Venous stasis ulcers
◆ Chronic venous insufficiency

Alert!
◆ Ulcers in an older adult caused by chronic venous insufficiency may take longer to heal.

Diagnosis
◆ Manual compression test detects a palpable impulse upon occlusion
◆ Trendelenburg's test helps detect incompetent vein valves
◆ Photoplethysmography characterizes venous blood flow
◆ Doppler ultrasonography detects backflow

Treatment
+ Antiembolism stockings
+ Regular exercise
+ Injection of sclerosing agent
+ Surgical ligation or stripping
+ Avoidance of wearing constrictive clothing
+ Avoidance of prolonged standing or sitting
+ Weight loss

Key nursing actions
+ After stripping and ligation or after injection of a sclerosing agent, administer analgesics.
+ Check circulation in toes.

Alert!
+ Watch for signs and symptoms of complications.

Characteristics of ventricular septal defect
+ Most common acyanotic congenital heart disorder
+ Opening in septum between ventricles allows blood to shunt between left and right ventricles
+ Causes ineffective heart pumping; increases heart failure risk
+ Prognosis good for defects that close or can be operated on

Causes
+ Fetal alcohol syndrome
+ Down syndrome
+ Renal anomalies

TREATMENT

To correct varicose veins, the underlying cause, such as an abdominal tumor or obesity, should be treated, if possible.

Antiembolism stockings or elastic bandages may be worn to counteract swelling by supporting the veins and improving circulation. A regular exercise program can promote muscular contraction to force blood through the veins and reduce venous pooling.

Small to medium-sized varicosities may be treated with an injection of a sclerosing agent and severe varicose veins may be corrected with surgical ligation or stripping. Phlebectomy, removing the varicose vein through small incision in the skin, may be performed in an outpatient setting.

The patient should be discouraged from wearing constrictive clothing that interferes with venous return. Elevating her legs above her heart whenever possible and avoiding prolonged standing or sitting will help to promote venous return and prevent venous pooling.

The obese patient should lose weight to reduce increased intra-abdominal pressure.

NURSING CONSIDERATIONS

+ After stripping and ligation or after injection of a sclerosing agent, administer analgesics, as ordered, to relieve pain.
+ Frequently check circulation in toes (color and temperature), and observe elastic bandages for bleeding. When ordered, rewrap bandages at least once per shift, wrapping from toe to thigh, with the leg elevated.

 CLINICAL ALERT Watch for signs and symptoms of complications, such as sensory loss in the leg (which could indicate saphenous nerve damage), calf pain (which could indicate thrombophlebitis), and fever (a sign of infection).

VENTRICULAR SEPTAL DEFECT

In a ventricular septal defect (VSD), the most common acyanotic congenital heart disorder, an opening in the septum between the ventricles allows blood to shunt between the left and right ventricles. This results in ineffective pumping of the heart and increases the risk of heart failure.

VSDs account for up to 30% of all congenital heart defects. The prognosis is good for defects that close spontaneously or are correctable surgically, but poor for untreated defects, which are sometimes fatal in children by age 1, usually from secondary complications.

CAUSES

A VSD may be associated with fetal alcohol syndrome, Down syndrome and other autosomal trisomies, renal anomalies, patent ductus arteriosus and coarctation of the aorta, and prematurity.

PATHOPHYSIOLOGY

In infants with a VSD, the ventricular septum fails to close completely by 8 weeks' gestation. VSDs are located in the membranous or muscular portion of the ventricular septum and vary in size. Some defects close spontaneously; in other defects, the septum is entirely absent, creating a single ventricle. Small VSDs are likely to close spontaneously. Large VSDs should be surgically repaired before pulmonary vascular disease occurs or while it's still reversible.

A VSD isn't readily apparent at birth because right and left pressures are approximately equal and pulmonary artery resistance is elevated. Alveoli aren't completely opened, so blood doesn't shunt through the defect. As the pulmonary vasculature gradually relaxes, between 4 and 8 weeks after birth, right ventricular pressure decreases, allowing blood to shunt from the left to the right ventricle. Initially, large VSD shunts cause left atrial and left ventricular hypertrophy. Later, an uncorrected VSD causes right ventricular hypertrophy due to increasing pulmonary resistance. Eventually, right- and left-sided heart failure and cyanosis (from reversal of the shunt direction) occur. Fixed pulmonary hypertension may occur much later in life with right-to-left shunting (Eisenmenger's syndrome), causing cyanosis and clubbing of the nail beds.

SIGNS AND SYMPTOMS

Infants with a large VSD and subsequent heart failure are generally thin and small and gain weight slowly.

A loud, harsh, widely transmitted systolic murmur may be heard best along the left sternal border at the third or fourth intercostal space, caused by abnormal blood flow through the VSD. A loud widely split pulmonic component of S_2 is caused by an increased pressure gradient across the VSD. Turbulent blood flow between the ventricles through a small VSD causes a palpable thrill. Hypertrophy of the heart causes displacement of the point of maximal impulse toward the left.

 CLINICAL ALERT Typically in infants, the apical impulse is palpated over the fourth intercostal space, just to the left of the midclavicular line. In children older than age 7, it's palpated over the fifth intercostal space. When the heart is enlarged, the apical beat is displaced to the left or downward.

The infant generally has a prominent anterior chest secondary to cardiac hypertrophy and liver, heart, and spleen enlargement because of systemic congestion. Heart failure results in feeding difficulties, diaphoresis, tachycardia, and rapid, grunting respirations. Pulmonary hypertension causes cyanosis and clubbing if the right-to-left shunting occurs later in life.

COMPLICATIONS

Complications of a VSD may include pulmonary hypertension, infective endocarditis, pneumonia, heart failure, Eisenmenger's syndrome, and aortic insufficiency (if the aortic valve is involved).

DIAGNOSIS

Certain tests help diagnose a VSD in patients. Chest X-rays appear normal in small defects. In large VSDs, the X-ray may show cardiomegaly, left atrial and left ventricular enlargement, and prominent vascular markings.

While small VSDs may show a normal electrocardiography, in large VSDs it may show left and right ventricular hypertrophy, suggestive of pulmonary hypertension. To detect a VSD in the septum, estimate the size of the left-to-right shunt, suggest pulmonary hypertension, and identify associated lesions and complications an echocardiography should be used.

Another useful test is a cardiac catheterization, which determines the size and exact location of the VSD and the extent of pulmonary hypertension. It also detects

How it happens

+ Alveoli aren't opened, so blood doesn't shunt through defect
+ 4 to 8 weeks after birth, right ventricular pressure decreases
+ Large VSD shunts cause left atrial and left ventricular hypertrophy
+ Eventually causes right- and left-sided heart failure and cyanosis

Key signs and symptoms

+ Infants generally thin and small; gain weight slowly
+ Loud, harsh, widely transmitted systolic murmur
+ Loud widely split pulmonic component of S_2
+ Palpable thrill

Alert!

+ In infants, the apical impulse is palpated over the fourth intercostal space, just to the left of the midclavicular line.
+ In children older than age 7, it's palpated over the fifth intercostal space.

Complications

+ Pulmonary hypertension
+ Infective endocarditis
+ Pneumonia
+ Heart failure

Diagnosis

+ Chest X-rays appear normal in small defects
+ Echocardiography can find VSD in septum
+ Cardiac catheterization determines size and exact location of VSD and extent of pulmonary hypertension; detects defects and calculates degree of shunting

Treatment

+ Early surgical correction
+ Placement of a permanent pacemaker after VSD repair
+ Surgical closure using sutures
+ Pulmonary artery banding
+ Digoxin
+ Sodium restriction

Key nursing actions

+ Parent teaching is vital to prevent complications until the child is scheduled for surgery or the defect closes.
+ Tell the parents how to give medications and how to recognize adverse effects.
+ Stress the importance of prophylactic antibiotics before and after surgery.

After surgery

+ Check oxygenation.
+ Monitor pacemaker effectiveness.

associated defects and calculates the degree of shunting by comparing the blood oxygen saturation in each ventricle. The oxygen saturation of the right ventricle is greater than normal because oxygenated blood is shunted from the left to the right ventricle.

TREATMENT

Early surgical correction for a large VSD, usually with a patch graft, is performed before heart failure and irreversible pulmonary vascular disease develop.

Placement of a permanent pacemaker may be necessary after VSD repair if complete heart block develops from interference with the bundle of His during surgery. Small defects may be surgically closed using sutures; however, they may not be surgically repaired if the patient has normal pulmonary artery pressure and a small shunt.

Pulmonary artery banding is used to normalize pressures and flow distal to the band and to prevent pulmonary vascular disease if the child has other defects and will benefit from delaying surgery.

Before surgery, digoxin (Lanoxin), sodium restriction, and diuretics help prevent heart failure. Prophylactic antibiotics before and after surgery prevent infective endocarditis.

NURSING CONSIDERATIONS

Although the parents of an infant with a VSD commonly suspect something is wrong with their child before diagnosis, they need psychological support to help them accept the reality of a serious cardiac disorder. Because surgery may take place months after diagnosis, parent teaching is vital to prevent complications until the child is scheduled for surgery or the defect closes. Thorough explanations of all tests are also essential.

+ Instruct the parents to watch for signs of heart failure, such as poor feeding, sweating, and heavy breathing.
+ If the child is receiving digoxin or other medications, tell the parents how to give it and how to recognize adverse effects. Caution them to keep medications out of the reach of all children.
+ Teach the parents to recognize and report early signs of infection and to avoid exposing the child to people with obvious infections.
+ Encourage the parents to let the child engage in normal activities.
+ Stress the importance of prophylactic antibiotics before and after surgery.

After surgery to correct the VSD

+ Monitor vital signs and intake and output. Maintain the infant's body temperature with an overbed warmer. Give catecholamines, nitroprusside (Nipride), and diuretics, as ordered, and analgesics as needed.
+ Monitor central venous pressure, intra-arterial blood pressure, and left atrial or pulmonary artery pressure readings. Assess heart rate and rhythm for signs of conduction block.
+ Check oxygenation, particularly in a child who requires mechanical ventilation. Suction as needed to maintain a patent airway and to prevent atelectasis and pneumonia.
+ Monitor pacemaker effectiveness, if needed. Watch for signs of failure, such as bradycardia and hypotension.
+ Reassure the parents, and allow them to participate in their child's care.

Respiratory system

The respiratory system's major function is gas exchange, in which air enters the body on inhalation (inspiration); travels throughout the respiratory passages, exchanging oxygen for carbon dioxide at the tissue level; and expels carbon dioxide on exhalation (expiration).

The upper airway — composed of the nose, mouth, pharynx, and larynx — allows airflow into the lungs. This area is responsible for warming, humidifying, and filtering the air, thereby protecting the lower airway from foreign matter.

The lower airway consists of the trachea, mainstem bronchi, secondary bronchi, bronchioles, and terminal bronchioles. These structures are anatomic dead spaces and function only as passageways for moving air into and out of the lungs. Distal to each terminal bronchiole is the acinus, which consists of respiratory bronchioles, alveolar ducts, and alveolar sacs. The bronchioles and ducts function as conduits, and the alveoli are the chief units of gas exchange. These final subdivisions of the bronchial tree make up the lobules — the functional units of the lungs. (See *Structure of the lobule*, page 230.)

In addition to warming, humidifying, and filtering inspired air, the lower airway protects the lungs with several defense mechanisms. Clearance mechanisms include the cough reflex and mucociliary system. The mucociliary system produces mucus, trapping foreign particles. Foreign matter is then swept to the upper airway for expectoration by specialized fingerlike projections called cilia. A breakdown in the epithelium of the lungs or the mucociliary system can cause the defense mechanisms to malfunction, and pollutants and irritants then enter and inflame the lungs. The lower airway also provides immunologic protection and initiates pulmonary injury responses.

The external component of respiration (ventilation or breathing) delivers inspired air to the lower respiratory tract and alveoli. Contraction and relaxation of the respiratory muscles moves air into and out of the lungs.

Normal expiration is passive; the inspiratory muscles cease to contract, and the elastic recoil of the lungs and the chest wall causes them to contract again. These

Key facts about the respiratory system

- Major function is gas exchange
- Upper airway allows airflow into lungs; warm, humidify, filter air
- Lower airway consists of trachea, mainstem bronchi, secondary bronchi, bronchioles, terminal bronchioles
- Structures are anatomic dead spaces, function only as passageways for moving air into and out of the lungs
- Distal to terminal bronchioles are acinus — respiratory bronchioles, alveolar ducts, alveolar sacs
- Bronchioles and ducts function as conduits
- Alveoli: chief units of gas exchange
- Clearance mechanisms: cough reflex and mucociliary system

Structure of the lobule

Each lobule contains terminal bronchioles and the acinus. The acinus consists of respiratory bronchioles and the alveolar sacs.

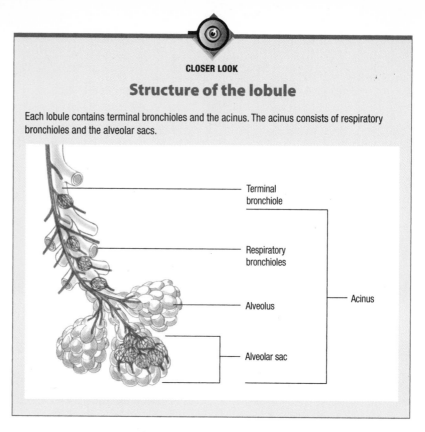

Terminal bronchiole

Respiratory bronchioles

Alveolus

Acinus

Alveolar sac

Key facts about the respiratory system
(continued)

+ Lower airway protects lungs with defense mechanisms
+ Respiration delivers inspired air to lower respiratory tract and alveoli
+ Contraction and relaxation of respiratory muscles moves air into and out of lungs
+ Normal expiration is passive
+ Adult lung contains 300 million alveoli; each supplied by many capillaries
+ To reach capillary lumen, oxygen must cross alveolar capillary membrane
+ The pulmonary alveoli promote gas exchange by diffusion
+ Circulating blood delivers oxygen to cells for metabolism and transports metabolic wastes and CO_2 back to lungs
+ CO_2 reaches alveolar capillaries, diffuses into the alveoli; removed from the alveoli during exhalation

actions raise the pressure within the lungs to above atmospheric pressure, moving air from the lungs to the atmosphere.

An adult lung contains an estimated 300 million alveoli; each alveolus is supplied by many capillaries. To reach the capillary lumen, oxygen must cross the alveolar capillary membrane.

The pulmonary alveoli promote gas exchange by diffusion — the passage of gas molecules through respiratory membranes. In diffusion, oxygen passes to the blood, and carbon dioxide, a by-product of cellular metabolism, passes out of the blood and is channeled away.

Circulating blood delivers oxygen to the cells of the body for metabolism and transports metabolic wastes and carbon dioxide from the tissues back to the lungs. When oxygenated arterial blood reaches tissue capillaries, the oxygen diffuses from the blood into the cells because of an oxygen tension gradient. The amount of oxygen available to cells depends on the concentration of hemoglobin (the principal carrier of oxygen) in the blood, the regional blood flow, the arterial oxygen content, and cardiac output.

Because circulation is continuous, carbon dioxide doesn't usually accumulate in tissues. Carbon dioxide produced during cellular respiration diffuses from tissues to regional capillaries and is transported by the systemic venous circulation. When carbon dioxide reaches the alveolar capillaries, it diffuses into the alveoli, where the partial pressure of carbon dioxide ($PaCO_2$) is lower. Carbon dioxide is removed from the alveoli during exhalation.

For effective gas exchange, ventilation and perfusion at the alveolar level must match closely. (See *Understanding ventilation and perfusion*.)

CLOSER LOOK

Understanding ventilation and perfusion

Effective gas exchange depends on the relationship between ventilation and perfusion, expressed as the V̇/Q̇ ratio. The diagrams below show what happens when the V̇/Q̇ ratio is normal and abnormal.

NORMAL VENTILATION AND PERFUSION

When the V̇/Q̇ ratio is matched, unoxygenated blood from the venous system returns to the right ventricle through the pulmonary artery to the lungs, carrying carbon dioxide. The arteries branch into the alveolar capillaries, where gas exchange occurs.

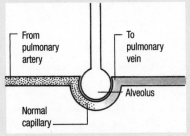

INADEQUATE PERFUSION (DEAD-SPACE VENTILATION)

When the V̇/Q̇ ratio is high, ventilation is normal, but alveolar perfusion is reduced or absent (illustrated by the perfusion blockage). This results from a perfusion defect, such as pulmonary embolism or a disorder that decreases cardiac output.

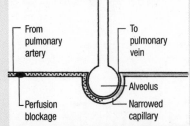

INADEQUATE VENTILATION (SHUNT)

When the V̇/Q̇ ratio is low, pulmonary circulation is adequate, but oxygen is inadequate for normal diffusion (illustrated by the ventilation blockage). A portion of the blood flowing through the pulmonary vessels doesn't become oxygenated.

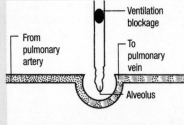

INADEQUATE VENTILATION AND PERFUSION (SILENT UNIT)

The silent unit indicates an absence of ventilation and perfusion to the lung area (illustrated by blockages in perfusion and ventilation). The silent unit may try to compensate for this V̇/Q̇ imbalance by delivering blood flow to better-ventilated lung areas.

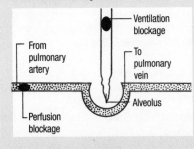

KEY

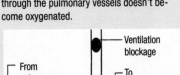

▓▓▓: Blood with CO_2 ▬▬▬ Blood with O_2 ▓▬▬ Blood with CO_2 and O_2

The ratio of ventilation to perfusion is called the *V̇/Q̇ ratio*. A V̇/Q̇ mismatch can result from ventilation-perfusion dysfunction or altered lung mechanics.

The amount of air carrying oxygen that reaches the lungs depends on lung volume and capacity, compliance, and resistance to airflow. Changes in compliance can occur in either the lung or the chest wall. Destruction of the lung's elastic fibers, which occurs in acute respiratory distress syndrome, decreases lung compli-

V̇/Q̇ ratios

+ Normal V̇/Q̇: unoxygenated blood returns to the right ventricle carrying carbon dioxide; gas exchange occurs
+ Inadequate ventilation: V̇/Q̇ ratio is low; pulmonary circulation is adequate; oxygen is inadequate for normal diffusion
+ Inadequate perfusion: V̇/Q̇ ratio is high; ventilation is normal; alveolar perfusion is reduced or absent
+ Inadequate V̇/Q̇: absence of ventilation and perfusion to the lung area

Key facts about the respiratory system
(continued)

+ Ratio of ventilation to perfusion is V̇/Q̇ ratio
+ Amount of air carrying oxygen that reaches lungs depends on lung volume and capacity, compliance, and resistance to airflow

Key facts about the respiratory system
(continued)

+ Respiration also controlled neurologically by lateral medulla oblongata of brain stem
+ Stimulation of lower pontine apneustic center produces forceful inspiratory gasps alternating with weak expiration
+ Chemoreceptors respond to pH of arterial blood, $Paco_2$, and Pao_2

ance. The lungs become stiff, making breathing difficult. The alveolar capillary membrane may also be affected, causing hypoxia. Chest wall compliance is affected by disorders causing thoracic deformity, muscle spasm, and abdominal distention.

Respiration is also controlled neurologically by the lateral medulla oblongata of the brain stem. Impulses travel down the phrenic nerves to the diaphragm and then down the intercostal nerves to the intercostal muscles between the ribs. The rate and depth of respiration are controlled similarly.

Apneustic and pneumotaxic centers in the pons of the midbrain influence the pattern of breathing. Stimulation of the lower pontine apneustic center (by trauma, tumor, or stroke) produces forceful inspiratory gasps alternating with weak expiration. This pattern doesn't occur if the vagi are intact. The apneustic center continually excites the medullary inspiratory center and thus facilitates inspiration. Signals from the pneumotaxic center and afferent impulses from the vagus nerve inhibit the apneustic center and "turn off" inspiration.

In addition, chemoreceptors respond to the pH of arterial blood, $Paco_2$, and the partial pressure of arterial oxygen (Pao_2). Central chemoreceptors respond indirectly to arterial blood by sensing changes in the pH of the cerebrospinal fluid (CSF). $Paco_2$ also helps regulate ventilation by impacting the pH of CSF. If $Paco_2$ is high, the respiratory rate increases; if $Paco_2$ is low, the respiratory rate decreases. Information from peripheral chemoreceptors in the carotid and aortic bodies also responds to decreased Pao_2 and pH. Either of these changes results in increased respiratory drive within minutes.

PATHOPHYSIOLOGIC CHANGES

Pathophysiologic manifestations of respiratory disease may stem from atelectasis, bronchiectasis, cyanosis, and hypoxemia.

ATELECTASIS

Atelectasis

+ Occurs when alveolar sacs or entire lung segments expand incompletely, producing partial or complete lung collapse
+ Allows unoxygenated blood to pass, resulting in hypoxia
+ May be chronic or acute
+ Commonly occurs in patients undergoing upper abdominal or thoracic surgery
+ Two major causes of collapse: absorptional atelectasis, compression atelectasis

Atelectasis occurs when the alveolar sacs or entire lung segments expand incompletely, producing a partial or complete lung collapse. This phenomenon removes certain regions of the lung from gas exchange, allowing unoxygenated blood to pass unchanged through these regions and resulting in hypoxia. Atelectasis may be chronic or acute, and commonly occurs in patients undergoing upper abdominal or thoracic surgery. There are two major causes of collapse due to atelectasis: absorptional atelectasis, secondary to bronchial or bronchiolar obstruction, and compression atelectasis.

Absorption atelectasis

Absorption atelectasis

+ Occurs when alveolar sacs or entire lung segments expand incompletely, producing partial or complete lung collapse

Bronchial occlusion, which prevents air from entering the alveoli distal to the obstruction, can cause absorption atelectasis—the air present in the alveoli is absorbed gradually into the bloodstream and eventually the alveoli collapse. This may result from intrinsic or extrinsic bronchial obstruction. The most common intrinsic cause is retained secretions or exudate-forming mucus plugs. Disorders, such as cystic fibrosis, chronic bronchitis, or pneumonia, increase the risk of absorption atelectasis. Extrinsic bronchial atelectasis usually results from occlusion caused by foreign bodies, bronchogenic carcinoma, and scar tissue.

Impaired production of surfactant can also cause absorption atelectasis. Increasing surface tension of the alveolus due to reduced surfactant leads to collapse.

Compression atelectasis

Compression atelectasis results from external compression, which drives the air out and causes the lung to collapse. This may result from upper abdominal surgical incisions, rib fractures, pleuritic chest pain, tight chest dressings, and obesity (which elevates the diaphragm and reduces tidal volume). These situations inhibit full lung expansion or make deep breathing painful, thus resulting in this disorder.

BRONCHIECTASIS

Bronchiectasis is marked by chronic abnormal dilation of the bronchi and destruction of the bronchial walls and can occur throughout the tracheobronchial tree. It may also be confined to a single segment or lobe. This disorder is usually bilateral in nature and involves the basilar segments of the lower lobes.

There are three forms of bronchiectasis: cylindrical, fusiform (varicose), and saccular (cystic). (See *Forms of bronchiectasis.*)

It results from conditions associated with repeated damage to bronchial walls with abnormal mucociliary clearance, which causes a breakdown of supporting tissue adjacent to the airways.

Such conditions include cystic fibrosis, immune disorders (agammaglobulinemia), recurrent bacterial infections that were inadequately treated (tuberculosis), and complications of measles, pneumonia, pertussis, or influenza. Other examples include an obstruction (from a foreign body, tumor, or stenosis) with recurrent infection, inhalation of corrosive gas, or repeated aspiration of gastric juices into the lungs. Congenital anomalies, such as bronchomalacia, congenital bronchiectasis, and Kartagener's syndrome, and rare disorders, such as immotile cilia syndrome, may also cause bronchiectasis.

Compression atelectasis

◆ Results from external compression: upper abdominal surgical incisions, rib fractures, tight chest dressings, obesity
◆ Inhibits full lung expansion or makes deep breathing painful

Bronchiectasis

◆ Marked by chronic abnormal dilation of bronchi and destruction of bronchial walls
◆ Can occur throughout tracheobronchial tree or may be confined to one segment or lobe
◆ Involves basilar segments of lower lobes
◆ Three forms: cylindrical, fusiform, and saccular
◆ Sputum stagnates in dilated bronchi and leads to infection

Forms of bronchiectasis

The three types of bronchiectasis are cylindrical, fusiform (varicose), and saccular (cystic). In cylindrical bronchiectasis, bronchioles are usually symmetrically dilated, whereas in fusiform bronchiectasis, bronchioles are deformed. In saccular bronchiectasis, large bronchi become enlarged and balloonlike.

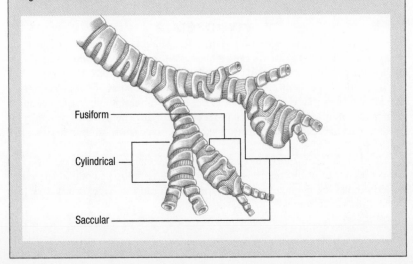

Fusiform

Cylindrical

Saccular

Cyanosis

+ Bluish discoloration of skin and mucous membranes
+ Indicates decreased oxygen saturation of hemoglobin in arterial blood
+ Peripheral cyanosis best visualized by examining nail bed
+ Caused by desaturation with oxygen or reduced hemoglobin
+ Develops when 5 g of hemoglobin is desaturated
+ Noncyanotic individual doesn't always have adequate oxygenation
+ Patient may seem cyanotic even if oxygenation is adequate
+ Cyanosis must be interpreted in relation to patient's underlying pathophysiology
+ Analysis of arterial blood gases may confirm diagnosis

Alert!

+ Best indicators of cyanosis in patients with black or dark complexions is oral mucosa and conjunctivae of the eyes.

Hypoxemia

+ Reduced oxygenation of arterial blood; hypoxia in blood
+ Caused by respiratory alterations
+ Hypoxia can result from low cardiac output, cyanide poisoning, and alterations in respiration
+ Can lead to tissue hypoxia
+ Can be caused by decreased oxygen content of inspired gas, hypoventilation, diffusion abnormalities, abnormal $\dot{V}/\dot{Q}$ ratios, and pulmonary right-to-left shunts
+ Physiologic mechanism for each cause varies

In patients with bronchiectasis, sputum stagnates in the dilated bronchi and leads to secondary infection, characterized by inflammation and leukocytic accumulations. Additional debris collects within and occludes the bronchi. Increasing pressure from the retained secretions induces mucosal injury.

CYANOSIS

Cyanosis is a bluish discoloration of the skin and mucous membranes. In most populations, it's readily detectable by a visible blue tinge on the nail beds and lips. Central cyanosis indicates decreased oxygen saturation of hemoglobin in arterial blood, which is best observed in the buccal mucous membranes and the lips. Peripheral cyanosis, a slowed blood circulation of the fingers and toes, is best visualized by examining the nail bed area.

 CLINICAL ALERT In patients with black or dark complexions, cyanosis may not be evident in the lip area or the nail beds. A better indicator in these individuals is the membranes of the oral mucosa (buccal mucous membranes) and of the conjunctivae of the eyes.

Cyanosis is caused by desaturation with oxygen or reduced hemoglobin amounts. It develops when 5 g of hemoglobin is desaturated, even if hemoglobin counts are adequate or reduced. Conditions that result in cyanosis include decreased arterial oxygenation (indicated by low PaO_2), pulmonary or cardiac right-to-left shunts, decreased cardiac output, anxiety, and a cold environment.

An individual who isn't cyanotic doesn't necessarily have adequate oxygenation. Inadequate tissue oxygenation occurs in severe anemia, resulting in inadequate hemoglobin concentration. It also occurs in carbon monoxide poisoning, in which hemoglobin binds to carbon monoxide instead of to oxygen. Although assessment doesn't reveal cyanosis, oxygenation is inadequate.

Another patient may appear cyanotic even though oxygenation is adequate — as in polycythemia, an abnormal increase in the red blood cell count. Because the hemoglobin count is increased and oxygenation occurs at a normal rate, the patient may still present with cyanosis.

Cyanosis as a presenting condition must be interpreted in relation to the patient's underlying pathophysiology. Diagnosis of inadequate oxygenation may be confirmed by analyzing arterial blood gases and measuring PaO_2.

HYPOXEMIA

Hypoxemia is reduced oxygenation of the arterial blood, evidenced by reduced PaO_2 of arterial blood gases. It's caused by respiratory alterations, whereas hypoxia is diminished tissue oxygenation at the cellular level that may be caused by conditions affecting other body systems that are unrelated to alterations of pulmonary function. Low cardiac output or cyanide poisoning can result in hypoxia, in addition to alterations in respiration. Hypoxia can occur anywhere in the body. If hypoxia occurs in the blood, it's termed hypoxemia. Hypoxemia can lead to tissue hypoxia.

Hypoxemia can be caused by decreased oxygen content of inspired gas, hypoventilation, diffusion abnormalities, abnormal $\dot{V}/\dot{Q}$ ratios, and pulmonary right-to-left shunts. The physiologic mechanism for each cause of hypoxemia varies. (See *Major causes of hypoxemia.*)

Major causes of hypoxemia

This chart lists the major causes of hypoxemia and contributing factors.

MAJOR CAUSE	CONTRIBUTING FACTORS
Decrease in inspired oxygen	High altitudes, inhaling poorly oxygenated gases, or breathing in an enclosed space
Hypoventilation	Respiratory center inappropriately stimulated (such as by oversedation, overdosage, or neurologic damage), chronic obstructive pulmonary disease
Alveolar capillary diffusion abnormality	Emphysema, conditions resulting in fibrosis, or pulmonary edema
Ventilation-perfusion mismatch	Asthma, chronic bronchitis, or pneumonia
Shunting	Acute respiratory distress syndrome, idiopathic respiratory distress syndrome of the newborn, or atelectasis

▼ *LIFE-THREATENING DISORDER*

ACUTE RESPIRATORY DISTRESS SYNDROME

Acute respiratory distress syndrome (ARDS) is a form of pulmonary edema that can quickly lead to acute respiratory failure. Also known as shock lung, stiff lung, white lung, wet lung, or Da Nang lung, ARDS may follow direct or indirect injury to the lung. However, its diagnosis is difficult, and death can occur within 48 hours of onset if not promptly diagnosed and treated. A differential diagnosis needs to rule out cardiogenic pulmonary edema, pulmonary vasculitis, and diffuse pulmonary hemorrhage. Patients who recover may have little or no permanent lung damage.

CAUSES

Trauma is the most common cause of ARDS, possibly because trauma-related factors, such as fat emboli, sepsis, shock, pulmonary contusions, and multiple transfusions, increase the likelihood of microemboli developing.

Other common causes of ARDS include anaphylaxis, aspiration of gastric contents, diffuse pneumonia (especially viral), drug overdose (for example, heroin, aspirin, and ethchlorvynol), idiosyncratic drug reaction (to ampicillin and hydrochlorothiazide), inhalation of noxious gases (such as nitrous oxide, ammonia, and chlorine), near-drowning, and oxygen toxicity.

Less common causes of ARDS include coronary artery bypass grafting, hemodialysis, leukemia, acute miliary tuberculosis, pancreatitis, thrombotic thrombocytopenic purpura, uremia, and venous air embolism.

Major causes

+ Decrease in inspired oxygen
+ Hypoventilation
+ Alveolar capillary diffusion abnormality
+ Ventilation-perfusion mismatch
+ Shunting

Characteristics of ARDS

+ Life-threatening disorder
+ Form of pulmonary edema; can lead to acute respiratory failure
+ May follow injury to the lung
+ Diagnosis is difficult, death can occur in 48 hours
+ Differential diagnosis needs to rule out cardiogenic pulmonary edema, pulmonary vasculitis, diffuse pulmonary hemorrhage
+ Patients who recover may have little or no lung damage

Causes

+ Trauma
+ Anaphylaxis
+ Aspiration of gastric contents
+ Diffuse pneumonia
+ Drug overdose or reaction
+ Inhalation of noxious gases
+ Near-drowning
+ Oxygen toxicity
+ Coronary artery bypass grafting

How it happens

+ Cellular and biochemical changes triggered by specific causative agents
+ Injury causes production of various cytokines, which promote cellular activation, chemotaxis, and adhesion
+ Activated cells produce inflammatory mediators, initiate complement cascade, intravascular coagulation, and fibrinolysis
+ Cellular triggers cause increased vascular permeability to proteins
+ Elevated capillary pressure greatly increases interstitial and alveolar edema
+ Alveolar closing pressure exceeds pulmonary pressures and alveolar closure and collapse begin
+ Fluid accumulation in the lung interstitium, the alveolar spaces, and small airways causes lungs to stiffen
+ Resulting injury reduces normal blood flow to the lungs
+ Substances inflame and damage alveolar membrane and increase capillary permeability
+ Proteins, blood cells, and fluid leak, increasing interstitial pressure, causing pulmonary edema

PATHOPHYSIOLOGY

Injury in ARDS involves the alveolar and pulmonary capillary epithelium. A cascade of cellular and biochemical changes is triggered by the specific causative agent. When initiated, this injury triggers neutrophils, macrophages, monocytes, and lymphocytes to produce various cytokines. The cytokines promote cellular activation, chemotaxis, and adhesion. The activated cells produce inflammatory mediators, including oxidants, proteases, kinins, growth factors, and neuropeptides, which initiate the complement cascade, intravascular coagulation, and fibrinolysis.

These cellular triggers result in increased vascular permeability to proteins, affecting the hydrostatic pressure gradient of the capillary. Elevated capillary pressure, such as that resulting from fluid overload or cardiac dysfunction in sepsis, increases interstitial and alveolar edema, which is evident in dependent lung areas and can be visualized as whitened areas on chest X-rays. Alveolar closing pressure then exceeds pulmonary pressures, and alveolar closure and collapse begin.

In ARDS, fluid accumulation in the lung interstitium, the alveolar spaces, and the small airways causes the lungs to stiffen, thus impairing ventilation and reducing oxygenation of the pulmonary capillary blood. The resulting injury reduces normal blood flow to the lungs. Damage can occur directly—by aspiration of gastric contents and inhalation of noxious gases—or indirectly—from chemical mediators released in response to systemic disease.

Platelets begin to aggregate and release substances, such as serotonin, bradykinin, and histamine, which attract and activate neutrophils. These substances inflame and damage the alveolar membrane and later increase capillary permeability. In the early stages, signs and symptoms may be undetectable.

Capillary permeability

Additional chemotactic factors released include endotoxins (such as those present in septic states), tumor necrosis factor, and interleukin-1. The activated neutrophils release several inflammatory mediators and platelet aggravating factors that damage the alveolar capillary membrane and increase capillary permeability.

Histamines and other inflammatory substances increase capillary permeability, allowing fluids to move into the interstitial space. Consequently, the patient experiences tachypnea, dyspnea, and tachycardia. As capillary permeability increases, proteins, blood cells, and more fluid leak out, increasing interstitial osmotic pressure and causing pulmonary edema. Tachycardia, dyspnea, and cyanosis may occur. Hypoxia (usually unresponsive to increasing fraction of inspired oxygen), decreased pulmonary compliance, crackles, and rhonchi develop. The resulting pulmonary edema and hemorrhage significantly reduce lung compliance and impair alveolar ventilation.

The fluid in the alveoli and decreased blood flow damage surfactant in the alveoli. This reduces the ability of alveolar cells to produce more surfactant. Without surfactant, alveoli and bronchioles fill with fluid or collapse, gas exchange is impaired, and the lungs are much less compliant. Ventilation of the alveoli is further decreased. The burden of ventilation and gas exchange shifts to uninvolved areas of the lung, and pulmonary blood flow is shunted from right to left. The work of breathing is increased, and the patient may develop thick, frothy sputum and marked hypoxemia with increasing respiratory distress.

Mediators released by neutrophils and macrophages also cause varying degrees of pulmonary vasoconstriction, resulting in pulmonary hypertension. The result of these changes is a ventilation-perfusion mismatch. Although the patient responds with an increased respiratory rate, sufficient oxygen can't cross the alveolar capillary membrane. Carbon dioxide continues to cross easily and is lost with every exhalation. As oxygen and carbon dioxide levels in the blood decrease, the patient develops increasing tachypnea, hypoxemia, and hypocapnia (low partial pressure of arterial carbon dioxide [$PaCO_2$]).

Pulmonary edema worsens, and hyaline membranes form. Inflammation leads to fibrosis, which further impedes gas exchange. Fibrosis progressively obliterates alveoli, respiratory bronchioles, and the interstitium. Functional residual capacity decreases, and shunting becomes more serious. Hypoxemia leads to metabolic acidosis. At this stage, the patient develops increasing $PaCO_2$, decreasing pH and partial pressure of arterial oxygen (PaO_2), decreasing bicarbonate (HCO_3^- levels, and mental confusion. (See *Looking at acute respiratory distress syndrome,* page 238.)

The end result is respiratory failure. Systemically, neutrophils and inflammatory mediators cause generalized endothelial damage and increased capillary permeability throughout the body. Multiple organ dysfunction syndrome (MODS) occurs as the cascade of mediators affects each system. Death may occur from the influence of ARDS and MODS.

SIGNS AND SYMPTOMS

ARDS initially produces rapid, shallow breathing and dyspnea, which occur hours to days after the initial injury in response to decreasing oxygen levels in the blood. An increased rate of ventilation due to hypoxemia develops. Intercostal and suprasternal retractions develop due to the increased effort required to expand the stiff lung. Crackles and rhonchi are audible and result from fluid accumulation in the lungs. Restlessness, apprehension, and mental sluggishness occur as the result of hypoxic brain cells. Motor dysfunction occurs as hypoxia progresses. Tachycardia signals the heart's effort to deliver more oxygen to the cells and vital organs. Respiratory acidosis occurs as carbon dioxide accumulates in the blood and oxygen levels decrease. Metabolic acidosis eventually results from failure of compensatory mechanisms.

COMPLICATIONS

Possible complications of ARDS include hypotension, decreased urine output, metabolic acidosis, respiratory acidosis, MODS, ventricular fibrillation, and ventricular standstill.

DIAGNOSIS

Arterial blood gas (ABG) analysis with the patient breathing room air initially reveals a reduced PaO_2 (less than 60 mm Hg) and a decreased $PaCO_2$ (less than 35 mm Hg). Hypoxemia, despite increased supplemental oxygen, is the hallmark of ARDS; the resulting blood pH reflects respiratory alkalosis. As ARDS worsens, ABG values show respiratory acidosis evidenced by an increasing $PaCO_2$ (over 45 mm Hg), metabolic acidosis evidenced by a decreasing HCO_3^- (less than 22 mEq/L), and a declining PaO_2 despite oxygen therapy.

Pulmonary artery catheterization helps identify the cause of pulmonary edema (cardiac versus noncardiac) by measuring pulmonary artery wedge pressure (PAWP); allows collection of pulmonary artery blood, which shows decreased oxygen saturation, reflecting tissue hypoxia; measures pulmonary artery pressure; measures cardiac output by thermodilution techniques; and provides information to allow calculation of the percentages of blood shunted through the lungs.

Serial chest X-rays in early stages show bilateral infiltrates. In later stages, lung fields with a ground-glass appearance and "white-outs" of both lung fields (with irreversible hypoxia) may be observed. To differentiate ARDS from heart failure,

How it happens
(continued)

✦ Resulting edema and hemorrhage impair alveolar ventilation and damage alveoli surfactant
✦ Edema worsens, generalized endothelial damage and capillary permeability occur throughout body; continuing cascade causes death

Key signs and symptoms

✦ Rapid, shallow breathing, dyspnea, increased ventilation rate
✦ Intercostal and suprasternal retractions
✦ Crackles and rhonchi
✦ Restlessness, apprehension, and mental sluggishness

Complications

✦ Hypotension
✦ Decreased urine output
✦ Respiratory acidosis

Diagnosis

✦ ABG analysis with patient breathing room air reveals reduced PaO_2 and decreased $PaCO_2$
✦ Hypoxemia (hallmark of ARDS)
✦ ABG values show respiratory acidosis, metabolic acidosis, and declining PaO_2 despite oxygen therapy

Looking at acute respiratory distress syndrome

These diagrams show the process and progress of acute respiratory distress syndrome.

In phase 1, injury reduces normal blood flow to the lungs. Platelets aggregate and release histamine (H), serotonin (S), and bradykinin (B).

In phase 4, decreased blood flow and fluids in the alveoli damage surfactant and impair the cell's ability to produce more. The alveoli then collapse, thus impairing gas exchange.

Phases of ARDS

✦ Phase 1: Injury reduces normal blood flow to the lungs
✦ Phase 2: Released substances inflame and damage alveolar capillary membrane; fluids shift into interstitial space
✦ Phase 3: Capillary permeability increases and proteins and fluids leak out
✦ Phase 4: Decreased blood flow and fluids in the alveoli damage surfactant; alveoli collapse, impairing gas exchange
✦ Phase 5: Oxygenation is impaired; blood oxygen and carbon dioxide levels are low
✦ Phase 6: Pulmonary edema worsens; inflammation leads to fibrosis

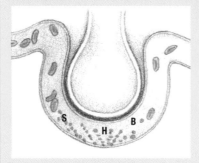

In phase 2, the released substances inflame and damage the alveolar capillary membrane, increasing capillary permeability. Fluids then shift into the interstitial space.

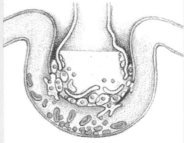

In phase 5, oxygenation is impaired, but carbon dioxide easily crosses the alveolar capillary membrane and is expired. Blood oxygen and carbon dioxide levels are low.

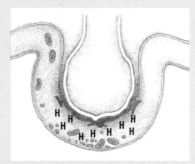

In phase 3, capillary permeability increases and proteins and fluids leak out, increasing interstitial osmotic pressure and causing pulmonary edema.

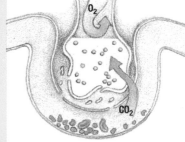

In phase 6, pulmonary edema worsens and inflammation leads to fibrosis. Gas exchange is further impeded.

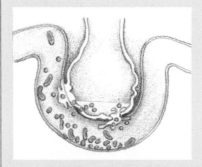

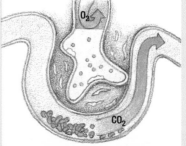

note that the normal cardiac silhouette appears diffuse. Bilateral infiltrates tend to be more peripheral and patchy, as opposed to the usual perihilar "bat wing" appearance of cardiogenic pulmonary edema; and there are fewer pleural effusions.

Sputum analysis, including Gram stain and culture and sensitivity, identifies causative organisms.

Blood cultures identify infectious organisms. Toxicology testing screens for drug ingestion. Serum amylase rules out pancreatitis.

TREATMENT

Therapy is focused on correcting the causes of ARDS and preventing progression of hypoxemia and respiratory acidosis. Supportive medical care consists of administration of humidified oxygen by a tight-fitting mask, which allows for the use of continuous positive airway pressure. Hypoxemia that doesn't respond adequately to the above measures requires ventilatory support with intubation, volume ventilation, and positive end-expiratory pressure (PEEP). Pressure-controlled inverse ratio ventilation reverses the conventional inspiration-to-expiration ratio and minimizes the risk of barotrauma. Mechanical breaths are pressure-limited to prevent increased damage to the alveoli. Permissive hypercapnia limits peak inspiratory pressure. Although carbon dioxide removal is compromised, treatment isn't given for subsequent changes in blood hydrogen and oxygen concentration.

Sedatives, opioids, or neuromuscular blockers, such as pancuronium, may be given during mechanical ventilation to minimize restlessness, oxygen consumption, and carbon dioxide production and to facilitate ventilation. Treatment with sodium bicarbonate may be necessary to reverse severe metabolic acidosis. Vasopressor and I.V. fluid administration may be required to maintain blood pressure by treating hypovolemia. Antimicrobial drugs treat nonviral infections.

Other supportive measure include diuretics to reduce interstitial and pulmonary edema, correction of electrolyte and acid-base imbalances to maintain cellular integrity, particularly the sodium-potassium pump, and fluid restriction to prevent increase of interstitial and alveolar edema.

NURSING CONSIDERATIONS

ARDS requires careful monitoring and supportive care.

✦ Frequently assess the patient's respiratory status. Be alert for retractions on inspiration. Note the rate, rhythm, and depth of respirations; watch for dyspnea and the use of accessory muscles of respiration. On auscultation, listen for adventitious or diminished breath sounds. Check for clear, frothy sputum, which may indicate pulmonary edema.

✦ Observe and document the hypoxemic patient's neurologic status (level of consciousness and mental sluggishness).

✦ Maintain a patent airway by suctioning, using sterile, nontraumatic technique. Ensure adequate humidification to help liquefy tenacious secretions.

✦ Closely monitor the patient's heart rate and blood pressure. Watch for arrhythmias that may result from hypoxemia, acid-base disturbances, or electrolyte imbalances. With pulmonary artery catheterization, know the desired PAWP level. Check readings often, and watch for decreasing mixed venous oxygen saturation.

✦ Monitor serum electrolytes and correct imbalances. Measure intake and output; weigh the patient daily.

✦ Check ventilator settings frequently, and empty condensate from tubing promptly to ensure maximum oxygen delivery. Monitor ABG studies; check for metabolic and respiratory acidosis and PaO_2 changes. The patient with severe hy-

Treatment

✦ Correct causes of ARDS; prevent progression of hypoxemia and respiratory acidosis
✦ Humidified oxygen by a tight-fitting mask
✦ Ventilatory support with intubation, volume ventilation, PEEP
✦ Pressure-controlled inverse ratio ventilation
✦ Sedatives, opioids, sodium bicarbonate

Key nursing actions

✦ Frequently assess the patient's respiratory status. Check for clear, frothy sputum.
✦ Document the hypoxemic patient's neurologic status.
✦ Maintain a patent airway by suctioning, using sterile, nontraumatic technique.
✦ Monitor the patient's heart rate and blood pressure often; watch for decreasing mixed venous oxygen saturation.
✦ Monitor serum electrolytes and correct imbalances. Measure intake and output; weigh the patient daily.
✦ Monitor peak pressures during ventilation.

Key nursing actions
(continued)

+ Check ventilator settings, and empty condensate often.
+ Check for hypotension, tachycardia, and decreased urine output. Suction as needed.
+ Reposition the patient often and record increase in secretions, temperature, or hypotension.

poxemia may need controlled mechanical ventilation with positive pressure. Give sedatives as needed to reduce restlessness.

+ Because PEEP may decrease cardiac output, check for hypotension, tachycardia, and decreased urine output. Suction only as needed to maintain PEEP or use an in-line suctioning apparatus. Reposition the patient often and record an increase in secretions, temperature, or hypotension that may indicate a deteriorating condition. Monitor peak pressures during ventilation. Because of stiff, noncompliant lungs, the patient is at high risk for barotrauma (pneumothorax), evidenced by increased peak pressures, decreased breath sounds on one side, and restlessness.

+ Monitor nutrition, maintain joint mobility, and prevent skin breakdown. Accurately record caloric intake. Give tube feedings and parenteral nutrition, as ordered. Perform passive range-of-motion exercises or help the patient perform active exercises, if possible. Provide meticulous skin care. Plan patient care to allow periods of uninterrupted sleep.

+ Provide emotional support. Warn the patient who's recovering from ARDS that recovery will take some time and that he'll feel weak for a while.

+ Watch for and immediately report all respiratory changes in the patient with injuries that may adversely affect the lungs (especially during the 2- to 3-day period after the injury, when the patient may appear to be improving).

▼ *LIFE-THREATENING DISORDER*

ACUTE RESPIRATORY FAILURE

When the lungs can't adequately maintain arterial oxygenation or eliminate carbon dioxide, acute respiratory failure (ARF) results, which can lead to tissue hypoxia. In patients with essentially normal lung tissue, ARF usually means partial pressure of arterial carbon dioxide ($PaCO_2$) above 50 mm Hg and partial pressure of arterial oxygen (PaO_2) below 50 mm Hg. These limits, however, don't apply to patients with chronic obstructive pulmonary disease (COPD), who typically have a consistently high $PaCO_2$ and low PaO_2. In patients with COPD, only acute deterioration in arterial blood gas (ABG) values, with corresponding clinical deterioration, indicates ARF.

CAUSES

ARF may develop in COPD patients from any condition that increases the work of breathing and decreases the respiratory drive. These conditions may result from respiratory tract infections (such as bronchitis or pneumonia), bronchospasm, or accumulated secretions secondary to cough suppression. Other common causes are related to ventilatory failure, in which the brain fails to direct respiration, and gas exchange failure, in which respiratory structures fail to function properly.

Other causes of ARF include central nervous system (CNS) depression due to head trauma or injudicious use of sedatives, opioids, tranquilizers, or oxygen and cardiovascular disorders such as myocardial infarction, heart failure, or pulmonary emboli. ARF also results from airway irritants, such as smoke and fumes, endocrine or metabolic disorders, such as myxedema or metabolic acidosis, and thoracic abnormalities, such as chest trauma, pneumothorax, and thoracic or abdominal surgery.

Characteristics of ARF

+ Life-threatening; lungs can't maintain arterial oxygenation or eliminate carbon dioxide
+ Can lead to tissue hypoxia
+ $PaCO_2$ above 50 mm Hg and PaO_2 below 50 mm Hg in normal patients; high $PaCO_2$ and low PaO_2 in patients with COPD
+ Acute deterioration in ABG values, with clinical deterioration, indicates ARF in COPD patients

Causes

+ Respiratory tract infections, bronchospasm, accumulated secretions, ventilatory failure, gas exchange failure in COPD
+ CNS depression
+ Airway irritants
+ Endocrine or metabolic disorders
+ Thoracic abnormalities

PATHOPHYSIOLOGY

Respiratory failure results from impaired gas exchange. Conditions associated with alveolar hypoventilation, ventilation-perfusion ($\dot{V}/\dot{Q}$) mismatch, and intrapulmonary (right-to-left) shunting can cause ARF if left untreated.

Decreased oxygen saturation may result from alveolar hypoventilation, in which chronic airway obstruction reduces alveolar minute ventilation. PaO_2 levels fall and $PaCO_2$ levels rise, resulting in hypoxemia.

Hypoventilation can occur from a decrease in the rate or duration of inspiratory signal from the respiratory center, such as with CNS conditions or trauma or CNS-depressant drugs. Neuromuscular diseases, such as poliomyelitis or amyotrophic lateral sclerosis, can result in alveolar hypoventilation if the condition affects normal contraction of the respiratory muscles. The most common cause of alveolar hypoventilation is airway obstruction, commonly seen with COPD (emphysema or bronchitis).

The most common cause of hypoxemia — $\dot{V}/\dot{Q}$ imbalance — occurs when such conditions as pulmonary embolism or acute respiratory distress syndrome interrupt normal gas exchange in a specific lung region. Too little ventilation with normal blood flow or too little blood flow with normal ventilation may cause the imbalance, resulting in decreased PaO_2 levels and, thus, hypoxemia.

Decreased fraction of inspired oxygen (FIO_2) is also a cause of respiratory failure, although it's uncommon. Hypoxemia results from inspired air that doesn't contain adequate oxygen to establish an adequate gradient for diffusion into the blood — for example, at high altitudes or in confined spaces.

The hypoxemia and hypercapnia characteristics of respiratory failure stimulate strong compensatory responses by all body systems, including the respiratory system, cardiovascular system, and CNS. In response to hypoxemia, for example, the sympathetic nervous system triggers vasoconstriction, increases peripheral resistance, and increases the heart rate. Untreated $\dot{V}/\dot{Q}$ imbalances can lead to right-to-left shunting in which blood passes from the heart's right side to its left without being oxygenated.

Tissue hypoxemia occurs, resulting in anaerobic metabolism and lactic acidosis. Respiratory acidosis occurs from hypercapnia. Heart rate increases, stroke volume increases, and heart failure may occur. Cyanosis occurs because of increased amounts of unoxygenated blood. Hypoxia of the kidneys results in the release of erythropoietin from renal cells, which causes the bone marrow to increase red blood cell production — an attempt by the body to increase the blood's oxygen-carrying capacity.

The body responds to hypercapnia with cerebral depression, hypotension, circulatory failure, and increased heart rate and cardiac output. Hypoxemia, hypercapnia, or both cause the brain's respiratory control center first to increase respiratory depth (tidal volume) and then to increase the respiratory rate. As respiratory failure worsens, intercostal, supraclavicular, and suprasternal retractions may also occur.

SIGNS AND SYMPTOMS

Specific symptoms vary with the underlying cause of ARF. Respiratory rate may be increased, decreased, or normal depending on the cause. Respirations may be shallow, deep, or alternate between the two. Air hunger may occur. Cyanosis may be present, depending on the hemoglobin level and arterial oxygenation. Auscultation of the chest may reveal crackles, rhonchi, wheezing, or diminished breath sounds.

How it happens

- Impaired gas exchange from alveolar hypoventilation, $\dot{V}/\dot{Q}$ mismatch, and right-to-left shunting results in hypoxemia and hypercapnia
- Hypoxemia and hypercapnia stimulate compensatory responses by all body systems
- Body responds with cerebral depression, hypotension, circulatory failure, and increased heart rate and cardiac output
- Respiratory failure worsens
- Anaerobic metabolism and lactic acidosis result from tissue hypoxemia
- Respiratory acidosis occurs from hypercapnia

Key signs and symptoms

- Respiratory rate: increased, decreased, or normal
- Respirations: shallow, deep, or alternating
- Cyanosis
- Crackles, rhonchi, wheezing
- Diminished breath sounds
- Restlessness, confusion
- Diminished tendon reflexes
- Coma
- Tachycardia, arrhythmias
- Pulmonary hypertension
- Distended jugular veins

When hypoxemia and hypercapnia occur, the patient may show evidence of restlessness, confusion, loss of concentration, irritability, tremulousness, diminished tendon reflexes, papilledema, and coma.

Tachycardia, with increased cardiac output and mildly elevated blood pressure secondary to adrenal release of catecholamine, occurs early in response to low PaO_2. With myocardial hypoxia, arrhythmias may develop. Pulmonary hypertension, secondary to pulmonary capillary vasoconstriction, may cause increased pressures on the right side of the heart, distended jugular veins, an enlarged liver, and peripheral edema.

COMPLICATIONS

Complications
+ Tissue hypoxia
+ Metabolic acidosis
+ Cardiac arrest

Tissue hypoxia, metabolic acidosis, and cardiac arrest are among possible complications.

DIAGNOSIS

Diagnosis
+ ABG analysis shows lower-than-normal pH compared with previous levels
+ Chest X-rays identify underlying conditions
+ ECG demonstrates ventricular arrhythmias or right ventricular hypertrophy
+ Pulse oximetry shows decreasing arterial oxygen saturation
+ Blood cultures identify pathogens
+ Pulmonary artery catheterization helps distinguish cause

ABG analysis indicates respiratory failure by deteriorating values and a pH below 7.35. Patients with COPD may have a lower than normal pH compared with previous levels.

Chest X-rays identify pulmonary diseases or conditions, such as emphysema, atelectasis, lesions, pneumothorax, infiltrates, and effusions.

Electrocardiography (ECG) can reveal ventricular arrhythmias (indicating myocardial hypoxia) or right ventricular hypertrophy (indicating cor pulmonale). And pulse oximetry reveals decreasing arterial oxygen saturation.

White blood cell count detects the underlying infection. Abnormally low hemoglobin and hematocrit levels signal blood loss, which indicates decreased oxygen-carrying capacity. Hypokalemia may result from compensatory hyperventilation, the body's attempt to correct acidosis. Hypochloremia usually occurs in metabolic alkalosis.

Blood cultures may identify pathogens.

Pulmonary artery catheterization helps to distinguish pulmonary and cardiovascular causes of ARF and monitors hemodynamic pressures.

TREATMENT

Treatment
+ Cautious oxygen therapy
+ Mechanical ventilation, high-frequency ventilation
+ Antibiotics, bronchodilators
+ Corticosteroids
+ Fluid restrictions
+ Positive inotropic agents
+ Vasopressors
+ Diuretics

The patient needs cautious oxygen therapy to promote oxygenation and raise PaO_2. Mechanical ventilation with an endotracheal or a tracheostomy tube may be necessary to provide adequate oxygenation and reverse acidosis. High-frequency ventilation may be initiated if the patient doesn't respond to treatment, to force the airways open, promoting oxygenation and preventing alveoli collapse. Treatment routinely includes antibiotics to treat infection, bronchodilators to maintain airway patency, and corticosteroids to decrease inflammation.

If the patient has cor pulmonale and decreased cardiac output, fluid restrictions to reduce volume and cardiac workload, positive inotropic agents to increase cardiac output, vasopressors to maintain blood pressure, and diuretics to reduce edema and fluid overload may be ordered.

NURSING CONSIDERATIONS

+ Because the patient with ARF is usually treated in an intensive care unit (ICU), orient him to the environment, procedures, and routines to minimize his anxiety.
+ To reverse hypoxemia, administer oxygen at appropriate concentrations to maintain PaO_2 at a minimum of 50 to 60 mm Hg. Patients with COPD usually require

only small amounts of supplemental oxygen. Watch for a positive response, such as improvement in the patient's breathing, color, and ABG results.

✦ Maintain a patent airway. If the patient is retaining carbon dioxide, encourage him to cough and to breathe deeply. Teach him to use pursed-lip and diaphragmatic breathing to control dyspnea. If the patient is alert, have him use an incentive spirometer; if he's intubated and lethargic, turn him every 1 to 2 hours. Use postural drainage and chest physiotherapy to help clear secretions.

✦ In an intubated patient, suction the trachea as needed after hyperoxygenation. Observe for change in quantity, consistency, and color of sputum. Provide humidification to liquefy secretions.

✦ Observe the patient closely for respiratory arrest. Auscultate for chest sounds. Monitor ABG levels and report changes immediately.

✦ Monitor and record serum electrolyte levels carefully, and correct imbalances; monitor fluid balance by recording intake and output or daily weight.

✦ Check the cardiac monitor for arrhythmias.

If the patient requires mechanical ventilation

✦ Check ventilator settings, cuff pressures, and ABG values often because the FIO_2 setting depends on ABG levels. Draw samples for ABG analysis 20 to 30 minutes after every FIO_2 change or check with oximetry.

✦ Prevent infection by using sterile technique while suctioning.

✦ Stress ulcers are common in intubated ICU patients. Check gastric secretions for evidence of bleeding if the patient has a nasogastric tube or complains of epigastric tenderness, nausea, or vomiting. Monitor hemoglobin level and hematocrit; check stools for occult blood. Administer antacids, histamine$_2$-receptor antagonists, or sucralfate, as ordered.

✦ Prevent tracheal erosion, which can result from artificial airway cuff overinflation. Use the minimal leak technique and a cuffed tube with high residual volume (low pressure cuff), a foam cuff, or a pressure-regulating valve on the cuff.

✦ To prevent oral or vocal cord trauma, make sure the endotracheal tube is positioned midline.

✦ To prevent nasal necrosis, keep the nasotracheal tube midline within the nostrils and provide good hygiene. Loosen the tape periodically to prevent skin breakdown. Avoid excessive movement of tubes; make sure the ventilator tubing is adequately supported.

ASTHMA

Asthma is a chronic inflammatory airway disorder characterized by airflow obstruction and airway hyperresponsiveness to a multiplicity of stimuli. This widespread but variable airflow obstruction is caused by bronchospasm, edema of the airway mucosa, and increased mucus production with plugging and airway remodeling. It's a type of chronic obstructive pulmonary disease (COPD), a long-term pulmonary disease characterized by increased airflow resistance; other types of COPD include chronic bronchitis and emphysema.

 CLINICAL ALERT Although asthma strikes at any age, about 50% of patients are younger than age 10; twice as many boys as girls are affected in this age-group. One-third of patients ages 10 to 30 develop asthma, and the incidence is the same in both sexes in this age-group. Moreover, approximately one-third of all patients share the disease with at least one immediate family member.

Key nursing actions

✦ Administer oxygen to maintain Pao_2 at 50 to 60 mm Hg. Watch for a positive response.
✦ Maintain a patent airway.
✦ Observe for change in sputum.
✦ Observe for respiratory arrest.
✦ Monitor and record serum electrolyte levels, and correct imbalances; monitor fluid balance.
✦ Check the cardiac monitor for arrhythmias.
✦ Check ventilator settings, cuff pressures, and ABG values.
✦ Use sterile technique while suctioning.

Characteristics of asthma

✦ Chronic inflammatory disorder
✦ Airflow obstruction and hyperresponsiveness to various stimuli
✦ Obstruction caused by bronchospasm, edema of airway mucosa, and increased mucus production with plugging and airway remodeling
✦ COPD characterized by increased airflow resistance
✦ Caused by sensitivity to allergens
✦ Extrinsic asthma begins in childhood
✦ Typically, patients sensitive to specific external allergens

Alert!

✦ 50% of asthmatics are younger than age 10; twice as many boys as girls are affected in this group.

Characteristics of asthma
(continued)

+ Intrinsic asthma reacts to internal, nonallergenic factors
+ External substances not implicated

Alert!

+ Extrinsic asthma is commonly accompanied by other hereditary allergies.

Causes

Extrinsic allergens
+ Pollen
+ Animal dander
+ House dust or mold
+ Kapok or feather pillows

Intrinsic allergens
+ Irritants
+ Emotional stress
+ Fatigue

How it happens

+ Locus of chromosome 11 contains an abnormal gene
+ Environmental factors interact with inherited factors
+ Bronchial linings overreact to stimuli; when exposed to antigen IgE antibody joins with antigen
+ Mast cells degranulate, release mediators, and release histamine and leukotrienes
+ Histamine causes swelling in smooth muscles
+ Mucous membranes become inflamed, irritated, and swollen
+ Leukotrienes cause swelling in bronchi; enhance histamine effect
+ Wheeze during coughing occurs

Asthma may result from sensitivity to extrinsic or intrinsic allergens. Extrinsic, or atopic, asthma begins in childhood; typically, patients are sensitive to specific external allergens.

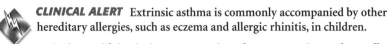 **CLINICAL ALERT** Extrinsic asthma is commonly accompanied by other hereditary allergies, such as eczema and allergic rhinitis, in children.

Patients with intrinsic, or nonatopic, asthma react to internal, nonallergenic factors; external substances can't be implicated in patients with intrinsic asthma. Most episodes occur after a severe respiratory tract infection, especially in adults. However, many patients with asthma, especially children, have intrinsic and extrinsic asthma.

A significant number of adults acquire an allergic form of asthma or exacerbation of existing asthma from exposure to agents in the workplace. Irritants, such as chemicals in flour, acid anhydrides, toluene diisocyanate, screw flies, river flies, and excreta of dust mites in carpet, have been identified as agents that trigger asthma.

CAUSES

Extrinsic allergens include pollen, animal dander, house dust or mold, kapok or feather pillows, food additives containing sulfites, and other sensitizing substances.

Intrinsic allergens include irritants, emotional stress, fatigue, endocrine changes, temperature variations, humidity variations, exposure to noxious fumes, anxiety, coughing or laughing, and genetic factors.

PATHOPHYSIOLOGY

Two genetic influences are identified with asthma, namely the ability of an individual to develop asthma (atopy) and the tendency to develop hyperresponsiveness of the airways independent of atopy. A locus of chromosome 11 associated with atopy contains an abnormal gene that encodes a part of the immunoglobulin (Ig) E receptor. Environmental factors interact with inherited factors to cause asthmatic reactions with associated bronchospasms.

In asthma, bronchial linings overreact to various stimuli, causing episodic smooth-muscle spasms that severely constrict the airways. (See *Pathophysiology of asthma.*)

IgE antibodies, attached to histamine-containing mast cells and receptors on cell membranes, initiate intrinsic asthma attacks. When exposed to an antigen, such as pollen, the IgE antibody combines with the antigen.

On subsequent exposure to the antigen, mast cells degranulate and release mediators. Mast cells in the lung interstitium are stimulated to release histamine and leukotrienes. Histamine attaches to receptor sites in the larger bronchi, where it causes swelling in smooth muscles. Mucous membranes become inflamed, irritated, and swollen. The patient may experience dyspnea, prolonged expiration, and an increased respiratory rate.

Leukotrienes attach to receptor sites in the smaller bronchi and cause local swelling of the smooth muscle. Leukotrienes also cause prostaglandins to travel through the bloodstream to the lungs, where they enhance histamine's effect. A wheeze may be audible during coughing—the higher the pitch, the narrower the bronchial lumen. Histamine stimulates the mucous membranes to secrete excessive mucus, further narrowing the bronchial lumen. Goblet cells secrete viscous mucus that's difficult to cough up, resulting in coughing, rhonchi, increased-pitch wheezing, and increased respiratory distress. Mucosal edema and thickened secretions further block the airways. (See *Looking at a bronchiole in asthma,* page 246.)

CLOSER LOOK

Pathophysiology of asthma

In asthma, hyperresponsiveness of the airways and bronchospasms occur. These illustrations show the progression of an asthma attack.

✦ Histamine (H) attaches to receptor sites in larger bronchi, causing swelling of the smooth muscles.

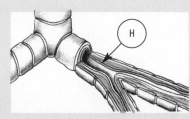

✦ Leukotrienes (L) attach to receptor sites in the smaller bronchi and cause swelling of smooth muscle there. Leukotrienes also cause prostaglandins to travel through the bloodstream to the lungs, where they enhance histamine's effects.

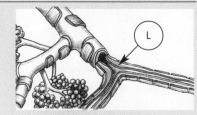

✦ Histamine stimulates the mucous membranes to secrete excessive mucus, further narrowing the bronchial lumen. On inhalation, the narrowed bronchial lumen can still expand slightly; however, on exhalation, the increased intrathoracic pressure closes the bronchial lumen completely.

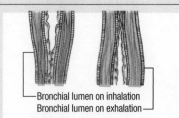

Bronchial lumen on inhalation
Bronchial lumen on exhalation

✦ Mucus fills lung bases, inhibiting alveolar ventilation. Blood is shunted to alveoli in other parts of the lungs, but it still can't compensate for diminished ventilation.

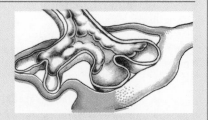

How it happens
(continued)

✦ Histamine stimulates excessive mucus secretion
✦ Goblet cells secrete viscous mucus—difficult to cough up
✦ Mucosal edema and thickened secretions further block airways
✦ On inhalation, narrowed bronchial lumen can still expand slightly
✦ On exhalation, increased intrathoracic pressure closes bronchial lumen completely
✦ Air enters but can't escape
✦ Patient develops a barrel chest; mucus fills lung bases
✦ Blood shunted to alveoli in other lung parts
✦ Intrapleural and alveolar gas pressures rise

On inhalation, the narrowed bronchial lumen can still expand slightly, allowing air to reach the alveoli. On exhalation, increased intrathoracic pressure closes the bronchial lumen completely. Air enters but can't escape. The patient develops a barrel chest and hyperresonance to percussion.

Mucus fills the lung bases, inhibiting alveolar ventilation. Blood is shunted to alveoli in other lung parts, but still can't compensate for diminished ventilation.

Hyperventilation is triggered by lung receptors to increase lung volume because of trapped air and obstructions. Intrapleural and alveolar gas pressures rise, causing a decreased perfusion of alveoli. Increased alveolar gas pressure, decreased ventilation, and decreased perfusion result in uneven ventilation-perfusion ratios and mismatching within different lung segments.

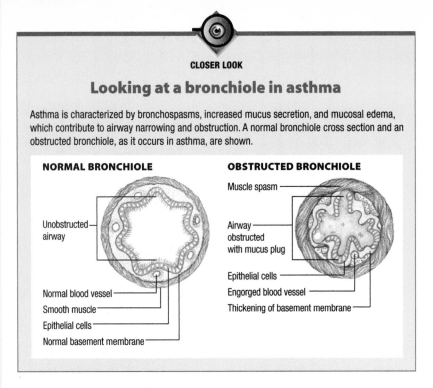

CLOSER LOOK

Looking at a bronchiole in asthma

Asthma is characterized by bronchospasms, increased mucus secretion, and mucosal edema, which contribute to airway narrowing and obstruction. A normal bronchiole cross section and an obstructed bronchiole, as it occurs in asthma, are shown.

NORMAL BRONCHIOLE

Unobstructed airway

Normal blood vessel
Smooth muscle
Epithelial cells
Normal basement membrane

OBSTRUCTED BRONCHIOLE

Muscle spasm

Airway obstructed with mucus plug

Epithelial cells
Engorged blood vessel
Thickening of basement membrane

How it happens
(continued)

+ Uneven ventilation-perfusion ratios and mismatching within different lung segments result
+ Hypoxia triggers hyperventilation by respiratory center stimulation
+ Respiratory alkalosis results
+ Ventilation and perfusion remain inadequate; CO_2 retention develops
+ Respiratory acidosis results
+ Respiratory failure occurs
+ Becomes life-threatening as no air becomes audible upon auscultation and $PaCO_2$ rises to over 70 mm Hg

Key signs and symptoms

+ Sudden dyspnea
+ Wheezing
+ Tightness in chest
+ Coughing that produces thick, clear, or yellow sputum
+ Tachypnea
+ Rapid pulse
+ Profuse perspiration
+ Hyperresonant lung fields
+ Diminished breath sounds

Hypoxia triggers hyperventilation by respiratory center stimulation, which in turn decreases partial pressure of arterial carbon dioxide ($PaCO_2$) and increases pH, resulting in respiratory alkalosis. As the airway obstruction increases in severity, more alveoli are affected. Ventilation and perfusion remain inadequate, and carbon dioxide retention develops. Respiratory acidosis results, and respiratory failure occurs.

If status asthmaticus occurs, hypoxia worsens and expiratory flows and volumes decrease even further. If treatment isn't initiated, the patient begins to tire out. (See *Averting an asthma attack.*)

Acidosis develops as $PaCO_2$ increases. The situation becomes life-threatening as no air becomes audible upon auscultation (a silent chest) and $PaCO_2$ rises to over 70 mm Hg.

SIGNS AND SYMPTOMS

Extrinsic asthma is usually accompanied by signs and symptoms of atopy (type I IgE-mediated allergy), such as eczema and allergic rhinitis. It commonly follows a severe respiratory tract infection, especially in adults.

An acute asthma attack begins dramatically, with simultaneous onset of severe multiple symptoms, or insidiously, with gradually increasing respiratory distress. Asthma that occurs with cyanosis, confusion, and lethargy indicates the onset of life-threatening status asthmaticus and respiratory failure.

Signs and symptoms of asthma include sudden dyspnea, wheezing, and tightness in the chest, coughing that produces thick, clear, or yellow sputum, tachypnea, along with use of accessory respiratory muscles, rapid pulse, profuse perspiration, hyperresonant lung fields, and diminished breath sounds.

In 1997, the National Heart, Lung, and Blood Institute of the National Institutes of Health identified four levels of asthma severity based on the frequency of symp-

Averting an asthma attack

This flowchart shows pathophysiologic changes that occur with asthma. Treatments and interventions show where the physiologic cascade would be altered to stop an asthma attack.

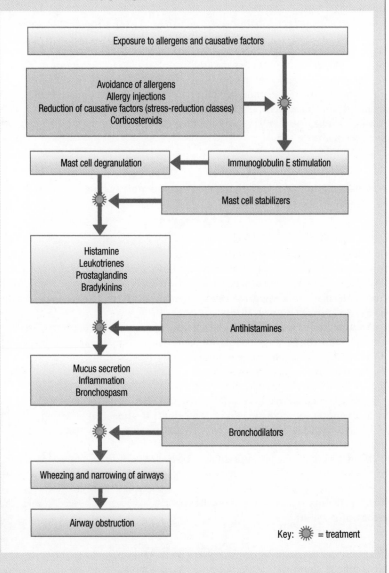

Medications used to treat asthma

✦ Mast cell stabilizers
✦ Antihistamines
✦ Bronchodilators

toms and exacerbations, effects on activity level, and lung function study results: mild intermittent, mild persistent, moderate persistent, and severe persistent.

In mild intermittent asthma, symptoms occur fewer than two times per week; the patient is asymptomatic with normal peak expiratory flow (PEF) between exacerbations. He experiences brief exacerbations (from a few hours to a few days) that vary in intensity. Nighttime symptoms occur fewer than two times per month. Lung function studies show forced expiratory volume in 1 second (FEV_1) or PEF greater than 80% of normal values; PEF may vary by less than 20%.

In mild persistent asthma, symptoms occur more than 2 times per week, but less than once per day; exacerbations may affect activity. Nighttime symptoms occur more than 2 times per month. Lung function studies show FEV_1 or PEF greater than 80% of normal values; PEF may vary by 20% to 30%.

In moderate persistent asthma, symptoms occur daily. Exacerbations occur more than 2 times per week and may last for days; exacerbations affect activity. Bronchodilator therapy is used daily. Nighttime symptoms occur more than once per week. Lung function studies show FEV_1 or PEF 60% to 80% of normal values; PEF may vary by greater than 30%.

In severe persistent asthma, symptoms occur continuously. Exacerbations occur frequently and limit physical activity. Nighttime symptoms occur frequently. Lung function studies show FEV_1 or PEF less than 60% of normal values; PEF may vary by more than 30%.

COMPLICATIONS

Asthma can produce status asthmaticus and respiratory failure.

DIAGNOSIS

Pulmonary function studies reveal signs of airway obstructive disease, low-normal or decreased vital capacity, and increased total lung and residual capacities. Pulmonary function may be normal between attacks. Partial pressure of arterial oxygen (PaO_2) and $PaCO_2$ are usually decreased, except in severe asthma, when $PaCO_2$ may be normal or increased, indicating severe bronchial obstruction. Serum IgE levels may increase from an allergic reaction.

Sputum analysis may indicate the presence of Curschmann's spirals (casts of airways), Charcot-Leyden crystals, and eosinophils. Complete blood count with differential reveals an increased eosinophil count.

Chest X-rays can be used to diagnose or monitor the progress of asthma and may show hyperinflation with areas of atelectasis.

Arterial blood gas (ABG) analysis detects hypoxemia (decreased PaO_2; decreased, normal, or increasing $PaCO_2$) and guides treatment. Skin testing may identify specific allergens. Results read in 1 or 2 days detect an early reaction; and after 4 or 5 days, a late reaction.

Bronchial challenge testing evaluates the clinical significance of allergens identified by skin testing.

Electrocardiography (ECG) shows sinus tachycardia during an attack; a severe attack may show signs of cor pulmonale (right axis deviation, peaked P wave) that resolve after the attack.

TREATMENT

Drug therapy for asthma is typically based on the severity of disease. Correcting asthma typically involves prevention, by identifying and avoiding precipitating factors, such as environmental allergens or irritants, which is the best treatment.

Desensitization to specific antigens is helpful if the stimuli can't be removed entirely and decreases the severity of attacks of asthma with future exposure.

Bronchodilators—including the xanthines (theophylline and aminophylline) and the beta$_2$-adrenergic agonists (albuterol and terbutaline)—decrease bronchoconstriction, reduce bronchial airway edema, and increase pulmonary ventilation. The anti-inflammatory and immunosuppressive effects of corticosteroids (such as hydrocortisone sodium succinate, prednisone, methylprednisolone, and beclomethasone) decrease inflammation and edema of the airways.

Mast cell stabilizers (cromolyn and nedocromil) are effective in patients with atopic asthma who have seasonal disease. Given prophylactically, they block the acute obstructive effects of antigen exposure by inhibiting the degranulation of mast cells, thereby preventing the release of chemicals responsible for anaphylaxis.

Leukotriene modifiers, such as zileuton (Zyflo), and leukotriene receptor antagonists (LTRAs), such as montelukast (Singulair) and zafirlukast (Accolate), inhibit the potent bronchoconstriction and inflammatory effects of the cysteinyl leukotrienes. LTRAs can be used as adjunctive therapy to avoid high-dose inhaled corticosteroids. Although this class of medications doesn't replace inhaled corticosteroids as first-line anti-inflammatory treatment, it can be used successfully in cases where poor compliance with inhaled corticosteroid use is suspected.

Anticholinergic bronchodilators, such as ipratropium, block acetylcholine, another chemical mediator

Low-flow humidified oxygen may be needed to treat dyspnea, cyanosis, and hypoxemia. However, the amount delivered should maintain Pao$_2$ between 65 and 85 mm Hg, as determined by ABG analysis.

Mechanical ventilation may be necessary if the patient doesn't respond to initial ventilatory support and drugs, or develops respiratory failure.

Relaxation exercises, such as yoga, help increase circulation and help a patient recover from an asthma attack.

NURSING CONSIDERATIONS

During an acute attack

✦ First, assess the severity of asthma.
✦ Administer the prescribed treatments, and assess the patient's response.
✦ Place the patient in high Fowler's position. Encourage pursed-lip and diaphragmatic breathing. Help him to relax.
✦ Monitor the patient's vital signs. Keep in mind that developing or increasing tachypnea may indicate worsening asthma or drug toxicity. Hypertension may indicate asthma-related hypoxemia.
✦ Administer prescribed humidified oxygen by nasal cannula at 2 L/minute to ease breathing and to increase arterial oxygen saturation (Sao$_2$). Later, adjust oxygen according to the patient's vital signs and ABG levels.
✦ Anticipate intubation and mechanical ventilation if the patient fails to maintain adequate oxygenation.
✦ Monitor serum theophylline levels to ensure they're in the therapeutic range. Observe the patient for signs and symptoms of theophylline toxicity (vomiting, diarrhea, and headache) as well as for signs of a subtherapeutic dosage (respiratory distress and increased wheezing).
✦ Observe the frequency and severity of the patient's cough, and note whether it's productive. Then auscultate his lungs, noting adventitious or absent breath sounds. If his cough isn't productive and rhonchi are present, teach him effective coughing techniques. If he can tolerate postural drainage and chest percussion, perform these procedures to clear secretions. Suction an intubated patient as needed.

Treatment
✦ Drug therapy
✦ Desensitization to antigens
✦ Bronchodilators
✦ Corticosteroids
✦ Mast cell stabilizers
✦ LTRAs
✦ Anticholinergic bronchodilators
✦ Low-flow humidified oxygen

Key nursing actions

During an acute attack
✦ Assess the severity of asthma.
✦ Administer prescribed treatments; assess the patient's response.
✦ Place the patient in high Fowler's position. Encourage pursed-lip and diaphragmatic breathing.
✦ Monitor the patient's vital signs. Keep in mind that developing or increasing tachypnea may indicate worsening asthma or drug toxicity.
✦ Administer prescribed humidified oxygen by nasal cannula at 2 L/minute to ease breathing and to increase Sao$_2$.
✦ Observe the frequency and severity of the patient's cough, and note whether it's productive.

Key nursing actions

During long-term care

+ Monitor the patient's respiratory status to detect baseline changes, to assess response to treatment, and to prevent or detect complications.
+ Auscultate the lungs frequently, noting the degree of wheezing and quality of air movement.
+ Review ABG levels, pulmonary function test results, and SaO_2 readings.
+ Control exercise-induced asthma by instructing the patient to use a bronchodilator or cromolyn 30 minutes before exercise.

During patient education

+ Teach the patient and his family to avoid known allergens and irritants.
+ Teach the patient how to use a metered-dose inhaler.
+ Explain how to use a peak flow meter to measure the degree of airway obstruction. Tell him to keep a record of peak flow readings.

Characteristics of chronic bronchitis

+ Inflammation of the bronchi caused by irritants or infection
+ Acute or chronic
+ In chronic bronchitis, hypersecretion of mucus and chronic productive cough last for 3 months of the year and occur for at least 2 consecutive years

---

+ Treat dehydration with I.V. fluids then oral fluids, to help loosen secretions.
+ If conservative treatment fails to improve the airway obstruction, anticipate bronchoscopy or bronchial lavage when a lobe or larger area collapses.

During long-term care

+ Monitor the patient's respiratory status to detect baseline changes, to assess response to treatment, and to prevent or detect complications.
+ Auscultate the lungs frequently, noting the degree of wheezing and quality of air movement.
+ Review ABG levels, pulmonary function test results, and SaO_2 readings.
+ If the patient is taking systemic corticosteroids, observe for complications, such as elevated blood glucose levels and friable skin and bruising. Cushingoid effects resulting from long-term use of corticosteroids may be minimized by alternate-day dosage or use of prescribed inhaled corticosteroids.
+ If the patient is taking corticosteroids by inhaler, watch for signs of candidal infection in the mouth and pharynx. Using an extender device and rinsing the mouth afterward may prevent this.
+ Observe the patient's anxiety level. Keep in mind that measures that reduce hypoxemia and breathlessness should help relieve anxiety.
+ Keep the room temperature comfortable and use an air conditioner or a fan in hot, humid weather.
+ Control exercise-induced asthma by instructing the patient to use a bronchodilator or cromolyn 30 minutes before exercise. Also, instruct him to use pursed-lip breathing while exercising.

During patient education

+ Teach the patient and his family to avoid known allergens and irritants.
+ Describe prescribed drugs, including their names, dosages, actions, adverse effects, and special instructions.
+ Teach the patient how to use a metered-dose inhaler. If he has difficulty using an inhaler, he may need an extender device to optimize drug delivery and lower the risk of candidal infection with orally inhaled corticosteroids.
+ Explain how to use a peak flow meter to measure the degree of airway obstruction. Tell him to keep a record of peak flow readings and to bring it to medical appointments. Explain the importance of calling the physician at once if the peak flow drops suddenly (may signal severe respiratory problems).
+ Tell the patient to notify the physician if he develops a fever above 100° F (37.8° C), chest pain, shortness of breath without coughing or exercising, or uncontrollable coughing. An uncontrollable attack requires immediate attention.
+ Teach the patient diaphragmatic and pursed-lip breathing as well as effective coughing techniques.
+ Urge the patient to drink at least 3 qt (3 L) of fluids daily to help loosen secretions and maintain hydration.

CHRONIC BRONCHITIS

Chronic bronchitis is inflammation of the bronchi caused by irritants or infection. A form of chronic obstructive pulmonary disease (COPD), bronchitis may be classified as acute or chronic. In chronic bronchitis, hypersecretion of mucus and chronic productive cough last for 3 months of the year and occur for at least 2 consecutive years. The distinguishing characteristic of bronchitis is airflow obstruction.

 CLINICAL ALERT COPD is more prevalent in urban than rural environments, and is also related to occupational factors (mineral or organic dusts).

 CLINICAL ALERT Children of parents who smoke are at higher risk for respiratory tract infection that can lead to chronic bronchitis.

CAUSES

Common causes of chronic bronchitis include exposure to irritants, cigarette smoking, genetic predisposition, exposure to organic or inorganic dusts, exposure to noxious gases, and respiratory tract infection.

PATHOPHYSIOLOGY

Chronic bronchitis occurs when irritants are inhaled for a prolonged time. The irritants inflame the tracheobronchial tree, leading to increased mucus production and a narrowed or blocked airway. As the inflammation continues, changes in the cells lining the respiratory tract result in resistance of the small airways and severe ventilation-perfusion ($\dot{V}/\dot{Q}$) imbalance, which decreases arterial oxygenation.

Chronic bronchitis results in hypertrophy and hyperplasia of the mucous glands, increased goblet cells, ciliary damage, squamous metaplasia of the columnar epithelium, and chronic leukocytic and lymphocytic infiltration of bronchial walls. (See *Changes in chronic bronchitis,* page 252.)

Hypersecretion of the goblet cells blocks the free movement of the cilia, which normally sweep dust, irritants, and mucus away from the airways. With mucus and debris accumulating in the airway, the defenses are altered, and the individual is prone to respiratory tract infections.

Additional effects include widespread inflammation, airway narrowing, and mucus within the airways. Bronchial walls become inflamed and thickened from edema and accumulation of inflammatory cells, and the effects of smooth-muscle bronchospasm further narrow the lumen. Initially, only large bronchi are involved but, eventually, all airways are affected. Airways become obstructed and closure occurs, especially on expiration. The gas is then trapped in the distal portion of the lung. Hypoventilation occurs, leading to a $\dot{V}/\dot{Q}$ mismatch and resultant hypoxemia.

Hypoxemia and hypercapnia occur secondary to hypoventilation. Pulmonary vascular resistance (PVR) increases as inflammatory and compensatory vasoconstriction in hypoventilated areas narrows the pulmonary arteries. Increased PVR leads to increased afterload of the right ventricle. With repeated inflammatory episodes, scarring of the airways occurs, and permanent structural changes develop. Respiratory infections can trigger acute exacerbations, and respiratory failure can occur.

Patients with chronic bronchitis have a diminished respiratory drive. The resulting chronic hypoxia causes the kidneys to produce erythropoietin, which stimulates excessive red blood cell production and leads to polycythemia. Although hemoglobin levels are high, the amount of reduced (not fully oxygenated) hemoglobin in contact with oxygen is low; therefore, cyanosis occurs.

Alert!

◆ COPD is more prevalent in urban than rural environments and is also related to occupational factors.
◆ Children of parents who smoke are at higher risk for respiratory tract infection that can lead to chronic bronchitis.

Causes

◆ Exposure to irritants
◆ Cigarette smoking
◆ Genetic predisposition
◆ Organic or inorganic dusts
◆ Noxious gases
◆ Respiratory tract infection

How it happens

◆ Irritants inhaled for prolonged time
◆ Inflamed tracheobronchial tree leads to increased mucus production and narrowed or blocked airway
◆ Respiratory changes result in $\dot{V}/\dot{Q}$ imbalance
◆ Results in hypertrophy and hyperplasia of mucous glands, increased goblet cells, ciliary damage, squamous metaplasia of columnar epithelium, and chronic leukocytic or lymphocytic infiltration of bronchial walls
◆ Hypersecretion of goblet cells blocks movement of the cilia
◆ Individual is prone to respiratory tract infections

CLOSER LOOK

Changes in chronic bronchitis

In chronic bronchitis, irritants inflame the tracheobronchial tree over time, leading to increased mucus production and a narrowed or blocked airway. As the inflammation continues, goblet and epithelial cells hypertrophy. Because the natural defense mechanisms are blocked, the airways accumulate debris in the respiratory tract. These illustrations show these changes.

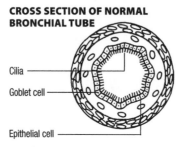

CROSS SECTION OF NORMAL BRONCHIAL TUBE

Cilia

Goblet cell

Epithelial cell

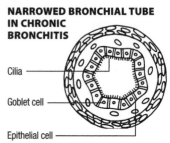

NARROWED BRONCHIAL TUBE IN CHRONIC BRONCHITIS

Cilia

Goblet cell

Epithelial cell

Key signs and symptoms

+ Gray, white, or yellow sputum
+ Dyspnea
+ Cyanosis
+ Use of accessory muscles for breathing
+ Tachypnea
+ Pedal edema
+ Jugular vein distention
+ Weight gain
+ Wheezing
+ Prolonged expiratory time
+ Rhonchi
+ Pulmonary hypertension

Complications

+ Recurrent respiratory tract infections
+ Cor pulmonale
+ Pulmonary hypertension
+ Heart failure
+ Acute respiratory failure

SIGNS AND SYMPTOMS

Signs and symptoms of chronic bronchitis may include copious gray, white, or yellow sputum due to hypersecretion of goblet cells, productive cough to expectorate mucus produced by the lungs, and dyspnea due to airflow obstruction to the lower tracheobronchial tree. Other symptoms include cyanosis related to diminished oxygenation and cellular hypoxia (reduced oxygen is supplied to the tissues), use of accessory muscles for breathing due to compensated attempts to supply the cells with increased oxygen, and tachypnea due to hypoxia.

Palpation may disclose pedal edema and jugular vein distention due to right-sided heart failure. The patient may report weight gain due to edema.

Auscultation findings include wheezing due to air moving through narrowed respiratory passages, prolonged expiratory time due to the body's attempt to keep airways patent, and rhonchi due to air moving through narrow, mucus-filled passages.

Pulmonary hypertension caused by involvement of small pulmonary arteries is due to inflammation in the bronchial walls and spasms of pulmonary blood vessels from hypoxia.

COMPLICATIONS

Possible complications of chronic bronchitis include recurrent respiratory tract infections; cor pulmonale (right ventricular hypertrophy with right-sided heart failure) due to increased right ventricular end-diastolic pressure; pulmonary hypertension; heart failure, resulting in increased venous pressure, liver engorgement, and dependent edema; and acute respiratory failure.

DIAGNOSIS

Chest X-rays may show hyperinflation and increased bronchovascular markings. Pulmonary function studies indicate increased residual volume, decreased vital capacity and forced expiratory flow, and normal static compliance and diffusing capacity. Arterial blood gas analysis (ABGs)reveals decreased partial pressure of arterial oxygen and normal or increased partial pressure of arterial carbon dioxide. Sputum analysis may reveal many microorganisms and neutrophils. Electrocardiography may show atrial arrhythmias; peaked P waves in leads II, III, and aV_F; and, occasionally, right ventricular hypertrophy.

TREATMENT

The most effective treatment is avoidance of air pollutants, smoking cessation, and avoidance of second-hand smoke. Antibiotics can be used to treat recurring infections. Bronchodilators may relieve bronchospasms and facilitate mucociliary clearance. Adequate hydration is essential to liquefy secretions. Chest physiotherapy may be needed to mobilize secretions. Ultrasonic or mechanical nebulizers may help to loosen and mobilize secretions. Occasionally, a patient responds to corticosteroids to combat inflammation. Diuretics may be used to reduce edema. Oxygen may be necessary to treat hypoxia.

NURSING CONSIDERATIONS

+ If the patient smokes, encourage him to stop. Provide him with smoking-cessation resources or counseling if necessary.
+ Assess the patient for changes in baseline respiratory function. Evaluate sputum quality and quantity, restlessness, increased tachypnea, and altered breath sounds. Report changes immediately.
+ Perform chest physiotherapy, including postural drainage as well as chest percussion and vibration for involved lobes, several times daily, as needed.
+ Weigh the patient three times weekly, and assess for edema.
+ Provide the patient with a high-calorie, protein-rich diet. Offer small, frequent meals to conserve the patient's energy and prevent fatigue.
+ Make sure the patient receives adequate fluids (at least 3 qt [3 L] per day) to loosen secretions.
+ Schedule respiratory therapy at least 1 hour before or after meals. Provide mouth care after bronchodilator inhalation therapy.
+ Advise the patient to avoid crowds and people with known infections and to obtain influenza and pneumococcal immunizations.
+ Urge the patient to avoid inhaled irritants, such as automobile exhaust fumes, aerosol sprays, and industrial pollutants.
+ Warn the patient that exposures to blasts of cold air may precipitate bronchospasm. Suggest that he avoid cold, windy weather or that he cover his mouth and nose with a scarf or mask if he must go outside.

CHRONIC OBSTRUCTIVE PULMONARY DISEASE

Chronic obstructive pulmonary disease (COPD), also called chronic obstructive lung disease, results from emphysema, chronic bronchitis, asthma, or a combination of these disorders. Usually, more than one of these underlying conditions coexist; bronchitis and emphysema typically occur together. (See "Asthma," page 243; "Chronic bronchitis," page 250; and "Emphysema," page 256, for a review of these conditions.)

Diagnosis

+ Chext X-rays show hyperinflation and increased bronchovascular markings,
+ Pulmonary function test reveals increased residual volume, decreased vital capacity, forced expiratory flow, normal static compliance and diffusing capacity
+ ABGs show decreased Pa_{O_2} and normal or increased Pa_{CO_2}

Treatment

+ Avoidance of air pollutants
+ Bronchodilators
+ Chest physiotherapy
+ Ultrasonic or mechanical nebulizers
+ Corticosteroids

Key nursing actions

+ Encourage smoking-cessation.
+ Perform chest physiotherapy.
+ Warn the patient that exposures to blasts of cold air may precipitate bronchospasm.
+ Provide adequate fluid intake.

Characteristics of COPD

+ Results from emphysema, chronic bronchitis, asthma, or combination
+ Most common lung disease
+ Affects 17 million Americans; incidence increasing

Causes

+ Cigarette smoking; air pollution
+ Respiratory tract infections
+ Allergies
+ Familial and hereditary factors

How it happens

+ Ciliary action and macrophage function impaired; causes airway inflammation
+ Increased mucus production
+ Destruction of alveolar septa
+ Mucus plugs and narrowed airways cause air trapping

Key signs and symptoms

+ Reduced ability to perform exercises or do strenuous work
+ Productive cough
+ Dyspnea on minimal exertion
+ Frequent respiratory tract infections

Complications

+ Cor pulmonale
+ Severe respiratory failure
+ Death

Diagnosis

+ ABG analysis shows degree of hypoxia
+ Chest X-rays support diagnosis
+ Pulmonary function studies support diagnosis
+ ECG shows arrhythmias

Treatment

+ Bronchodilators
+ Effective coughing
+ Postural drainage and chest physiotherapy
+ Low oxygen concentrations
+ Antibiotics

COPD is the most common lung disease and affects an estimated 17 million Americans; the incidence is increasing. The disease doesn't always produce symptoms and may cause only minimal disability. However, COPD worsens with time.

CAUSES

Common causes of COPD may include cigarette smoking, recurrent or chronic respiratory tract infections, air pollution, allergies, and familial and hereditary factors such as an alpha$_1$-antitrypsin deficiency.

PATHOPHYSIOLOGY

Smoking, one of the major causes of COPD, impairs ciliary action and macrophage function and causes inflammation in the airways, increased mucus production, destruction of alveolar septa, and peribronchiolar fibrosis. Early inflammatory changes may reverse if the patient stops smoking before lung disease becomes extensive.

The mucus plugs and narrowed airways cause air trapping, as in chronic bronchitis and emphysema. Hyperinflation occurs to the alveoli on expiration. On inspiration, airways enlarge, allowing air to pass beyond the obstruction; on expiration, airways narrow and gas flow is prevented. Air trapping (also called *ball valving*) occurs commonly in asthma and chronic bronchitis. (See *Air trapping in chronic obstructive pulmonary disease.*)

SIGNS AND SYMPTOMS

Signs and symptoms of COPD may include reduced ability to perform exercises or do strenuous work because of diminished pulmonary reserve, productive cough due to stimulation of the reflex by mucus, dyspnea on minimal exertion, frequent respiratory tract infections, intermittent or continuous hypoxemia, grossly abnormal pulmonary function studies, and thoracic deformities.

COMPLICATIONS

Possible complications of COPD include overwhelming disability, cor pulmonale, severe respiratory failure, and death.

DIAGNOSIS

Arterial blood gas (ABG) analysis determines oxygen need by indicating the degree of hypoxia and helps avoid carbon dioxide narcosis. Chest X-rays support the underlying diagnosis. Pulmonary function studies support the diagnosis of the underlying condition. Electrocardiography (ECG) may show arrhythmias consistent with hypoxemia.

TREATMENT

Most patients are treated with bronchodilators to alleviate bronchospasms and enhance mucociliary clearance of secretions. Teach the patient about effective coughing to remove secretions. If the patient with copious secretions has difficulty mobilizing them, teach the family postural drainage and chest physiotherapy to help mobilize secretions.

Administer low oxygen concentrations as needed. High flow rates of oxygen can lead to narcosis. Administer antibiotics to allow for treatment of respiratory tract

Air trapping in chronic obstructive pulmonary disease

In chronic obstructive pulmonary disease, mucus plugs and narrowed airways trap air (also called *ball valving*). During inspiration, the airways enlarge and gas enters; on expiration, the airways narrow and air can't escape. This commonly occurs in asthma and chronic bronchitis.

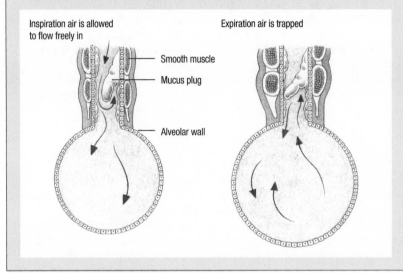

Inspiration air is allowed to flow freely in

Expiration air is trapped

Smooth muscle

Mucus plug

Alveolar wall

infections. Provide smoking cessation counseling or refer him to a program. Educate the patient on the benefits of increased fluid intake and the use of a humidifier to thin secretions.

NURSING CONSIDERATIONS

✦ Urge the patient to stop smoking. Provide smoking-cessation counseling or refer him to a program. Avoid other respiratory irritants, such as second-hand smoke, aerosol spray products, and outdoor air pollution. An air conditioner with an air filter in his home may be helpful.

✦ The patient is usually treated with beta$_2$-adrenergic-agonist bronchodilators (albuterol or salmeterol), anticholinergic bronchodilators (ipratropium), and corticosteroids (beclomethasone or triamcinolone). These are usually given by metered-dose inhaler, requiring that the patient be taught the correct administration technique.

✦ Administer antibiotics, as ordered, to treat respiratory infections. Stress the need to complete the prescribed course of antibiotic therapy. Teach the patient and his family how to recognize early signs of infection; warn him to avoid contact with people with respiratory infections. Encourage good oral hygiene to help prevent infection. Pneumococcal and annual influenza vaccinations are important preventive measures.

✦ To strengthen the muscles of respiration, teach the patient to take slow, deep breaths and exhale through pursed lips.

Key nursing actions

✦ Urge the patient to stop smoking and to avoid other respiratory irritants.

✦ Teach the correct use of a metered-dose inhaler.

✦ Administer antibiotics, as ordered, to treat respiratory infections. Teach the patient and his family how to recognize early signs of infection.

✦ Teach the patient to take slow, deep breaths and exhale through pursed lips.

Key nursing actions
(continued)

+ Teach the patient how to cough effectively.
+ Perform ABG analysis to determine the patient's oxygen needs and to avoid carbon dioxide narcosis.
+ Emphasize the importance of a balanced diet.
+ Help the patient and his family adjust their lifestyles to accommodate the limitations imposed by this disease.
+ As COPD progresses, encourage the patient to discuss his fears.
+ Assist in the early detection of COPD by urging the patient to have periodic physical examinations.

Characteristics of emphysema

+ Form of COPD
+ Abnormal, permanent enlargement of the acini with destruction of alveolar walls
+ Results from tissue changes
+ Marked by airflow limitation, lack of elastic recoil in the lungs
+ More prevalent in males

Alert!

+ Aging is a risk factor for emphysema.

Causes

+ AAT deficiency
+ Smoking

+ To help mobilize secretions, teach the patient how to cough effectively. If the patient with copious secretions has difficulty mobilizing secretions, teach his family how to perform postural drainage and chest physiotherapy. If secretions are thick, urge the patient to drink 12 to 15 glasses of fluid per day. A home humidifier may be beneficial, particularly in the winter.

+ Perform ABG analysis to determine the patient's oxygen needs and to avoid carbon dioxide narcosis. If the patient is to continue oxygen therapy at home, teach him how to use the equipment correctly. The patient with COPD rarely requires more than 2 to 3 L/minute to maintain adequate oxygenation. Higher flow rates can further increase partial pressure of arterial oxygen, but the patient whose ventilatory drive is largely based on hypoxemia commonly develops markedly increased partial pressure of arterial carbon dioxide tensions. In this patient, chemoreceptors in the brain are relatively insensitive to the increase in carbon dioxide. Teach the patient and his family that excessive oxygen therapy may eliminate the hypoxic respiratory drive, causing confusion and drowsiness, signs of carbon dioxide narcosis.

+ Emphasize the importance of a balanced diet. Because the patient may tire easily when eating, suggest that he eat frequent, small meals and consider using oxygen, administered by nasal cannula, during meals.

+ Help the patient and his family adjust their lifestyles to accommodate the limitations imposed by this debilitating chronic disease. Instruct the patient to allow for daily rest periods and to exercise daily as his physician directs.

+ As COPD progresses, encourage the patient to discuss his fears.

+ To help prevent COPD, advise the patient not to smoke, especially if he has a family history of COPD or if his disease is in its early stages.

+ Assist in the early detection of COPD by urging the patient to have periodic physical examinations, including spirometry and medical evaluation of a chronic cough, and to seek treatment for recurring respiratory infections promptly.

EMPHYSEMA

Emphysema, a form of chronic obstructive pulmonary disease, is the abnormal, permanent enlargement of the acini accompanied by destruction of alveolar walls. Obstruction results from tissue changes rather than mucus production, which occurs with asthma and chronic bronchitis. The distinguishing characteristic of emphysema is airflow limitation caused by lack of elastic recoil in the lungs.

Emphysema appears to be more prevalent in males than in females; about 65% of patients with well-defined emphysema are men and 35% are women.

 CLINICAL ALERT Aging is a risk factor for emphysema. Senile emphysema results from degenerative changes; stretching occurs without destruction in the smooth muscle. Connective tissue isn't usually affected.

CAUSES

Emphysema is usually caused by alpha$_1$-antitrypsin (AAT) deficiency and cigarette smoking.

PATHOPHYSIOLOGY

Primary emphysema has been linked to an inherited deficiency of the enzyme AAT, a major component of alpha$_1$-globulin. AAT inhibits the activation of several proteolytic enzymes; deficiency of this enzyme is an autosomal recessive trait that pre-

CLOSER LOOK

A look at abnormal alveoli

In the patient with emphysema, recurrent pulmonary inflammation damages and eventually destroys the alveolar walls, creating large air spaces. The damaged alveoli can't recoil normally after expanding; therefore, bronchioles collapse on expiration, trapping air in the lungs and causing overdistention. As the alveolar walls are destroyed, the lungs become enlarged, and the total lung capacity and residual volume then increase. Changes that occur during emphysema are shown here.

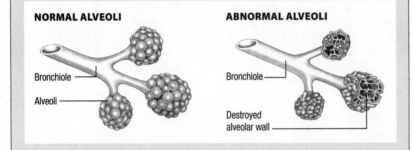

disposes an individual to develop emphysema because proteolysis in lung tissues isn't inhibited. Homozygous individuals have up to an 80% chance of developing lung disease; people who smoke have a greater chance of developing emphysema. Patients who develop emphysema before or during their early 40s and those who are nonsmokers are believed to have an AAT deficiency.

In emphysema, recurrent inflammation is associated with the release of proteolytic enzymes from lung cells. This causes irreversible enlargement of the air spaces distal to the terminal bronchioles. Enlargement of air spaces destroys the alveolar walls, which results in a breakdown of elasticity and loss of fibrous and muscle tissue, thus making the lungs less compliant.

In normal breathing, the air moves into and out of the lungs to meet metabolic needs. A change in airway size compromises the lungs' ability to circulate sufficient air. In patients with emphysema, recurrent pulmonary inflammation damages and eventually destroys the alveolar walls, creating large air spaces. (See *A look at abnormal alveoli.*)

The alveolar septa are initially destroyed, eliminating a portion of the capillary bed and increasing air volume in the acinus. This breakdown leaves the alveoli unable to recoil normally after expanding and results in bronchiolar collapse on expiration. The damaged or destroyed alveolar walls can't support the airways to keep them open. (See *Air trapping in emphysema,* page 258.)

The amount of air that can be expired passively is diminished, thus trapping air in the lungs and leading to overdistention. Hyperinflation of the alveoli produces bullae (air spaces) adjacent to the pleura (blebs). Septal destruction also decreases airway calibration. Part of each inspiration is trapped because of increased residual volume and decreased calibration. Septal destruction may affect only the respiratory bronchioles and alveolar ducts, leaving alveolar sacs intact (centriacinar emphysema), or it can involve the entire acinus (panacinar emphysema), with damage more random and involving the lower lobes of the lungs.

Abnormal alveoli
+ Can't recoil normally after expanding
+ Cause bronchioles to collapse on expiration
+ As walls are destroyed, lungs become enlarged
+ Total lung capacity and residual volume increase

How it happens
+ Recurrent pulmonary inflammation damages and destroys alveolar walls
+ Large air spaces created
+ Amount of air expired passively is diminished, trapping air
+ Hyperinflation of alveoli produces bullae adjacent to pleura
+ Septal destruction decreases airway calibration
+ Damage occurs to respiratory bronchioles, alveolar ducts
+ Can involve entire acinus with damage more random and involving lower lobes
+ Pulmonary capillary destruction usually allows ventilation to perfusion match
+ Total lung capacity and residual volume increase

CLOSER LOOK

Air trapping in emphysema

After alveolar walls are damaged or destroyed, they can't support and keep the airways open. The alveolar walls then lose their capability of elastic recoil. Collapse then occurs on expiration, as shown here.

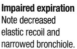

Normal expiration
Note normal recoil and the open bronchiole.

Impaired expiration
Note decreased elastic recoil and narrowed bronchiole.

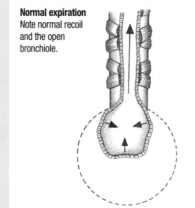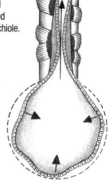

Alert!
+ Panacinar emphysema tends to occur in elderly people with an AAT deficiency.
+ Centriacinar emphysema occurs in smokers with chronic bronchitis.

Key signs and symptoms
+ Shortness of breath; chronic cough
+ Anorexia and feeling of malaise
+ Barrel-chest
+ Breathing through pursed lips
+ Decreased tactile fremitus and chest expansion
+ Hyperresonance
+ Decreased breath sounds

Complications
+ Cor pulmonale
+ Respiratory failure
+ Recurrent respiratory tract infections

 CLINICAL ALERT Panacinar emphysema tends to occur in elderly people with an AAT deficiency, whereas centriacinar emphysema occurs in smokers with chronic bronchitis.

Associated pulmonary capillary destruction usually allows a patient with severe emphysema to match ventilation to perfusion. This process prevents the development of cyanosis. The lungs are usually enlarged; therefore, the total lung capacity and residual volume increase.

SIGNS AND SYMPTOMS
The health history may reveal that the patient is a long-time smoker. The patient may report shortness of breath and a chronic cough. The history may also reveal anorexia with resultant weight loss and a general feeling of malaise.

Inspection may show a barrel-chested patient who breathes through pursed lips and uses accessory muscles. You may notice peripheral cyanosis, clubbed fingers and toes, and tachypnea.

Palpation may reveal decreased tactile fremitus and decreased chest expansion. Percussion may detect hyperresonance. On auscultation, you may hear decreased breath sounds, crackles and wheezing during inspiration, a prolonged expiratory phase with grunting respirations, and distant heart sounds.

COMPLICATIONS
Possible complications of emphysema include right ventricular hypertrophy (cor pulmonale), respiratory failure, and recurrent respiratory tract infections.

DIAGNOSIS

Chest X-rays in advanced disease may show a flattened diaphragm, reduced vascular markings at the lung periphery, overaeration of the lungs, a vertical heart, enlarged anteroposterior chest diameter, and a large retrosternal air space.

Pulmonary function studies indicate increased residual volume and total lung capacity, reduced diffusing capacity, and increased inspiratory flow.

Arterial blood gas analysis usually reveals reduced partial pressure of arterial oxygen and a normal partial pressure of arterial carbon dioxide until late in the disease process.

Electrocardiography may show tall, symmetrical P waves in leads II, III, and aV_F; a vertical QRS axis and signs of right ventricular hypertrophy are seen late in the disease.

Complete blood count usually reveals an increased hemoglobin level late in the disease when the patient has persistent, severe hypoxia.

TREATMENT

Correcting emphysema starts with avoiding smoking and air pollution to preserve remaining alveoli. Drugs prescribed include bronchodilators, such as beta-adrenergic blockers, albuterol, and ipratropium, to reverse bronchospasms and promote mucociliary clearance, antibiotics to treat respiratory tract infections, polyvalent pneumococcal vaccine to prevent pneumococcal pneumonia, and adequate hydration to liquefy secretions.

Other medications include mucolytics to thin secretions and aid in mucus expectoration, aerosolized or systemic corticosteroids, and the flu vaccine to prevent influenza.

Some patients may require oxygen therapy at low settings to correct hypoxia. They may also require transtracheal catheterization to enable the patient to receive oxygen therapy at home. Some patients undergo lung-volume reduction surgery. (Nonfunctional parts of the lung [tissue filled with disease providing little ventilation or perfusion] are surgically removed; removal allows more functional lung tissue to expand and the diaphragm to return to its normally elevated position.)

NURSING CONSIDERATIONS

✦ If the patient smokes, encourage him to stop. Provide him with smoking-cessation resources or counseling if necessary.
✦ Assess for changes in baseline respiratory function. Evaluate sputum quality and quantity, restlessness, increased tachypnea, and altered breath sounds. Report changes immediately.
✦ As needed, perform chest physiotherapy, including postural drainage and chest percussion and vibration for involved lobes, several times daily.
✦ Weigh the patient three times weekly, and assess for edema.
✦ Provide the patient with a high-calorie, protein-rich diet. Offer small, frequent meals to conserve his energy and prevent fatigue.
✦ Make sure the patient receives adequate fluids (at least 3 qt [3 L] per day) to loosen secretions.
✦ Schedule respiratory therapy at least 1 hour before or after meals. Provide mouth care after bronchodilator inhalation therapy.
✦ Advise the patient to avoid crowds and people with known infections and to obtain influenza and pneumococcal immunizations.
✦ Urge the patient to avoid inhaled irritants, such as automobile exhaust fumes, aerosol sprays, and industrial pollutants.

Diagnosis
✦ Chest X-ray shows flattened diaphragm, reduced vascular markings at lung periphery, overaeration of the lungs, vertical heart, enlarged anteroposterior chest diameter, and large retrosternal air space
✦ Pulmonary function studies reveal reduced diffusing capacity and increased inspiratory flow
✦ ABG analysis reveals reduced Pao_2

Treatment
✦ Avoid smoking and air pollution
✦ Bronchodilators
✦ Antibiotics
✦ Polyvalent pneumococcal vaccine
✦ Adequate hydration
✦ Mucolytics
✦ Aerosolized or systemic corticosteroids

Key nursing actions
✦ Assess for changes in baseline respiratory function.
✦ As needed, perform chest physiotherapy several times daily.
✦ Weigh the patient three times weekly and assess for edema.
✦ Make sure the patient receives adequate fluids to loosen secretions.
✦ Schedule respiratory therapy at least 1 hour before or after meals.
✦ Warn the patient that exposure to blasts of cold air may precipitate bronchospasm.

Alert!

✦ Inform the patient about signs and symptoms that suggest ruptured alveolar blebs and bullae.

Characteristics of pleural effusion and empyema

✦ Pleural effusion: excess fluid in pleural space
✦ Empyema: accumulation of pus and necrotic tissue in pleural space; blood and chyle may also collect in this space

Causes

Transudative
✦ Heart failure
✦ Hepatic disease with ascites
✦ Peritoneal dialysis

Exudative
✦ TB
✦ Subphrenic abscess
✦ Bacterial or fungal pneumonitis

Empyema
✦ Idiopathic infection
✦ Pneumonitis
✦ Carcinoma

How it happens

✦ Transudative pleural effusion occurs from excessive hydrostatic pressure in visceral pleural capillaries
✦ Ultrafiltrate of plasma containing low protein concentrations results
✦ Exudative pleural effusions occur when capillaries exhibit increased permeability
✦ Empyema associated with infection in pleural space

✦ Warn the patient that exposure to blasts of cold air may precipitate bronchospasm. Suggest that he avoid cold, windy weather or that he cover his mouth and nose with a scarf or mask if he must go outside.

 CLINICAL ALERT Inform the patient about signs and symptoms that suggest ruptured alveolar blebs and bullae. Explain the seriousness of possible spontaneous pneumothorax. Urge him to notify the physician if he feels sudden, sharp pleuritic pain exacerbated by chest movement, breathing, or coughing.

✦ For family members of the patient with familial emphysema, recommend a blood test for AAT deficiency. If a deficiency is found, stress the importance of not smoking and avoiding areas (if possible) where smoking is permitted.

PLEURAL EFFUSION AND EMPYEMA

Pleural effusion is excess fluid in the pleural space. Normally, this space contains a small amount of extracellular fluid that lubricates the pleural surfaces. Increased production or inadequate removal of this fluid results in pleural effusion. Empyema is the accumulation of pus and necrotic tissue in the pleural space. Blood (hemothorax) and chyle (chylothorax) may also collect in this space.

CAUSES

Transudative pleural effusions commonly result from heart failure, hepatic disease with ascites, peritoneal dialysis, hypoalbuminemia, and disorders resulting in overexpanded intravascular volume.

Exudative pleural effusions occur with tuberculosis (TB), subphrenic abscess, pancreatitis, bacterial or fungal pneumonitis or empyema, malignancy, pulmonary embolism with or without infarction, collagen disease (lupus erythematosus [LE] and rheumatoid arthritis), myxedema, and chest trauma.

Empyema may result from idiopathic infection or may be related to pneumonitis, carcinoma, perforation, or esophageal rupture.

PATHOPHYSIOLOGY

The balance of osmotic and hydrostatic pressures in parietal pleural capillaries normally results in fluid movement into the pleural space. Balanced pressures in visceral pleural capillaries promote reabsorption of this fluid. Excessive hydrostatic pressure or decreased osmotic pressure can cause excess fluid to pass across intact capillaries. The result is a transudative pleural effusion, an ultrafiltrate of plasma containing low concentrations of protein.

Exudative pleural effusions result when capillaries exhibit increased permeability with or without changes in hydrostatic and colloid osmotic pressures, allowing protein-rich fluid to leak into the pleural space.

Empyema is usually associated with an infection in the pleural space, which results from an extension of an infection of nearby structures.

SIGNS AND SYMPTOMS

Patients with pleural effusion characteristically experience symptoms related to the underlying pathologic condition. Most patients with large effusions, particularly those with underlying pulmonary disease, complain of dyspnea. Those with effusions associated with pleurisy complain of pleuritic chest pain. Other clinical features depend on the cause of the effusion. Patients with empyema also develop fever and malaise.

COMPLICATIONS

Complications of pleural effusion may include impaired ventilation and pleurisy. Complications of empyema may include pleurisy, pericarditis, and septicemia.

DIAGNOSIS

Auscultation of the chest reveals decreased breath sounds; percussion detects dullness over the effused area, which doesn't change with breathing. Chest X-ray shows radiopaque fluid in dependent regions. However, diagnosis also requires other tests to distinguish transudative from exudative effusions and to help pinpoint the underlying disorder. The most useful test is thoracentesis, in which aspirated pleural fluid is analyzed.

Transudative effusion usually has a specific gravity lower than 1.015 and contains less than 3 g/dl of protein. Exudative effusion has a ratio of protein in the fluid to serum of greater than or equal to 0.5, pleural fluid lactate dehydrogenase (LD) of greater than or equal to 200 IU, and a ratio of LD in pleural fluid to LD in serum of greater than or equal to 0.6.

Aspirated fluid in empyema contains acute inflammatory white blood cells and microorganisms and shows leukocytosis. Fluid in empyema and rheumatoid arthritis, which can be the cause of an exudative pleural effusion, shows an extremely decreased pleural fluid glucose level.

In addition, if a pleural effusion results from esophageal rupture or pancreatitis, fluid amylase levels are usually higher than serum levels. Aspirated fluid may be tested for LE cells, antinuclear antibodies, and neoplastic cells. It may also be analyzed for color and consistency; acid-fast bacillus, fungal, and bacterial cultures; and triglycerides (in chylothorax). Cell analysis shows leukocytosis in empyema. A negative tuberculin skin test strongly rules against TB as the cause. In exudative pleural effusions in which thoracentesis isn't definitive, pleural biopsy may be done. It's particularly useful for confirming TB or malignancy.

TREATMENT

Depending on the amount of fluid present, symptomatic effusion may require thoracentesis to remove fluid or careful monitoring of the patient's own reabsorption of the fluid. Hemothorax requires drainage to prevent fibrothorax formation. Pleural effusions associated with lung cancer typically reaccumulate quickly. If a chest tube is inserted to drain the fluid, a sclerosing agent, such as talc, may be injected through the tube to cause adhesions between the parietal and visceral pleura, thereby obliterating the potential space for fluid to recollect.

Treatment of empyema requires insertion of one or more chest tubes after thoracentesis, to allow drainage of purulent material, and possibly decortication (surgical removal of the thick coating over the lung) or rib resection to allow open drainage and lung expansion. Empyema also requires parenteral antibiotics. Associated hypoxia requires oxygen administration.

Key signs and symptoms

+ Dyspnea
+ Pleuritic chest pain
+ Fever and malaise

Complications

Pleural effusion
+ Impaired ventilation
+ Pleurisy

Empyema
+ Pleurisy
+ Pericarditis
+ Septicemia

Diagnosis

+ Decreased breath sounds
+ Dullness over effused area
+ Chest X-ray shows fluid
+ Pleural fluid analysis distinguishes transudative from exudative effusion

Treatment

Pleural effusion
+ Thoracentesis
+ Drainage
+ Chest tube
+ Sclerosing agent

Empyema
+ Chest tubes after thoracentesis
+ Decortication
+ Rib resection
+ Parenteral antibiotics
+ Oxygen administration

Key nursing actions

✦ Explain thoracentesis to the patient.
✦ Reassure the patient during thoracentesis. Remind him to breathe normally.
✦ Encourage the patient to perform deep-breathing exercises to promote lung expansion.
✦ Provide meticulous chest tube care, and use sterile technique for changing dressings around the tube insertion site in empyema.

Characteristics of pneumothorax

✦ Life-threatening disorder
✦ Accumulation of air in the pleural cavity
✦ Leads to partial or complete lung collapse
✦ Types include open, closed, and tension

Causes

Open
✦ Penetrating chest injury
✦ Insertion of a central venous catheter
✦ Chest surgery
✦ Transbronchial biopsy

Closed
✦ Blunt chest trauma
✦ Air leakage from ruptured blebs
✦ Interstitial lung disease

Tension
✦ Penetrating chest wound treated with an airtight dressing
✦ Fractured ribs
✦ Mechanical ventilation

NURSING CONSIDERATIONS

✦ **Explain thoracentesis to the patient.** Before the procedure, tell the patient to expect a stinging sensation from the local anesthetic and a feeling of pressure when the needle is inserted. Instruct him to tell you immediately if he feels uncomfortable or has trouble breathing during the procedure.
✦ **Reassure the patient during thoracentesis.** Remind him to breathe normally and avoid sudden movements, such as coughing or sighing. Monitor vital signs, and watch for syncope. If fluid is removed too quickly, the patient may experience bradycardia, hypotension, pain, pulmonary edema, or even cardiac arrest. Watch for respiratory distress or pneumothorax (sudden onset of dyspnea and cyanosis) after thoracentesis.
✦ Administer oxygen and, in empyema, antibiotics, as ordered.
✦ **Encourage the patient to perform deep-breathing exercises to promote lung expansion.** Use an incentive spirometer to promote deep breathing.
✦ **Provide meticulous chest tube care, and use sterile technique for changing dressings around the tube insertion site in empyema.** Ensure tube patency by watching for fluctuations of fluid in the underwater-seal chamber. Watch for bubbling in the water-seal chamber, indicating the presence of air in the pleural spaces. Record the amount, color, and consistency of tube drainage.
✦ If the patient has open drainage through a rib resection or intercostal tube, use hand and dressing precautions. Because weeks of such drainage are usually necessary to obliterate the space, make visiting nurse referrals for the patient who will be discharged with the tube in place.
✦ If pleural effusion is a complication of pneumonia or influenza, advise prompt medical attention for chest colds.

▼ **LIFE-THREATENING DISORDER**

PNEUMOTHORAX

Pneumothorax is an accumulation of air in the pleural cavity that leads to partial or complete lung collapse. When the air between the visceral and parietal pleurae collects and accumulates, increasing tension in the pleural cavity can cause the lung to progressively collapse. Air is trapped in the intrapleural space and determines the degree of lung collapse. Venous return to the heart may be impeded to cause a life-threatening condition called tension pneumothorax.

The most common types of pneumothorax are open, closed, and tension.

CAUSES

Common causes of open pneumothorax include penetrating chest injury (gunshot or stab wound), insertion of a central venous catheter, chest surgery, transbronchial biopsy, and thoracentesis, or closed pleural biopsy.

Causes of closed pneumothorax include blunt chest trauma, air leakage from ruptured blebs, rupture resulting from barotrauma caused by high intrathoracic pressures during mechanical ventilation, tubercular or cancerous lesions that erode into the pleural space, and interstitial lung disease, such as eosinophilic granuloma.

Tension pneumothorax may be caused by a penetrating chest wound treated with an airtight dressing, fractured ribs, mechanical ventilation, high-level positive end-expiratory pressure that causes alveolar blebs to rupture, and chest tube occlusion or malfunction.

PATHOPHYSIOLOGY

A rupture in the visceral or parietal pleura and chest wall causes air to accumulate and separate the visceral and parietal pleurae. Negative pressure is destroyed, and the elastic recoil forces are affected. The lung recoils by collapsing toward the hilus.

Open pneumothorax (also called a *sucking chest wound* or *communicating pneumothorax*) results when atmospheric air (positive pressure) flows directly into the pleural cavity (negative pressure). As the air pressure in the pleural cavity becomes positive, the lung collapses on the affected side, resulting in decreased total lung capacity, vital capacity, and lung compliance. Ventilation-perfusion imbalances lead to hypoxia.

Closed pneumothorax occurs when air enters the pleural space from within the lung, causing increased pleural pressure, which prevents lung expansion during normal inspiration. Spontaneous pneumothorax is another type of closed pneumothorax.

 CLINICAL ALERT Spontaneous pneumothorax is common in older patients with chronic pulmonary disease, but it may also occur in healthy, tall, young adults.

Both types of closed pneumothorax can result in a collapsed lung with hypoxia and decreased total lung capacity, vital capacity, and lung compliance. The range of lung collapse is between 5% and 95%.

Tension pneumothorax results when air in the pleural space is under higher pressure than air in the adjacent lung. The air enters the pleural space from the site of pleural rupture, which acts as a one-way valve. Air is allowed to enter into the pleural space on inspiration, but can't escape as the rupture site closes on expiration. More air enters on inspiration, and air pressure begins to exceed barometric pressure. Increasing air pressure pushes against the recoiled lung, causing compression atelectasis. Air also presses against the mediastinum, compressing and displacing the heart and great vessels. The air can't escape, and the accumulating pressure causes the lung to collapse. As air continues to accumulate and intrapleural pressures increase, the mediastinum shifts away from the affected side and decreases venous return. This forces the heart, trachea, esophagus, and great vessels to the unaffected side, compressing the heart and the contralateral lung. Without immediate treatment, this emergency can rapidly become fatal. (See *Understanding tension pneumothorax,* page 264.)

SIGNS AND SYMPTOMS

The cardinal features of pneumothorax are sudden, sharp pleuritic pain, exacerbated by chest movement, breathing, and coughing; asymmetrical chest wall movement due to lung collapse; and cyanosis and shortness of breath due to hypoxia.

Other signs and symptoms include respiratory distress and decreased vocal fremitus related to lung collapse.

Auscultation reveals absent breath sounds on the affected side due to lung collapse, chest rigidity on the affected side due to decreased expansion, and tachycardia due to hypoxia.

Palpation may reveal crackling beneath the skin (subcutaneous emphysema), which is due to air leaking into the tissues.

Tension pneumothorax produces the most severe respiratory symptoms, including decreased cardiac output; hypotension due to decreased cardiac output; compensatory tachycardia; tachypnea due to hypoxia; lung collapse due to air or blood in the intrapleural space; mediastinal shift due to increasing tension; tracheal devi-

How it happens

Open pneumothorax

- ✦ Atmospheric air flows directly into pleural cavity; air pressure in cavity becomes positive
- ✦ Lung collapses on affected side
- ✦ Decreased total lung capacity, vital capacity, and compliance occurs
- ✦ Ventilation-perfusion imbalances lead to hypoxia

Closed pneumothorax

- ✦ Air enters pleural space from lung
- ✦ Pleural pressure increases
- ✦ Prevents lung expansion during normal inspiration

Tension pneumothorax

- ✦ Air in pleural space under higher pressure than air in adjacent lung
- ✦ Air enters the pleural space from site of rupture, can't escape
- ✦ Pressure begins to exceed barometric pressure
- ✦ Air compresses and displaces heart and great vessels
- ✦ Accumulating pressure causes lung to collapse

Alert!

- ✦ Spontaneous pneumothorax is common in older patients with chronic pulmonary disease, but it may occur in young patients.

Key signs and symptoms

- ✦ Sudden, sharp pleuritic pain
- ✦ Asymmetrical chest wall movement
- ✦ Cyanosis, shortness of breath
- ✦ Tension pneumothorax: decreased cardiac output, hypotension, lung collapse, distended jugular veins

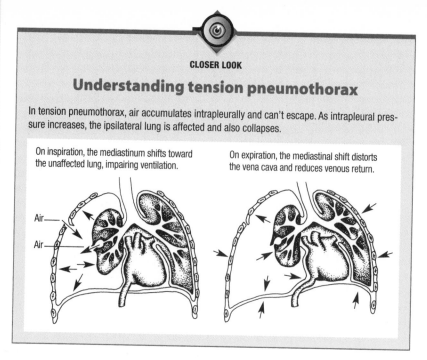

CLOSER LOOK

Understanding tension pneumothorax

In tension pneumothorax, air accumulates intrapleurally and can't escape. As intrapleural pressure increases, the ipsilateral lung is affected and also collapses.

On inspiration, the mediastinum shifts toward the unaffected lung, impairing ventilation.

On expiration, the mediastinal shift distorts the vena cava and reduces venous return.

Air

Air

Complications
+ Decreased cardiac output
+ Hypoxemia
+ Cardiac arrest

Diagnosis
+ Chest X-rays confirm diagnosis
+ ABG analysis may reveal hypoxemia, respiratory acidosis, and hypercapnia

Treatment
Spontaneous pneumothorax with less than 30% of lung collapse
+ Bed rest
+ Monitoring of blood pressure, pulse, and respiratory rate
+ Oxygen
+ Aspiration of air with a large-bore needle attached to a syringe

Pneumothorax with more than 30% of lung collapse
+ Placement of thoracostomy tube
+ Thoracotomy
+ Pleurectomy

ation to the opposite side; distended jugular veins due to intrapleural pressure, mediastinal shift, and increased cardiovascular pressure; pallor related to decreased cardiac output; anxiety related to hypoxia; and weak and rapid pulse due to decreased cardiac output.

COMPLICATIONS

Possible complications of pneumothorax include decreased cardiac output, hypoxemia, and cardiac arrest.

DIAGNOSIS

Chest X-rays confirm the diagnosis by revealing air in the pleural space and, possibly, a mediastinal shift.

Arterial blood gas analysis may reveal hypoxemia, possibly with respiratory acidosis and hypercapnia. Partial pressure of arterial oxygen levels may decrease at first, but typically return to normal within 24 hours.

TREATMENT

Treatment depends on the type of pneumothorax.

Spontaneous pneumothorax with less than 30% of lung collapse, no signs of increased pleural pressure, and no dyspnea or indications of physiologic compromise, may be corrected with bed rest to conserve energy and reduce oxygenation demands; monitoring of blood pressure and pulse for early detection of physiologic compromise; monitoring of respiratory rate to detect early signs of respiratory compromise; oxygen administration to enhance oxygenation; and possibly, aspiration of air with a large-bore needle attached to a syringe to restore negative pressure within the pleural space.

Correction of pneumothorax with more than 30% of lung collapse may include placement of thoracostomy tube in the second or third intercostal space in the midclavicular line with connection to underwater-seal and low-pressure suction to try to reexpand the lung by restoring negative intrapleural pressure.

If the spontaneous pneumothorax is recurring, thoracotomy and pleurectomy may be performed, which causes the lung to adhere to the parietal pleura.

Open (traumatic) pneumothorax may be corrected with chest tube drainage to reexpand the lung and may require surgical repair of the lung.

Correction of tension pneumothorax typically involves immediate treatment with large-bore needle insertion into the pleural space through the second intercostal space to reexpand the lung, insertion of a thoracostomy tube, and analgesics to promote comfort and encourage deep breathing and coughing.

NURSING CONSIDERATIONS

✦ Watch for pallor, gasping respirations, and sudden chest pain. Carefully monitor vital signs at least every hour for indications of shock, increasing respiratory distress, or mediastinal shift. Listen for breath sounds over both lungs. Falling blood pressure and rising pulse and respiratory rates may indicate tension pneumothorax, which could be fatal without prompt treatment.
✦ Urge the patient to control coughing and gasping during thoracotomy. However, after the chest tube is in place, encourage him to cough and breathe deeply (at least once per hour) to facilitate lung expansion.
✦ If the patient is undergoing chest tube drainage, watch for continuing air leakage (bubbling), indicating the lung defect has failed to close; this may require surgery. Also, watch for increasing subcutaneous emphysema by checking around the neck or at the tube insertion site for crackling beneath the skin. If the patient is on a ventilator, watch for difficulty in breathing in time with the ventilator as well as pressure changes on ventilator gauges.
✦ Change dressings around the chest tube insertion site as necessary. Be careful not to reposition or dislodge the tube. If the tube dislodges, place a petroleum gauze dressing over the opening immediately to prevent rapid lung collapse.
✦ Monitor vital signs frequently after thoracotomy. Also, for the first 24 hours, assess respiratory status by checking breath sounds hourly. Observe the chest tube site for leakage, noting the amount and color of drainage. Help the patient walk, as ordered (usually on the first postoperative day), to facilitate deep inspiration and lung expansion.
✦ To reassure the patient, explain what pneumothorax is, what causes it, and all diagnostic tests and procedures. Make him as comfortable as possible. (The patient with pneumothorax is usually most comfortable sitting upright.)

▼ *LIFE-THREATENING DISORDER*

PULMONARY EDEMA

Pulmonary edema is an accumulation of fluid in the extravascular spaces of the lungs. It's a common complication of cardiac disorders and may occur as a chronic condition or may develop quickly and rapidly become fatal.

CAUSES

Pulmonary edema is caused by left-sided heart failure due to arteriosclerosis, cardiomyopathy, hypertension, and valvular heart disease.

Factors that predispose the patient to pulmonary edema include barbiturate or opiate poisoning, cardiac failure, excess infusion of I.V. fluids or overly rapid infu-

---

Treatment

Open pneumothorax
✦ Chest tube drainage

Tension pneumothorax
✦ Large-bore needle insertion into the pleural space
✦ Insertion of thoracostomy tube
✦ Analgesics

Key nursing actions
✦ Watch for pallor, gasping respirations, and sudden chest pain.
✦ Urge the patient to control coughing and gasping during thoracotomy.
✦ If the patient is undergoing chest tube drainage, watch for continuing air leakage, indicating the lung defect has failed to close.
✦ To reassure the patient, explain what pneumothorax is, what causes it, and all diagnostic tests and procedures.

Characteristics of pulmonary edema
✦ Life-threatening disorder
✦ Accumulation of fluid in the extravascular spaces of lungs
✦ Complication of cardiac disorders
✦ May be chronic or develop quickly and rapidly become fatal

Causes
✦ Left-sided heart failure
✦ Barbiturate or opiate poisoning
✦ Cardiac failure
✦ Excess infusion of I.V. fluids or overly rapid infusion
✦ Inhalation of irritating gases

sion, impaired pulmonary lymphatic drainage (from Hodgkin's disease or oblitera-
tive lymphangitis after radiation), inhalation of irritating gases, mitral stenosis and
left atrial myxoma (which impairs left atrial emptying), pneumonia, and pulmonary veno-occlusive disease.

PATHOPHYSIOLOGY

Normally, pulmonary capillary hydrostatic pressure, capillary oncotic pressure,
capillary permeability, and lymphatic drainage are in balance. When this balance
changes or the lymphatic drainage system is obstructed, fluid infiltrates the lung
and pulmonary edema results. If pulmonary capillary hydrostatic pressure increases, the compromised left ventricle requires increased filling pressures to maintain
adequate cardiac output. These pressures are transmitted to the left atrium, pulmonary veins, and pulmonary capillary bed, forcing fluids and solutes from the intravascular compartment into the interstitium of the lungs. As the interstitium
overloads with fluid, fluid floods the peripheral alveoli and impairs gas exchange.

If colloid osmotic pressure decreases, the hydrostatic force that regulates intravascular fluids (the natural pulling force) is lost because there's no opposition.
Fluid flows freely into the interstitium and alveoli, impairing gas exchange and
leading to pulmonary edema. (See *Understanding pulmonary edema*.)

A blockage of the lymph vessels can result from compression by edema or tumor fibrotic tissue and by increased systemic venous pressure. Hydrostatic pressure
in the large pulmonary veins increases, the pulmonary lymphatic system can't
drain correctly into the pulmonary veins, and excess fluid moves into the interstitial space. Pulmonary edema then results from fluid accumulation.

Capillary injury, such as occurs in acute respiratory distress syndrome (ARDS)
or with inhalation of toxic gases, increases capillary permeability. The injury causes
plasma proteins and water to leak out of the capillary and move into the interstitium, increasing the interstitial oncotic pressure, which is normally low. As interstitial oncotic pressure begins to equal capillary oncotic pressure, the water begins to
move out of the capillary and into the lungs, resulting in pulmonary edema.

SIGNS AND SYMPTOMS

Signs and symptoms of early states of pulmonary edema reflect interstitial fluid accumulation and diminished lung compliance. They include dyspnea on exertion
due to hypoxia, paroxysmal nocturnal dyspnea due to decreased lung expansion,
orthopnea due to decreased ability of the diaphragm to expand, and a cough due to
stimulation of cough reflex by excessive fluid.

Clinical features include mild tachypnea due to hypoxia, increased blood pressure due to increased pulmonary pressures and decreased oxygenation, dependent
crackles as air moves through fluid in the lungs, jugular vein distention due to decreased cardiac output and increased pulmonary vascular resistance, and tachycardia due to hypoxia.

With severe pulmonary edema, the alveoli and bronchioles may fill with fluid
and intensify the early symptoms. Respirations become labored and rapid due to
hypoxia. Air moves through fluid in the lungs, diffuse crackles and coughing produce frothy, bloody sputum. Tachycardia increases due to hypoxemia. Arrhythmias
may occur due to hypoxic myocardium. Skin becomes cold and clammy due to peripheral vasoconstriction, diaphoretic due to decreased cardiac output and shock,
and cyanotic due to hypoxia. Blood pressure falls and pulse becomes thready as
cardiac output falls.

How it happens
+ Pressure balance changes or lymphatic drainage system obstructed
+ Fluid infiltrates lung
+ Can be caused by capillary hydrostatic pressure, colloid osmotic pressure decrease, or capillary injury

Key signs and symptoms
+ Dyspnea
+ Cough
+ Mild tachypnea
+ Increased blood pressure
+ Dependent crackles
+ Jugular vein distention
+ Tachycardia
+ Alveoli and bronchioles may fill with fluid
+ Frothy, bloody sputum
+ Arrhythmias

Understanding pulmonary edema

In pulmonary edema, diminished function of the left ventricle causes blood to back up into pulmonary veins and capillaries. The increasing capillary hydrostatic pressure pushes flu-id into the interstitial spaces and alveoli. These illustrations show a normal alveolus and an alveolus affected by pulmonary edema.

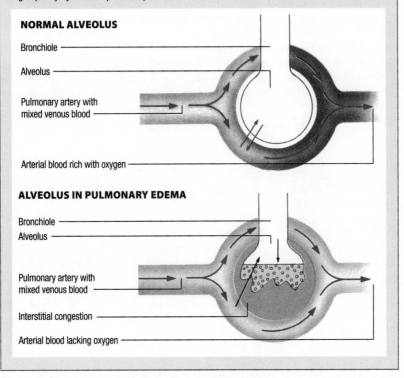

NORMAL ALVEOLUS
- Bronchiole
- Alveolus
- Pulmonary artery with mixed venous blood
- Arterial blood rich with oxygen

ALVEOLUS IN PULMONARY EDEMA
- Bronchiole
- Alveolus
- Pulmonary artery with mixed venous blood
- Interstitial congestion
- Arterial blood lacking oxygen

COMPLICATIONS

Possible complications of pulmonary edema include respiratory failure, respiratory acidosis, and cardiac arrest.

DIAGNOSIS

Arterial blood gas (ABG) analysis usually reveals hypoxemia with variable partial pressure of arterial carbon dioxide, depending on the patient's degree of fatigue. Respiratory acidosis may occur.

Chest X-rays show diffuse haziness of the lung fields and, usually, cardiomegaly and pleural effusion.

Pulse oximetry may reveal decreasing arterial oxygen saturation levels. Pulmonary artery catheterization identifies left-sided heart failure and helps rule out ARDS. Electrocardiography (ECG) may show previous or current myocardial infarction (MI).

Complications
+ Respiratory failure
+ Respiratory acidosis
+ Cardiac arrest

Diagnosis
+ ABG analysis usually reveals hypoxemia
+ Chest X-rays show diffuse haziness of lung
+ Pulse oximetry may reveal decreasing arterial oxygen saturation
+ Pulmonary artery catheterization identifies left-sided heart failure
+ ECG may show MI

Treatment

+ High concentrations of oxygen by nasal cannula
+ Assisted ventilation
+ Diuretics
+ Positive inotropic agents
+ Pressor agents
+ Antiarrhythmics
+ Arterial vasodilators

Key nursing actions

+ Carefully monitor the vulnerable patient for early signs of pulmonary edema.
+ Administer oxygen as ordered.
+ Monitor vital signs every 15 to 30 minutes while administering nitroprusside in dextrose 5% in water by I.V. drip.
+ Carefully record the time and amount of morphine given.

Characteristics of pulmonary embolism

+ Life-threatening disorder
+ Obstruction of pulmonary arterial bed by thrombus, heart valve growths, or foreign substance
+ Strikes estimated 6 million adults each year in the United States
+ Resulting pulmonary infarction may be mild, producing no symptoms
+ Massive embolism and accompanying infarction can be rapidly fatal

TREATMENT

Treatment measures for pulmonary edema are designed to reduce extravascular fluid, to improve gas exchange and myocardial function and, if possible, to correct underlying pathologic conditions.

Administration of high concentrations of oxygen by nasal cannula enhances gas exchange and improves oxygenation. Assisted ventilation improves oxygen delivery to the tissues and promotes acid-base balance. Diuretics, such as furosemide, and bumetanide increase urination which helps mobilize extravascular fluid.

Positive inotropic agents, such as digoxin and inamrinone, enhance contractility in myocardial dysfunction. Pressor agents enhance contractility and promote vasoconstriction in peripheral vessels. Antiarrhythmics are administered for arrhythmias related to decreased cardiac output. Arterial vasodilators such as nitroprusside decrease peripheral vascular resistance, preload, and afterload.

Morphine is used to reduce anxiety and dyspnea and to dilate the systemic venous bed, promoting blood flow from pulmonary circulation to the periphery.

NURSING CONSIDERATIONS

+ Carefully monitor the vulnerable patient for early signs of pulmonary edema, especially tachypnea, tachycardia, and abnormal breath sounds. Report abnormalities. Check for peripheral edema, which may also indicate that fluid level is accumulating in pulmonary tissue.
+ Administer oxygen as ordered.
+ Monitor vital signs every 15 to 30 minutes while administering nitroprusside in dextrose 5% in water by I.V. drip. Protect the nitroprusside solution from light by wrapping the bottle or bag with aluminum foil, and discard unused solution after 4 hours. Watch for arrhythmias in the patient receiving cardiac glycosides and for marked respiratory depression in the patient receiving morphine.
+ Assess the patient's condition frequently, and record his response to treatment. Monitor ABG levels, oral and I.V. fluid intake, urine output and, in the patient with a pulmonary artery catheter, pulmonary end-diastolic and wedge pressures. Check cardiac monitoring often. Report changes immediately.
+ Carefully record the time and amount of morphine given.
+ Reassure the patient, who will be frightened by decreased respiratory capability, in a calm voice, and explain all procedures. Provide emotional support to his family as well.

▼ *LIFE-THREATENING DISORDER*

PULMONARY EMBOLISM

The most common pulmonary complication in hospitalized patients, pulmonary embolism is an obstruction of the pulmonary arterial bed by a dislodged thrombus, heart valve growths, or a foreign substance. It strikes an estimated 6 million adults each year in the United States, resulting in 100,000 deaths. Although pulmonary infarction that results from embolism may be so mild as to produce no symptoms, massive embolism (more than 50% obstruction of pulmonary arterial circulation) and the accompanying infarction can be rapidly fatal.

CAUSES

Pulmonary embolism generally results from dislodged thrombi originating in the leg veins or pelvis. More than 50% of such thrombi arise in the deep veins of the legs. Other less common sources of thrombi are the pelvic veins, renal veins, hepatic vein, right side of the heart, and upper extremities.

Predisposing factors for pulmonary embolism include long-term immobility, chronic pulmonary disease, heart failure or atrial fibrillation, thrombophlebitis, polycythemia vera, thrombocytosis, autoimmune hemolytic anemia, sickle cell anemia, varicose veins, recent surgery, advanced age, pregnancy, lower-extremity fractures or surgery, burns, obesity, vascular injury, cancer, I.V. drug abuse, or hormonal contraceptives.

PATHOPHYSIOLOGY

Thrombus formation results directly from vascular wall damage, venostasis, or hypercoagulability of the blood. Trauma, clot dissolution, sudden muscle spasm, intravascular pressure changes, or a change in peripheral blood flow can cause the thrombus to loosen or fragment. Then the thrombus — now called an embolus — floats to the heart's right side and enters the lung through the pulmonary artery. There, the embolus may dissolve, continue to fragment, or grow.

By occluding the pulmonary artery, the embolus prevents alveoli from producing enough surfactant to maintain alveolar integrity. As a result, alveoli collapse and atelectasis develops. If the embolus enlarges, it may clog most or all of the pulmonary vessels and cause death.

Rarely, the emboli contain air, fat, bacteria, amniotic fluid, talc (from drugs intended for oral administration, which are injected I.V. by addicts), or tumor cells.

SIGNS AND SYMPTOMS

Total occlusion of the main pulmonary artery is rapidly fatal; smaller or fragmented emboli produce symptoms that vary with the size, number, and location. Usually, the first symptom of pulmonary embolism is dyspnea, which may be accompanied by anginal or pleuritic chest pain. Other clinical features include tachycardia, productive cough (sputum may be blood-tinged), low-grade fever, and pleural effusion. Less common signs include massive hemoptysis, splinting of the chest, leg edema and, with a large embolus, cyanosis, syncope, and distended neck veins.

In addition, pulmonary embolism may cause pleural friction rub and signs of circulatory collapse (weak, rapid pulse and hypotension) and of hypoxia (restlessness and anxiety).

COMPLICATIONS

Complications of pulmonary embolism may include pulmonary infarction, acute respiratory failure, death, and acute cor pulmonale.

DIAGNOSIS

The patient history should reveal predisposing conditions for pulmonary embolism. A triad of deep vein thrombosis (DVT) formation is stasis, endothelial injury, and hypercoagulability. Risk factors include long car or plane trips, cancer, pregnancy, hypercoagulability, previous DVTs, and pulmonary emboli.

Chest X-ray helps to rule out other pulmonary diseases; areas of atelectasis, elevated diaphragm and pleural effusion, prominent pulmonary artery and, occasion-

Causes

Causes of dislodged thrombi in legs or pelvis
+ Long-term immobility
+ Chronic pulmonary disease
+ Heart failure or atrial fibrillation
+ Thrombophlebitis
+ Autoimmune hemolytic anemia
+ Recent surgery
+ Hormonal contraceptives

How it happens
+ Thrombus formation occurs from vascular wall damage, venostasis, or hypercoagulability of blood
+ Embolus floats to heart's right side and enters lung through pulmonary artery
+ Embolus may dissolve, continue to fragment, or grow
+ Embolus prevents alveoli from maintaining integrity
+ Alveoli collapse and atelectasis develops
+ Embolus may clog most or all pulmonary vessels

Key signs and symptoms
+ Dyspnea
+ Anginal or pleuritic chest pain
+ Tachycardia
+ Productive cough
+ Pleural effusion
+ Massive hemoptysis

Complications
+ Pulmonary infarction
+ Acute respiratory failure
+ Death
+ Acute cor pulmonale

Diagnosis

- History of long car or plane trips, cancer, pregnancy, hypercoagulability, previous DVTs, pulmonary emboli
- Chest X-ray helps rule out other pulmonary diseases
- Lung scan shows perfusion defects beyond occluded vessels; doesn't rule out microemboli
- ECG helps distinguish from myocardial infarction
- Auscultation reveals a right ventricular S_3 gallop and increased intensity of a pulmonic component of S_2
- Crackles and a pleural rub at embolism site

Treatment

- Oxygen therapy
- Heparin
- Fibrinolytic therapy
- Vasopressors
- Antibiotics
- Surgery

ally, the characteristic wedge-shaped infiltrate suggestive of pulmonary infarction, or focal oligemia of blood vessels, are apparent.

Lung scan shows perfusion defects in areas beyond occluded vessels; however, it doesn't rule out microemboli.

Pulmonary angiography is the most definitive test, but requires a skilled angiographer and radiologic equipment; it also poses some risk to the patient. Its use depends on the uncertainty of the diagnosis and the need to avoid unnecessary anticoagulant therapy in a high-risk patient.

Electrocardiography (ECG) is inconclusive, but helps distinguish pulmonary embolism from myocardial infarction. In extensive embolism, the ECG may show right axis deviation; right bundle-branch block; tall, peaked P waves; depression of ST segments and T-wave inversions (indicative of right-sided heart strain); and supraventricular tachyarrhythmias. A pattern sometimes observed is S_1, Q_3, and T_3 (S wave in lead I, Q wave in lead III, and inverted T wave in lead III).

Auscultation occasionally reveals a right ventricular S_3 gallop and increased intensity of a pulmonic component of S_2. Also, crackles and a pleural rub may be heard at the embolism site.

Arterial blood gas (ABG) measurements showing decreased partial pressure of arterial oxygen and partial pressure of arterial carbon dioxide are characteristic, but don't always occur.

If pleural effusion is present, thoracentesis may rule out empyema, which indicates pneumonia.

TREATMENT

Treatment is designed to maintain adequate cardiovascular and pulmonary function during resolution of the obstruction and to prevent embolus recurrence. Because most emboli resolve within 10 to 14 days, treatment consists of oxygen therapy, as needed, and anticoagulation with heparin to inhibit new thrombus formation. Heparin therapy is monitored by daily coagulation studies (partial thromboplastin time [PTT]).

Patients with massive pulmonary embolism and shock may need fibrinolytic therapy with urokinase, streptokinase, or alteplase to enhance fibrinolysis of the pulmonary emboli and remaining thrombi. Emboli that cause hypotension may require the use of vasopressors. Treatment of septic emboli requires antibiotics, not anticoagulants, and evaluation for the infection's source, particularly endocarditis.

Surgery is performed on patients who can't take anticoagulants (because of recent surgery or blood dyscrasia), or who have recurrent emboli during anticoagulant therapy. Surgery (which shouldn't be performed without angiographic evidence of pulmonary embolism) consists of vena cava ligation, plication, or insertion of a device (umbrella filter) to filter blood returning to the heart and lungs. To prevent postoperative venous thromboembolism, a combination of heparin and dihydroergotamine may be given.

NURSING CONSIDERATIONS

- Give oxygen by nasal cannula or mask. Check ABG levels if the patient develops fresh emboli or worsening dyspnea. Be prepared to provide endotracheal intubation with assisted ventilation if breathing is severely compromised.
- Administer heparin, as ordered, through I.V. push or continuous drip. Monitor coagulation studies daily. Effective heparin therapy raises the PTT to more than $1\frac{1}{2}$ times normal. Watch closely for nosebleed, petechiae, and other signs of abnor-

mal bleeding; check stool for occult blood. Tell the patient to prevent bleeding by shaving with an electric razor and by brushing his teeth with a soft toothbrush.

✦ After the patient is stable, encourage him to move about often, and assist with isometric and range-of-motion exercises. Check pedal pulses, temperature, and color of his feet to detect venostasis. Never vigorously massage the patient's legs. Offer diversional activities to promote rest and relieve restlessness.

✦ Help the patient walk as soon as possible after surgery to prevent venostasis.

✦ Maintain adequate nutrition and fluid balance to promote healing.

✦ Report frequent pleuritic chest pain, so that analgesics can be prescribed. Also, incentive spirometry can assist in deep breathing.

✦ Warn the patient not to cross his legs or sit with his legs in a dependent position for prolonged periods; this promotes thrombus formation.

✦ To relieve anxiety, explain procedures and treatments. Encourage the patient's family to participate in his care.

✦ The patient usually takes an oral anticoagulant (warfarin) for 3 to 6 months after a pulmonary embolism. Advise him to watch for signs of bleeding (bloody stool, blood in urine, and large ecchymoses), to take the prescribed medication exactly as ordered, not to change dosages without consulting his physician, and to avoid taking additional medication (even for headaches or colds). Stress the importance of follow-up laboratory tests (prothrombin time) to monitor anticoagulant therapy.

✦ To prevent pulmonary emboli, encourage early ambulation in the patient predisposed to this condition. With close medical supervision, low-dose heparin may be used prophylactically.

✦ Low-molecular-weight heparin may be given to prevent pulmonary embolism in the high-risk patient.

Key nursing actions

✦ Give oxygen by nasal cannula or mask. Be prepared to provide endotracheal intubation with assisted ventilation if breathing is severely compromised.

✦ Administer heparin, as ordered.

✦ Help the patient walk as soon as possible after surgery to prevent venostasis.

✦ Warn the patient not to cross his legs or sit with his legs in a dependent position for prolonged periods.

✦ To prevent pulmonary emboli, encourage early ambulation in the patient predisposed to this condition.

Nervous system

Key facts about the nervous system

- ✦ Coordinates and organizes functions of all body systems
- ✦ Has three main divisions: CNS, peripheral nervous system, ANS
- ✦ Neurons transmit nerve impulses through body
- ✦ Most neurons have several dendrites, only one axon
- ✦ Three types: sensory, motor, and interneurons
- ✦ Nervous system disorders can cause signs and symptoms in any body system; hard to diagnose

The nervous system coordinates and organizes the functions of all body systems. This intricate network of interlocking receptors and transmitters is a dynamic system that controls and regulates every mental and physical function. It has three main divisions:

✦ *central nervous system (CNS)* — the brain and spinal cord (see *Reviewing the central nervous system*)

✦ *peripheral nervous system* — the motor and sensory nerves, which carry messages between the CNS and remote parts of the body (see *Reviewing the peripheral nervous system*, pages 274 and 275)

✦ *autonomic nervous system (ANS)* — part of the peripheral nervous system, regulates involuntary functions of the internal organs.

The fundamental unit that participates in all nervous system activity is the neuron, a highly specialized cell that receives and transmits electrochemical nerve impulses through delicate, threadlike fibers that extend from the central cell body. Axons carry impulses away from the cell body; dendrites carry impulses to it. Most neurons have several dendrites but only one axon.

✦ Sensory (or afferent) neurons transmit impulses from receptors to the spinal cord or the brain.

✦ Motor (or efferent) neurons transmit impulses from the CNS to regulate the activity of muscles or glands.

✦ Interneurons, also known as connecting or association neurons, carry signals through complex pathways between sensory and motor neurons. Interneurons account for 99% of all the neurons in the nervous system.

From birth to death, the nervous system efficiently organizes and controls the smallest action, thought, or feeling; monitors communication and the instinct for survival; and allows introspection, wonder, abstract thought, and self-awareness. Together, the CNS and peripheral nervous system keep a person alert, awake, oriented, and able to move about freely without discomfort and with all body systems working to maintain homeostasis.

Reviewing the central nervous system

The central nervous system includes the brain and spinal cord. The brain consists of the cerebrum, cerebellum, brain stem, and primitive structures that lie below the cerebrum: the diencephalon, limbic system, and reticular activating system (RAS). The spinal cord is the primary pathway for messages between peripheral areas of the body and the brain. It also mediates reflexes.

CEREBRUM

The left and right cerebral hemispheres are joined by the corpus callosum, a mass of nerve fibers that allows communication between corresponding centers in the right and left hemispheres. Each hemisphere is divided into four lobes, based on anatomic landmarks and functional differences. The lobes are named for the cranial bones that lie over them (frontal, temporal, parietal, and occipital):

✦ *frontal lobe* — influences personality, judgment, abstract reasoning, social behavior, language expression, and movement (in the motor portion)

✦ *temporal lobe* — controls hearing, language comprehension, and storage and recall of memories (although memories are stored throughout the brain)

✦ *parietal lobe* — interprets and integrates sensations, including pain, temperature, and touch; also interprets size, shape, distance, and texture (The parietal lobe of the nondominant hemisphere, usually the right, is especially important for awareness of body schema [shape].)

✦ *occipital lobe* — functions primarily in interpreting visual stimuli.

The cerebral cortex, the thin surface layer of the cerebrum, is composed of gray matter (unmyelinated cell bodies). The surface of the cerebrum has convolutions (gyri) and creases or fissures (sulci).

CEREBELLUM

The cerebellum, which also has two hemispheres, maintains muscle tone, coordinates muscle movement, and controls balance.

BRAIN STEM

Composed of the pons, midbrain, and medulla oblongata, the brain stem relays messages between upper and lower levels of the nervous system. The cranial nerves originate from the pons, midbrain, and medulla oblongata:

✦ *pons* — connects the cerebellum with the cerebrum and the midbrain to the medulla oblongata, and contains one of the respiratory centers

✦ *midbrain* — mediates the auditory and visual reflexes

✦ *medulla oblongata* — regulates respiratory, vasomotor, and cardiac function.

PRIMITIVE STRUCTURES

The diencephalon contains the thalamus and hypothalamus, which lie beneath the cerebral hemispheres. The thalamus relays all sensory stimuli (except olfactory) as they ascend to the cerebral cortex. Thalamic functions include primitive awareness of pain, screening of incoming stimuli, and focusing of attention. The hypothalamus controls or affects body temperature, appetite, water balance, pituitary secretions, emotions, and autonomic functions, including sleep and wake cycles.

The limbic system lies deep within the temporal lobe. It initiates primitive drives (hunger, aggression, and sexual and emotional arousal) and screens all sensory messages traveling to the cerebral cortex.

The RAS, a diffuse network of hyperexcitable neurons fanning out from the brain stem through the cerebral cortex, screens all incoming sensory information and channels it to appropriate areas of the brain for interpretation. RAS activity also stimulates wakefulness.

SPINAL CORD

The spinal cord joins the brain stem at the level of the foramen magnum and terminates near the second lumbar vertebra.

A cross section of the spinal cord reveals a central H-shaped mass of gray matter divided into dorsal (posterior) and ventral (anterior) horns. Gray matter in the dorsal horns relays sensory (afferent) impulses; in the ventral horns, motor (efferent) impulses. White matter (myelinated axons of sensory and motor nerves) surrounds these horns and forms the ascending and descending tracts.

Reviewing the CNS

✦ Cerebrum — frontal lobe, temporal lobe, parietal lobe, occipital lobe
✦ Cerebellum — maintains muscle tone, coordination
✦ Brain stem — pons, midbrain, medulla oblongata
✦ Primitive structures — thalamus, hypothalamus, limbic system, RAS
✦ Spinal cord — relays sensory, motor impulses

Reviewing the peripheral nervous system

The peripheral nervous system consists of the cranial nerves (CN), the spinal nerves, and the autonomic nervous system (ANS).

CRANIAL NERVES

The 12 pairs of cranial nerves transmit motor or sensory messages, or both, primarily between the brain or brain stem and the head and neck. All cranial nerves, except for the olfactory and optic nerves, originate from the midbrain, pons, or medulla oblongata. The cranial nerves are sensory, motor, or mixed (both sensory and motor):

- olfactory (CN I) — Sensory: smell
- optic (CN II) — Sensory: vision
- oculomotor (CN III) — Motor: extraocular eye movement (superior, medial, and inferior lateral), pupillary constriction, and upper eyelid elevation
- trochlear (CN IV) — Motor: extraocular eye movement (inferior medial)
- trigeminal (CN V) — Sensory: transmitting stimuli from face and head, corneal reflex; Motor: chewing, biting, and lateral jaw movements
- abducens (CN VI) — Motor: extraocular eye movement (lateral)
- facial (CN VII) — Sensory: taste receptors (anterior two-thirds of tongue); Motor: Facial muscle movement, including muscles of expression (those in the forehead and around the eyes and mouth)
- acoustic (CN VIII) — Sensory: hearing, sense of balance
- glossopharyngeal (CN IX) — Motor: swallowing movements; Sensory: sensations of throat; taste receptors (posterior one-third of tongue)
- vagus (CN X) — Motor: movement of palate, swallowing, gag reflex; activity of the thoracic and abdominal viscera, such as heart rate and peristalsis; Sensory: sensations of throat, larynx, and thoracic and abdominal viscera (heart, lungs, bronchi, and GI tract)
- spinal accessory (CN XI) — Motor: shoulder movement, head rotation
- hypoglossal (CN XII) — Motor: tongue movement.

SPINAL NERVES

The 31 pairs of spinal nerves are named according to the vertebra immediately below their exit point from the spinal cord. Each spinal nerve consists of afferent (sensory) and efferent (motor) neurons, which carry messages to and from particular body regions, called dermatomes.

AUTONOMIC NERVOUS SYSTEM

The ANS innervates all internal organs. Sometimes known as the *visceral efferent nerves,* autonomic nerves carry messages to the viscera from the brain stem and neuroendocrine system. The ANS has two major divisions: the sympathetic (thoracolumbar) nervous system and the parasympathetic (craniosacral) nervous system.

Sympathetic nervous system

Sympathetic nerves exit the spinal cord between the levels of the first thoracic and second lumbar vertebrae; hence the name thoracolumbar. These preganglionic neurons enter small relay stations (ganglia) near the cord. The ganglia form a chain that disseminates the impulse to postganglionic neurons, which reach many organs and glands, and can produce widespread, generalized responses.

The physiologic effects of sympathetic activity include:

- vasoconstriction
- elevated blood pressure
- enhanced blood flow to skeletal muscles
- increased heart rate and contractility
- heightened respiratory rate
- smooth-muscle relaxation of the bronchioles, GI tract, and urinary tract
- sphincter contraction
- pupillary dilation and ciliary muscle relaxation
- increased sweat gland secretion
- reduced pancreatic secretion.

Parasympathetic nervous system

The fibers of the parasympathetic, or craniosacral, nervous system leave the central nervous system (CNS) by way of the cranial nerves from the midbrain and medulla and with the spinal nerves between the second and fourth sacral vertebrae (S2 to S4).

After leaving the CNS, the long preganglionic fiber of each parasympathetic nerve travels to a ganglion near a particular organ

---

Reviewing the peripheral nervous system

- Cranial nerves — 12 pairs: olfactory, optic, oculomotor, trochlear, trigeminal, abducens, facial, acoustic, glossopharyngeal, vagus, spinal accessory, hypoglossal
- Spinal nerves — 31 pairs with sensory and motor neurons
- ANS — innervates internal organs; sympathetic nervous system and parasympathetic nervous system

Reviewing the peripheral nervous system *(continued)*

or gland, and the short postganglionic fiber enters the organ or gland. Parasympathetic nerves have a specific response involving only one organ or gland.

The physiologic effects of parasympathetic system activity include:
♦ reduced heart rate, contractility, and conduction velocity
♦ bronchial smooth-muscle constriction
♦ increased GI tract tone and peristalsis with sphincter relaxation

♦ urinary system sphincter relaxation and increased bladder tone
♦ vasodilation of external genitalia, causing erection
♦ pupillary constriction
♦ increased pancreatic, salivary, and lacrimal secretions.

The parasympathetic system has little effect on mental or metabolic activity.

Thus, any disorder affecting the nervous system can cause signs and symptoms in any and all body systems. Patients with nervous system disorders commonly have signs and symptoms that are elusive, subtle, and sometimes latent.

PATHOPHYSIOLOGIC CHANGES

Typically, disorders of the nervous system involve some alteration in arousal, cognition, movement, muscle tone, homeostatic mechanisms, or pain. Most disorders cause more than one alteration, and the close intercommunication between the CNS and peripheral nervous system means that one alteration may lead to another.

AROUSAL

Arousal refers to the level of consciousness or state of awareness. A person who's aware of himself and the environment and can respond to the environment in specific ways is said to be fully conscious. Full consciousness requires that the reticular activating system (RAS), higher systems in the cerebral cortex, and thalamic connections be intact and functioning properly. Several mechanisms can alter arousal:
♦ direct destruction of the RAS and its pathways
♦ destruction of the brain stem, either directly by invasion or indirectly by impairment of its blood supply
♦ compression of the RAS by a disease process, either from direct pressure or compression as structures expand or herniate.

Those mechanisms may result from structural, metabolic, or psychogenic disturbances:
♦ Structural changes include infections, vascular problems, neoplasms, trauma, and developmental and degenerative conditions. They're usually identified by their location relative to the tentorial plate, the double fold of dura that supports the temporal and occipital lobes and separates the cerebral hemispheres from the brain stem and cerebellum. Those above the tentorial plate are called supratentorial, whereas those below are called infratentorial.
♦ Metabolic changes that affect the nervous system include hypoxia, electrolyte disturbances, hypoglycemia, drugs, and toxins (endogenous and exogenous). Essentially any systemic disease can affect the nervous system.
♦ Psychogenic changes are commonly associated with mental and psychiatric illnesses. Ongoing research has linked neuroanatomy and neurophysiology of the

Pathophysiologic changes

♦ Typically involve alteration in arousal, cognition, movement, muscle tone, homeostatic mechanisms, or pain
♦ Most cause more than one alteration
♦ One alteration may lead to another

Key facts about arousal

♦ Level of consciousness or state of awareness

Several mechanisms can alter arousal
♦ Direct destruction of RAS and pathways
♦ Destruction of brain stem
♦ Compression of RAS by disease process
♦ Mechanisms may result from structural, metabolic, or psychogenic disturbances

6 stages of altered arousal

✦ Usually begins with interruption or disruption in diencephalon
✦ Patient shows evidence of dullness, confusion, lethargy, and stupor
✦ Continued decreases result from midbrain dysfunction
✦ Coma results if medulla and pons effected
✦ Patient will progress through rostral-caudal progression
✦ Levels: confusion, disorientation, lethargy, obtundation, stupor, coma

5 neurologic function areas used to identify cause

✦ Level of consciousness
✦ Pattern of breathing
✦ Pupillary changes
✦ Eye movement and reflex responses
✦ Motor responses

Key facts about cognition

✦ Ability to be aware, perceive, reason, judge, remember, use intuition
✦ Reflects higher functioning of cerebral cortex
✦ Alteration results from direct or indirect destruction
✦ May manifest as agnosia, aphasia, or dysphasia

CNS and supporting structures, including neurotransmitters, with certain psychiatric illnesses. For example, dysfunction of the limbic system has been associated with schizophrenia, depression, and anxiety disorders.

Decreased arousal may be a result of diffuse or localized dysfunction in supratentorial areas:
✦ Diffuse dysfunction reflects damage to the cerebral cortex or underlying subcortical white matter. Disease is the most common cause of diffuse dysfunction; other causes include neoplasms, closed head trauma with subsequent bleeding, and pus accumulation.
✦ Localized dysfunction reflects mechanical forces on the thalamus or hypothalamus. Masses (such as bleeding, infarction, emboli, and tumors) may directly impinge on the deep diencephalic structures, or herniation may compress them.

Six stages of altered arousal

An alteration in arousal usually begins with some interruption or disruption in the diencephalon. When this occurs, the patient shows evidence of dullness, confusion, lethargy, and stupor. Continued decreases in arousal result from midbrain dysfunction and are evidenced by a deepening of the stupor. Eventually, if the medulla and pons are affected, coma results.

A patient may move back and forth between stages or levels of arousal, depending on the cause of the altered arousal state, initiation of treatment, and response to the treatment. Typically, if the underlying problem isn't or can't be corrected, then the patient will progress through the various stages of decreased consciousness, termed rostral-caudal progression.

Six levels of altered arousal or consciousness have been identified. (See *Stages of altered arousal.*)

Typically, five areas of neurologic function are evaluated to help identify the cause of altered arousal:
✦ level of consciousness (LOC) (includes awareness and cognitive functioning, which reflect cerebral status)
✦ pattern of breathing (helps to localize the cause to the cerebral hemisphere or brain stem)
✦ pupillary changes (reflects the level of brain stem function; the brain stem areas that control arousal are anatomically next to the areas that control the pupils)
✦ eye movement and reflex responses (help identify the level of brain stem dysfunction and its mechanism, such as destruction or compression)
✦ motor responses (help identify the level, side, and severity of brain dysfunction).

COGNITION

Cognition is the ability to be aware and to perceive, reason, judge, remember, and to use intuition. It reflects higher functioning of the cerebral cortex, including the frontal, parietal, and temporal lobes, and portions of the brain stem. Typically, an alteration in cognition results from direct destruction by ischemia and hypoxia or from indirect destruction by compression or the effects of toxins and chemicals.

Altered cognition may manifest as agnosia, aphasia, or dysphasia:
✦ Agnosia is a defect in the ability to recognize the form or nature of objects. Usually, agnosia involves only one sense—hearing, vision, or touch.
✦ Aphasia is loss of the ability to comprehend or produce language.
✦ Dysphasia is impaired ability to comprehend or use symbols in either verbal or written language, or to produce language.

Stages of altered arousal

This chart highlights the six levels or stages of altered arousal and their manifestations.

STAGE	MANIFESTATIONS
Confusion	✦ Loss of ability to think rapidly and clearly ✦ Impaired judgment and decision making
Disorientation	✦ Beginning loss of consciousness ✦ Disorientation to time progresses to include disorientation to place ✦ Impaired memory ✦ Lack of recognition of self (last to go)
Lethargy	✦ Limited spontaneous movement or speech ✦ Easy to arouse by normal speech or touch ✦ Possible disorientation to time, place, or person
Obtundation	✦ Mild to moderate reduction in arousal ✦ Limited responsiveness to environment ✦ Ability to fall asleep easily without verbal or tactile stimulation from others ✦ Ability to answer questions with minimum response
Stupor	✦ State of deep sleep or unresponsiveness ✦ Arousable (motor or verbal response only to vigorous and repeated stimulation) ✦ Withdrawal or grabbing response to stimulation
Coma	✦ Lack of motor or verbal response to external environment or any stimuli ✦ No response to noxious stimuli such as deep pain ✦ Can't be aroused by any stimulus

Altered arousal stages
✦ Confusion
✦ Disorientation
✦ Lethargy
✦ Obtundation
✦ Stupor
✦ Coma

Dysphasia typically arises from the left cerebral hemisphere, usually the frontotemporal region. However, different types of dysphasia occur, depending on the specific area of the brain involved. For example, a dysfunction in the posteroinferior frontal lobe (Broca's area) causes a motor dysphasia in which the patient can't find the words to speak and has difficulty writing and repeating words. Dysfunction in the pathways connecting the primary auditory area to the auditory association areas in the middle third of the left superior temporal gyrus causes a form of dysphasia called word deafness: the patient has fluent speech, but comprehension of the spoken word and ability to repeat speech are impaired. Rather than words, the patient hears only noise that has no meaning, yet reading comprehension and writing ability are intact.

Dementia
Dementia is the loss of more than one intellectual or cognitive function, which interferes with the ability to function in daily life. The patient may experience a problem with orientation, general knowledge and information, vigilance (attentiveness, alertness, and watchfulness), recent memory, remote memory, concept formulation, abstraction (the ability to generalize about nonconcrete thoughts and ideas), reasoning, or language use.

Key facts about dementia
✦ Loss of more than one intellectual or cognitive function
✦ Affects orientation, general knowledge and information, vigilance (attentiveness, alertness, and watchfulness), recent memory, remote memory, concept formulation, abstraction, reasoning, language use

Key facts about dementia
(continued)

+ Underlying mechanism is defect in neuronal circuitry
+ Extent of dysfunction reflects total quantity of neurons lost
+ Associated processes: degeneration, cerebrovascular disorders, compression, effects of toxins, metabolic conditions, biochemical imbalances, demyelinization, infection
+ Three major types: amnestic, intentional, cognitive

The underlying mechanism is a defect in the neuronal circuitry of the brain. The extent of dysfunction reflects the total quantity of neurons lost and the area where this loss occurred. Processes that have been associated with dementia include degeneration, cerebrovascular disorders, compression, effects of toxins, metabolic conditions, biochemical imbalances, demyelinization, and infection.

Three major types of dementia have been identified: amnestic, intentional, and cognitive. Each type affects a specific area of the brain, resulting in characteristic impairments:

+ Amnestic dementia typically results from defective neuronal circuitry in the temporal lobe. Characteristically, the patient exhibits difficulty in naming things, loss of recent memory, and loss of language comprehension.
+ Intentional dementia results from a defect in the frontal lobe. The patient is easily distracted and, although able to follow simple commands, can't carry out such sequential executive functions as planning, initiating, and regulating behavior or achieving specific goals. The patient may exhibit personality changes and a flat affect. Possibly appearing accident prone, he may lose motor function, as evidenced by a wide shuffling gait, small steps, muscle rigidity, abnormal reflexes, incontinence of bowel and bladder and, possibly, total immobility.
+ Cognitive dementia reflects dysfunctional neuronal circuitry in the cerebral cortex. Typically, the patient loses remote memory, language comprehension, and mathematical skills, and has difficulty with visual-spatial relationships.

MOVEMENT

Movement involves a complex array of activities controlled by the cerebral cortex, the pyramidal system, the extrapyramidal system, and the motor units (the axon of the lower motor neuron from the anterior horn cell of the spinal cord and the muscles innervated by it). A problem in any one of these areas can affect movement. (See *Reviewing motor impulse transmission.*)

For movement to occur, the muscles must change their state from one of contraction to relaxation or vice versa. A change in muscle innervation anywhere along the motor pathway will affect movement. Certain neurotransmitters, such as dopamine, play a role in altered movement.

Alterations in movement typically include excessive movement (hyperkinesia) or decreased movement (hypokinesia). Hyperkinesia is a broad category that includes many different types of abnormal movements. Each type of hyperkinesia is associated with a specific underlying pathophysiologic mechanism affecting the brain or motor pathway. (See *Types of hyperkinesia,* pages 280 and 281.)

Hypokinesia usually involves loss of voluntary control, even though peripheral nerve and muscle functions are intact. The types of hypokinesia include paresis, akinesia, bradykinesia, and loss of associated movement.

Paresis

Paresis is a partial loss of motor function (paralysis) and muscle power, which the patient will commonly describe as weakness. Paresis can result from the dysfunction of:

+ the upper motor neurons in the cerebral cortex, subcortical white matter, internal capsule, brain stem, or spinal cord
+ the lower motor neurons in the brain stem motor nuclei and anterior horn of the spinal cord, or problems with their axons as they travel to the skeletal muscle
+ the motor units affecting the muscle fibers or the neuromuscular junction.

Key facts about movement

+ Involves activities controlled by cerebral cortex, pyramidal system, extrapyramidal system, motor units
+ Problem in any one area can affect movement
+ Muscles must contract and relax for movement
+ Alterations typically include hyperkinesia, hypokinesia

Key facts about paresis

+ Partial paralysis, muscle power loss
+ Can result from dysfunction of upper motor neurons, lower motor neurons, motor units

Reviewing motor impulse transmission

Motor impulses that originate in the motor cortex of the frontal lobe travel through upper motor neurons of the pyramidal or extrapyramidal tract to the lower motor neurons of the peripheral nervous system.

In the pyramidal tract, most impulses from the motor cortex travel through the internal capsule to the medulla, where they cross (decussate) to the opposite side and continue down the spinal cord as the lateral corticospinal tract, ending in the anterior horn of the gray matter at a specific spinal cord level. Some fibers don't cross in the medulla but continue down the anterior corticospinal tract and cross near the level of termination in the anterior horn. The fibers of the pyramidal tract are considered upper motor neurons. In the anterior horn of the spinal cord, upper motor neurons relay impulses to the lower motor neurons, which carry them via the spinal and peripheral nerves to the muscles, producing a motor response.

Motor impulses that regulate involuntary muscle tone and muscle control travel along the extrapyramidal tract from the premotor area of the frontal lobe to the pons of the brain stem, where they cross to the opposite side. The impulses then travel down the spinal cord to the anterior horn, where they're relayed to lower motor neurons for ultimate delivery to the muscles.

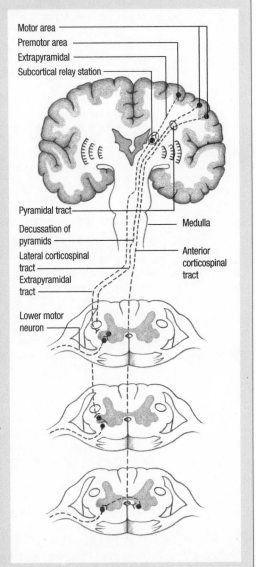

Transmitting motor impulses

+ Originate in motor cortex of frontal lobe and travel through upper motor neurons
+ In pyramidal tract, most travel through internal capsule to the medulla
+ Some fibers don't cross medulla but cross near level of termination
+ Motor impulses that regulate muscles travel along extrapyramidal tract

Upper motor neurons

Upper motor neuron dysfunction reflects an interruption in the pyramidal tract and consequent decreased activation of the lower motor neurons innervating one or more areas of the body. Upper motor neuron dysfunction usually affects more than one muscle group and generally affects distal muscle groups more severely than proximal groups. Onset of spastic muscle tone over several days to weeks commonly accompanies upper motor neuron paresis, unless the dysfunction is

Types of hyperkinesia
+ Akathisia
+ Asterixis
+ Athetosis
+ Ballism
+ Chorea
+ Hyperactivity
+ Intentional cerebellar tremor
+ Myoclonus
+ Parkinsonian tremor
+ Wandering

Types of hyperkinesia

This chart summarizes some of the most common types of hyperkinesias, their manifestations, and the underlying mechanisms involved in their development.

TYPE	MANIFESTATIONS	MECHANISMS
Akathisia	+ Ranges from mildly-compulsive movement (usually the legs) to severely-frenzied motion + Partly voluntary, with ability to suppress for short periods + Relief obtained by performing motion	Possible association with impaired dopaminergic transmission
Asterixis	+ Irregular flapping-hand movement + More prominent when arms outstretched	Believed to result from buildup of toxins not broken down by the liver (such as ammonia)
Athetosis	+ Slow, sinuous, irregular movements in the distal extremities + Characteristic hand posture + Slow, fluctuating grimaces	Believed to result from injury to the putamen of the basal ganglion
Ballism	+ Severe, wild, flinging, stereotypical limb movements + Present when awake or asleep + Usually on one side of the body	Injury to subthalamus nucleus, causing inhibition of the nucleus
Chorea	+ Random, irregular, involuntary, rapid contractions of muscle groups + Nonrepetitive + Diminishes with rest, disappears during sleep + Increases during emotional stress or attempts at voluntary movement	Excess concentration or heightened sensitivity to dopamine in the basal ganglia
Hyperactivity	+ Prolonged, generalized, increased activity + Mainly involuntary but possibly subject to voluntary control + Continual changes in body posture or excessive performance of a simple activity at inappropriate times	Possibly due to injury to frontal lobe and reticular activating system
Intentional cerebellar tremor	+ Tremor secondary to movement + Most severe when nearing end of the movement	Errors in feedback from the periphery and goal-directed movement due to disease of dentate nucleus and superior cerebellar peduncle
Myoclonus	+ Shocklike contractions + Throwing limb movements + Random occurrence + Triggered by startle + Present even during sleep	Irritability of nervous system and spontaneous discharge of neurons in the cerebral cortex, cerebellum, RAS and spinal cord

Types of hyperkinesia *(continued)*

TYPE	MANIFESTATIONS	MECHANISMS
Parkinsonian tremor	✦ Regular, rhythmic, slow flexion and extension contraction ✦ Primarily affects metacarpopha-langeal and wrist joints ✦ Disappears with voluntary movement	Loss of inhibitory effects of dopamine in basal ganglia
Wandering	✦ Moving about without attention to environment	Possibly due to bilateral injury to globus pallidus or putamen

acute. In acute dysfunction, flaccid tone and loss of deep tendon reflexes indicates spinal shock, caused by a severe, acute lesion below the foramen magnum. Incoordination associated with upper motor neuron paresis manifests as slow coarse movement with abnormal rhythm.

Lower motor neurons

Lower motor neurons are of two basic types: large (alpha) and small (gamma). Dysfunction of the large motor neurons of the anterior horn of the spinal cord, the motor nuclei of the brain stem, and their axons, causes impairment of voluntary and involuntary movement. The extent of paresis is directly correlated to the number of large motor neurons affected. If only a small portion of the neurons are involved, paresis occurs; if all motor units are affected, the result is paralysis.

The small motor neurons play two necessary roles in movement: maintaining muscle tone and protecting the muscle from injury. Usually when the large motor neurons are affected, dysfunction of the small motor neurons causes reduced or absent muscle tone, flaccid paresis, and paralysis.

Motor units

The muscles innervated by motor neurons in the anterior horn of the spinal cord may also be affected. Paresis results from a decrease in the number or force of activated muscle fibers in the motor unit. The action potential of each motor unit decreases so that additional motor units are needed more quickly to produce the power necessary to move the muscle. Dysfunction of the neuromuscular junction causes paresis in a similar fashion; however, the functional capability of the motor units to function is lost, not the actual number of units.

Akinesia

Akinesia is a partial or complete loss of voluntary and associated movements as well as a disturbance in the time needed to perform a movement. Commonly caused by dysfunction of the extrapyramidal tract, it's associated with dopamine deficiency at the synapse or a defect in the postsynaptic receptors for dopamine.

Bradykinesia

Bradykinesia refers to slow voluntary movements that are labored, deliberate, and hard to initiate. The patient has difficulty performing movements consecutively

Key facts about lower motor neurons

✦ Two types: small (alpha) and large (gamma)
✦ Extent of paresis correlates to number of large lower motor neurons affected
✦ Maintain muscle tone and protect the muscle from injury

Key facts about motor units

✦ Paresis results from decrease in the number or force of activated muscle fibers in the motor unit
✦ In dysfunction of the neuromuscular junction, functional capability of motor units is lost

Akinesia

✦ Partial or complete loss of voluntary and associated movements and a disturbance in the time needed to perform movement
✦ Dysfunction of the extrapyramidal tract
✦ Associated with dopamine deficiency or receptor dysfunction

Bradykinesia

✦ Slow voluntary movements
✦ Difficulty performing movements consecutively or at same time
✦ Disturbance in time to perform movement

Key facts about loss of associated neurons

✦ Involves alterations in movement accompanying skill, grace, balance

Muscle tone

✦ Involves complex activities controlled by cerebral cortex, pyramidal system, extrapyramidal system, motor units
✦ Slight resistance in response to passive movement
✦ Two major types of altered muscle tone: hypotonia and hypertonia

Key facts about hypotonia

✦ Reflects cerebellar damage; rarely may result from pyramidal tract damage
✦ May involve decrease in muscle spindle activity
✦ Flaccidity generally occurs with loss of nerve impulses for maintaining muscle tone
✦ May be localized or generalized
✦ Flaccid muscles become limp and atrophy

Key facts about hypertonia

✦ Increased resistance to passive movement
✦ Four types: spasticity, paratonia, dystonia, rigidity
✦ Usually leads to atrophy of unused muscles
✦ If motor reflex arc remains functional but uninhibited; overstimulated muscles may hypertrophy

and at the same time. Like akinesia, bradykinesia involves a disturbance in the time needed to perform a movement.

Loss of associated neurons

Movement involves not only the innervation of specific muscles to accomplish an action, but also the work of other innervated muscles that enhance the action. Loss of associated neurons involves alterations in movement that accompany the usual habitual voluntary movements for skill, grace, and balance. For example, when a person expresses emotion, the muscles of the face change and the posture relaxes. Loss of associated neurons involving emotional expression would result in a flat, blank expression and a stiff posture. Loss of associated neurons necessary for locomotion would result in a decrease in arm and shoulder movement, hip swinging, and rotation of the cervical spine.

MUSCLE TONE

Like movement, muscle tone involves complex activities controlled by the cerebral cortex, pyramidal system, extrapyramidal system, and motor units. Normal muscle tone is the slight resistance that occurs in response to passive movement. When one muscle contracts, reciprocal muscles relax to permit movement with only minimal resistance. For example, when the elbow is flexed, the biceps muscle contracts and feels firm and the triceps muscle is somewhat relaxed and soft; with continued flexion, the biceps relax and the triceps contract. Thus, when a joint is moved through range of motion, the resistance is normally smooth, even, and constant.

The two major types of altered muscle tone are hypotonia (decreased muscle tone) and hypertonia (increased muscle tone).

Hypotonia

Hypotonia (also referred to as muscle flaccidity) typically reflects cerebellar damage, but rarely it may result from pure pyramidal tract damage.

Hypotonia is thought to involve a decrease in muscle spindle activity because of a decrease in neuron excitability. Flaccidity generally occurs with loss of nerve impulses from the motor unit responsible for maintaining muscle tone.

It may be localized to a limb or muscle group, or it may be generalized, affecting the entire body. Flaccid muscles can be moved rapidly with little or no resistance; eventually they become limp and atrophy.

Hypertonia

Hypertonia is increased resistance to passive movement, and there are four types:
✦ Spasticity is hyperexcitability of stretch reflexes caused by damage to the lateral corticospinal tract and the motor, premotor, and supplementary motor areas. (See *How spasticity develops.*)
✦ Paratonia (gegenhalten) is variance in resistance to passive movement in direct proportion to the force applied; the cause is frontal lobe injury.
✦ Dystonia is sustained, involuntary twisting movements resulting from slow muscle contraction; the cause is lack of appropriate inhibition of reciprocal muscles.
✦ Rigidity, or constant, involuntary muscle contraction, is resistance in both flexion and extension; the causes are damage to basal ganglion (cog-wheel or lead-pipe rigidity) or loss of cerebral cortex inhibition or cerebellar control (gamma and alpha rigidity).

How spasticity develops

Motor activity is controlled by pyramidal and extrapyramidal tracts that originate in the motor cortex, basal ganglia, brain stem, and spinal cord. Nerve fibers from the various tracts converge and synapse at the anterior horn of the spinal cord. Together they maintain segmental muscle tone by modulating the stretch reflex arc. This arc, shown in a simplified version below, is basically a negative feedback loop in which muscle stretch (stimulation) causes reflexive contraction (inhibition), thus maintaining muscle length and tone.

Damage to certain tracts results in loss of inhibition and disruption of the stretch reflex arc. Uninhibited muscle stretch produces exaggerated, uncontrolled muscle activity, accentuating the reflex arc, and eventually resulting in spasticity.

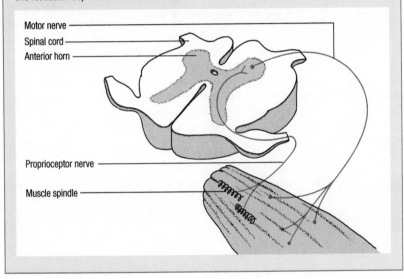

Motor nerve
Spinal cord
Anterior horn

Proprioceptor nerve

Muscle spindle

Spasticity
◆ Stretch reflex arc is made up of motor cortex, basal ganglia, brain stem, and spinal cord
◆ Damage to certain tracts results in loss of inhibition and disruption of stretch reflex arc
◆ Uninhibited stretch produces exaggerated, uncontrolled muscle activity
◆ Spasticity develops

Hypertonia usually leads to atrophy of unused muscles. However, in some cases, if the motor reflex arc remains functional but isn't inhibited by the higher centers, the overstimulated muscles may hypertrophy.

HOMEOSTATIC MECHANISMS

For proper function, the brain must maintain and regulate pressure inside the skull (intracranial pressure [ICP]) as it also maintains the flow of oxygen (O_2) and nutrients to its tissues. Both of these are accomplished by balancing changes in blood flow and cerebrospinal fluid (CSF) volume.

Constriction and dilation of the cerebral blood vessels help to regulate ICP and delivery of nutrients to the brain. These vessels respond to changes in concentrations of carbon dioxide (CO_2), O_2, and hydrogen ions (H^+). For example, if the CO_2 concentration in blood increases, the gas combines with body fluids to form carbonic acid, which eventually releases H^+. An increase in H^+ concentration causes the cerebral vessels to dilate, increasing blood flow to the brain, cerebral perfusion and, subsequently, causing a drop in H^+ concentration. A decrease in O_2 concentration also stimulates cerebral vasodilation, increasing blood flow and O_2 delivery to the brain.

Homeostatic mechanisms
◆ Brain regulates ICP, maintains O_2 and nutrient flow to tissues by balancing changes in blood flow and CSF volume
◆ Constriction and dilation of blood vessels help to regulate ICP
◆ Decrease in O_2 concentration stimulates cerebral vasodilation

Key facts about increased ICP

+ May result from any condition altering normal intracranial component balance
+ Body uses compensatory mechanisms to maintain homeostasis and lower ICP
+ If mechanisms are overwhelmed, ICP continues to rise
+ Cerebral perfusion pressure falls and cerebral blood flow decreases
+ Ischemia leads to cellular hypoxia
+ Vasodilation of cerebral blood vessels causes ICP to increase further
+ Compression of brain tissue and cerebral vessels impairs cerebral blood flow
+ Brain begins to shift under extreme pressure and may herniate
+ Cerebral ischemia and hypoxia worsen

Key facts about cerebral edema

+ Increase in fluid content of brain tissue leading to increase in ICF or ECF volume
+ May result from initial injury to brain tissue or in response to cerebral ischemia, hypoxia, hypercapnia
+ Classified in four types: vasogenic, cytotoxic, ischemic, interstitial

If these normal autoregulatory mechanisms fail, the abnormal blood chemistry stimulates the sympathetic nervous system to cause vasoconstriction of the large and medium-sized cerebral arteries. This helps to prevent increases in blood pressure from reaching the smaller cerebral vessels.

CSF volume remains relatively constant. However, if ICP rises, even as little as 5 mm Hg, the arachnoid villi open and excess CSF drains into the venous system.

The blood-brain barrier also helps to maintain homeostasis in the brain. This barrier is composed of tight junctions between the endothelial cells of the cerebral vessels and neuroglial cells and is relatively impermeable to most substances. However, some substances required for metabolism pass through the blood-brain barrier, depending on their size, solubility, and electrical charge. This barrier also regulates water flow from the blood, thereby helping to maintain the volume within the skull.

Increased ICP

The pressure exerted by the brain tissue, CSF, and cerebral blood (intracranial components) against the skull is ICP. The skull is a rigid structure; therefore, a change in the volume of the intracranial contents triggers a reciprocal change in one or more of the intracranial components to maintain a consistent pressure. Any condition that alters the normal balance of the intracranial components — including increased brain volume, increased blood volume, or increased CSF volume — can increase ICP.

Initially the body uses its compensatory mechanisms (described above) to attempt to maintain homeostasis and lower ICP. However, if these mechanisms become overwhelmed and are no longer effective, ICP continues to rise. Cerebral perfusion pressure falls and cerebral blood flow decreases. Ischemia leads to cellular hypoxia, which initiates vasodilation of cerebral blood vessels in an attempt to increase cerebral blood flow. Unfortunately, this only causes the ICP to increase further. As the pressure continues to rise, compression of brain tissue and cerebral vessels further impairs cerebral blood flow.

If ICP continues to rise, the brain begins to shift under the extreme pressure and may herniate to an area of lesser pressure. When the herniating brain tissue's blood supply is compromised, cerebral ischemia and hypoxia worsen. The herniation increases pressure in the area where the pressure was lower, thus impairing its blood supply. As ICP approaches systemic blood pressure, cerebral perfusion slows even more, ceasing when ICP equals systemic blood pressure. (See *What happens when ICP rises.*)

Cerebral edema

Cerebral edema is an increase in the fluid content of brain tissue that leads to an increase in the intracellular fluid (ICF) or extracellular fluid (ECF) volume. Cerebral edema may result from an initial injury to the brain tissue or it may develop in response to cerebral ischemia, hypoxia, and hypercapnia.

Cerebral edema is classified in four types — vasogenic, cytotoxic, ischemic, or interstitial — depending on the underlying mechanism responsible for the increased fluid content.

+ *Vasogenic* — Injury to the vasculature increases capillary permeability and disruption of blood-brain barrier; leakage of plasma proteins into the extracellular spaces pulls water into the brain parenchyma.
+ *Cytotoxic (metabolic)* — Toxins cause failure of the active transport mechanisms. Loss of intracellular potassium and influx of sodium (and water) cause cells in the brain to swell.

What happens when ICP rises

Intracranial pressure (ICP) is the pressure exerted within the intact skull by the intracranial volume — about 10% blood, 10% cerebrospinal fluid (CSF), and 80% brain tissue. The rigid skull has little space for expansion of these substances.

The brain compensates for increases in ICP by regulating the volume of the three substances in the following ways:

✦ limiting blood flow to the head

✦ displacing CSF into the spinal canal
✦ increasing absorption or decreasing production of CSF — withdrawing water from brain tissue and excreting it through the kidneys.

When compensatory mechanisms become overworked, small changes in volume lead to large changes in pressure. This chart will help you understand the pathophysiology of increased ICP.

What happens when ICP rises

✦ Brain insult
✦ Slight increase in ICP
✦ Attempt at regulation of ICP
✦ Slight increase in cerebral perfusion pressure
✦ Loss of autoregulatory mechanism
✦ Passive dilation
✦ Increased cerebral blood flow, venous congestion
✦ Further increase in ICP
✦ Cellular hypoxia
✦ Uncal or cortical herniation and further increase in ICP
✦ Brain death

BRAIN INSULT

Trauma (contusion, laceration, intracranial hemorrhage)
Cerebral edema (after surgery, stroke, infection, hypoxia)
Hydrocephalus
Space-occupying lesion (tumor, abscess)

↓

Slight increase in ICP

↓

Attempt at normal regulation of ICP: decreased blood flow to head

↓

Slight increase in cerebral perfusion pressure

↓

If ICP remains high: Loss of autoregulatory mechanism
(constriction or dilation of cerebral blood vessels)

↓

Passive dilation

↓

Increased cerebral blood flow, venous congestion

↓

Further increase of ICP

↓

Cellular hypoxia

↓   ↓

Uncal or cortical herniation   Further increase in ICP

↓

Brain death

◆ *Ischemic*—Due to cerebral infarction and initially confined to intracellular compartment; after several days, released lysosomes from necrosed cells disrupt blood-brain barrier.

◆ *Interstitial*—Movement of CSF from ventricles to extracellular spaces increases brain volume.

Regardless of the type of cerebral edema, blood vessels become distorted and brain tissue is displaced, ultimately leading to herniation.

PAIN

Pain is the result of a complex series of steps from a site of injury to the brain, which interprets the stimuli as pain. Pain that originates outside the nervous system is termed nociceptive pain; pain in the nervous system is neurogenic or neuropathic pain.

Nociception

Nociception begins when noxious stimuli reach pain fibers. Sensory receptors called *nociceptors*—which are free nerve endings in the tissues—are stimulated by various agents, such as chemicals, temperature, or mechanical pressure. If a stimulus is sufficiently strong, impulses travel via the afferent nerve fibers along sensory pathways to the spinal cord, where they initiate autonomic and motor reflexes. The information also continues to travel to the brain, which perceives it as pain. Several theories have been developed in an attempt to explain pain. (See *Theories of pain.*)

Nociception consists of four steps: transduction, transmission, modulation, and perception.

Transduction

Transduction is the conversion of noxious stimuli into electrical impulses and subsequent depolarization of the nerve membrane. These electrical impulses are created by algesic substances that sensitize the nociceptors and are released at the site of injury or inflammation. Examples include hydrogen ions and potassium ions, serotonin, histamine, prostaglandins, bradykinin, and substance P.

Transmission

A-delta fibers and C fibers transmit pain sensations from the tissues to the CNS.

A-delta fibers are small diameter, lightly myelinated fibers. Mechanical or thermal stimuli elicit a rapid or fast response. These fibers transmit localized, sharp, stinging, or pinpricking type pain sensations. A-delta fibers connect with secondary neuron groupings on the dorsal horn of the spinal cord.

C fibers are smaller and unmyelinated. They connect with second order neurons in lamina I and II (the latter includes the substantia gelatinosa, an area in which pain is modulated). C fibers respond to chemical stimuli, rather than heat or pressure, triggering a slow pain response, usually within 1 second. This dull ache or burning sensation isn't localized and leads to two responses: an acute response transmitted immediately through fast pain pathways, which prompts the person to evade the stimulus, and lingering pain transmitted through slow pathways, which persists or worsens.

The A-delta and C fibers carry the pain signal from the peripheral tissues to the dorsal horn of the spinal cord. Excitatory and inhibitory interneurons and projection cells (neurons that connect pathways in the cerebral cortex of the CNS and peripheral nervous system) carry the signal to the brain by way of crossed and uncrossed pathways. An example of a crossed pathway is the spinothalamic tract,

---

Pain

◆ Result of complex series of steps from a site of injury to brain
◆ Stimuli interpreted as pain

Nociception

◆ Begins when noxious stimuli reach pain fibers
◆ Nociceptors are stimulated by external agents
◆ If sufficiently strong, impulses travel to spinal cord and initiate autonomic and motor reflexes
◆ Information also goes to brain; perceived as pain
◆ Four steps: transduction, transmission, modulation, perception

Transduction

◆ Conversion of noxious stimuli into electrical impulses and subsequent depolarization of the nerve membrane

Transmission

◆ A-delta and C fibers transmit pain sensations from the tissues to CNS
◆ A-delta fibers transmit localized, sharp, stinging, or pinpricking sensations
◆ C fibers transmit a slow pain response; dull ache isn't localized and leads to acute response or lingering pain
◆ Both fibers carry pain signal to the dorsal horn of spinal cord

Theories of pain

Over the years numerous theories have attempted to explain the sensation of pain and describe how it occurs. This chart highlights some of the major theories about pain.

THEORY	MAJOR ASSUMPTIONS	COMMENT
Specificity	✦ There are four types of cutaneous sensation: touch, warmth, cold, and pain. Each results from stimulation of specific skin receptor sites and neural pathways. ✦ Specific pain neurons transmit pain sensation along specific pain fibers. ✦ At synapses in the substantia gelatinosa, pain impulses cross to the opposite side of the cord and ascend the specific pain pathways of the spinothalamic tract to the thalamus and the pain receptor areas of the cerebral cortex.	✦ Focuses on the direct relationship between the pain stimulus and perception; doesn't account for adaptation to pain and the psychosocial factors modulating it.
Intensity	✦ Pain results from excessive stimulation of sensory receptors. Disorders or processes causing pain create an intense summation of nonnoxious stimuli.	✦ Doesn't explain existence of intense stimuli not perceived as pain.
Pattern	✦ Nonspecific receptors transmit specific patterns (characterized by the length of the pain sensation, the amount of involved tissue, and the summation of impulses) from the skin to the spinal cord, leading to pain perception.	✦ Includes some components of the intensity theory; pain possibly a response to intense stimulation of the sensory receptors regardless of receptor type or pathway.
Neuromatrix	✦ Sensations are imprinted in the brain (a pattern theory). Sensory inputs may trigger a pattern of sensation from the neuromatrix (a proposed network of neurons looping between the thalamus and the cortex, and the cortex and the limbic system). ✦ Sensation pattern is possible without the sensory trigger.	✦ Explains existence of phantom pain.
Gate control	✦ Pain is transmitted from skin via the small diameter A-delta and C fibers to cells of the substantia gelatinosa in the dorsal horn, where interconnections between other sensory pathways exist. Stimulation of the large-diameter, fast, myelinated A-beta and A-alpha fibers closes the gate, which restricts transmission of the impulse to the central nervous system (CNS) and diminishes pain perception.	✦ Provides the basis for use of massage and electrical stimulation in pain management; being used to develop additional theories and models.

(continued)

Theories of pain

✦ Specificity: focuses on direct relationship between pain stimulus and perception
✦ Intensity: doesn't explain existence of intense pain stimuli not perceived as pain
✦ Pattern: pain possibly a response to intense stimulation of the sensory receptors regardless of receptor type or pathway
✦ Neuromatrix: explains existence of phantom pain

Theories of pain
(continued)

✦ Gate control: provides basis for use of massage and electrical stimulation in pain management
✦ Melzak-Casey conceptual model of pain: takes into account the powerful role of psychological functioning in determining quality and intensity of pain

Theories of pain *(continued)*

THEORY	MAJOR ASSUMPTIONS	COMMENT
Gate control *(continued)*	✦ Large-fiber stimulation is possible through massage, scratching or rubbing the skin, or through electrical stimulation. Concurrent firing of pain and touch paths reduces transmission and perception of the pain impulses but not of touch impulses. ✦ An increase in small-fiber activity inhibits the substantia gelatinosa cells, "opening the gate" and increasing pain transmission and perception. ✦ Substantia gelatinosa acts as a gate-control system to inhibit the flow of nerve impulses from peripheral fibers to the CNS. ✦ Central T cells act as a CNS control to stimulate selective brain processes that influence the gate-control system. Inhibition of T cells closes the gate; pain impulses aren't transmitted to the brain. ✦ T cell activation of neural mechanisms in the brain is responsible for pain perception and response; transmitters partly regulate the release of substance P, the peptide that conveys pain information. Pain modulation is also partly controlled by the neurotransmitters, enkephalin and serotonin. ✦ Persistent pain initiates a gradual decline in the fraction of impulses that pass through the various gates. ✦ Descending efferent impulses from the brain may be responsible for closing, partially opening, or completely opening the gate.	
Melzack-Casey Conceptual Model of Pain	✦ Three major psychological dimensions of pain: sensory-discriminative from thalamus and somatosensory cortex, motivational-affective from the reticular formation, and cognitive-evaluative. ✦ Interactions among the three produce descending inhibitory influences that alter pain input to the dorsal horn and ultimately modify the sensory pain experience and motivational-affective dimensions. ✦ Pain is localized and identified by its characteristics, evaluated by past experiences, and undergoes further cognitive processing. The complex sensory, motivational, and cognitive interactions determine motor activities and behaviors associated with the pain experience.	✦ Takes into account the powerful role of psychological functioning in determining the quality and intensity of pain.

which enters the brain stem and ends in the thalamus. Sensory impulses travel from the medial and lateral lemniscus (tract) to the thalamus and brain stem. From the thalamus, other neurons carry the information to the sensory cortex, where pain is perceived and understood.

Another example of a crossed pathway is the ascending spinoreticulothalamic tract, which is responsible for the psychological components of pain and arousal. At this site, neurons synapse with interneurons before they cross to the opposite side of the cord and make their way to the medulla and, eventually, the reticular activating system, mesencephalon, and thalamus. Impulses then are transmitted to the cerebral cortex, limbic system, and basal ganglia.

After stimuli are delivered, responses from the brain must be relayed back to the original site. Several pathways carry the information in the dorsolateral white columns to the dorsal horn of the spinal cord. Some corticospinal tract neurons end in the dorsal horn and allow the brain to pay selective attention to certain stimuli while ignoring others. This allows transmission of the primary signal while suppressing the tendency for signals to spread to adjacent neurons.

Modulation

Modulation refers to modifications in pain transmission. Some neurons from the cerebral cortex and brain stem activate inhibitory processes, thus modifying the transmission. Substances — such as serotonin from the mesencephalon, norepinephrine from the pons, and endorphins from the brain and spinal cord — inhibit pain transmission by decreasing the release of nociceptive neurotransmitters. Spinal reflexes involving motor neurons may initiate a protective action such as withdrawal from a pinprick or may enhance the pain, as when trauma causes a muscle spasm in the injured area.

Perception

Perception is the end result of pain transduction, transmission, and modulation. It encompasses the emotional, sensory, and subjective aspects of the pain experience. Pain perception is thought to occur in the cortical structures of the somatosensory cortex and limbic system. Alertness, arousal, and motivation are believed to result from the action of the reticular activating system and limbic system. Cardiovascular responses and typical fight or flight responses are thought to involve the medulla and hypothalamus.

The following three variables contribute to the wide variety of individual pain experiences:

+ *pain threshold* — level of intensity at which a stimulus is perceived as pain
+ *perceptual dominance* — existence of pain at another location that's given more attention
+ *pain tolerance* — duration or intensity of pain to be endured before a response is initiated.

Neurogenic pain

Neurogenic pain is associated with neural injury. Pain results from spontaneous discharges from the damaged nerves, spontaneous dorsal root activity, or degeneration of modulating mechanisms. Neurogenic pain doesn't activate nociceptors, and there's no typical pathway for transmission.

Modulation

+ Modifications in pain transmission (serotonin, endorphins)
+ Some neurons activate inhibitory processes and modify transmission
+ Spinal reflexes involving motor neurons may initiate a protective action

Perception

+ End result of pain transduction, transmission, and modulation
+ Encompasses emotional, sensory, and subjective aspects of pain experience
+ Occurs in cortical structures of the somatosensory cortex and limbic system
+ Three variables: pain threshold, perceptual dominance, pain tolerance

Neurogenic pain

+ Associated with neural injury
+ Results from spontaneous discharges from damaged nerves, spontaneous dorsal root activity, or degeneration of modulating mechanisms
+ Doesn't activate nociceptors
+ No typical pathway for transmission

Characteristics of Alzheimer's disease

+ Degenerative disorder of cerebral cortex, especially frontal lobe
+ Accounts for more than 50% of dementia cases
+ Found in elderly population
+ Primary progressive dementia has poor prognosis

Causes

+ Exact cause unknown

Neurochemical factors

+ Deficiencies in acetylcholine, somatostatin, substance P, and norepinephrine

Environmental factors

+ Repeated head trauma
+ Exposure to aluminum or manganese

Genetic factors

+ Family history
+ Down syndrome

How it happens

+ Brain tissue exhibits neurofibrillatory tangles, neuritic plaques, granulovascular changes
+ Structural changes: cortical atrophy, ventricular dilation, amyloid deposits around cortical blood vessels, and reduced brain volume

Key signs and symptoms

+ Reflect neurologic abnormalities associated with the disease
+ Loss of memory
+ Flattening of affect and personality
+ Deterioration of personal hygiene
+ Progressive impaired communication

ALZHEIMER'S DISEASE

Alzheimer's disease is a degenerative disorder of the cerebral cortex, especially the frontal lobe, which accounts for more than one-half of dementia cases. Although primarily found in the elderly population, 1% to 10% of cases have their onset in middle age.

Because this is a primary progressive dementia, the prognosis for a patient with this disease is poor.

CAUSES

The exact cause of Alzheimer's disease is unknown. Several factors have been associated with its development. These include *neurochemical* factors, such as deficiencies in the neurotransmitters acetylcholine, somatostatin, substance P, and norepinephrine. *Environmental* factors include repeated head trauma and exposure to aluminum or manganese. *Genetic* factors include the autosomal dominant form of Alzheimer's disease associated with early onset and death, and the established risk factors of a family history of the disease or the presence of Down syndrome in the patient.

PATHOPHYSIOLOGY

The brain tissue of patients with Alzheimer's disease exhibits three distinct and characteristic features. These are neurofibrillatory tangles (fibrous proteins), neuritic plaques (composed of degenerating axons and dendrites), and granulovascular changes.

Additional structural changes include cortical atrophy, ventricular dilation, deposition of amyloid (a glycoprotein) around the cortical blood vessels, and reduced brain volume. Also found is a selective loss of cholinergic neurons in the pathways to the frontal lobes and hippocampus, areas that are important for memory and cognitive functions. Examination of the brain after death commonly reveals an atrophic brain, often weighing less than 1,000 g (normal, 1,380 g).

SIGNS AND SYMPTOMS

The typical signs and symptoms reflect neurologic abnormalities associated with the disease. The patient experiences a gradual loss of recent and remote memory, loss of sense of smell, and flattening of affect and personality. Initially, the patient undergoes imperceptible changes like difficulty with learning new information, the deterioration of personal hygiene, and inability to concentrate.

Gradually, the patient has increasing difficulty with abstraction and judgment. Progressive impaired communication and a severe deterioration in memory, language, and motor function, result in a loss of coordination and an inability to write or speak. Personality changes, wanderings, and nocturnal awakenings are common. Patients also exhibit a loss of eye contact, fearful look, and signs of anxiety such as wringing of hands. The patient experiences acute confusion, agitation, compulsiveness, or fearfulness when overwhelmed with anxiety. Eventually, the patient becomes disoriented, and emotional lability and deterioration of physical and intellectual ability progress.

COMPLICATIONS

The most common complications include injury secondary to violent behavior or wandering, pneumonia and other infections, malnutrition, dehydration, aspiration, and death.

DIAGNOSIS

Alzheimer's disease is diagnosed by exclusion; that is, by ruling out other disorders as the cause for the patient's signs and symptoms. The only true way to confirm Alzheimer's disease is by finding pathological changes in the brain at autopsy. However, the following diagnostic tests may be useful.

Positron emission tomography (PET) scan shows changes in the metabolism of the cerebral cortex. Computed tomography (CT) scan shows evidence of early brain atrophy in excess of that which occurs in normal aging. Magnetic resonance imaging (MRI) shows no lesion as the cause of the dementia. EEG shows evidence of slowed brain waves in the later stages of the disease. Cerebral blood flow studies show abnormalities in blood flow.

TREATMENT

No cure or definitive treatment exists for Alzheimer's disease. Therapy may include cerebral vasodilators, such as ergoloid mesylates, isoxsuprine, and cyclandelate to enhance cerebral circulation. Hyperbaric oxygen is administered to increase oxygenation to the brain. Psychostimulants such as methylphenidate are administered to enhance the patient's mood. Antidepressants are given if depression exacerbates the dementia. Tacrine, an anticholinesterase agent, is given to help improve memory deficits. Choline salts, lecithin, physostigmine, or an experimental agent, such as enkephalins or naloxone, may be administered to possibly slow the disease process.

NURSING CONSIDERATIONS

Overall care is focused on supporting the patient's remaining abilities and compensating for those he has lost.
✦ Establish an effective communication system with the patient and his family to help them adjust to the patient's altered cognitive abilities.
✦ Offer emotional support to the patient and his family. Behavior problems may be worsened by excess stimulation or change in established routine. Teach them about the disease, and refer them to social service and community resources for legal and financial advice and support.
✦ Anxiety may cause the patient to become agitated or fearful. Intervene by helping him focus on another activity.
✦ Provide the patient with a safe environment. Encourage him to exercise, as ordered, to help maintain mobility.

AMYOTROPHIC LATERAL SCLEROSIS

Commonly called *Lou Gehrig disease,* after the New York Yankees first baseman who died of this disorder, amyotrophic lateral sclerosis (ALS) is the most common of the motor neuron diseases causing muscular atrophy. Other motor neuron diseases include progressive muscular atrophy and progressive bulbar palsy. Onset usually occurs between ages 40 and 70. A chronic, progressively debilitating disease, ALS may be fatal in less than 1 year or continue for 10 years or more, depending on

Complications
✦ Injury from violent behavior
✦ Pneumonia and other infections
✦ Malnutrition

Diagnosis
✦ Diagnosed by exclusion
✦ PET scan shows changes in metabolism of cerebral cortex
✦ CT scan shows evidence of early brain atrophy
✦ MRI shows no lesion as cause of dementia

Treatment
✦ No cure or definitive treatment
✦ Cerebral vasodilators
✦ Hyperbaric oxygen
✦ Psychostimulants
✦ Antidepressants

Key nursing actions
✦ Focus on supporting the patient's remaining abilities.
✦ Establish a communication system with the patient and his family.
✦ Provide the patient with a safe environment.

Characteristics of ALS
✦ Also known as *Lou Gehrig disease*
✦ Most common motor neuron disease causing muscular atrophy
✦ Onset between ages 40 and 70
✦ Chronic, progressively debilitating disease
✦ May be fatal in less than 1 year
✦ Affects three times as many men as women

Causes

- Exact cause unknown
- 5% to 10% have autosomal dominant trait

Theories

- Slow-acting virus
- Nutritional deficiency related to enzyme metabolism

How it happens

- Progressively destroys upper and lower motor neurons
- Intellectual and sensory functions aren't affected
- Some think glutamate accumulates to toxic levels at synapses
- Affected motor units no longer innervated
- Progressive degeneration of axons causes loss of myelin
- Nonfunctional scar tissue replaces normal neuronal tissue

Key signs and symptoms

- Fasciculations
- Loss of functioning motor units
- Impaired speech
- Difficulty swallowing and breathing
- Choking

Complications

- Respiratory infections and failure
- Aspiration

Diagnosis

- No tests specific to ALS
- Electromyography shows abnormal electrical activity in involved muscle
- Muscle biopsy shows atrophic fibers between normal fibers
- Nerve conduction studies normal

the muscles affected. More than 30,000 Americans have ALS; about 5,000 new cases are diagnosed each year; and the disease affects three times as many men as women.

CAUSES

The exact cause of ALS is unknown, but about 5% to 10% of cases have a genetic component—an autosomal dominant trait that affects men and women equally.

Several mechanisms have been postulated, including a slow-acting virus, a nutritional deficiency related to a disturbance in enzyme metabolism, a metabolic interference in nucleic acid production by the nerve fibers, and autoimmune disorders that affect immune complexes in the renal glomerulus and basement membrane.

Precipitating factors for acute deterioration include severe stress, such as myocardial infarction, trauma, viral infections, and physical exhaustion.

PATHOPHYSIOLOGY

ALS progressively destroys the upper and lower motor neurons. It doesn't affect cranial nerves III, IV, and VI, and therefore some facial movements, such as blinking, persist. Intellectual and sensory functions aren't affected.

Some believe that glutamate—the primary excitatory neurotransmitter of the central nervous system—accumulates to toxic levels at the synapses. The affected motor units are no longer innervated and progressive degeneration of axons causes loss of myelin. Some nearby motor nerves may sprout axons in an attempt to maintain function but, ultimately, nonfunctional scar tissue replaces normal neuronal tissue.

SIGNS AND SYMPTOMS

Typical signs and symptoms of ALS include fasciculations accompanied by spasticity, atrophy, and weakness, due to degeneration of the upper and lower motor neurons, and loss of functioning motor units, especially in the muscles of the forearms and the hands. Other signs include impaired speech, difficulty chewing and swallowing, choking, and excessive drooling from degeneration of cranial nerves V, IX, X, and XII. The patient has difficulty breathing, especially if the brain stem is affected. Inspection reveals muscle atrophy due to loss of innervation.

Mental deterioration doesn't usually occur, but patients may become depressed as a reaction to the disease. Progressive bulbar palsy may cause crying spells or inappropriate laughter.

COMPLICATIONS

The most common complications include respiratory infections, respiratory failure, aspiration, and complications of physical immobility, such as pressure ulcers and contractures.

DIAGNOSIS

Although no diagnostic tests are specific to ALS, the following may aid in the diagnosis.

Electromyography shows abnormalities of electrical activity in involved muscles. Muscle biopsy shows atrophic fibers interspersed between normal fibers. Nerve conduction studies show normal results. Computed tomography scan and EEG show normal results and thus rule out multiple sclerosis, spinal cord neoplasm, polyarteritis, syringomyelia, myasthenia gravis, progressive muscular dystrophy, and progressive stroke.

TREATMENT

ALS has no cure. Treatment is supportive and may include diazepam, dantrolene, or baclofen for decreasing spasticity, and quinidine to relieve painful muscle cramps. Thyrotropin-releasing hormone (I.V. or intrathecally) is administered to temporarily improve motor function (successful only in some patients). Riluzole may increase quality of life and is administered to modulate glutamate activity and slow disease progression. Respiratory, speech, and physical therapy are scheduled to maintain function as much as possible. Psychological support should be offered to assist with coping with this progressive, fatal illness.

NURSING CONSIDERATIONS

Remember that because mental status remains intact while progressive physical degeneration takes place, the patient acutely perceives every change. This threatens the patient's relationships, career, income, muscle coordination, sexuality, and energy.

✦ Implement a rehabilitation program designed to maintain independence as long as possible.

✦ Help the patient obtain assistive equipment, such as a walker and a wheelchair. Arrange for a visiting nurse to oversee the patient's status, provide support, and teach the family about the illness.

✦ Depending on the patient's muscular capacity, assist with bathing, personal hygiene, and transfers from wheelchair to bed. Help establish a regular bowel and bladder routine.

✦ To help the patient handle an increased accumulation of secretions and dysphagia, teach him to suction himself. He should have a suction machine handy at home to reduce the fear of choking.

✦ To prevent skin breakdown, provide good skin care when the patient is bedridden. Turn him often, keep his skin clean and dry, and use pressure-reducing devices such as an alternating air mattress.

✦ If the patient has trouble swallowing, give him soft, solid foods and position him upright during meals. Gastrostomy or nasogastric tube feedings may be necessary if he can no longer swallow. Teach the family (or the patient if he can still feed himself) how to administer gastrostomy feedings.

✦ Provide emotional support. A discussion of directives regarding health care decisions should be instituted before the patient becomes unable to communicate his wishes. Prepare the patient and family members for his eventual death, and encourage the start of the grieving process. Patients with ALS may benefit from a hospice program or the local ALS support group chapter.

ARTERIOVENOUS MALFORMATIONS

Arteriovenous malformations (AVMs) are tangled masses of thin-walled, dilated blood vessels between arteries and veins that don't connect by capillaries. AVMs are common in the brain, primarily in the posterior portion of the cerebral hemispheres. Abnormal channels between the arterial and venous system mix oxygenat-

Treatment

✦ No cure; treatment supportive
✦ Diazepam
✦ Dantrolene
✦ Baclofen
✦ Quinidine
✦ Thyrotropin-releasing hormone
✦ Riluzole
✦ Respiratory, speech, and physical therapy

Key nursing actions

✦ Implement a rehabilitation program designed to maintain independence as long as possible.
✦ Help the patient obtain assistive equipment.
✦ If necessary, assist the patient with bathing, personal hygiene, and transfers from wheelchair to bed.
✦ Provide good skin care when the patient is bedridden.
✦ If the patient has trouble swallowing, give him soft, solid foods and sit him upright for meals.
✦ Provide emotional support. Prepare the patient and his family members for his eventual death.

Characteristics of AVMs

✦ Tangled masses of thin-walled, dilated blood vessels between arteries and veins
✦ Common in brain
✦ Prevent adequate perfusion of brain tissue
✦ Range in size
✦ More than one commonly present
✦ Males and females affected equally
✦ Most are present at birth
✦ Symptoms typically don't occur until age 10 to 20

Causes
+ May be congenital or acquired from penetrating injuries

How it happens
+ Vessels of AVM very thin; fed by one or more arteries
+ Appear dilated and torturous
+ Aneurysm may develop
+ Shunting can deprive surrounding tissue of adequate blood flow
+ Vessels may ooze blood or rupture into brain or subarachnoid space

Key signs and symptoms
+ Few unless AVM is large, leaks, or ruptures
+ Chronic mild headache and confusion from AVM dilation
+ Seizures
+ Systolic bruit over carotid artery, mastoid process, or orbit
+ Focal neurologic deficits

Complications
+ Depend on severity
+ Aneurysm development or rupture
+ Hemorrhage
+ Hydrocephalus

Diagnosis
+ Cerebral arteriogram confirms presence, evaluates blood flow
+ Doppler ultrasonography indicates abnormal, turbulent blood flow

ed and unoxygenated blood and thereby prevent adequate perfusion of brain tissue.

AVMs range in size from a few millimeters to large malformations extending from the cerebral cortex to the ventricles. Commonly more than one AVM is present. Males and females are affected equally, and some evidence exists that AVMs occur in families. Most AVMs are present at birth; however, symptoms typically don't occur until the person is age 10 to 20.

CAUSES
Causes of AVMs may be congenital, due to a hereditary defect, or acquired from penetrating injuries such as trauma.

PATHOPHYSIOLOGY
AVMs lack the typical structural characteristics of the blood vessels. The vessels of an AVM are very thin; one or more arteries feed into the AVM, causing it to appear dilated and torturous. The typically high-pressured arterial flow moves into the venous system through the connecting channels to increase venous pressure, engorging and dilating the venous structures. An aneurysm may develop. If the AVM is large enough, the shunting can deprive the surrounding tissue of adequate blood flow. Additionally, the thin-walled vessels may ooze small amounts of blood or rupture, causing hemorrhage into the brain or subarachnoid space.

SIGNS AND SYMPTOMS
Typically, the patient experiences few, if any, signs and symptoms unless the AVM is large, leaks, or ruptures. Possible signs and symptoms include chronic mild headache and confusion from AVM dilation, vessel engorgement, and increased pressure. Seizures occur secondary to compression of the surrounding tissues by the engorged vessels. Auscultation reveals systolic bruit over carotid artery, mastoid process, or orbit, indicating turbulent blood flow. Focal neurologic deficits are seen (depending on the location of the AVM) resulting from compression and diminished perfusion.

The patient may report symptoms of intracranial (intracerebral, subarachnoid, or subdural) hemorrhage, including sudden severe headache, seizures, confusion, lethargy, and meningeal irritation from bleeding into the brain tissue or subarachnoid space. The patient may develop hydrocephalus from AVM extension into the ventricular lining.

COMPLICATIONS
Complications depend on the severity (location and size) of the AVM. They include aneurysm development and subsequent rupture, hemorrhage (intracerebral, subarachnoid, or subdural, depending on the location of the AVM), and hydrocephalus.

DIAGNOSIS
Cerebral arteriogram confirms the presence of AVMs and evaluates blood flow. Doppler ultrasonography of the cerebrovascular system indicates abnormal, turbulent blood flow.

TREATMENT

Treatment can be supportive, corrective, or both. Support measures include aneurysm precautions to prevent possible rupture. Surgery options — block dissection, laser, or ligation — are prescribed to repair the communicating channels and remove the feeding vessels. If surgery isn't possible, embolization or radiation therapy is recommended to close the communicating channels and feeder vessels and thus reduce the blood flow to the AVM.

NURSING CONSIDERATIONS

✦ Monitor vital signs frequently.
✦ Control hypertension and seizure activity as well as other activity or stress that could elevate the patient's systemic blood pressure by administering drug therapy as ordered, conducting ongoing neurologic assessments, and maintaining a quiet, therapeutic environment.
✦ If the AVM has ruptured, work to control elevated intracranial pressure (ICP) and intracranial hemorrhage. The patient with a ruptured AVM may have intracerebral or intraventricular bleeding; bleeding into the subarachnoid, subdural, or epidural space; or bleeding into the brain itself, usually causing a concurrent elevation in ICP.

CEREBRAL PALSY

The most common cause of crippling in children, cerebral palsy (CP) is a group of neuromuscular disorders caused by prenatal, perinatal, or postnatal damage to the upper motor neurons. Although nonprogressive, these disorders may become more obvious as an affected infant grows.

The three major types of CP — spastic, athetoid, and ataxic — may occur alone or in combination. Motor impairment may be minimal (sometimes apparent only during physical activities such as running) or severely disabling. Common associated defects are seizures, speech disorders, and mental retardation.

CP occurs in an estimated 7,000 live births every year. Incidence is highest in premature infants (anoxia plays the greatest role in contributing to CP) and in those who are small for gestational age. Almost one-half of the children with CP are mentally retarded, approximately one-fourth have seizure disorders, and more than three-fourths have impaired speech. Additionally, children with CP commonly have dental abnormalities, vision and hearing defects, and reading disabilities.

CP is more common in whites than in other ethnic groups. The prognosis varies. Treatment may make a near-normal life possible for children with mild impairment. Those with severe impairment require special services and schooling.

CAUSES

The exact cause of CP is unknown; however, conditions resulting in cerebral anoxia, hemorrhage, or other central nervous system damage are probably responsible. Potential causes vary with time of damage.

Prenatal causes include maternal infection (especially rubella), exposure to radiation, anoxia, toxemia, maternal diabetes, abnormal placental attachment, malnutrition, and isoimmunization.

Perinatal and birth factors may include forceps delivery, breech presentation, placenta previa, abruptio placentae, depressed maternal vital signs from general or spinal anesthesia, prolapsed cord with delay in blood delivery to the head, prema-

---

Treatment
✦ Supportive therapies
✦ Aneurysm precautions
✦ Surgery
✦ Radiation therapy

Key nursing actions
✦ Monitor vital signs frequently.
✦ Control hypertension and seizure activity.
✦ If the AVM has ruptured, work to control elevated ICP and intracranial hemorrhage.

Characteristics of CP
✦ Most common cause of crippling in children
✦ Group of neuromuscular disorders caused by prenatal, perinatal, or postnatal damage to upper motor neurons
✦ Nonprogressive but may become more obvious with age
✦ Spastic, athetoid, and ataxic
✦ Motor impairment may be minimal or severely disabling
✦ Associated defects: speech disorders, mental retardation, seizures
✦ Occurs in 7,000 live births per year

Causes
✦ Exact cause unknown
✦ Cerebral anoxia, hemorrhage, or CNS damage probably responsible

Prenatal
✦ Maternal infection
✦ Exposure to radiation
✦ Maternal diabetes
✦ Abnormal placental attachment

Perinatal and birth
✦ Forceps delivery
✦ Breech presentation
✦ Premature birth

Causes

Postnatal
- Kernicterus
- Brain infection or tumor
- Head trauma

How it happens

- Lesion or abnormality causes structural or functional defects
- Impaired motor function or cognition results
- Problems may not be apparent until months after birth

Key signs and symptoms

- Excessive lethargy or irritability
- Weak sucking reflex
- Delayed motor development
- Inability to meet major developmental milestones

Complications

- Contractures
- Skin breakdown; ulcer formation
- Muscle atrophy
- Seizure disorders
- Speech, hearing, and vision problems
- Mental retardation

Diagnosis

- No specific diagnostic tests
- Neurologic screening excludes other conditions
- Developmental screening reveals milestone delays
- Vision and hearing screening for degree of impairment

Alert!

- Suspect CP whenever an infant exhibits an alteration in neurologic function during clinical observation.

ture birth, prolonged or unusually rapid labor, multiple births (especially infants born last), and infection or trauma during infancy.

Postnatal causes include kernicterus resulting from erythroblastosis fetalis, brain infection or tumor, head trauma, prolonged anoxia, cerebral circulatory anomalies causing blood vessel rupture, and systemic disease resulting in cerebral thrombosis or embolus.

PATHOPHYSIOLOGY

In the early stages of brain development, a lesion or abnormality causes structural and functional defects that in turn cause impaired motor function or cognition. Even though the defects are present at birth, problems may not be apparent until months later, when the axons have become myelinated and the basal ganglia are mature.

SIGNS AND SYMPTOMS

Shortly after birth, the infant with CP may exhibit some typical signs and symptoms, including excessive lethargy or irritability, high-pitched cry, poor head control, and weak sucking reflex.

Additional physical findings that may suggest CP include delayed motor development and the inability to meet major developmental milestones. Inspection reveals an abnormal head circumference, typically smaller than normal for age (because the head grows as the brain grows). The patient exhibits abnormal postures, such as straightening legs when on back, toes down, and holding his head higher than normal when prone due to arching of back. The patient has abnormal reflexes (neonatal reflexes lasting longer than expected, extreme reflexes, or clonus) and abnormal muscle tone and performance (scooting on back to crawl, toe-first walking).

Each type of CP typically produces a distinctive set of clinical features, although some children display a mixed form of the disease. (See *Assessing signs of cerebral palsy.*)

COMPLICATIONS

Complications depend on the type of CP and the severity of the involvement. Possible complications include contractures; skin breakdown and ulcer formation; muscle atrophy; malnutrition; seizure disorders; speech, hearing, and vision problems; language and perceptual deficits; mental retardation; dental problems; and respiratory difficulties, including aspiration from poor gag and swallowing reflexes.

DIAGNOSIS

No diagnostic tests are specific to CP. However, neurologic screening excludes other possible conditions, such as infection, spina bifida, or muscular dystrophy.

Developmental screening reveals delay in achieving milestones. Vision and hearing screening demonstrates degree of impairment. EEG identifies the source of seizure activity.

CLINICAL ALERT Suspect CP whenever an infant exhibits an alteration in neurologic function during clinical observation. This may include difficulty in sucking or moving voluntarily. Infants particularly at risk include those with a low birth weight, low Apgar score at 5 minutes, seizures, and metabolic disturbances. However, all infants should have a screening test for CP as a regular part of their 6-month checkup.

Assessing signs of cerebral palsy

Each type of cerebral palsy (CP) is manifested by specific signs. This chart highlights the major signs and symptoms associated with each type of CP. The manifestations reflect impaired upper motor neuron function and disruption of the normal stretch reflex.

TYPE OF CEREBRAL PALSY	SIGNS AND SYMPTOMS
Spastic CP (due to impairment of the pyramidal tract [most common type])	◆ Hyperactive deep tendon reflexes ◆ Increased stretch reflexes ◆ Rapid alternating muscle contraction and relaxation ◆ Muscle weakness ◆ Underdevelopment of affected limbs ◆ Muscle contraction in response to manipulation ◆ Tendency toward contractures ◆ Walking on toes with a scissors gait, crossing one foot in front of the other
Athetoid CP (due to impairment of the extrapyramidal tract)	◆ Involuntary movements usually affecting arms more severely than legs, including: – grimacing – wormlike writhing – dystonia – sharp jerks ◆ Difficulty with speech due to involuntary facial movements ◆ Increasing severity of movements during stress; decreased with relaxation and disappearing entirely during sleep
Ataxic CP (due to impairment of the extrapyramidal tract)	◆ Disturbed balance ◆ Incoordination (especially of the arms) ◆ Hypoactive reflexes ◆ Nystagmus ◆ Muscle weakness ◆ Tremor ◆ Lack of leg movement during infancy ◆ Wide gait as the child begins to walk ◆ Sudden or fine movements impossible (due to ataxia)
Mixed CP	◆ Spasticity and athetoid movements ◆ Ataxic and athetoid movements (resulting in severe impairment)

Assessing signs of CP
Spastic CP
✦ Hyperactive deep tendon reflexes
✦ Rapid muscle contractions and weakness
✦ Walking on toes with scissors gate

Athetoid CP
✦ Involuntary movements
✦ Speech difficulties

Ataxic CP
✦ Disturbed balance
✦ Incoordination
✦ Hypoactive reflex

Mixed CP
✦ Characteristics of multiple types

TREATMENT

CP can't be cured, but proper treatment can help affected children reach their full potential within the limits set by this disorder. Such treatment requires a comprehensive and cooperative effort, involving physicians, nurses, teachers, psychologists, the child's family, and occupational, physical, and speech therapists. Home care is usually possible.

Treatment typically includes braces, casts, or splints and special appliances, such as adapted eating utensils and a low toilet seat with arms, to help the child perform activities of daily living independently.

An artificial urinary sphincter may be indicated for the incontinent child who can use the hand controls. Range-of-motion (ROM) exercises minimize contrac-

Treatment
✦ No cure
✦ Home care usually possible
✦ Braces, casts, or splints
✦ Special appliances
✦ Artificial urinary sphincter
✦ ROM exercises
✦ Muscle relaxants
✦ Surgery
✦ Rehabilitation

tures and anticonvulsants control seizures. Muscle relaxants may be used (sometimes) to reduce spasticity. Surgery may be indicated to decrease spasticity or correct contractures. Muscle transfer or tendon lengthening surgery may also be indicated to improve function of joints.

Rehabilitation, including occupational, physical, and speech therapy, maintains or improves functional abilities.

NURSING CONSIDERATIONS

A child with CP may be hospitalized for surgery or treatment of complications.

✦ Speak slowly and distinctly. Encourage the child to ask for things he wants. Listen patiently and don't rush him.
✦ Plan a high-calorie diet that's adequate to meet the child's high energy needs.
✦ During meals, maintain a quiet, unhurried atmosphere with as few distractions as possible. The child should be encouraged to feed himself and may need special utensils and a chair with a solid footrest. Teach him to place food far back in his mouth to facilitate swallowing.
✦ Encourage the child to chew food thoroughly, drink through a straw, and suck on lollipops to develop the muscle control needed to minimize drooling.
✦ Allow the child to wash and dress independently, assisting only as needed. The child may need clothing modifications.
✦ Give all care in an unhurried manner; otherwise, muscle spasticity may increase.
✦ Encourage the child and his family to participate in the care plan so they can continue it at home.
✦ Care for associated hearing or vision disturbances, as necessary.
✦ Give frequent mouth and dental care, as necessary.
✦ Reduce muscle spasms that increase postoperative pain by moving and turning the child carefully after surgery; provide analgesics as needed.
✦ After orthopedic surgery, provide good cast care. Wash and dry the skin at the edge of the cast frequently. Reposition the child often, check for foul odor, and ventilate under the cast with a cool-air blow-dryer. Use a flashlight to check for skin breakdown beneath the cast. Help the child relax, perhaps by giving a warm bath, before reapplying a bivalved cast.

To help the parents
✦ Encourage them to set realistic individual goals.
✦ Assist in planning crafts and other activities.
✦ Stress the child's need to develop peer relationships; warn the parents against being overprotective.
✦ Identify and deal with family stress. The parents may feel unreasonable guilt about their child's disability and may need psychological counseling.
✦ Refer the parents to supportive community organizations. For more information, tell them to contact the United Cerebral Palsy Association or their local chapter.

CREUTZFELDT-JAKOB DISEASE

Creutzfeldt-Jakob disease (CJD) is a rare, rapidly-progressive viral disease that attacks the central nervous system (CNS), causing dementia and neurologic signs and symptoms, such as myoclonic jerking, ataxia, aphasia, visual disturbances, and paralysis. It generally affects adults ages 40 to 65 and occurs in more than 50 countries. Males and females are affected equally. CJD is always fatal. A new variant of CJD (vCJD) emerged in Europe in 1996. (See *Understanding vCJD*.)

Key nursing actions
✦ Speak slowly and distinctly. Encourage the child to ask for things he wants.
✦ Plan a high-calorie diet that's adequate to meet the child's high energy needs.
✦ During meals, maintain a quiet, unhurried atmosphere with as few distractions as possible.
✦ Teach him to place food far back in his mouth to facilitate swallowing.
✦ Encourage the child to chew food thoroughly, drink through a straw, and suck on lollipops to develop the muscle control needed to minimize drooling.
✦ Give all care in an unhurried manner; otherwise, muscle spasticity may increase.
✦ After orthopedic surgery, provide good cast care.

Helping parents
✦ Encourage them to set realistic individual goals.
✦ Assist in planning crafts and other activities.
✦ Stress the child's need to develop peer relationships.
✦ Refer the parents to supportive community organizations.

Characteristics of CJD
✦ Rare, rapidly progressive viral disease that attacks CNS
✦ Causes dementia and neurologic signs and symptoms
✦ Generally affects adults ages 40 to 65; occurs in more than 50 countries
✦ Always fatal

Understanding vCJD

As with conventional Creutzfeldt-Jakob disease (CJD), the new variant of the disease (vCJD) is a rare, fatal neurodegenerative disease. Most cases have been reported in the United Kingdom. Researchers believe vCJD is most likely caused by exposure to bovine spongiform encephalopathy (BSE) — fatal brain disease in cattle also known as *mad cow disease* — via ingestion of beef products from cattle with BSE.

The disease affects patients at a much younger age (younger than age 55) than conventional CJD, and the duration of the illness is much longer (14 months).

Regulations have been established in Europe to control outbreaks of BSE in cattle and to prevent contaminated meat from entering the food supply. The Centers for Disease Control and Prevention and the World Health Organization are still exploring vCJD and its relationship to BSE.

CAUSES

The causative organism is difficult to identify because no foreign ribonucleic acid (RNA) or deoxyribonucleic acid (DNA) has been linked to the disease. Most cases are sporadic; 5% to 15% are familial, with an autosomal dominant pattern of inheritance. Although CJD isn't transmitted by normal casual contact, human-to-human transmission can occur as a result of certain medical procedures, such as corneal and cadaveric dura mater grafts. Isolated cases are attributed to treatment during childhood with human growth hormone and to improperly decontaminated neurosurgical instruments and brain electrodes.

PATHOPHYSIOLOGY

CJD is believed to be caused by a specific protein called a *prion*. These modified proteins are resistant to proteolytic digestion and aggregate in the brain to produce rodlike particles. The accumulation of these modified cellular proteins results in neuronal degeneration and spongiform changes in brain tissue.

SIGNS AND SYMPTOMS

Early signs and symptoms of mental impairment may include slowness in thinking, difficulty concentrating, impaired judgment, and memory loss. Dementia is progressive and occurs early. With disease progression and mental deterioration, involuntary movements, such as muscle twitching, trembling, and peculiar body movements, and vision disturbances appear. Hallucinations are also common. Duration of the typical illness is 4 months.

COMPLICATIONS

Complications may include severe, progressive dementia, CNS abnormalities, and death.

DIAGNOSIS

CJD must be considered for anyone experiencing signs of progressive dementia. Neurologic examination is the most effective tool in diagnosing CJD. Difficulty with rapid alternating movements and point-to-point movements are typically evident early in the disease.

Causes
+ No foreign RNA or DNA linked to disease; most cases sporadic
+ 5% to 15% familial, with autosomal dominant inheritance
+ Can occur from medical procedures
+ Isolated cases attributed to human growth hormone, improperly decontaminated instruments, brain electrodes

How it happens
+ Believed to be caused by a prion resistant to proteolytic digestion and aggregate in brain
+ Accumulation of modified cellular proteins causes neuronal degeneration and spongiform changes in brain

Key signs and symptoms
+ Slowness in thinking
+ Difficulty concentrating
+ Impaired judgment
+ Memory loss
+ Progressive dementia
+ Involuntary movements
+ Typical illness duration is 4 months

Complications
+ Severe, progressive dementia
+ CNS abnormalities
+ Death

Diagnosis
+ Considered for anyone experiencing signs of progressive dementia
+ Neurologic examination
+ Difficulty with rapid alternating movements
+ EEG may show changes in brain wave activity

Treatment

+ No cure; progress can't be slowed
+ Palliative care provided

Key nursing actions

+ Offer emotional support to the patient and his family.
+ Contact social services and hospice, as appropriate, to assist the family with their needs.
+ Encourage the patient and his family to discuss and complete an advance directive.

Alert!

+ To prevent disease transmission, use caution when handling body fluids from patients suspected of having CJD.

Characteristics of Guillain-Barré syndrome

+ Life-threatening disorder
+ Acute, rapidly progressive, potentially fatal form of polyneuritis
+ Occurs most commonly between ages 30 and 50
+ Affects both genders equally
+ Recovery spontaneous and complete in about 95% of patients
+ Occurs in three phases: acute, plateau, recovery

Causes

+ Precise cause unknown
+ May be cell-mediated immune response to virus
+ 50% of patients have recent history of minor febrile illness
+ Signs of infection subside before neurologic features appear

---

An EEG may also be performed to assess the patient for typical changes in brain wave activity. Computed tomography scan, magnetic resonance imaging of the brain, and lumbar puncture may be useful in ruling out other disorders that cause dementia. Definitive diagnosis isn't usually obtained until an autopsy is done and brain tissue is examined.

TREATMENT

No cure has been found for CJD, and its progress can't be slowed. Palliative care is provided to make the patient comfortable and to ease symptoms.

NURSING CONSIDERATIONS

+ Offer emotional support to the patient and his family. Teach them about the disease, and assist them through the grieving process. Refer the patient and his family to CJD support groups, and encourage participation.
+ Contact social services and hospice, as appropriate, to assist the family with their needs.
+ Encourage the patient and his family to discuss and complete an advance directive.

 CLINICAL ALERT To prevent disease transmission, use caution when handling body fluids and other materials from patients suspected of having CJD.

▼ *LIFE-THREATENING DISORDER*

GUILLAIN-BARRÉ SYNDROME

Also known as *infectious polyneuritis, Landry's syndrome,* or *acute idiopathic polyneuritis,* Guillain-Barré syndrome is an acute, rapidly progressive, and potentially fatal form of polyneuritis that causes muscle weakness and mild distal sensory loss.

This syndrome can occur at any age but is most common between ages 30 and 50. It affects both sexes equally. Recovery is spontaneous and complete in about 95% of patients, although mild motor or reflex deficits may persist in the feet and legs. The prognosis is best when symptoms clear within 20 days after onset.

This syndrome occurs in three phases. The *acute* phase begins with the onset of the first definitive symptom and ends 1 to 3 weeks later. Further deterioration doesn't occur after the acute phase. The *plateau* phase lasts several days to 2 weeks. The *recovery* phase is believed to coincide with remyelinization and regrowth of axonal processes. It extends over 4 to 6 months, but may last up to 3 years if the disease is severe.

CAUSES

The precise cause of Guillain-Barré syndrome is unknown, but it may be a cell-mediated immune response to a virus.

About 50% of patients with Guillain-Barré syndrome have a recent history of minor febrile illness, usually an upper respiratory tract infection or, less commonly, gastroenteritis. When infection precedes the onset of Guillain-Barré syndrome, signs of infection subside before neurologic features appear.

Other possible precipitating factors include surgery, rabies or swine influenza vaccination, Hodgkin's or other malignant disease, and systemic lupus erythematosus.

PATHOPHYSIOLOGY

The major pathologic manifestation is segmental demyelination of the peripheral nerves. This prevents normal transmission of electrical impulses along the sensorimotor nerve roots. Because this syndrome causes inflammation and degenerative changes in both the posterior (sensory) and the anterior (motor) nerve roots, signs of sensory and motor losses occur simultaneously. (See *Understanding sensorimotor nerve degeneration,* page 302.) Additionally, autonomic nerve transmission may be impaired.

SIGNS AND SYMPTOMS

Symptoms are progressive and include symmetrical muscle weakness (major neurologic sign) appearing in the legs first (ascending type) and then extending to the arms and facial nerves within 24 to 72 hours, from impaired anterior nerve root transmission. Muscle weakness develops in the arms first (descending type) or in the arms and legs simultaneously, from impaired anterior nerve root transmission. In milder forms of the disease, muscle weakness is absent or affects only the cranial nerves. Another common neurologic sign is paresthesia, sometimes preceding muscle weakness but vanishing quickly, from impairment of the dorsal nerve root transmission. Other clinical features may include diplegia, possibly with ophthalmoplegia (ocular paralysis), from impaired motor nerve root transmission and involvement of cranial nerves III, IV, and VI, dysphagia or dysarthria and, less commonly, weakness of the muscles supplied by cranial nerve XI (spinal accessory nerve). Hypotonia and areflexia occur from interruption of the reflex arc.

COMPLICATIONS

Because of the patient's inability to use his muscles, complications can occur. Common complications include thrombophlebitis, pressure ulcers, muscle wasting, sepsis, joint contractures, aspiration, respiratory tract infections, mechanical respiratory failure, sinus tachycardia or bradycardia, hypertension and orthostatic hypotension, and loss of bladder and bowel sphincter control.

DIAGNOSIS

Cerebrospinal fluid (CSF) analysis by lumbar puncture reveals elevated protein levels, peaking in 4 to 6 weeks, probably as a result of widespread inflammation of the nerve roots; the CSF white blood cell count remains normal, but in severe disease, CSF pressure may rise above normal.

Complete blood count shows leukocytosis with immature forms early in the illness, and then quickly returns to normal. Electromyography possibly shows repeated firing of the same motor unit, instead of widespread sectional stimulation. Nerve conduction velocities show slowing soon after paralysis develops. Serum immunoglobulin levels reveal elevated levels from inflammatory response.

TREATMENT

Primarily supportive, treatments include endotracheal (ET) intubation or tracheotomy if respiratory muscle involvement causes difficulty in clearing secretions.

A trial dose (7 days) of prednisone is given to reduce inflammatory response if the disease is relentlessly progressive; if prednisone produces no noticeable improvement, the drug is discontinued.

Plasmapheresis is useful during the initial phase but of no benefit if begun 2 weeks after onset.

How it happens

+ Segmental demyelination of peripheral nerves
+ Simultaneous sensory and motor losses
+ Autonomic nerve transmission impairment

Key signs and symptoms

+ Symmetrical muscle weakness
+ Paresthesia
+ Diplegia
+ Ophthalmoplegia
+ Hypotonia

Complications

+ Thrombophlebitis
+ Pressure ulcers
+ Muscle wasting
+ Sepsis
+ Joint contractures
+ Respiratory tract infections

Diagnosis

+ CSF analysis by lumbar puncture reveals elevated protein levels
+ Electromyography possibly shows repeated firing of same motor unit
+ Nerve conduction velocities show slowing
+ Serum immunoglobulin levels elevated

Treatment

+ Primarily supportive
+ ET intubation or tracheotomy
+ Prednisone
+ Plasmapheresis
+ Propranolol

Sensorimotor nerve degeneration

✦ Myelin sheath degenerates, causing inflammation, swelling, and patchy demyelination
✦ Nodes of Ranvier widen, delaying and impairing transmission
✦ Patient may experience tingling and numbness

Key nursing actions

✦ Watch for ascending sensory loss, which precedes motor loss.
✦ Assess and treat respiratory dysfunction.
✦ Because neuromuscular disease results in primary hypoventilation with hypoxemia and hypercapnia, watch for partial Pao_2 below 70 mm Hg, which signals respiratory failure.
✦ Auscultate breath sounds, turn and position the patient, and encourage coughing and deep breathing.
✦ If respiratory failure is imminent, establish an emergency airway with an ET tube.
✦ Give meticulous skin care to prevent skin breakdown and contractures. Establish a strict turning schedule.
✦ Perform passive ROM exercises within the patient's pain limits.

CLOSER LOOK

Understanding sensorimotor nerve degeneration

Guillain-Barré syndrome attacks the peripheral nerves so that they can't transmit messages to the brain correctly.

WHAT GOES WRONG

The myelin sheath degenerates for unknown reasons. This sheath covers the nerve axons and conducts electrical impulses along the nerve pathways. Degeneration brings inflammation, swelling, and patchy demyelination. As this disorder destroys myelin, the nodes of Ranvier (at the junction of the myelin sheaths) widen. This delays and impairs impulse transmission along the dorsal and anterior nerve roots.

Because the dorsal nerve roots handle sensory function, the patient may experience tingling and numbness. Similarly, because the anterior nerve roots are responsible for motor function, impairment causes varying weakness, immobility, and paralysis.

Continuous electrocardiogram monitoring alerts for possible arrhythmias from autonomic dysfunction; propranolol treats tachycardia and hypertension, atropine treats bradycardia; and volume replacement is required for severe hypotension.

NURSING CONSIDERATIONS

Monitoring the patient for escalation of symptoms is of special concern.
✦ Watch for ascending sensory loss, which precedes motor loss. Also, monitor vital signs and level of consciousness.
✦ Assess and treat respiratory dysfunction. If respiratory muscles are weak, take serial vital capacity recordings. Use a respirometer with a mouthpiece or a face mask for bedside testing.
✦ Obtain arterial blood gas measurements. Because neuromuscular disease results in primary hypoventilation with hypoxemia and hypercapnia, watch for partial pressure of arterial oxygen (Pao_2) below 70 mm Hg, which signals respiratory failure. Be alert for signs of rising partial pressure of arterial carbon dioxide (confusion, tachypnea).
✦ Auscultate breath sounds, turn and position the patient, and encourage coughing and deep breathing. Begin respiratory support at the first sign of dyspnea (in adults, vital capacity less than 800 ml; in children, less than 12 ml/kg body weight) or with decreasing Pao_2.
✦ If respiratory failure is imminent, establish an emergency airway with an ET tube.
✦ Give meticulous skin care to prevent skin breakdown and contractures. Establish a strict turning schedule; inspect the skin (especially sacrum, heels, and ankles) for breakdown, and reposition the patient every 2 hours. After each position change, stimulate circulation by carefully massaging pressure points. Also, use foam, gel, or alternating pressure pads at points of contact.
✦ Perform passive ROM exercises within the patient's pain limits, perhaps using a Hubbard tank. (Although this disease doesn't produce pain, exercising little-used muscles will.) Remember that the proximal muscle group of the thighs, shoulders, and trunk will be the most tender and will cause the most pain on passive movement and turning. When the patient's condition stabilizes, change to gentle stretching and active assistance exercises.

✦ To prevent aspiration, test the gag reflex, and elevate the head of the bed before giving the patient anything to eat. If the gag reflex is absent, give nasogastric feedings until this reflex returns.

✦ As the patient regains strength and can tolerate a vertical position, be alert for orthostatic hypotension. Monitor his blood pressure and pulse during tilting periods and, if necessary, apply toe-to-groin elastic bandages or an abdominal binder to prevent orthostatic hypotension.

✦ If the patient has severe paralysis and is expected to have a long recovery period, a gastrostomy tube may be necessary to provide adequate nourishment.

✦ Inspect the patient's legs regularly for signs of thrombophlebitis (localized pain, tenderness, erythema, edema, and positive Homans' sign), a common complication of Guillain-Barré syndrome. To prevent thrombophlebitis, apply antiembolism stockings and give prophylactic anticoagulants, as ordered.

✦ If the patient has facial paralysis, give eye and mouth care every 4 hours. Protect the corneas with isotonic eye drops and conical eye shields.

✦ Watch for urine retention. Measure and record intake and output every 8 hours, and offer the bedpan every 3 to 4 hours. Encourage adequate fluid intake of 2 qt (2 L)/day, unless contraindicated. If urine retention develops, begin intermittent catheterization, as ordered. Because the abdominal muscles are weak, the patient may need manual pressure on the bladder (Credé's method) before he can urinate.

✦ To prevent and relieve constipation, offer prune juice and a high-bulk diet. If necessary, give daily or alternate-day suppositories (glycerin or bisacodyl) or enemas, as ordered.

✦ Before discharge, prepare a home care plan. Teach the patient how to transfer from bed to wheelchair, from wheelchair to toilet or tub, and how to walk short distances with a walker or a cane. Teach the family how to help him eat, compensating for facial weakness and how to help him avoid skin breakdown. Stress the need for a regular bowel and bladder routine. Refer the patient for physical therapy as needed.

HEADACHE

The most common patient complaint, headache usually occurs as a symptom of an underlying disorder. Ninety percent of all headaches are vascular, muscle contraction, or a combination; 10% are due to underlying intracranial, systemic, or psychological disorders. Migraine headaches, probably the most intensely studied, are throbbing, vascular headaches that usually begin to appear in childhood or adolescence and recur throughout adulthood. Affecting up to 10% of Americans, they're more common in females and have a strong familial incidence.

CAUSES

Most chronic headaches result from tension (muscle contraction), which may be caused by emotional stress or fatigue, menstruation, and environmental stimuli (noise, crowds, or bright lights).

Other possible causes include glaucoma; inflammation of the eyes or mucosa of the nasal or paranasal sinuses; diseases of the scalp, teeth, extracranial arteries, or external or middle ear; vasodilators (nitrates, alcohol, and histamine); systemic disease; hypertension; increased intracranial pressure (ICP); head trauma or tumor; and intracranial bleeding, abscess, or aneurysm.

Characteristics of headache

✦ Usually occurs as a symptom of an underlying disorder

✦ 90% are vascular, muscle contraction, or combination

✦ 10% due to underlying intracranial, systemic, psychological disorders

Migraine headaches

✦ Throbbing, vascular headaches

✦ Begin in childhood and recur throughout adulthood

✦ More common in females

✦ Strong familial incidence

Causes

✦ Tension

✦ Glaucoma

✦ Inflammation of eyes or nasal or paranasal sinus mucosa

✦ Diseases of scalp, teeth, extracranial arteries, external or middle ear

✦ Vasodilators

✦ Systemic disease

✦ Head trauma or tumor

✦ Intracranial bleeding, abscess, or aneurysm

How it happens

+ Associated with constriction and dilation of intracranial and extracranial arteries
+ During migraine, biochemical abnormalities thought to occur
+ Pain may emanate from skin, scalp, muscles, arteries, and veins; cranial nerves V, VII, IX, and X; or cervical nerves 1, 2, and 3

4 headache phases

+ Normal
+ Vasoconstriction (aura)
+ Parenchymal artery dilation
+ Vasodilation (headache)

Key signs and symptoms

Migraine
+ Initially produces unilateral, pulsating pain; later more generalized
+ Preceded by a scintillating scotoma, hemianopsia, unilateral paresthesia, or speech disorders
+ Patient may experience irritability, anorexia, nausea, vomiting, and photophobia

Muscle contraction and traction-inflammatory vascular headaches
+ Produce dull, persistent ache
+ Tender spots on head and neck
+ Feeling of tightness around head
+ "Hat-band" distribution
+ Pain severe and unrelenting
+ May result in neurologic deficits if caused by bleeding
+ If caused by tumor, pain most severe when patient awakens

Complications

+ Misdiagnosis
+ Status migraines
+ Drug dependence

PATHOPHYSIOLOGY

Headaches are believed to be associated with constriction and dilation of intracranial and extracranial arteries. During a migraine attack, certain biochemical abnormalities, including local leakage of a vasodilator polypeptide called neurokinin through the dilated arteries and a decrease in the plasma level of serotonin are thought to occur.

Headache pain may emanate from the pain-sensitive structures of the skin, scalp, muscles, arteries, and veins; cranial nerves V, VII, IX, and X; or cervical nerves 1, 2, and 3. Intracranial mechanisms of headaches include traction or displacement of arteries, venous sinuses, or venous tributaries and inflammation or direct pressure on the cranial nerves with afferent pain fibers.

Four headache phases

The evolution of a headache has four distinct phases.
+ *Normal*—Cerebral and temporal arteries are innervated extracranially; parenchymal arteries are noninnervated.
+ *Vasoconstriction (aura)*—Stress-related neurogenic local vasoconstriction of innervated cerebral arteries reduces cerebral blood flow (localized ischemia). Systematically, the prostaglandin thromboxane causes increased platelet aggregation and release of serotonin, a potent vasoconstrictor and, possibly, other vasoactive substances.
+ *Parenchymal artery dilation*—Noninnervated parenchymal vessels dilate in response to local acidosis and anoxia (ischemia). Neurogenic or biologic factors may cause preformed arteriovenous shunts to open. Increased blood flow, increased internal pressure, and enhanced pulsations short-circuit the normal nutritive capillaries and cause pain.
+ *Vasodilation (headache)*—Compensatory mechanisms cause marked vasodilation of the innervated arteries resulting in headache. Systemic platelet aggregation decreases, and falling serotonin levels result in vasodilation. A painful, sterile perivascular inflammation develops and persists into a postheadache phase.

SIGNS AND SYMPTOMS

Initially, migraine headaches usually produce unilateral, pulsating pain, which later becomes more generalized. They're commonly preceded by a scintillating scotoma, hemianopsia, unilateral paresthesia, or speech disorders. The patient may experience irritability, anorexia, nausea, vomiting, and photophobia. (See *Clinical features of migraine headaches*.)

Both muscle contraction and traction-inflammatory vascular headaches produce a dull, persistent ache, tender spots on the head and neck, and a feeling of tightness around the head, with a characteristic "hat-band" distribution. The pain is typically severe and unrelenting. If caused by intracranial bleeding, headache may result in neurologic deficits, such as paresthesia and muscle weakness; opioids may fail to relieve pain in these cases. If caused by a tumor, pain is most severe when the patient awakens.

COMPLICATIONS

Complications may include misdiagnosis, status migraines, drug dependence, disruption of lifestyle, and worsening of existing hypertension.

Clinical features of migraine headaches

TYPE	SIGNS AND SYMPTOMS
Common migraine (most prevalent)	
Usually occurs on weekends and holidays	✦ Prodromal symptoms, including fatigue, nausea, vomiting, and fluid imbalance, that precede headache by about 1 day ✦ Sensitivity to light and noise (most prominent feature) ✦ Headache pain (unilateral or bilateral, aching or throbbing)
Classic migraine	
Usually occurs in compulsive personalities and within families	✦ Prodromal symptoms, including vision disturbances, such as zigzag lines and bright lights (most common), sensory disturbances (tingling of face, lips, and hands), or motor disturbances (staggering gait) ✦ Recurrent, periodic headaches
Hemiplegic and ophthalmoplegic migraine (rare)	
Usually occurs in young adults	✦ Severe, unilateral pain ✦ Extraocular muscle palsies (involving third cranial nerve) and ptosis ✦ With repeated headaches, possible permanent third cranial nerve injury ✦ In hemiplegic migraine, neurologic deficits (hemiparesis, hemiplegia) that may persist after headache subsides
Basilar artery migraine	
Occurs in young women before menses	✦ Prodromal symptoms, including partial vision loss followed by vertigo, ataxia, dysarthria, tinnitus and, sometimes, tingling of fingers and toes that lasts from several minutes to almost an hour ✦ Headache pain, severe occipital throbbing, vomiting

DIAGNOSIS

Diagnosis requires a history of recurrent headaches and physical examination of the head and neck. Such examination includes percussion, auscultation for bruits, inspection for signs of infection, and palpation for defects, crepitus, or tender spots (especially after trauma). Definitive diagnosis also requires a complete neurologic examination, assessment for other systemic diseases, and a psychosocial evaluation when such factors are suspected.

Diagnostic tests include cervical spine and sinus X-rays, EEG, computed tomography scan — performed before lumbar puncture to rule out increased ICP — or magnetic resonance imaging. A lumbar puncture isn't done if there's evidence of increased ICP or if a brain tumor is suspected because rapidly reducing pressure by removing spinal fluid can cause brain herniation.

TREATMENT

Depending on the type of headache, analgesics — ranging from aspirin to codeine or meperidine — may provide symptomatic relief. Other measures include identifi-

Clinical features of migraine

Common
✦ Prodromal symptoms, light and noise sensitivity, headache pain

Classic
✦ Prodromal symptoms; recurrent, periodic headache

Hemiplegic and ophthalmoplegic
✦ Severe pain
✦ Extraocular muscle palsies
✦ Possible nerve injury
✦ Neurologic deficits

Basilar artery
✦ Prodromal symptoms
✦ Headache pain
✦ Nausea and vomiting
✦ Occipital throbbing

Diagnosis
✦ Requires history of recurrent headaches
✦ Physical examination
✦ Complete neurologic examination
✦ Assessment for systemic diseases, psychosocial evaluation
✦ Cervical spine and sinus X-rays

Treatment
✦ Analgesics
✦ Identification and elimination of causative factors
✦ Psychotherapy
✦ Muscle relaxants

Treatment

Migraine
+ Ergotamine alone or with caffeine
+ Metoclopramide
+ Naproxen
+ Sumatriptan drugs
+ Preventative drugs

Key nursing actions
+ Headaches seldom require hospitalization unless caused by a serious disorder.
+ Obtain complete patient history.
+ Using the history as a guide, help the patient avoid exacerbating factors.
+ Instruct the patient to take the prescribed medication at the onset of migraine symptoms.
+ The patient with a migraine headache usually needs to be hospitalized only if nausea and vomiting are severe enough to induce dehydration and possible shock.

Characteristics of head trauma
+ Life-threatening disorder
+ Any traumatic insult to brain causing physical, intellectual, emotional, social, vocational changes
+ Children 6 months to 2 years, people 15 to 24, and elderly people are at highest risk
+ Generally categorized as closed or open trauma
+ Mortality has declined with advances
+ Technology has increased effectiveness of rehabilitation

cation and elimination of causative factors and, possibly, psychotherapy for headaches caused by emotional stress. Chronic tension headaches may also require muscle relaxants.

For migraine headaches, ergotamine alone or with caffeine may be an effective treatment. Remember that these medications can't be taken by pregnant women because they stimulate uterine contractions. These drugs and others, such as metoclopramide or naproxen, work best when taken early in the course of an attack. If nausea and vomiting make oral administration impossible, drugs may be given as rectal suppositories.

Drugs in the class of sumatriptan are considered by many clinicians to be the drug of choice for acute migraine attacks or cluster headaches. Drugs that can help prevent migraine headaches include propranolol, atenolol, clonidine, and amitriptyline.

NURSING CONSIDERATIONS

Headaches seldom require hospitalization unless caused by a serious disorder. If that's the case, direct your care to the underlying problem.
+ Obtain a complete patient history, including duration and location of the headache, time of day it usually begins, nature of the pain, concurrence with other symptoms such as blurred vision, medications taken such as oral contraceptives, prolonged fasting, and precipitating factors, such as tension, menstruation, loud noises, menopause, or alcohol. Exacerbating factors can also be assessed through ongoing observation of the patient's personality, habits, activities of daily living, family relationships, coping mechanisms, and relaxation activities.
+ Using the history as a guide, help the patient avoid exacerbating factors. Advise her to lie down in a dark, quiet room during an attack and to place ice packs on her forehead or a cold cloth over her eyes.
+ Instruct the patient to take the prescribed medication at the onset of migraine symptoms, to prevent dehydration by drinking plenty of fluids after nausea and vomiting subside, and to use other headache relief measures.
+ The patient with a migraine headache usually needs to be hospitalized only if nausea and vomiting are severe enough to induce dehydration and possible shock.
+ Avoid repeated use of opioids if possible.

▼ *LIFE-THREATENING DISORDER*

HEAD TRAUMA

Head trauma describes any traumatic insult to the brain that results in physical, intellectual, emotional, social, or vocational changes. Young children ages 6 months to 2 years, people ages 15 to 24, and elderly people are at highest risk for head trauma. The risk for men is double the risk for women.

Head trauma is generally categorized as closed or open trauma. Closed trauma, or blunt trauma as it's sometimes called, is more common. It typically occurs when the head strikes a hard surface or a rapidly moving object strikes the head. The dura is intact, and no brain tissue is exposed to the external environment. In open trauma, as the name suggests, an opening in the scalp, skull, meninges, or brain tissue, including the dura, exposes the cranial contents to the environment, and the risk of infection is high.

Mortality from head trauma has declined with advances in preventive measures, such as seat belts and airbags, quicker response and transport times, and improved treatment, including the development of regional trauma centers. Advances in technology have increased the effectiveness of rehabilitative services, even for patients with severe head injuries.

CAUSES

Causes of head trauma may include transportation or automobile accident (number one cause), falls, sports-related accidents, and crime and assaults.

PATHOPHYSIOLOGY

The brain is shielded by the cranial vault (hair, skin, bone, meninges, and cerebrospinal fluid [CSF]), which intercepts the force of a physical blow. Below a certain level of force (the absorption capacity), the cranial vault prevents energy from affecting the brain. The degree of traumatic head injury usually is proportional to the amount of force reaching the cranial tissues. Furthermore, unless ruled out, neck injuries should be presumed present in patients with traumatic head injury.

Closed trauma is typically a sudden acceleration-deceleration or *coup-contrecoup* injury. In coup-contrecoup, the head hits a relatively stationary object, injuring cranial tissues near the point of impact (*coup*); then the remaining force pushes the brain against the opposite side of the skull, causing a second impact and injury (*contrecoup*). Contusions and lacerations may also occur during contrecoup as the brain's soft tissues slide over the rough bone of the cranial cavity. In addition, the cerebrum may endure rotational shear, damaging the upper midbrain and areas of the frontal, temporal, and occipital lobes.

Open trauma may penetrate the scalp, skull, meninges, or brain. Open head injuries are usually associated with skull fractures, and bone fragments commonly cause hematomas and meningeal tears with consequent loss of CSF.

SIGNS AND SYMPTOMS

Types of head trauma include concussion, contusion, epidural hematoma, subdural hematoma, intracerebral hematoma, and skull fractures. Each is associated with specific signs and symptoms. (See *Types of head trauma,* pages 308 to 311.)

COMPLICATIONS

Complications may include intracranial pressure (ICP), infection (open trauma), respiratory depression and failure, and brain herniation.

DIAGNOSIS

Each type of head trauma is associated with specific diagnostic findings. (See *Types of head trauma,* pages 308 to 311.)

TREATMENT

Surgical treatment includes evacuation of the hematoma or a craniotomy to elevate or remove fragments that have been driven into the brain, and to extract foreign bodies and necrotic tissue, thereby reducing the risk of infection and further brain damage from fractures.

Supportive treatment includes close observation to detect changes in neurologic status suggesting further damage or expanding hematoma, cleaning and debridement of any wounds associated with skull fractures, and diuretics such as mannitol to reduce cerebral edema.

(*Text continues on page 310.*)

Causes
◆ Automobile accidents
◆ Falls
◆ Sports-related accidents
◆ Crime and assaults

How it happens
Closed trauma
◆ Typically sudden coup-contrecoup injury
◆ Head hits relatively stationary object, injuring cranial tissues near point of impact (*coup*)
◆ Remaining force pushes brain against the opposite side of skull, causing second injury (*contrecoup*)
◆ Contusions and lacerations may occur during contrecoup

Open trauma
◆ May penetrate scalp, skull, meninges, or brain
◆ Associated with skull fractures
◆ Bone fragments cause hematomas, meningeal tears, loss of CSF

Key signs and symptoms
◆ Each type of trauma has specific signs and symptoms

Complications
◆ ICP
◆ Infection (open trauma)
◆ Respiratory failure

Diagnosis
◆ Each type has specific findings

Treatment
◆ Evacuation of hematoma
◆ Craniotomy
◆ Observation
◆ Analgesics

Key facts about concussion

◆ Most common head injury
◆ Symptoms include short term loss of consciousness and vomiting
◆ CT scan reveals no sign of fracture, bleeding, or other nervous system lesion

Key facts about contusion

◆ Most result from arterial bleeding
◆ Most commonly affects people 20 to 40 years old
◆ Symptoms include severe scalp wounds, labored respiration, and loss of consciousness
◆ CT scan shows changes in tissue density
◆ EEG recordings reveal progressive abnormalities

Types of head trauma

This chart summarizes the signs and symptoms and diagnostic test findings for the different types of head trauma.

TYPE	DESCRIPTION
Concussion (closed head injury)	◆ A blow to the head hard enough to make the brain hit the skull but not hard enough to cause a cerebral contusion; causes temporary neural dysfunction. ◆ Is by far the most common head injury. ◆ Recovery is usually complete within 24 to 48 hours. ◆ Repeated injuries exact a cumulative toll on the brain.
Contusion (bruising of brain tissue; more serious than concussion)	◆ Most commonly affects people ages 20 to 40. ◆ Most result from arterial bleeding. ◆ Blood commonly accumulates between skull and dura. Injury to middle meningeal artery in parietotemporal area is most common and is usually accompanied by linear skull fractures in temporal region over middle meningeal artery. ◆ Less commonly arises from dural venous sinuses. ◆ Normal nerve function is disrupted in the bruised area.
Epidural hematoma	◆ Acceleration-deceleration or *coup-contrecoup* injuries disrupt normal nerve functions in bruised area. ◆ Injury is directly beneath the site of impact when the brain rebounds against the skull from the force of a blow (a beating with a blunt instrument, for example), when the force of the blow drives the brain against the opposite side of the skull, or when the head is hurled forward and stopped abruptly (as in an automobile accident when a driver's head strikes the windshield). ◆ Brain continues moving and slaps against the skull (acceleration), then rebounds (deceleration). Brain may strike bony prominences inside the skull (especially the sphenoidal ridges), causing intracranial hemorrhage or hematoma that may result in tentorial herniation.

SIGNS AND SYMPTOMS	DIAGNOSTIC TEST FINDINGS
✦ Short-term loss of consciousness secondary to disruption of reticular activating system (RAS), possibly due to abrupt pressure changes in the areas responsible for consciousness, changes in polarity of the neurons, ischemia, or structural distortion of neurons ✦ Vomiting from localized injury and compression ✦ Anterograde and retrograde amnesia (patient can't recall events immediately after the injury or events that led up to the traumatic incident) correlating with severity of injury; all related to disruption of RAS ✦ Irritability or lethargy from localized injury and compression ✦ Behavior out of character due to focal injury ✦ Complaints of dizziness, nausea, or severe headache due to focal injury and compression	✦ Computed tomography (CT) scan reveals no sign of fracture, bleeding, or other nervous system lesion.
✦ Severe scalp wounds from direct injury ✦ Labored respiration and loss of consciousness secondary to increased pressure from bruising ✦ Drowsiness, confusion, disorientation, agitation, or violence from increased intracranial pressure (ICP) associated with trauma ✦ Hemiparesis related to interrupted blood flow to the site of injury ✦ Decorticate or decerebrate posturing from cortical damage or hemispheric dysfunction ✦ Unequal pupillary response from brain stem involvement	✦ CT scan shows changes in tissue density, possible displacement of the surrounding structures, and evidence of ischemic tissue, hematomas, and fractures. ✦ EEG directly over area of contusion reveals progressive abnormalities by appearance of high-amplitude theta and delta waves.
✦ Brief period of unconsciousness after injury reflecting the concussive effects of head trauma, followed by a lucid interval varying from 10 to 15 minutes to hours or, rarely, days ✦ Severe headache ✦ Progressive loss of consciousness and deterioration in neurologic signs resulting from expanding lesion and extrusion of medial portion of temporal lobe through tentorial opening ✦ Compression of brain stem by temporal lobe causing clinical manifestations of intracranial hypertension ✦ Deterioration in level of consciousness resulting from compression of brain stem reticular formation as temporal lobe herniates on its upper portion ✦ Respirations, initially deep and labored, becoming shallow and irregular as brain stem is impacted ✦ Contralateral motor deficits reflecting compression of corticospinal tracts that pass through the brain stem ✦ Ipsilateral (same-side) pupillary dilation due to compression of third cranial nerve ✦ Seizures possible from high ICP ✦ Continued bleeding leading to progressive neurologic degeneration, evidenced by bilateral pupillary dilation, bilateral decerebrate response, increased systemic blood pressure, decreased pulse, and profound coma with irregular respiratory patterns	✦ CT scan or magnetic resonance imaging (MRI) identifies abnormal masses or structural shifts within the cranium.

Key facts about epidural hematoma

✦ Injury is directly beneath the site of impact
✦ Brain moves and slaps against skull, then rebounds
✦ Symptoms include brief period of unconsciousness after injury and severe headache
✦ CT scan or MRI identifies abnormal masses or structural shifts in cranium

(continued)

Key facts about subdural hematoma

✦ Meningeal hemorrhages
✦ May be acute, subacute, or chronic
✦ Acute hematoma is a surgical emergency
✦ Symptoms similar to epidural hematoma but slower in onset
✦ CT scan, X-rays, and arteriography reveal mass and altered blood flow
✦ CSF is yellow and has low protein

Key facts about intracerebral hematoma

✦ Traumatic or spontaneous disruption of cerebral vessels in brain parenchyma causes neurologic defects
✦ Frontal and temporal lobes are common sites
✦ Symptoms include immediate unresponsiveness or lucid period before lapsing into a coma
✦ CT scan or cerebral arteriograpy identifies bleeding site
✦ CSF pressure elevated

Types of head trauma *(continued)*

TYPE	DESCRIPTION
Subdural hematoma	✦ Meningeal hemorrhages, resulting from accumulation of blood in subdural space (between dura mater and arachnoid) are most common. ✦ May be acute, subacute, or chronic; unilateral or bilateral. ✦ Usually associated with torn connecting veins in cerebral cortex; rarely from arteries. ✦ Acute hematoma is a surgical emergency.
Intracerebral hematoma	✦ Subacute hematomas have better prognosis because venous bleeding tends to be slower. ✦ Traumatic or spontaneous disruption of cerebral vessels in brain parenchyma causes neurologic deficits, depending on site and amount of bleeding. ✦ Shear forces from brain movement frequently cause vessel laceration and hemorrhage into the parenchyma. ✦ Frontal and temporal lobes are common sites. Trauma is associated with few intracerebral hematomas; most caused by result of hypertension.
Skull fractures	✦ There are four types of skull fractures: linear, comminuted, depressed, and basilar. ✦ Fractures of anterior and middle fossae are associated with severe head trauma and are more common than those of posterior fossa. ✦ Blow to the head causes one or more of these types. May not be problematic unless brain is exposed or bone fragments are driven into neural tissue.

Administration of analgesics, such as acetaminophen and codeine (for severe headache), to relieve complaints of headache, and anticonvulsants, such as phenytoin, to prevent and treat seizures may be necessary.

Respiratory support is indicated, including mechanical ventilation and endotracheal intubation for respiratory failure from brain stem involvement.

Prophylactic antibiotics are administered to prevent the onset of meningitis from CSF leakage associated with skull fractures.

SIGNS AND SYMPTOMS	DIAGNOSTIC TEST FINDINGS
✦ Similar to epidural hematoma but significantly slower in onset because bleeding is typically of venous origin	✦ CT scan, X-rays, and arteriography reveal mass and altered blood flow in the area, confirming hematoma. ✦ CT scan or MRI reveals evidence of masses and tissue shifting. ✦ CSF is yellow and has relatively low protein (chronic subdural hematoma).
✦ Unresponsive immediately or experiencing a lucid period before lapsing into a coma from increasing ICP and mass effect of hemorrhage ✦ Possible motor deficits and decorticate or decerebrate responses from compression of corticospinal tracts and brain stem	✦ CT scan or cerebral arteriography identifies bleeding site. CSF pressure elevated; fluid may appear bloody or xanthochromic (yellow or straw-colored) from hemoglobin breakdown.
✦ May not produce symptoms, depending on underlying brain trauma ✦ Discontinuity and displacement of bone structure with severe fracture ✦ Motor sensory and cranial nerve dysfunction with associated facial fractures ✦ Persons with anterior fossa basilar skull fractures may have periorbital ecchymosis (raccoon eyes), anosmia (loss of smell due to first cranial nerve involvement) and pupil abnormalities (second and third cranial nerve involvement) ✦ Cerebrospinal fluid (CSF) rhinorrhea (leakage through nose), CSF otorrhea (leakage from the ear), hemotympanum (blood accumulation at the tympanic membrane), ecchymosis over the mastoid bone (Battle's sign), and facial paralysis (seventh cranial nerve injury) accompany middle fossa basilar skull fractures ✦ Signs of medullary dysfunction, such as cardiovascular and respiratory failure, accompany posterior fossa basilar skull fracture	✦ CT scan and MRI reveal intracranial hemorrhage from ruptured blood vessels and swelling. ✦ Skull X-ray may reveal fracture. ✦ Lumbar puncture contraindicated by expanding lesions.

NURSING CONSIDERATIONS

✦ Obtain a thorough history of the injury from the patient (if he isn't suffering from amnesia), family members, eyewitnesses, or emergency medical services personnel. Ask whether the patient lost consciousness.

✦ Monitor vital signs and check for additional injuries. Palpate the skull for tenderness or hematomas.

✦ If the patient has an altered level of consciousness (LOC) or if a neurologic examination reveals abnormalities, observe the patient in the emergency department. Check vital signs, LOC, and pupil size every 15 minutes. The patient who's stable

Key facts about skull fractures

✦ Four types: linear, comminuted, depressed, and basilar
✦ Blow to the head causes one or more of the types
✦ Symptoms include discontinuity and displacement of bone structure with severe fracture
✦ CT scan and MRI reveal intracranial hemorrhage
✦ Skull X-ray reveals fracture

Key nursing actions

✦ Obtain a thorough history of the injury from the patient, family members, eyewitnesses, or emergency medical services personnel.
✦ Monitor vital signs, and check for additional injuries.
✦ If the patient has an altered LOC or if a neurologic examination reveals abnormalities, observe the patient in the emergency department.

Key nursing actions
(continued)

✦ After the patient is stabilized, clean and dress any superficial scalp wounds.

✦ If it's determined that the patient can be discharged, instruct the patient to be alert for worsening of headache, vomiting, and signs of an ear bleed or CSF leak.

For serious head injuries

✦ Establish and maintain a patent airway; nasal airways are contraindicated in patients who may have a basilar skull fracture.

✦ Look for CSF draining from the patient's ears, nose, or mouth. Check pillowcases and linens for CSF leaks.

✦ If spinal injury is ruled out, position the patient with a head injury so that secretions can drain properly.

✦ Take seizure precautions, but don't restrain the patient.

✦ Don't give the patient opioids or sedatives.

✦ Restrict total fluid intake to 1,200 to 1,500 ml/day to reduce fluid volume and intracerebral swelling.

Characteristics of Huntington's disease

✦ Hereditary disorder

✦ Degeneration of cerebral cortex and basal ganglia causes chronic progressive chorea, cognitive deterioration, dementia

✦ Occurs between ages 25 and 55

✦ 2% of cases occur in children; 5% occur as late as age 60

✦ Death usually results in 10 to 15 years from suicide, heart failure, pneumonia

---

after 4 or more hours of observation can be discharged (with a head injury instruction sheet) in the care of a responsible adult.

✦ After the patient is stabilized, clean and dress any superficial scalp wounds. (If the skin has been broken, tetanus prophylaxis may be in order.) Assist with suturing if necessary.

✦ If it's determined that the patient can be discharged, instruct the patient to be alert for worsening of headache, vomiting, signs of an ear bleed or CSF leak. Be sure to also include instructions for waking the patient every few hours during the night for observation of mental state and administration of medication.

For the patient with more serious head injuries

✦ Establish and maintain a patent airway; nasal airways are contraindicated in patients who may have a basilar skull fracture. Intubation may be necessary. Suction the patient through the mouth, not the nose, to prevent introducing bacteria if a CSF leak is present.

✦ Assist with diagnostic tests, including a complete neurologic examination, a computed tomography scan, and other studies.

✦ Look for CSF draining from the patient's ears, nose, or mouth. Check pillowcases and linens for CSF leaks and look for a halo sign. If the patient's nose is draining CSF, wipe it — don't let him blow it. If an ear is draining, cover it lightly with sterile gauze — don't pack it.

✦ If spinal injury is ruled out, position the patient with a head injury so that secretions can drain properly. Elevate the head of the bed 30 degrees if intracerebral injury is suspected.

✦ Take seizure precautions, but don't restrain the patient. Agitated behavior may be due to hypoxia or increased ICP, so check for these symptoms. Speak in a calm, reassuring voice, and touch the patient gently. Don't make any sudden, unexpected moves.

✦ Don't give the patient opioids or sedatives because they may depress respirations, increase carbon dioxide levels, lead to increased ICP, and mask changes in neurologic status. Give acetaminophen or another mild analgesic for pain, as ordered.

✦ Restrict total fluid intake to 1,200 to 1,500 ml/day to reduce fluid volume and intracerebral swelling.

✦ Type and crossmatch blood for a patient suspected of having an intracerebral hemorrhage. Such a patient may need a blood transfusion and, possibly, a craniotomy to control bleeding and to aspirate blood.

HUNTINGTON'S DISEASE

Also called *Huntington's chorea, hereditary chorea, chronic progressive chorea,* and *adult chorea,* Huntington's disease is a hereditary disorder in which degeneration of the cerebral cortex and basal ganglia causes chronic progressive chorea (involuntary and irregular movements) and cognitive deterioration, ending in dementia.

Huntington's disease usually strikes people between ages 25 and 55 (the average age is 35), affecting men and women equally. However, 2% of cases occur in children, and 5% occur as late as age 60. Death usually results 10 to 15 years after onset from suicide, heart failure, or pneumonia.

CAUSES

The cause of this disorder is unknown. However, it's transmitted as an autosomal dominant trait, which either gender can transmit and inherit. Each child of an affected parent has a 50% chance of inheriting it; the child who doesn't inherit it can't transmit it. Huntington's disease is prevalent in areas where affected families have lived for several generations because of hereditary transmission and delayed expression. Genetic testing is now available to families with a known history of the disease.

PATHOPHYSIOLOGY

Huntington's disease involves a disturbance in neurotransmitter substances, primarily gamma-aminobutyric acid (GABA) and dopamine. In the basal ganglia, frontal cortex, and cerebellum, GABA neurons are destroyed and replaced by glial cells. The consequent deficiency of GABA (an inhibitory neurotransmitter) results in a relative excess of dopamine and abnormal neurotransmission along the affected pathways.

SIGNS AND SYMPTOMS

The onset of this disease is insidious. The patient eventually becomes totally dependent—emotionally and physically—through loss of musculoskeletal control.

Neurologic manifestations include progressively severe choreic movements, which are due to the relative excess of dopamine. Such movements are rapid, typically violent, and purposeless.

Choreic movements are initially unilateral and more prominent in the face and arms than in the legs. They progress from mild fidgeting to grimacing, tongue smacking, dysarthria (indistinct speech), emotion-related athetoid (slow, twisting, snakelike) movements (especially of the hands) from injury to the basal ganglion, and torticollis due to shortening of neck muscles.

The patient also exhibits bradykinesia (slow movement), commonly accompanied by rigidity, and impairment of both voluntary and involuntary movement due to the combination of chorea, bradykinesia, and normal muscle strength.

Dysphagia occurs in most patients in the advanced stages. Dysarthria may be complicated by perseveration (persistent repetition of a reply), oral apraxia (difficulty coordinating movement of the mouth), and aprosody (inability to accurately reproduce or interpret the tone of language).

Cognitive signs and symptoms may include dementia, an early indication of the disease, from dysfunction of the subcortex without significant impairment of immediate memory. The patient experiences problems with recent memory due to retrieval rather than encoding problems, deficits of executive function (planning, organizing, regulating, and programming) from frontal lobe involvement, and impaired impulse control.

The patient may also exhibit psychiatric symptoms, typically before movement problems occur. Psychiatric symptoms may include depression and possible mania (earliest symptom) related to altered levels of dopamine and GABA, and personality changes including irritability, lability, impulsiveness, and aggressive behavior.

COMPLICATIONS

Common complications of Huntington's disease include choking, aspiration, pneumonia, heart failure, and infections.

Causes
+ Cause unknown
+ Transmitted as autosomal dominant trait
+ Prevalent where affected families have lived for several generations
+ Genetic testing now available to families with known history

How it happens
+ Involves disturbance in neurotransmitter substances
+ GABA neurons destroyed and replaced by glial cells
+ Deficiency of GABA causes excess of dopamine and abnormal neurotransmission along affected pathways

Key signs and symptoms
+ Onset insidious
+ Progressively severe choreic movements
+ Bradykinesia
+ Rigidity
+ Impairment of voluntary and involuntary movement
+ Dysphagia
+ Dysarthria
+ Perseveration

Complications
+ Choking
+ Aspiration
+ Pneumonia
+ Heart failure
+ Infections

Diagnosis

+ Genetic testing reveals autosomal dominant trait
+ PET scan confirms disorder
+ CT scan shows brain atrophy
+ MRI shows ventricular enlargement

Treatment

+ No known cure exists
+ Symptom-based, supportive, and protective treatment
+ Haloperidol or diazepam
+ Psychotherapy

Key nursing actions

+ Patient comfort and support are the primary considerations.
+ Provide physical support by attending to the patient's basic needs.
+ Stay alert for possible suicide attempts.
+ If the patient has difficulty walking, provide a walker to help him maintain his balance.
+ Make sure that affected families receive genetic counseling.

Characteristics of intracranial aneurysm

+ Weakness in wall of cerebral artery causes localized dilation
+ Most common form is berry aneurysm
+ Usually arise at arterial junction in Circle of Willis
+ Cerebral aneurysms rupture and cause subarachnoid hemorrhage.
+ Incidence slightly higher in women in their 40s and 50s
+ Occurs at any age in either gender
+ 50% of patients die immediately

DIAGNOSIS

Genetic testing reveals autosomal dominant trait. Positron emission tomography (PET) scan confirms disorder. Computed tomography (CT) scan shows brain atrophy, and magnetic resonance imaging (MRI) shows ventricular enlargement.

TREATMENT

No known cure exists for Huntington's disease. Treatment is symptom-based, supportive, and protective. It may include haloperidol or diazepam to modify choreic movements and control behavioral manifestations and depression. Psychotherapy may be helpful to decrease anxiety and stress and manage psychiatric symptoms. Institutionalization is commonly necessary to manage progressive mental deterioration and self-care deficits.

NURSING CONSIDERATIONS

Patient comfort and support are the primary considerations.
+ Provide physical support by attending to the patient's basic needs, such as hygiene, skin care, bowel and bladder care, and nutrition. Increase this support as mental and physical deterioration make the patient increasingly immobile.
+ Offer emotional support to the patient and his family. Teach them about the disease, and listen to their concerns and special problems. Keep in mind the patient's dysarthria, and allow him extra time to express himself, thereby decreasing frustration. Teach the family to participate in the patient's care.
+ Stay alert for possible suicide attempts. Control the patient's environment to protect him from suicide or other self-inflicted injury. Pad the side rails of the bed but avoid restraints, which may cause the patient to injure himself with violent, uncontrolled movements.
+ If the patient has difficulty walking, provide a walker to help him maintain his balance.
+ Make sure that affected families receive genetic counseling. All affected family members should realize that each of their offspring has a 50% chance of inheriting this disease.
+ Refer people at risk who desire genetic testing to centers specializing in care of patients with Huntington's disease, where psychosocial support is available.
+ Refer the patient and his family to appropriate community organizations.
+ For more information about this degenerative disease, refer the patient and his family to the Huntington's Disease Association.

▼ *LIFE-THREATENING DISORDER*

INTRACRANIAL ANEURYSM

In an intracranial, or cerebral, aneurysm a weakness in the wall of a cerebral artery causes localized dilation. Its most common form is the berry aneurysm, a saclike outpouching in a cerebral artery. Cerebral aneurysms usually arise at an arterial junction in the Circle of Willis, the circular anastomosis forming the major cerebral arteries at the base of the brain. (See *Most common sites of cerebral aneurysm.*)

Cerebral aneurysms commonly rupture and cause subarachnoid hemorrhage.

The incidence is slightly higher in women than in men, especially those in their late 40s or early to mid-50s, but a cerebral aneurysm may occur at any age in either sex. The prognosis is guarded. About 50% of patients who suffer a subarachnoid hemorrhage die immediately. Of those who survive untreated, 40% die from the ef-

Most common sites of cerebral aneurysm

Cerebral aneurysms usually arise at the arterial bifurcation in the Circle of Willis and its branch-es. This illustration shows the most common sites around this circle

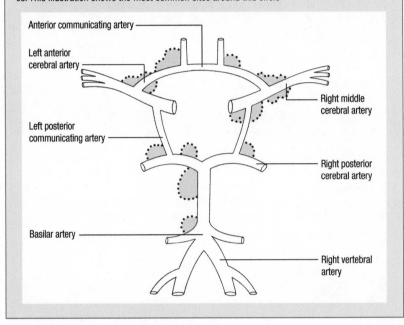

fects of hemorrhage and another 20% die later from recurring hemorrhage. New treatments are improving the prognosis.

CAUSES

Intracranial aneurysm results from a congenital defect of the vessel wall, head trauma, hypertensive vascular disease, advancing age, infection, or atherosclerosis, which can weaken the vessel wall.

PATHOPHYSIOLOGY

Blood flow exerts pressure against a congenitally weak arterial wall, stretching it like an overblown balloon and making it likely to rupture. Such a rupture is followed by a subarachnoid hemorrhage, in which blood spills into the space normally occupied by cerebrospinal fluid. Sometimes, blood also spills into brain tissue, where a clot can cause potentially fatal increased intracranial pressure (ICP) and brain tissue damage.

SIGNS AND SYMPTOMS

Occasionally, the patient may exhibit premonitory symptoms resulting from oozing of blood into the subarachnoid space. These symptoms include headache, intermittent nausea, nuchal rigidity, and stiff back and legs.

Causes
+ Congenital defect of vessel wall
+ Head trauma
+ Hypertensive vascular disease
+ Advancing age
+ Infection
+ Atherosclerosis

How it happens
+ Blood flow exerts pressure against congenitally weak arterial wall, making it likely to rupture
+ Rupture followed by subarachnoid hemorrhage
+ Blood spills into brain tissue
+ Clot can cause potentially fatal increased ICP, brain tissue damage

Key signs and symptoms
+ Headache
+ Intermittent nausea
+ Nuchal rigidity
+ Stiff back and legs

Key signs and symptoms
(continued)

- Projectile vomiting
- Altered LOC
- Back and leg pain
- Fever
- Restlessness
- Irritability

Grading

- Grade I: minimal bleeding
- Grade II: mild bleeding
- Grade III: moderate bleeding
- Grade IV: severe bleeding
- Grade V: moribund

Complications

- Subarachnoid hemorrhage and brain tissue infarction
- Cerebral vasospasm
- Rebleeding
- Meningeal irritation

Diagnosis

- Cerebral angiography reveals altered cerebral blood flow, vessel lumen dilation, differences in arterial filling
- CT scan reveals subarachnoid or ventricular bleeding
- MRI shows cerebral blood flow void
- Skull X-rays may reveal calcified wall of aneurysm and areas of bone erosion

---

Determining severity of an intracranial aneurysm rupture

The severity of symptoms varies from patient to patient, depending on the site and amount of bleeding. Five grades characterize a ruptured cerebral aneurysm:

- *Grade I: minimal bleeding* — The patient is alert with no neurologic deficit; he may have a slight headache and nuchal rigidity.
- *Grade II: mild bleeding* — The patient is alert, with a mild to severe headache and nuchal rigidity; he may have third-nerve palsy.
- *Grade III: moderate bleeding* — The patient is confused or drowsy, with nuchal rigidity and, possibly, a mild focal deficit.
- *Grade IV: severe bleeding* — The patient is stuporous, with nuchal rigidity and, possibly, mild to severe hemiparesis.
- *Grade V: moribund (often fatal)* — If the rupture is nonfatal, the patient is in a deep coma or decerebrate.

Usually, however, the rupture occurs abruptly and without warning, causing sudden severe headache caused by increased pressure from bleeding into a closed space, nausea and projectile vomiting related to increased pressure, and an altered level of consciousness (LOC), including deep coma, depending on the severity and location of bleeding, from increased pressure caused by increased cerebral blood volume.

Bleeding causes meningeal irritation, resulting in nuchal rigidity, back and leg pain, fever, restlessness, irritability, occasional seizures, photophobia, and blurred vision, secondary to bleeding into the meninges. Bleeding into the brain tissue causes hemiparesis, hemisensory defects, dysphagia, and visual defects.

Diplopia, ptosis, dilated pupil, and inability to rotate the eye are caused by compression on the oculomotor nerve if the aneurysm is near the internal carotid artery.

Typically, the severity of a ruptured intracranial aneurysm is graded according to the patient's signs and symptoms. (See *Determining severity of an intracranial aneurysm rupture.*)

COMPLICATIONS

Potentially fatal complications after rupture of an aneurysm include subarachnoid hemorrhage and brain tissue infarction. Cerebral vasospasm, probably the most common cause of death after rupture, occurs in about 40% of all patients after subarachnoid hemorrhage occurs.

Other possible complications include rebleeding, which usually occurs within the first 7 days but can occur anytime within the first 6 months; meningeal irritation from blood in the subarachnoid space and hydrocephalus, which can occur weeks or even months after rupture if blood obstructs the fourth ventricle.

DIAGNOSIS

Cerebral angiography reveals altered cerebral blood flow, vessel lumen dilation, and differences in arterial filling. Computed tomography (CT) scan reveals subarachnoid or ventricular bleeding with blood in subarachnoid space and displaced midline structures. Magnetic resonance imaging (MRI) shows a cerebral blood flow void. Skull X-rays may reveal the calcified wall of the aneurysm and areas of bone erosion.

TREATMENT

Treatment to reduce the risk of rupture if it hasn't occurred may include bed rest in a quiet, darkened room with minimal stimulation, and avoidance of coffee and other stimulants, to reduce the risk of blood pressure elevation. Codeine or another analgesic as needed to maintain rest and minimize risk of pressure changes.

Medications may include hydralazine or another antihypertensive agent, if the patient is hypertensive, and phenobarbital or another sedative to prevent agitation leading to hypertension.

Other treatment may include surgical repair by clipping, ligation, or wrapping (before or after rupture) usually 7 to 10 days after the initial bleed. Prescribed medications may include calcium channel blockers to decrease spasm and subsequent rebleeding, corticosteroids to manage headache in subarachnoid hemorrhage, phenytoin or another anticonvulsant to prevent or treat seizures secondary to pressure and tissue irritation from bleeding, and aminocaproic acid, an inhibitor of fibrinolysis, to minimize the risk of rebleeding by delaying blood clot lysis (this drug's effectiveness is under dispute).

NURSING CONSIDERATIONS

An accurate neurologic assessment, good patient care, patient and family teaching, and psychological support can speed recovery and reduce complications.
✦ During initial treatment after hemorrhage, establish and maintain a patent airway. Position the patient to promote pulmonary drainage and prevent upper airway obstruction. If he's intubated, administering 100% oxygen before suctioning to remove secretions will prevent hypoxia and vasodilation from carbon dioxide accumulation. Suction no longer than 20 seconds to avoid increased intracranial pressure (ICP). Give frequent nose and mouth care.
✦ Impose aneurysm precautions to minimize the risk of rebleed and to avoid increased ICP. Such precautions include bed rest in a quiet, darkened room (keep the head of the bed flat or less than 30 degrees, as ordered); limited visitation; avoidance of strenuous physical activity and straining with bowel movements; and restricted fluid intake. Be sure to explain why these restrictive measures are necessary.

Preventive measures and good patient care can minimize other complications
✦ Turn the patient often. Encourage occasional deep breathing and leg movement. Warn him to avoid all unnecessary physical activity. Assist with active range-of-motion (ROM) exercises; if he is paralyzed, perform regular passive ROM exercises.
✦ Monitor arterial blood gas levels, LOC, and vital signs often, and measure intake and output. Avoid taking the patient's temperature rectally because vagus nerve stimulation may cause cardiac arrest.
✦ Watch for danger signals, such as decreased LOC, unilateral enlarged pupil, onset or worsening of hemiparesis or motor deficit, increased blood pressure, slowed pulse, worsening of headache or sudden onset of a headache, renewed or worsened nuchal rigidity, and renewed or persistent vomiting, that may indicate an enlarging aneurysm, rebleeding, intracranial clot, vasospasm, or other complications. Intermittent signs such as restlessness, extremity weakness, and speech alterations can also indicate increasing ICP.
✦ Give fluids, as ordered, and monitor I.V. infusions to avoid increased ICP.
✦ If the patient has facial weakness, assess the gag reflex and assist him during meals, placing food in the unaffected side of his mouth. If he can't swallow, insert a nasogastric tube, as ordered, and give all tube feedings slowly. Prevent skin break-

Treatment
✦ Bed rest with minimal stimulation
✦ Avoidance of stimulants
✦ Antihypertensive agents
✦ Sedatives
✦ Surgical repair by clipping, ligation, or wrapping
✦ Calcium channel blockers
✦ Corticosteroids
✦ Anticonvulsants
✦ Aminocaproic acid

Key nursing actions
✦ Establish and maintain a patent airway. If the patient is intubated, administering 100% oxygen before suctioning to remove secretions will prevent hypoxia and vasodilation from carbon dioxide accumulation.
✦ Impose aneurysm precautions to minimize the risk of rebleed and to avoid increased ICP.

Preventive measures help minimize other complications
✦ Turn the patient often.
✦ Monitor arterial blood gas levels, LOC, and vital signs often, and measure intake and output.
✦ Watch for danger signals, such as decreased LOC, unilateral enlarged pupil, and onset or worsening of hemiparesis or motor deficit.
✦ Give fluids, as ordered, and monitor I.V. infusions to avoid increased ICP.

Key nursing actions
(continued)

✦ If the patient has facial weakness, assess the gag reflex and assist him during meals, placing food in the unaffected side of his mouth.

✦ To minimize stress, encourage relaxation techniques.

✦ Administer aminocaproic acid I.V. orally, or as ordered at least every 2 hours to maintain therapeutic blood levels. Monitor the patient for adverse reactions, such as nausea, diarrhea, and phlebitis.

✦ If the patient can't speak, establish a simple means of communication or use cards or a notepad.

✦ Before discharge, make a referral to a visiting nurse or a rehabilitation center when necessary.

down by taping the tube so it doesn't press against the nostril. If the patient can eat, provide a high-fiber diet to prevent straining at stool, which can increase ICP. Get an order for a stool softener, such as dioctyl sodium sulfosuccinate, or a mild laxative, and administer as ordered. Don't force fluids. Implement a bowel program based on previous habits. If the patient is receiving steroids, check stools for blood.

✦ With third or facial cranial nerve palsy, administer artificial tears or ointment to the affected eye and tape the eye shut at night to prevent corneal damage.

✦ To minimize stress, encourage relaxation techniques. If possible, avoid using restraints because they can cause agitation and raise ICP.

✦ Administer antihypertensives as ordered. Carefully monitor blood pressure and immediately report any significant change, but especially a rise in systolic pressure.

✦ Administer aminocaproic acid I.V. (in dextrose 5% in water), orally, or as ordered at least every 2 hours to maintain therapeutic blood levels. (Renal insufficiency may require a dosage adjustment.) Monitor the patient for adverse reactions, such as nausea and diarrhea (most common with oral administration) and phlebitis (most common with I.V. administration). Prevent deep vein thrombosis by applying antiembolism stockings or sequential compression sleeves.

✦ If the patient can't speak, establish a simple means of communication or use cards or a notepad. Try to limit conversation to topics that won't frustrate the patient. Encourage his family to speak to him in a normal tone, even if he doesn't seem to respond.

✦ Provide emotional support, and include the patient's family in his care as much as possible. Encourage family members to adopt a realistic attitude, but don't discourage hope.

✦ Before discharge, make a referral to a visiting nurse or a rehabilitation center when necessary, and teach the patient and his family how to recognize signs of rebleeding.

Characteristics of MS

✦ Causes demyelination of white matter of brain and spinal cord; damages nerve fibers and targets

✦ Characterized by exacerbations and remissions

✦ Symptoms appear between ages 20 and 40

✦ Prognosis varies — may progress rapidly or have long remissions

✦ Several types: elapsing, primary progressive, secondary progressive, progressive relapsing

MULTIPLE SCLEROSIS

Multiple sclerosis (MS) causes demyelination of the white matter of the brain and spinal cord and damage to nerve fibers and their targets. Characterized by exacerbations and remissions, MS is a major cause of chronic disability in young adults. It usually begins to produce symptoms between ages 20 and 40 (the average age of onset is 27). MS affects three women for every two men and five whites for every nonwhite. Incidence is generally higher among urban populations and upper socioeconomic groups. A family history of MS and living in a cold, damp climate increase the risk.

The prognosis varies. MS may progress rapidly, disabling the patient by early adulthood or causing death within months of onset. However, 70% of patients lead active, productive lives with prolonged remissions.

Several types of MS have been identified. Terms to describe MS types include:

✦ *elapsing-remitting* — clear relapses (or acute attacks or exacerbations) with full recovery or partial recovery and lasting disability (The disease doesn't worsen between the attacks.)

✦ *primary progressive* — steady progression from the onset with minor recovery or plateaus (This form is uncommon and may involve different brain and spinal cord damage than other forms.)

✦ *secondary progressive* — begins as a pattern of clear-cut relapses and recovery (This form becomes steadily progressive and worsens between acute attacks.)

✦ *progressive relapsing* — steadily progressive from the onset, but also has clear acute attacks. (This form is rare.)

CAUSES

The exact cause of MS is unknown, but current theories suggest that a slow-acting or latent viral infection triggers an autoimmune response. Other theories suggest that environmental and genetic factors may also be linked to MS.

Certain conditions appear to precede onset or exacerbation, including emotional stress, fatigue (physical or emotional), pregnancy, and acute respiratory infections.

PATHOPHYSIOLOGY

In MS, sporadic patches of axon demyelination and nerve fiber loss occur throughout the central nervous system, inducing widely disseminated and varied neurologic dysfunction. (See *How myelin breaks down*, page 320.)

New evidence of nerve fiber loss may provide an explanation for the invisible neurologic deficits experienced by many patients with MS. The axons determine the presence or absence of function; loss of myelin doesn't correlate with loss of function.

SIGNS AND SYMPTOMS

Signs and symptoms depend on the extent and site of myelin destruction, the extent of remyelination, and the adequacy of subsequent restored synaptic transmission. Flares may be transient, or they may last for hours or weeks, possibly waxing and waning with no predictable pattern, varying from day to day, and being bizarre and difficult for the patient to describe. Clinical effects may be so mild that the patient is unaware of them or so intense that they're debilitating. Typical first signs and symptoms related to conduction deficits and impaired impulse transmission along the nerve fiber include vision problems, fatigue, and sensory impairment, such as burning, pins and needles, and electrical sensations.

Other characteristic changes include:
✦ *ocular disturbances* — optic neuritis, diplopia, ophthalmoplegia, blurred vision, and nystagmus from impaired cranial nerve dysfunction and conduction deficits to the optic nerve
✦ *muscle dysfunction* — weakness, paralysis ranging from monoplegia to quadriplegia, spasticity, hyperreflexia, intention tremor, and gait ataxia from impaired motor reflex
✦ *urinary disturbances* — incontinence, frequency, urgency, and frequent infections from impaired transmission involving sphincter innervation
✦ *bowel disturbances* — involuntary evacuation or constipation from altered impulse transmission to internal sphincter
✦ *fatigue* — commonly the most debilitating symptom
✦ *speech problems* — poorly articulated or scanning speech and dysphagia from impaired transmission to the cranial nerves and sensory cortex.

COMPLICATIONS

Complications may include injuries from falls, urinary tract infection, constipation, joint contractures, pressure ulcers, rectal distention, pneumonia, and depression.

Causes
✦ Exact cause unknown
✦ Slow-acting and latent viral infection may trigger autoimmune response
✦ Environmental and genetic factors may play role
✦ Conditions may precede onset or exacerbation

How it happens
✦ Sporadic patches of axon demyelination and nerve fiber loss occur throughout CNS
✦ Induces neurologic dysfunction
✦ New evidence shows nerve fiber may be lost

Key signs and symptoms
✦ Depend on extent and site of myelin destruction, extent of remyelination, adequacy of restored synaptic transmission
✦ Flares may be transient or they may last for hours or weeks
✦ Flares wax and wane unpredictably
✦ Sensory impairment
✦ Ocular disturbances
✦ Muscle dysfunction

Complications
✦ Injuries from falls
✦ Urinary tract infection
✦ Constipation
✦ Joint contractures
✦ Pressure ulcers

Myelin break down

✦ Myelin sheath becomes inflamed
✦ Membrane layers break down into smaller components
✦ Damaged myelin sheath can't conduct normally
✦ Neurologic dysfunction occurs

CLOSER LOOK

How myelin breaks down

Myelin speeds electrical impulses to the brain for interpretation. This lipoprotein complex formed of glial cells or oligodendrocytes protects the neuron's axon much like the insulation on an electrical wire. Its high electrical resistance and low capacitance allow the myelin to conduct nerve impulses from one node of Ranvier to the next.

Myelin is susceptible to injury; for example, by hypoxemia, toxic chemicals, vascular insufficiencies, or autoimmune responses. The sheath becomes inflamed, and the membrane layers break down into smaller components that become well-circumscribed plaques (filled with microglial elements, macroglia, and lymphocytes). This process is called *demyelination*.

The damaged myelin sheath can't conduct normally. The partial loss or dispersion of the action potential causes neurologic dysfunction.

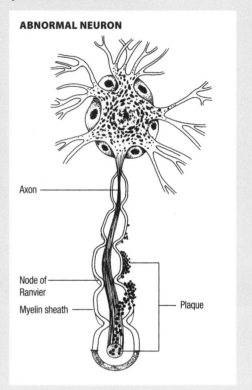

ABNORMAL NEURON

Axon

Node of Ranvier

Myelin sheath

Plaque

Diagnosis

✦ Early symptoms may be mild
✦ Evidence of two or more neurologic attacks
✦ Rule out other conditions
✦ MRI shows multifocal white matter lesions
✦ EEG shows abnormal brain waves in some
✦ Normal CSF protein, elevated IgG
✦ IgG reflects hyperactivity of immune system
✦ CSF white blood cell count elevated
✦ Slowed conduction of nerve impulses in most patients

DIAGNOSIS

Because early symptoms may be mild, years may elapse between onset and diagnosis. Diagnosis of this disorder requires evidence of two or more neurologic attacks. Periodic testing and close observation are necessary, perhaps for years, depending on the course of the disease. Spinal cord compression, foramen magnum tumor (which may mimic the exacerbations and remissions of MS), multiple small strokes, syphilis or another infection, thyroid disease, and chronic fatigue syndrome must be ruled out.

Magnetic resonance imaging (MRI) reveals multifocal white matter lesions.

EEG reveals abnormalities in brain waves in one-third of patients.

Lumbar puncture shows normal total cerebrospinal fluid (CSF) protein but elevated immunoglobulin (Ig) G (gamma globulin); IgG reflects hyperactivity of the immune system due to chronic demyelination. An elevated CSF IgG is significant only when serum IgG is normal. CSF white blood cell count may be elevated.

CSF electrophoresis detects bands of IgG in most patients, even when the percentage of IgG in CSF is normal. Presence of kappa light chains provides additional support to the diagnosis.

Evoked potential studies (visual, brain stem, auditory, and somatosensory) reveal slowed conduction of nerve impulses in most patients.

TREATMENT

The aim of treatment is threefold: Treat the acute exacerbation, treat the disease process, and treat the related signs and symptoms.

I.V. methylprednisolone followed by oral therapy reduces edema of the myelin sheath (speeds recovery from acute attacks). Other drugs, such as azathioprine or methotrexate and cyclophosphamide, may be used.

Immune system therapy consisting of interferon and glatiramer (a combination of four amino acids) reduces frequency and severity of relapses, and may possibly slow central nervous system damage.

Stretching and ROM exercises, coupled with correct positioning, may relieve the spasticity resulting from opposing muscle groups relaxing and contracting at the same time; helpful in relaxing muscles and maintaining function.

Baclofen and tizanidine may be used to treat spasticity. For severe spasticity, botulinum toxin injections, intrathecal injections, nerve blocks, and surgery may be necessary.

Frequent rest periods, aerobic exercise, and cooling techniques (air conditioning, breezes, water sprays) may minimize fatigue. Fatigue is characterized by an overwhelming feeling of exhaustion that can occur at any time of the day without warning. The cause is unknown. Changes in environmental conditions, such as heat and humidity, can aggravate fatigue.

Amantadine, pemoline, and methylphenidate have proven beneficial, as have antidepressants to manage fatigue.

Bladder problems (failure to store urine, failure to empty the bladder or, more commonly, both) are managed by such strategies as drinking cranberry juice or insertion of an indwelling catheter and suprapubic tubes. Intermittent self-catheterization and postvoid catheterization programs are helpful, as are anticholinergic medications in some patients.

Bowel problems (constipation and involuntary evacuation) are managed by such measures as increasing fiber intake, using bulking agents, and bowel-training strategies, such as daily suppositories and rectal stimulation.

Low-dose tricyclic antidepressants, phenytoin, or carbamazepine may manage sensory symptoms, such as pain, numbness, burning, and tingling sensations.

Adaptive devices and physical therapy assist with motor dysfunction, such as problems with balance, strength, and muscle coordination. Beta-adrenergic blockers, sedatives, or diuretics may be used to alleviate tremors. Speech therapy may manage dysarthria. Antihistamines, vision therapy, or exercises may minimize vertigo. Vision therapy or adaptive lenses may manage visual problems.

NURSING CONSIDERATIONS

Management considerations focus on educating the patient and his family.

✦ Assist with physical therapy. Increase patient comfort with massages and relaxing baths. Make sure the bath water isn't too hot because it may temporarily intensify otherwise subtle symptoms. Assist with active, resistive, and stretching exercises to maintain muscle tone and joint mobility, decrease spasticity, improve coordination, and boost morale.

✦ Educate the patient and his family concerning the chronic course of MS. Emphasize the need to avoid stress, infections, and fatigue and to maintain independence by developing new ways of performing daily activities. Be sure to tell the patient to avoid exposure to infections.

✦ Stress the importance of eating a nutritious, well-balanced diet that contains sufficient roughage and adequate fluids to prevent constipation.

Treatment

✦ Methylprednisolone
✦ Immune system therapy
✦ Stretching and ROM exercises
✦ Baclofen and tizanidine
✦ Botulinum toxin injections
✦ Intrathecal injections
✦ Nerve blocks
✦ Surgery
✦ Frequent rest periods
✦ Aerobic exercise
✦ Cooling techniques
✦ Antidepressants
✦ Bladder control measures

Key nursing actions

✦ Management considerations focus on educating the patient and his family.
✦ Assist with physical therapy. Increase patient comfort with massages and relaxing baths.
✦ Educate the patient and his family concerning the chronic course of MS.
✦ Stress the importance of eating a nutritious, well-balanced diet that contains sufficient roughage and adequate fluids to prevent constipation.

Key nursing actions
(continued)

✦ Evaluate the need for bowel and bladder training.
✦ Promote emotional stability.
✦ Inform the patient that exacerbations are unpredictable.

Characteristics of myasthenia gravis

✦ Causes sporadic, progressive weakness or abnormal fatigability of striated muscles
✦ Symptoms exacerbated by exercise
✦ Mainly affects muscles innervated by cranial nerves
✦ Unpredictible; no known cure
✦ Life-threatening when respiratory muscles involved
✦ Incidence peaks between ages 20 and 40
✦ Remission in 25% of patients

Causes

✦ Exact cause unknown
✦ Autoimmune disorder
✦ Blood cells and thymus gland produce antibodies that affect neuroreceptors

How it happens

✦ Causes a failure in nerve impulse transmission at neuromuscular junction
✦ Theory: antireceptor antibodies block, weaken, reduce number of acetylcholine receptors; impair muscle depolarization necessary for movement

Key signs and symptoms

✦ May occur gradually or suddenly
✦ Weak eye closure
✦ Muscle weakness

✦ Evaluate the need for bowel and bladder training during hospitalization. Encourage adequate fluid intake and regular urination. Eventually, the patient may require urinary drainage by self-catheterization or, in men, condom drainage. Teach the correct use of suppositories to help establish a regular bowel schedule.
✦ Promote emotional stability. Help the patient establish a daily routine to maintain optimal functioning. Activity level is regulated by tolerance level. Encourage regular rest periods to prevent fatigue and daily physical exercise.
✦ Inform the patient that exacerbations are unpredictable, necessitating physical and emotional adjustments in lifestyle.
✦ For more information, refer the patient to the National Multiple Sclerosis Society.

MYASTHENIA GRAVIS

Myasthenia gravis causes sporadic but progressive weakness and abnormal fatigability of striated (skeletal) muscles; symptoms are exacerbated by exercise and repeated movement, and relieved by anticholinesterase drugs. Usually, this disorder affects muscles innervated by the cranial nerves (face, lips, tongue, neck, and throat), but it can affect any muscle group.

Myasthenia gravis follows an unpredictable course of periodic exacerbations and remissions. There's no known cure. Drug treatment has improved the prognosis and allows patients to lead relatively normal lives, except during exacerbations. When the disease involves the respiratory system, it may be life-threatening.

Myasthenia gravis affects 1 in 25,000 people at any age, but incidence peaks between ages 20 and 40. It's three times more common in women than in men in this age group, but after age 40, the incidence is similar.

About 20% of infants born to mothers with myasthenia gravis have transient (or occasionally persistent) myasthenia. This disease may coexist with immune and thyroid disorders; 15% of patients with myasthenia gravis have thymomas. Remissions occur in about 25% of patients.

CAUSES

The exact cause of myasthenia gravis is unknown. Myasthenia gravis is thought to be an autoimmune disorder. For an unknown reason, the patient's blood cells and thymus gland produce antibodies that block, destroy, or weaken the neuroreceptors that transmit nerve impulses, causing a failure in transmission of nerve impulses at the neuromuscular junction.

PATHOPHYSIOLOGY

Myasthenia gravis causes a failure in transmission of nerve impulses at the neuromuscular junction. The site of action is the postsynaptic membrane. Theoretically, antireceptor antibodies block, weaken, or reduce the number of acetylcholine receptors available at each neuromuscular junction and thereby impair muscle depolarization necessary for movement. (See *Impaired transmission in myasthenia gravis*.)

SIGNS AND SYMPTOMS

Myasthenia gravis may occur gradually or suddenly. In many patients weak eye closure, ptosis, and diplopia are the first symptoms of impaired neuromuscular transmission to the cranial nerves supplying the eye muscles.

Patients report skeletal muscle weakness and fatigue, increasing through the day but decreasing with rest. In the early stages, easy fatigability of certain muscles may appear with no other findings. Later, it may be severe enough to cause paralysis.

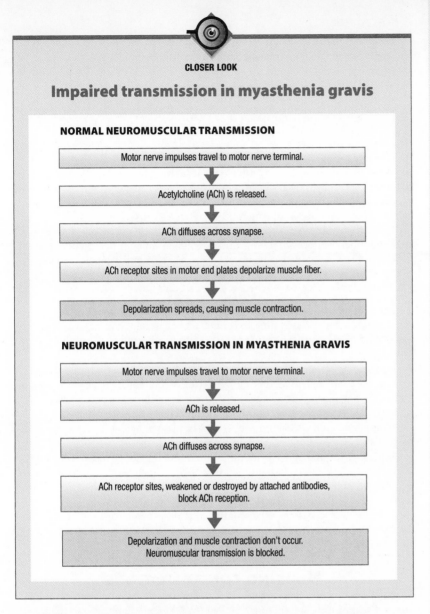

CLOSER LOOK

Impaired transmission in myasthenia gravis

NORMAL NEUROMUSCULAR TRANSMISSION

Motor nerve impulses travel to motor nerve terminal.

⬇

Acetylcholine (ACh) is released.

⬇

ACh diffuses across synapse.

⬇

ACh receptor sites in motor end plates depolarize muscle fiber.

⬇

Depolarization spreads, causing muscle contraction.

NEUROMUSCULAR TRANSMISSION IN MYASTHENIA GRAVIS

Motor nerve impulses travel to motor nerve terminal.

⬇

ACh is released.

⬇

ACh diffuses across synapse.

⬇

ACh receptor sites, weakened or destroyed by attached antibodies, block ACh reception.

⬇

Depolarization and muscle contraction don't occur. Neuromuscular transmission is blocked.

Muscle weakness is progressive and accompanies loss of function depending on muscle group affected, becoming more intense during menses and after emotional stress, prolonged exposure to sunlight or cold, or infections.

Myasthenic patients usually have a blank and expressionless facial appearance and nasal vocal tones secondary to impaired transmission of cranial nerves innervating the facial muscles.

They experience frequent nasal regurgitation of fluids and difficulty chewing and swallowing from cranial nerve involvement.

Their eyelids droop from weakness of facial and extraocular muscles, and the patient's head may tilt back for a proper field of vision. Neck muscles may become too weak to support the head without bobbing.

In patients with weakened respiratory muscles, decreased tidal volume and vital capacity from impaired transmission to the diaphragm make breathing difficult and predispose the patient to pneumonia and other respiratory tract infections.

Key signs and symptoms
(continued)

- ✦ Blank and expressionless facial appearance, nasal vocal tones
- ✦ Frequent nasal regurgitation
- ✦ Eyelids droop
- ✦ Head bobbing
- ✦ Decreased tidal volume and vital capacity
- ✦ Predisposed to pneumonia and respiratory tract infections

Complications
+ Respiratory distress
+ Pneumonia
+ Myasthenic crisis
+ Chewing and swallowing difficulties
+ Choking and food aspiration

Diagnosis
+ Tensilon test: temporary improved muscle function after injection of edrophonium or neostigmine
+ Electromyography shows progressive decrease in muscle fiber contraction
+ Serum antiacetylcholine antibody titer elevated
+ Chest X-ray may reveal thymoma

Treatment
+ Anticholinesterase drugs
+ Immunosuppressant therapy
+ Thymectomy
+ Tracheotomy
+ Positive-pressure ventilation
+ Vigorous suctioning

Key nursing actions
+ Careful baseline assessment, early recognition and treatment of potential crises, supportive measures, and thorough patient teaching can minimize exacerbations and complications.
+ Be alert for signs of an impending crisis.

Respiratory muscle weakness (myasthenic crisis) may be severe enough to require an emergency airway and mechanical ventilation.

COMPLICATIONS
Complications may include respiratory distress, pneumonia, myasthenic crisis, and chewing and swallowing difficulties, possibly leading to choking and food aspiration.

DIAGNOSIS
Tensilon test confirms diagnosis of myasthenia gravis, revealing temporarily improved muscle function within 30 to 60 seconds after I.V. injection of edrophonium or neostigmine and lasting up to 30 minutes.

Electromyography with repeated neural stimulation shows progressive decrease in muscle fiber contraction. Serum antiacetylcholine antibody titer may be elevated.

Chest X-ray reveals thymoma in approximately 15% of patients.

TREATMENT
Measures to relieve symptoms may include anticholinesterase drugs, such as neostigmine and pyridostigmine, to counteract fatigue and muscle weakness and allow about 80% of normal muscle function (drugs are less effective as disease worsens).

Immunosuppressant therapy with corticosteroids, azathioprine, cyclosporine, and cyclophosphamide is used in a progressive fashion (when the previous drug response is poor, the next one is used) to decrease the immune response toward acetylcholine receptors at the neuromuscular junction.

Immunoglobulin G during acute relapses or plasmapheresis in severe exacerbations is also used to suppress the immune system.

Some patients undergo a thymectomy to remove thymomas and possibly induce remission in some cases of adult- onset myasthenia. Tracheotomy, positive-pressure ventilation, and vigorous suctioning are required to remove secretions for treatment of acute exacerbations that cause severe respiratory distress.

Anticholinesterase drugs are discontinued in myasthenic crisis until respiratory function improves — myasthenic crisis requires immediate hospitalization and vigorous respiratory support.

NURSING CONSIDERATIONS
Careful baseline assessment, early recognition and treatment of potential crises, supportive measures, and thorough patient teaching can minimize exacerbations and complications. Continuity of care is essential.

+ Establish an accurate neurologic and respiratory baseline. Thereafter, monitor tidal volume and vital capacity regularly. The patient may need a ventilator and frequent suctioning to remove accumulating secretions.

+ Be alert for signs of an impending crisis (increased muscle weakness, respiratory distress, and difficulty in talking or chewing).

+ To prevent relapses, adhere closely to the ordered drug administration schedule. Be prepared to give atropine for anticholinesterase overdose or toxicity.

+ Plan exercise, meals, patient care, and activities to make the most of energy peaks. For example, give medication 20 to 30 minutes before meals to facilitate chewing or swallowing. Allow the patient to participate in his care.

+ When swallowing is difficult for the patient, give soft, solid foods instead of liquids to lessen the risk of choking.

✦ After a severe exacerbation, try to increase social activity as soon as possible.

✦ Patient teaching is essential because myasthenia gravis is usually a lifelong condition. Help the patient plan daily activities to coincide with energy peaks. Stress the need for frequent rest periods throughout the day. Emphasize that periodic remissions, exacerbations, and day-to-day fluctuations are common.

✦ Teach the patient how to recognize the adverse effects and signs of toxicity of anticholinesterase drugs (headaches, weakness, sweating, abdominal cramps, nausea, vomiting, diarrhea, excessive salivation, and bronchospasm) and corticosteroids (euphoria, insomnia, edema, and increased appetite).

✦ Warn the patient to avoid strenuous exercise, stress, infection, and needless exposure to the sun or cold. All of these things may worsen signs and symptoms. Wearing an eye patch or glasses with one frosted lens may help the patient with diplopia.

✦ For more information and an opportunity to meet other myasthenia gravis patients who lead full, productive lives, refer the patient to the Myasthenia Gravis Foundation.

PARKINSON'S DISEASE

Named for James Parkinson, the English physician who wrote the first accurate description of the disease in 1817, Parkinson's disease (also known as shaking palsy) characteristically produces progressive muscle rigidity, akinesia, and involuntary tremor. Deterioration is a progressive process. Death may result from complications, such as aspiration pneumonia or some other infection.

Parkinson's disease is one of the most common crippling diseases in the United States. It strikes 1 in every 100 people over age 60 and affects men more commonly than women. Roughly 60,000 new cases are diagnosed annually in the United States alone, and incidence is predicted to increase as the population ages.

CAUSES

The cause of Parkinson's disease is unknown. However, study of the extrapyramidal brain nuclei (corpus striatum, globus pallidus, substantia nigra) has established that a dopamine deficiency prevents affected brain cells from performing their normal inhibitory function in the central nervous system.

Some cases are caused by exposure to toxins, such as manganese dust or carbon monoxide, that destroy cells in the substantia nigra.

PATHOPHYSIOLOGY

Parkinson's disease is a degenerative process involving the dopaminergic neurons in the substantia nigra (the area of the basal ganglia that produces and stores the neurotransmitter dopamine). This area plays an important role in the extrapyramidal system, which controls posture and coordination of voluntary motor movements.

Normally, stimulation of the basal ganglia results in refined motor movement because acetylcholine (excitatory) and dopamine (inhibitory) release are balanced. Degeneration of the dopaminergic neurons and loss of available dopamine leads to an excess of excitatory acetylcholine at the synapse and consequent rigidity, tremors, and bradykinesia.

Other nondopaminergic neurons may be affected, possibly contributing to depression and the other nonmotor symptoms associated with this disease. Also, the basal ganglia are interconnected to the hypothalamus, potentially affecting autonomic and endocrine function as well.

Key nursing actions
(continued)

✦ Adhere closely to the ordered drug administration schedule.

✦ Plan exercise, meals, patient care, and activities.

✦ When swallowing is difficult for the patient, give soft, solid foods instead of liquids to lessen the risk of choking.

✦ Warn the patient to avoid strenuous exercise, infection, and needless sun or cold exposure.

Characteristics of Parkinson's disease

✦ Produces progressive muscle rigidity, akinesia, and involuntary tremor

✦ Progressive deterioration

✦ Strikes 1 in every 100 people older than age 60

✦ 60,000 new cases diagnosed annually in United States

Causes

✦ Cause unknown

✦ Dopamine deficiency prevents brain cells from performing normal inhibitory function in CNS

✦ Some due to exposure to toxins

How it happens

✦ Degenerative process involving the dopaminergic neurons in the substantia nigra

✦ Leads to excess of excitatory acetylcholine at synapse

✦ Nondopaminergic neurons may be affected

✦ Oxidative stress believed a factor

Current research on the pathogenesis of Parkinson's disease focuses on damage to the substantia nigra from oxidative stress. Oxidative stress is believed to diminish brain iron content, impair mitochondrial function, inhibit antioxidant and protective systems, reduce glutathione secretion, and damage lipids, proteins, and deoxyribonucleic acid. Brain cells are less capable of repairing oxidative damage than are other tissues.

SIGNS AND SYMPTOMS

The cardinal symptoms of Parkinson's disease are muscle rigidity, akinesia, and an insidious tremor beginning in the fingers (unilateral pill-roll tremor) that increases during stress or anxiety and decreases with purposeful movement and sleep, secondary to loss of inhibitory dopamine activity at the synapse.

Muscle rigidity results in resistance to passive muscle stretching, which may be uniform (lead-pipe rigidity) or jerky (cogwheel rigidity) secondary to depletion of dopamine.

Akinesia causes the patient to walk with difficulty (gait that lacks normal parallel motion and may be retropulsive or propulsive) from impaired dopamine action, and produces a high-pitched, monotone voice, drooling, the masklike facial expression, loss of posture control (the patient walks with body bent forward) from loss of motor control, and dysarthria, dysphagia, or both.

Occasionally, akinesia may also cause oculogyric crises (eyes are fixed upward, with involuntary tonic movements) or blepharospasm (eyelids are completely closed).

The patient experiences excessive sweating and decreased motility of GI and genitourinary smooth muscle from impaired autonomic transmission.

The patient may also experience orthostatic hypotension from impaired vascular smooth-muscle response and report oily skin secondary to inappropriate androgen production controlled by the hypothalamus pituitary axis.

COMPLICATIONS

Complications may include injury from falls because of impaired voluntary movements, and aspiration, urinary tract infections, and pressure ulcers as the patient becomes less mobile.

DIAGNOSIS

Generally, diagnostic tests are of little value in identifying Parkinson's disease. Diagnosis is based on the patient's age and history and on the characteristic clinical picture. However, urinalysis may support the diagnosis by revealing decreased dopamine levels.

A conclusive diagnosis is possible only after ruling out other causes of tremor, involutional depression, cerebral arteriosclerosis and, in patients under age 30, intracranial tumors, Wilson's disease, or phenothiazine or other drug toxicity.

TREATMENT

The aim of treatment is to relieve symptoms and keep the patient functional as long as possible. Treatment includes levodopa, a dopamine replacement most effective during early stages and given in increasing doses until symptoms are relieved or adverse effects appear. (Because adverse effects can be serious, levodopa is usually given in combination with carbidopa to halt peripheral dopamine synthesis.) Dopamine agonists may be used early in the disease or in combination with lev-

Key signs and symptoms
+ Muscle rigidity
+ Akinesia
+ Insidious tremor beginning in fingers; increases during stress; decreases with purposeful movement and sleep
+ Excessive sweating and decreased motility of GI, genitourinary smooth muscle
+ Orthostatic hypotension
+ Oily skin

Complications
+ Injury from falls
+ Aspiration
+ Urinary tract infections
+ Pressure ulcers

Diagnosis
+ Diagnosis based on patient's age, history, characteristic clinical picture
+ Urinalysis may reveal decreased dopamine
+ Rule out other causes of tremor

odopa to enhance response or decrease adverse effects (such as pramipexole, ropinirole, pergolide, bromocriptine).

Patients may be prescribed an alternative drug therapy, including anticholinergics, such as trihexyphenidyl; antihistamines, such as diphenhydramine; and amantadine, an antiviral agent, or selegiline, an enzyme-inhibiting agent, when levodopa is ineffective to conserve dopamine and enhance the therapeutic effect of levodopa.

Stereotactic neurosurgery is performed to prevent involuntary movement, which is most effective in young, otherwise healthy persons with unilateral tremor or muscle rigidity, when drug therapy fails to destroy the ventrolateral nucleus of the thalamus. Neurosurgery can only relieve symptoms, not cure the disease. Deep brain stimulation is an alternative for patients who fail conventional treatment, in which a neurostimulator and electrodes are implanted that stimulate the globus pallidus subthalamic nucleus to decrease tremors and allow normal function. Fetal cell transplantation is controversial. Fetal brain tissue is injected into the patient's brain, in the hope that injected cells will grow, allowing the brain to process dopamine, thereby halting or reducing the disease progression.

Physical therapy, including active and passive range-of-motion exercises, routine daily activities, walking, and baths and massage help relax muscles and complement drug treatment and neurosurgery, in an attempt to maintain normal muscle tone and function.

NURSING CONSIDERATIONS

Effectively caring for the patient with Parkinson's disease requires careful monitoring of drug treatment, emphasis on teaching self-reliance, and generous psychological support.

✦ Monitor drug treatment and adjust dosage, if necessary, to minimize adverse effects.

✦ If the patient has surgery, watch for signs of hemorrhage and increased intracranial pressure by frequently checking level of consciousness and vital signs.

✦ Encourage independence. The patient with excessive tremor may achieve partial control of his body by sitting on a chair and using its arms to steady himself. Advise the patient to change position slowly and dangle his legs before getting out of bed. Remember that fatigue may cause him to depend more on others.

✦ Help the patient overcome problems related to eating and elimination. For example, if he has difficulty eating, offer supplementary or small, frequent meals to increase caloric intake. Help establish a regular bowel routine by encouraging him to drink at least 2 qt (2 L) of liquids daily and eat high-fiber foods. He may need an elevated toilet seat to assist him from a standing to a sitting position.

✦ Give the patient and his family emotional support. Teach them about the disease, its progressive stages, and adverse drug effects. Show the family how to prevent pressure ulcers and contractures by proper positioning. Inform them of the dietary restrictions levodopa imposes, and explain household safety measures to prevent accidents. Help the patient and his family express their feelings and frustrations about the progressively debilitating effects of the disease. Establish long- and short-term treatment goals, and be aware of the patient's need for intellectual stimulation and diversion. Refer the patient and his family to the National Parkinson Foundation or the United Parkinson Foundation for more information.

Treatment
✦ Levodopa
✦ Anticholinergics
✦ Stereotactic neurosurgery
✦ Deep brain stimulation
✦ Fetal cell transplantation
✦ Physical therapy

Key nursing actions
✦ Monitor drug treatment and adjust dosage, if necessary.
✦ If the patient has surgery, watch for signs of hemorrhage and increased intracranial pressure by frequently checking level of consciousness and vital signs.
✦ Encourage independence.
✦ Help the patient overcome problems related to eating and elimination.
✦ Give the patient and his family emotional support. Teach them about the disease, its progressive stages, and adverse drug effects.

REYE'S SYNDROME

Reye's syndrome is an acute childhood illness that causes fatty infiltration of the liver with concurrent hyperammonemia, encephalopathy, and increased intracranial pressure (ICP). In addition, fatty infiltration of the kidneys, brain, and myocardium may occur. Reye's syndrome affects children from infancy to adolescence and occurs equally in boys and girls.

Prognosis depends on the severity of central nervous system depression. Until recently, mortality was as high as 90%. Today, ICP monitoring and, consequently, early treatment of increased ICP, along with other treatment measures, have reduced mortality to about 20%. Death is usually a result of cerebral edema or respiratory arrest. Comatose patients who survive may have residual brain damage.

Incidence commonly rises during influenza outbreaks and may be linked to the use of aspirin. Therefore, use of aspirin for children under age 15 isn't recommended.

CAUSES

Reye's syndrome typically begins within 1 to 3 days of an acute viral infection, such as an upper respiratory tract infection, type B influenza, or varicella (chickenpox).

PATHOPHYSIOLOGY

In Reye's syndrome, damaged hepatic mitochondria disrupt the urea cycle, which normally changes ammonia to urea for its excretion from the body. This results in hyperammonemia, hypoglycemia (in 15% of cases), and an increase in serum short-chain fatty acids, leading to encephalopathy. Simultaneously, fatty infiltration occurs in renal tubular cells, neuronal tissue, and muscle tissue, including the heart.

SIGNS AND SYMPTOMS

The severity of the child's signs and symptoms varies with the degree of encephalopathy and cerebral edema. In any case, Reye's syndrome develops in five stages. After the initial viral infection, a brief recovery period follows when the child doesn't seem seriously ill. A few days later, he develops intractable vomiting; lethargy; rapidly changing mental status (mild to severe agitation, confusion, irritability, and delirium); rising blood pressure, respiratory rate, and pulse rate; and hyperactive reflexes.

Reye's syndrome commonly progresses to coma. As coma deepens, seizures develop, followed by decreased tendon reflexes and, usually, respiratory failure.

COMPLICATIONS

Increased ICP, a serious complication, is now considered the result of an increased cerebral blood volume causing intracranial hypertension. Such swelling may develop because of acidosis, increased cerebral metabolic rate, and an impaired autoregulatory mechanism.

Other complications may include respiratory failure and death.

DIAGNOSIS

A history of a recent viral disorder with typical clinical features strongly suggests Reye's syndrome. An increased serum ammonia level, abnormal clotting studies, and hepatic dysfunction confirm it. Testing serum salicylate levels rules out aspirin use. Absence of jaundice despite increased liver aminotransferase levels rules out acute hepatic failure and hepatic encephalopathy.

Stages of treatment for Reye's syndrome

SIGNS AND SYMPTONS	BASELINE TREATMENT	BASELINE INTERVENTION
Stage I		
Vomiting, lethargy, hepatic dysfunction	✦ To decrease intracranial pressure (ICP) and brain edema, give I.V. fluids at two-thirds maintenance rate. Also give an osmotic diuretic or furosemide. ✦ To treat hypoprothrombinemia, give vitamin K; if vitamin K is unsuccessful, give fresh frozen plasma. ✦ Monitor serum ammonia and blood glucose levels and plasma osmolality every 4 to 8 hours to check progress.	✦ Monitor vital signs and check level of consciousness for increasing lethargy. Take vital signs more often as the patient's condition deteriorates. ✦ Monitor fluid intake and output to prevent fluid overload. Maintain urine output at 1 ml/kg/hr; plasma osmolality, 290 mOsm/kg; and blood glucose, 150 mg/ml. (Goal: Keep glucose level high, osmolality normal to high, and ammonia level low.) Also, restrict protein.
Stage II		
Hyperventilation, delirium, hepatic dysfunction, hyperactive reflexes	✦ Continue baseline treatment from stage I.	✦ Maintain seizure precautions. ✦ Immediately report any signs of coma that require invasive, supportive therapy, such as intubation. ✦ Keep head of bed at 30-degree angle.
Stage III		
Coma, hyperventilation, decorticate rigidity, hepatic dysfunction	✦ Continue baseline treatment from stage I and seizure treatment. ✦ Monitor ICP with a subarachnoid screw or other invasive device. ✦ Provide endotracheal intubation and mechanical ventilation to control partial pressure of arterial carbon dioxide ($Paco_2$) levels. A paralyzing agent, such as atracurium besylate or pancuronium I.V., may help maintain ventilation. ✦ Give mannitol I.V.	✦ Monitor ICP (should be less than 20 mm Hg before suctioning) or give a barbiturate I.V., as ordered; hyperventilate the patient as necessary. ✦ When ventilating the patient, maintain $Paco_2$ between 25 and 30 mm Hg and partial pressure of arterial oxygen between 80 and 100 mm Hg. ✦ Monitor cardiovascular status with a pulmonary artery catheter or central venous pressure line. ✦ Give good skin and mouth care and range-of-motion exercises.
Stage IV		
Deepening coma; decerebrate rigidity; large, fixed pupils; minimal hepatic dysfunction	✦ Continue baseline treatment from stage I and supportive care. ✦ If all previous measures fail, some pediatric centers use barbiturate coma, decompressive craniotomy, hypothermia, or exchange transfusion.	✦ Check patient for loss of reflexes and signs of flaccidity. ✦ Give the family the extra support they need, considering their child's poor prognosis.

Stages of treatment

Stage I
✦ Decrease ICP and brain edema
✦ Treat hypoprothrombinemia; give vitamin K
✦ Monitor serum ammonia and blood glucose levels

Stage II
✦ Continue treatments for stage 1
✦ Maintain seizure precautions

Stage III
✦ Continue treatment from stage 1 and seizure treatment
✦ Provide endotracheal intubation
✦ Give mannitol I.V.

Stage IV
✦ Continue baseline treatment from stage 1
✦ Continue supportive care
✦ Monitor serum ammonia and blood glucose levels

Stage V
✦ Continue baseline treatment
✦ Continue supportive care

Diagnosis

+ History of recent viral disorder
+ Increased serum ammonia level
+ Serum salicylate level rules out aspirin use
+ Absence of jaundice rules out hepatic failure and encephalopathy
+ High aspartate and alanine aminotransferase levels
+ Increased PT and PTT

Treatment

+ I.V. fluids
+ Vitamin K
+ Fresh frozen plasma
+ Mechanical ventilation

Key nursing actions

+ Advise parents to give nonsalicylate analgesics and antipyretics.

Characteristics of seizure disorder

+ Also known as *epilepsy*
+ Characterized by susceptibility to recurrent seizures
+ Primary: idiopathic without apparent structural changes in brain
+ Secondary: structural changes or metabolic alterations of neuronal membranes; causes increased automaticity
+ Affects 1% to 2% of the population

Causes

+ 50% are idiopathic
+ Birth trauma
+ Perinatal infection

Stages of treatment for Reye's syndrome (continued)

SIGNS AND SYMPTONS	BASELINE TREATMENT	BASELINE INTERVENTION
Stage V		
Seizures, loss of deep tendon reflexes, flaccidity, respiratory arrest, ammonia level above 300 mg/dl	+ Continue baseline treatment from stage 1; continue supportive care.	+ Help the family to face the patient's impending death.

Laboratory tests disclose elevated serum ammonia levels; normal or (in 15% of cases) low serum glucose levels; and increased serum fatty acid and lactate levels. Liver function studies indicate aspartate aminotransferase and alanine aminotransferase at twice the normal levels. Bilirubin levels are normal.

Coagulation studies demonstrate increased prothrombin time (PT) and partial thromboplastin time (PTT). Cerebrospinal fluid (CSF) analysis shows a white blood cell count of less than 10/µl; coma causes increased CSF pressure.

Liver biopsy reveals fatty droplets uniformly distributed throughout liver cells.

TREATMENT

For treatment guidelines, see *Stages of treatment for Reye's syndrome,* pages 329 and 330.

NURSING CONSIDERATIONS

Advise parents to give nonsalicylate analgesics and antipyretics such as acetaminophen. For more information, refer parents to the National Reye's Syndrome Foundation.

SEIZURE DISORDER

Seizure disorder, or *epilepsy,* is a condition of the brain characterized by susceptibility to recurrent seizures (paroxysmal events associated with abnormal electrical discharges of neurons in the brain). Primary seizure disorder or epilepsy is idiopathic without apparent structural changes in the brain. Secondary epilepsy, characterized by structural changes or metabolic alterations of the neuronal membranes, causes increased automaticity.

Epilepsy is believed to affect 1% to 2% of the population; approximately 2 million people have been diagnosed with epilepsy. The incidence is highest in childhood and old age. The prognosis is good if the patient adheres strictly to prescribed treatment.

CAUSES

About 50% of all seizure disorder cases are idiopathic; possible causes of other cases include birth trauma (inadequate oxygen supply to the brain, blood incompatibility, or hemorrhage); perinatal infection; anoxia; infectious diseases (meningitis, encephalitis, or brain abscess); ingestion of toxins (mercury, lead, or carbon monoxide); brain tumors; inherited disorders or degenerative disease, such as phenylketonuria or tuberous sclerosis; head injury or trauma; metabolic disorders, such as hypoglycemia and hypoparathyroidism; and stroke (hemorrhage, thrombosis, or embolism).

PATHOPHYSIOLOGY

Some neurons in the brain may depolarize easily or be hyperexcitable; this epileptogenic focus fires more readily than normal when stimulated. In these neurons, the membrane potential at rest is less negative or inhibitory connections are missing, possibly because of decreased gamma-aminobutyric acid activity or localized shifts in electrolytes.

On stimulation, the epileptogenic focus fires and spreads electric current to surrounding cells. These cells fire in turn and the impulse cascades to one side of the brain (a partial seizure), both sides of the brain (a generalized seizure), or cortical, subcortical, and brain stem areas.

The brain's metabolic demand for oxygen increases dramatically during a seizure. If this demand isn't met, hypoxia and brain damage ensue. Firing of inhibitory neurons causes the excitatory neurons to slow their firing and eventually stop. If this inhibitory action doesn't occur, the result is status epilepticus: one seizure occurring right after another and another; without treatment the anoxia is fatal.

SIGNS AND SYMPTOMS

The hallmark of epilepsy is recurring seizures, which can be classified as partial, generalized, status epilepticus, or unclassified (some patients may be affected by more than one type). (See *Seizure types*, page 332.)

COMPLICATIONS

Associated complications can occur during a seizure. These include anoxia from airway occlusion by the tongue or vomitus and traumatic injury. Such traumatic injury could result from a fall at the onset of a generalized tonic-clonic seizure; from the rapid, jerking movements that occur during or after a generalized tonic-clonic seizure; or from a fall or sudden movement sustained while the patient is confused or has an altered level of consciousness.

DIAGNOSIS

Clinically, the diagnosis of epilepsy is based on the occurrence of one or more seizures and proof or the assumption that the condition that caused them is still present. Diagnostic tests help support the findings.

✦ Computed tomography (CT) scan or magnetic resonance imaging (MRI) reveals abnormalities.

✦ EEG reveals paroxysmal abnormalities to confirm the diagnosis and provide evidence of the continuing tendency to have seizures. In tonic-clonic seizures, high, fast-voltage spikes are present in all leads; in absence seizures, rounded spike wave complexes are diagnostic. A negative EEG doesn't rule out epilepsy because the abnormalities occur intermittently.

✦ Skull X-ray may show evidence of fractures or shifting of the pineal gland, bony erosion, or separated sutures.

✦ Serum chemistry blood studies may reveal hypoglycemia, electrolyte imbalances, elevated liver enzymes, and elevated alcohol levels, providing clues to underlying conditions that increase the risk of seizure activity.

How it happens

✦ Some neurons in the brain may depolarize easily or be hyperexcitable

✦ On stimulation, epileptogenic focus fires and spreads electric current to surrounding cells

✦ Impulse cascades to one or both sides of brain or cortical, subcortical, brain stem areas

✦ Brain's metabolic demand increases dramatically during seizure

✦ Hypoxia and brain damage ensue without oxygen

✦ Firing of inhibitory neurons causes excitatory neurons to slow and stop

✦ If inhibitory action doesn't occur, result is status epilepticus

Key signs and symptoms

✦ Recurring seizures

Complications

✦ Anoxia

✦ Injury during seizure

Diagnosis

✦ Based on occurrence of one or more seizures; proof or assumption that cause still present

✦ CT scan or MRI reveals abnormalities

✦ EEG reveals paroxysmal abnormalities

✦ Tonic-clonic seizures, high, fast-voltage spikes present in all leads

✦ Absence seizures, rounded spike wave complexes are diagnostic

Types of seizures

Partial
✦ Simple partial: begins locally and may present with sensory symptoms
✦ Complex partial: alters consciousness; seizure lasts for 1 to 3 minutes

Generalized
✦ Absence: occurs most commonly in children; patient retains posture and continues preseizure activity without difficulty
✦ Myoclonic: brief, involuntary muscular jerks; consciousness isn't affected
✦ Generalized tonic-clonic: begins with a loud cry, precipated by air rushing from the lungs to the vocal cords; stops in 2 to 5 minutes
✦ Atonic: general loss of postural tone; temporary loss of consciousness

Status epilepticus
✦ Continuous seizure; accompanied by respiratory distress leading to hypoxia or anoxia

Unclassified
✦ Seizures that don't fit the other categories; lack of data to make definitive diagnosis

Seizure types

The various types of seizures — partial, generalized, status epilepticus, and unclassified — have distinct signs and symptoms.

PARTIAL SEIZURES
Arising from a localized area of the brain, partial seizures cause focal symptoms. These seizures are classified by their effect on consciousness and whether they spread throughout the motor pathway, causing a generalized seizure.

✦ A *simple partial seizure* begins locally and generally doesn't cause an alteration in consciousness. It may present with sensory symptoms (lights flashing, smells, hearing hallucinations), autonomic symptoms (sweating, flushing, pupil dilation), and psychic symptoms (dream states, anger, fear). The seizure lasts for a few seconds and occurs without preceding or provoking events. This type can be motor or sensory.

✦ A *complex partial seizure* alters consciousness. Amnesia for events that occur during and immediately after the seizure is a differentiating characteristic. During the seizure, the patient may follow simple commands. This seizure generally lasts for 1 to 3 minutes.

GENERALIZED SEIZURES
As the term suggests, generalized seizures cause a generalized electrical abnormality within the brain. They can be convulsive or nonconvulsive and include several types:

✦ *Absence seizures* occur most commonly in children, although they may affect adults. They usually begin with a brief change in level of consciousness, indicated by blinking or rolling of the eyes, a blank stare, and slight mouth movements. The patient retains his posture and continues preseizure activity without difficulty. Typically, each seizure lasts from 1 to 10 seconds. If not properly treated, seizures can recur as often as 100 times per day. An absence seizure is a nonconvulsive seizure, but it may progress to a generalized tonic-clonic seizure.

✦ *Myoclonic seizures* (bilateral massive epileptic myoclonus) are brief, involuntary muscular jerks of the body or extremities, which may be rhythmic. Consciousness isn't usually affected.

✦ *Generalized tonic-clonic seizures* typically begin with a loud cry, precipitated by air rushing from the lungs through the vocal cords. The patient then loses consciousness and falls to the ground. The body stiffens (tonic phase) and then alternates between episodes of muscle spasm and relaxation (clonic phase). Tongue biting, incontinence, labored breathing, apnea, and subsequent cyanosis may occur. The seizure stops in 2 to 5 minutes, when abnormal electrical conduction ceases. When the patient regains consciousness, he's confused and may have difficulty talking. If he can talk, he may complain of drowsiness, fatigue, headache, muscle soreness, and arm or leg weakness. He may fall into a deep sleep after the seizure.

✦ *Atonic seizures* are characterized by a general loss of postural tone and a temporary loss of consciousness. They occur in young children and are sometimes called "drop attacks" because they cause the child to fall.

STATUS EPILEPTICUS
Status epilepticus is a continuous seizure state that can occur in all seizure types. The most life-threatening example is generalized tonic-clonic status epilepticus, a continuous generalized tonic-clonic seizure. Status epilepticus is accompanied by respiratory distress leading to hypoxia or anoxia. It can result from abrupt withdrawal of anticonvulsant medications, hypoxic encephalopathy, acute head trauma, metabolic encephalopathy, or septicemia secondary to encephalitis or meningitis.

UNCLASSIFIED SEIZURES
This category is reserved for seizures that don't fit the characteristics of partial or generalized seizures or status epilepticus. Included are events that lack the data to make a more definitive diagnosis.

TREATMENT

Treatment consists of drug therapy specific to the type of seizure. The most commonly prescribed drugs include phenytoin, carbamazepine, phenobarbital, gabapentin, and primidone for generalized tonic-clonic seizures and complex partial seizures. I.V. fosphenytoin is an alternative to phenytoin that's just as effective, with a long half-life and minimal central nervous system depression. It's stable for 120 days at room temperature and compatible with many commonly used I.V. solutions. It also can be administered rapidly without the adverse cardiovascular effects that occur with phenytoin.

Valproic acid, clonazepam, and ethosuximide are commonly prescribed for absence seizures. Gabapentin and felbamate are newer anticonvulsant drugs.

Treatment may include surgical removal of a demonstrated focal lesion, if drug therapy is ineffective. Surgery is also performed to remove the underlying cause, such as a tumor, abscess, or vascular problem.

A vagus nerve stimulator implant may help reduce the incidence of focal seizure. The nerve is stimulated for approximately 30 seconds every 5 minutes. Emergency treatment usually consists of I.V. diazepam, lorazepam, phenytoin, or phenobarbital for status epilepticus and the administration of dextrose (when seizures are secondary to hypoglycemia) or thiamine (in chronic alcoholism or withdrawal).

NURSING CONSIDERATIONS

A key to support is a true understanding of the nature of epilepsy and of the misconceptions that surround it.

✦ Encourage the patient and his family to express their feelings about the patient's condition. Answer their questions, and help them cope by dispelling some of the myths about epilepsy, for example, the myth that epilepsy is contagious. Assure them that epilepsy is controllable for most patients who follow a prescribed regimen of medication and that most patients maintain a normal lifestyle.

Because drug therapy is the treatment of choice for most people with epilepsy, information about medications is invaluable.

✦ Stress the need for compliance with the prescribed drug schedule. Reinforce dosage instructions and stress the importance of taking medication regularly and at scheduled times. Caution the patient to monitor the quantity of medication he has so he doesn't run out of it.

✦ Warn against possible adverse effects — drowsiness, lethargy, hyperactivity, confusion, and visual and sleep disturbances — all of which indicate the need for dosage adjustment. Phenytoin therapy may lead to hyperplasia of the gums, which may be relieved by conscientious oral hygiene. Instruct the patient to report adverse effects immediately.

✦ When administering phenytoin I.V., use a large vein and monitor vital signs frequently. Avoid I.M. administration and mixing with dextrose solutions.

✦ Emphasize the importance of having anticonvulsant blood levels checked at regular intervals, even if the seizures are under control.

✦ Warn the patient against drinking alcoholic beverages.

✦ Know which social agencies in your community can help epileptic patients. Refer the patient to the Epilepsy Foundation of America for general information and to the state motor vehicle department for information about a driver's license.

The primary goals of the health care professional and family members caring for a patient having a seizure are protection from injury, protection from aspiration, and observation of the seizure activity. Generalized tonic-clonic seizures may

Treatment
✦ Drug therapy specific to type of seizure
✦ Vagus nerve stimulator implant
✦ Emergency drug treatment

Key nursing actions
✦ Encourage the patient and his family to express their feelings about the patient's condition.
✦ Because drug therapy is the treatment of choice for most people with epilepsy, information about medications is invaluable.
✦ When administering phenytoin I.V., use a large vein and monitor vital signs frequently.
✦ Emphasize the importance of having anticonvulsant blood levels checked at regular intervals, even if the seizures are under control.
✦ Warn the patient against drinking alcoholic beverages.
✦ Refer the patient to the Epilepsy Foundation of America.

Key nursing actions
(continued)

✦ Avoid restraining the patient during a seizure. Help the patient to a lying position and loosen any tight clothing.
✦ Don't restrain the patient during a complex partial seizure. Gently call his name and direct him away from the source of danger.

Characteristics of spinal cord trauma

✦ Include fractures, contusions, and compressions of vertebral column
✦ Damage may involve entire cord or be restricted to one-half
✦ Fractures of 5th, 6th, 7th cervical, 12th thoracic, 1st lumbar vertebrae most common

Causes

✦ Automobile accidents
✦ Falls
✦ Sports injuries
✦ Diving into shallow water

How it happens

✦ Hyperextension: acceleration-deceleration, sudden reduction in the anteroposterior diameter of spinal cord
✦ Hyperflexion: sudden and excessive force, propelling neck forward or causing exaggerated movement to one side
✦ Vertical compression: force applied from top of cranium along vertical axis
✦ Force causes microscopic hemorrhages in gray matter and pia-arachnoid; necrosis develops
✦ Collagen replaces normal tissue
✦ Scarring and meningeal thickening leaves nerves blocked

necessitate first aid. Show the patient's family members how to administer first aid correctly.

✦ Avoid restraining the patient during a seizure. Help the patient to a lying position, loosen any tight clothing, and place something flat and soft, such as a pillow, jacket, or hand, under his head. Clear the area of hard objects. Don't force anything into the patient's mouth if his teeth are clenched—a tongue blade or spoon could lacerate the mouth and lips or displace teeth, precipitating respiratory distress. However, if the patient's mouth is open, protect his tongue by placing a soft object (such as a folded cloth) between his teeth. Turn his head to provide an open airway. After the seizure subsides, reassure the patient that he's all right, orient him to time and place, and inform him that he has had a seizure.

✦ Don't restrain the patient during a complex partial seizure. Clear the area of hard objects. Protect him from injury by gently calling his name and directing him away from the source of danger. After the seizure passes, reassure him and tell him that he has just had a seizure.

SPINAL CORD TRAUMA

Spinal injuries include fractures, contusions, and compressions of the vertebral column, usually as the result of trauma to the head or neck. The real danger lies in spinal cord damage—cutting, pulling, twisting, or compression. Damage may involve the entire cord or be restricted to one-half, and it can occur at any level. Fractures of the 5th, 6th, or 7th cervical, 12th thoracic, and 1st lumbar vertebrae are most common.

CAUSES

The most serious spinal cord trauma typically results from automobile accidents, falls, sports injuries, diving into shallow water, and gunshot or stab wounds.

Less serious injuries commonly occur from lifting heavy objects and minor falls. Spinal dysfunction may also result from hyperparathyroidism and neoplastic lesions.

PATHOPHYSIOLOGY

Like head trauma, spinal cord trauma results from acceleration, deceleration, or other deforming forces usually applied from a distance.

Hyperextension occurs from acceleration-deceleration forces and sudden reduction in the anteroposterior diameter of the spinal cord.

Hyperflexion occurs from sudden and excessive force, propelling the neck forward or causing an exaggerated movement to one side.

Vertical compression occurs from force being applied from the top of the cranium along the vertical axis through the vertebra.

Rotational forces occur from twisting, which adds shearing forces.

Injury causes microscopic hemorrhages in the gray matter and pia-arachnoid. The hemorrhages gradually enlarge until all of the gray matter is filled with blood, which causes necrosis. From the gray matter, the blood enters the white matter, where it impedes the circulation within the spinal cord. Ensuing edema causes compression and decreases the blood supply. Thus, the spinal cord loses perfusion and becomes ischemic. The edema and hemorrhage are greatest at and approximately two segments above and below the injury. The edema temporarily adds to the patient's dysfunction by increasing pressure and compressing the nerves. Edema near the third to fifth cervical vertebrae may interfere with phrenic nerve impulse transmission to the diaphragm and inhibit respiratory function.

In the white matter, circulation usually returns to normal in approximately 24 hours. However, in the gray matter, an inflammatory reaction prevents restoration of circulation. Phagocytes appear at the site within 36 to 48 hours after the injury, macrophages engulf degenerating axons, and collagen replaces the normal tissue. Scarring and meningeal thickening leaves the nerves in the area blocked or tangled.

SIGNS AND SYMPTOMS

The patient typically complains of muscle spasm and back pain that worsens with movement. In cervical fractures, pain may cause point tenderness; in dorsal and lumbar fractures, it may radiate to other body areas such as the legs.

Physical assessment may reveal mild paresthesia to quadriplegia and shock, if the injury damages the spinal cord. In milder injury, such symptoms may be delayed several days or weeks. Specific signs and symptoms depend on injury type and degree. (See *Types of spinal cord injury,* page 336.)

COMPLICATIONS

Spinal injuries can be complicated by spinal cord damage, resulting in paralysis and even death. The extent of cord damage depends on the level of injury to the spinal column. Autonomic dysreflexia, spinal shock, and neurogenic shock are complications of spinal injuries. (See *Complications of spinal cord injury,* page 337.)

DIAGNOSIS

Spinal X-rays, the most important diagnostic measure, detect the fracture. Thorough neurologic evaluation locates the level of injury and detects cord damage. Lumbar puncture may show increased cerebrospinal fluid (CSF) pressure from a lesion or trauma in spinal compression. Computed tomography (CT) scan or magnetic resonance imaging (MRI) reveals spinal cord edema and compression and may reveal a spinal mass.

TREATMENT

The primary treatment after spinal injury is immediate immobilization to stabilize the spine and prevent cord damage. Cervical injuries require the use of sandbags on both sides of the patient's head, a hard cervical collar, or skeletal traction with skull tongs or a halo device.

High doses of methylprednisolone are administered to reduce inflammation with evidence of cord injury. Treatment of stable lumbar and dorsal fractures consists of bed rest on firm support (such as a bed board), analgesics, and muscle relaxants for several days until the fracture stabilizes.

A plaster cast or a turning frame is required to treat unstable dorsal or lumbar fracture. Laminectomy and spinal fusion is required for severe lumbar fractures.

Neurosurgery may relieve the pressure when the damage results in compression of the spinal column—if the cause of compression is a metastatic lesion, chemotherapy and radiation may relieve it.

Treatment of surface wounds accompanying the spinal injury requires tetanus prophylaxis unless the patient has had recent immunization.

Later treatment includes exercises to strengthen the back muscles, a back brace or corset to provide support while walking, and rehabilitation to maintain or improve functional level.

Key signs and symptoms

- ✦ Muscle spasm and back pain that worsens with movement
- ✦ Point tenderness or radiating pain
- ✦ Mild paresthesia to quadriplegia and shock
- ✦ Depend on injury type and degree

Complications

- ✦ Spinal cord damage
- ✦ Autonomic dysreflexia
- ✦ Spinal shock
- ✦ Neurogenic shock

Diagnosis

- ✦ Spinal X-rays detect fracture
- ✦ Neurologic evaluation of level of injury
- ✦ Lumbar puncture shows increased CSF pressure
- ✦ CT scan or MRI reveals spinal cord edema, compression, may reveal spinal mass

Treatment

- ✦ Immediate immobilization
- ✦ High doses of methylprednisolone
- ✦ Bed rest on firm support
- ✦ Analgesics
- ✦ Muscle relaxants
- ✦ Plaster cast or turning frame
- ✦ Laminectomy and spinal fusion
- ✦ Neurosurgery
- ✦ Treatment of surface wounds
- ✦ Physical therapy or rehabilitation
- ✦ Back brace or corset

Types of spinal cord injury

Complete transection
+ All tracks of spinal cord are disrupted
+ Complete and permanent loss

Incomplete transection: Central cord syndrome
+ Center portion of cord affected
+ Typically from hyperextension injury

Incomplete transection: Anterior cord syndrome
+ Occlusion of anterior spinal artery
+ Occulsion from pressure of bone fragments

Incomplete transection: Brown-Séquard's syndrome
+ Hemisection of cord affected
+ Most common in stabbing and gunshot wounds

Key nursing actions
+ In all spinal injuries, suspect cord damage until proven otherwise.
+ During the initial assessment and X-ray studies, immobilize the patient on a firm surface, with sandbags or a cervical immobilization device on both sides of his head.
+ If you must move the patient, get at least three other members of the staff to help you logroll him to avoid disturbing body alignment.

Types of spinal cord injury

Injury to the spinal cord can be classified as incomplete or complete. An incomplete spinal injury may be an anterior cord syndrome, central cord syndrome, or Brown-Séquard's syndrome, depending on the area of the cord affected. This chart highlights the characteristic signs and symptoms of each.

TYPE	DESCRIPTION	SIGNS AND SYMPTOMS
Complete transection	+ All tracts of the spinal cord completely disrupted + All functions involving the spinal cord below the level of transection lost + Complete and permanent loss	+ Loss of motor function (quadriplegia) with cervical cord transection; paraplegia with thoracic cord transection + Muscle flaccidity + Loss of all reflexes and sensory function below level of injury + Bladder and bowel atony + Paralytic ileus + Loss of vasomotor tone in lower body parts with low and unstable blood pressure + Loss of perspiration below level of injury + Dry pale skin + Respiratory impairment
Incomplete transection: Central cord syndrome	+ Center portion of cord affected + Typically from hyperextension injury	+ Motor deficits greater in upper than in lower extremities + Variable degree of bladder dysfunction
Incomplete transection: Anterior cord syndrome	+ Occlusion of anterior spinal artery + Occlusion from pressure of bone fragments	+ Loss of motor function below level of injury + Loss of pain and temperature sensations below level of injury + Intact touch, pressure, position, and vibration senses
Incomplete transection: Brown-Séquard's syndrome	+ Hemisection of cord affected + Most common in stabbing and gunshot wounds + Damage to cord on only one side	+ Ipsilateral paralysis or paresis below level of injury + Ipsilateral loss of touch, pressure, vibration, and position senses below level of injury + Contralateral loss of pain and temperature sensations below level of injury

NURSING CONSIDERATIONS

In all spinal injuries, suspect cord damage until proven otherwise.
+ During the initial assessment and X-ray studies, immobilize the patient on a firm surface, with sandbags or a cervical immobilization device on both sides of his head. Tell him not to move and avoid moving him yourself because hyperflexion can damage the cord. If you must move the patient, get at least three other members of the staff to help you logroll him to avoid disturbing body alignment.

Complications of spinal cord injury

Of the following three sets of complications, only autonomic dysreflexia requires emergency attention.

AUTONOMIC DYSREFLEXIA
Also known as *autonomic hyperreflexia*, autonomic dysreflexia is a serious medical condition that occurs after resolution of spinal shock. Emergency recognition and management are needed.

Autonomic dysreflexia should be suspected in the patient with:
+ spinal cord trauma at or above level T6
+ bradycardia
+ hypertension and a severe pounding headache
+ cold or goose-fleshed skin below the lesion.

Dysreflexia is caused by noxious stimuli, most commonly a distended bladder or skin lesion.

Treatment focuses on eliminating the stimulus; rapid identification and removal may avoid the need for pharmacologic control of the headache and hypertension.

SPINAL SHOCK
Spinal shock is the loss of autonomic, reflex, motor, and sensory activity below the level of the cord lesion. It occurs secondary to damage of the spinal cord.

Signs of spinal shock include:
+ flaccid paralysis
+ loss of deep tendon and perianal reflexes
+ loss of motor and sensory function.

Until spinal shock has resolved (usually 1 to 6 weeks after injury), the extent of actual cord damage can't be assessed. The earliest indicator of resolution is the return of reflex activity.

NEUROGENIC SHOCK
Neurogenic shock is an abnormal vasomotor response that occurs secondary to disruption of sympathetic impulses from the brain stem to the thoracolumbar area, and is seen most commonly in patients with cervical cord injury. This temporary loss of autonomic function below the level of injury causes cardiovascular changes.

Signs of neurogenic shock include:
+ orthostatic hypotension
+ bradycardia
+ loss of the ability to sweat below the level of the lesion.

Treatment depends on symptoms. Symptoms resolve when spinal cord edema resolves.

Key facts about spinal cord injury complications

Autonomic dysreflexia
+ Occurs after resolution of spinal shock
+ Emergency recognition and management are needed
+ Occurs from spinal cord trauma at or above level T6

Spinal shock
+ Occurs secondary to damage of spinal cord
+ Until it's resolved, extent of cord damage can't be assessed

Neurogenic shock
+ Abnormal vasomotor response
+ Temporary loss of autonomic function below the level of injury
+ Treatment depends on symptoms

Key nursing actions
(continued)
+ Throughout assessment, offer comfort and reassurance.
+ If the injury requires surgery, administer prophylactic antibiotics.
+ Explain traction methods to the patient and his family.
+ Turn the patient on his side during feedings to prevent aspiration. Create a relaxed atmosphere at mealtimes.
+ Watch closely for neurologic changes. Immediately report changes in skin sensation and loss of muscle strength.
+ Before discharge, instruct the patient about continuing analgesics or other medication.

+ Throughout assessment, offer comfort and reassurance. Remember, the fear of possible paralysis will be overwhelming. Talk to the patient quietly and calmly. Allow a family member who isn't too distraught to accompany him.
+ If the injury requires surgery, administer prophylactic antibiotics as ordered. Catheterize the patient, as ordered, to avoid urine retention, and monitor bowel elimination patterns to avoid impaction.
+ Explain traction methods to the patient and his family. Reassure them that traction devices don't penetrate the brain. If the patient has a halo or skull-tong traction device, clean pin sites daily, trim hair short, and provide analgesics for persistent headaches. During traction, turn the patient often to prevent pneumonia, embolism, and skin breakdown; perform passive range-of-motion exercises to maintain muscle tone. If available, use a CircOlectric bed or Stryker frame to facilitate turning and to prevent spinal cord injury.
+ Turn the patient on his side during feedings to prevent aspiration. Create a relaxed atmosphere at mealtimes.
+ Suggest appropriate diversionary activities to fill the patient's hours of immobility.
+ Watch closely for neurologic changes. Immediately report changes in skin sensation and loss of muscle strength — either of which might indicate pressure on the spinal cord, possibly because of edema or shifting bone fragments.

♦ Help the patient walk as soon as the physician allows; he'll probably need to wear a back brace.

♦ Before discharge, instruct the patient about continuing analgesics or other medication, and stress the importance of regular follow-up examinations.

♦ To help prevent a spinal injury from becoming a spinal cord injury, educate firemen, policemen, paramedics, and the general public about the proper way to handle such injuries.

STROKE

A stroke, also known as a *cerebrovascular accident* or *brain attack,* is a sudden impairment of cerebral circulation in one or more blood vessels. A stroke interrupts or diminishes oxygen supply, and commonly causes serious damage or necrosis in the brain tissues. The sooner the circulation returns to normal after a stroke, the better the chances are for a complete recovery. However, about one-half of the patients who survive a stroke remain permanently disabled and experience a recurrence within weeks, months, or years. It's the leading cause of admission to long-term care.

Stroke is the third most common cause of death in the United States and the most common cause of neurologic disability. It strikes more than 500,000 people per year and is fatal in approximately 50% of them.

 CLINICAL ALERT Although strokes may occur in younger people, most patients experiencing strokes are over age 65. In fact, the risk of stroke doubles with each passing decade after age 55.

 CLINICAL ALERT The incidence of stroke is higher in Blacks than in Whites. In fact, Blacks have a 60% higher risk of stroke than Whites or Hispanics of the same age. This is believed to be the result of an increased prevalence of hypertension in Blacks. In addition, strokes in Blacks usually result from disease in the small cerebral vessels, whereas strokes in Whites are typically the result of disease in the large carotid arteries. The mortality rate for Blacks from stroke is twice the rate for Whites.

CAUSES

Stroke typically results from cerebral thrombosis, embolism, or hemorrhage.

Thrombosis of the cerebral arteries supplying the brain or of the intracranial vessels occluding blood flow is the most common cause of stroke in middle-aged and elderly people. (See *Types of stroke.*)

Embolism from thrombus outside the brain, such as in the heart, aorta, or common carotid artery can occur at any age, especially among patients with a history of rheumatic heart disease, endocarditis, posttraumatic valvular disease, myocardial fibrillation and other cardiac arrhythmias, or after open heart surgery.

Hemorrhage from an intracranial artery or vein, such as from hypertension, ruptured aneurysm, arteriovenous malformations, trauma, hemorrhagic disorder, or septic embolism can also occur at any age.

Risk factors that have been identified as predisposing a patient to stroke include hypertension; family history of stroke; a history of transient ischemic attacks (TIAs) (see *Understanding TIAs,* page 340); cardiac disease, including arrhythmias, coronary artery disease, acute myocardial infarction, dilated cardiomyopathy, and valvular disease; diabetes; familial hyperlipidemia; cigarette smoking; increased alcohol intake; obesity; sedentary lifestyle; and use of hormonal contraceptives.

Types of stroke

Strokes are typically classified as ischemic or hemorrhagic depending on the underlying cause. This chart describes the major types of stroke.

TYPE OF STROKE	DESCRIPTION
Ischemic: Thrombotic	✦ Most common cause of stroke ✦ Commonly the result of atherosclerosis; also associated with hypertension, smoking, and diabetes ✦ Thrombus in extracranial or intracranial vessel blocks blood flow to the cerebral cortex ✦ Carotid artery most commonly affected extracranial vessel ✦ Common intracranial sites include bifurcation of carotid arteries, distal intracranial portion of vertebral arteries, and proximal basilar arteries ✦ May occur during sleep or shortly after awakening, during surgery, or after a myocardial infarction
Ischemic: Embolic	✦ Second most common type of stroke ✦ Embolus from heart or extracranial artery floats into cerebral bloodstream and lodges in middle cerebral artery or branches ✦ Embolus commonly originates during atrial fibrillation ✦ Typically occurs during activity ✦ Develops rapidly
Ischemic: Lacunar	✦ Subtype of thrombotic stroke ✦ Hypertension creates cavities deep in white matter of the brain, affecting the internal capsule, basal ganglia, thalamus, and pons ✦ Lipid coated lining of the small penetrating arteries thickens and weakens wall, causing microaneurysms and dissections
Hemorrhagic	✦ Third most common type of stroke ✦ Typically caused by hypertension or rupture of aneurysm ✦ Diminished blood supply to area supplied by ruptured artery and compression by accumulated blood

PATHOPHYSIOLOGY

Regardless of the cause, the underlying event is deprivation of oxygen and nutrients. Normally, if the arteries become blocked, autoregulatory mechanisms help maintain cerebral circulation until collateral circulation develops to deliver blood to the affected area. If the compensatory mechanisms become overworked or cerebral blood flow remains impaired for more than a few minutes, oxygen deprivation leads to infarction of brain tissue. The brain cells cease to function because they can neither store glucose or glycogen for use nor engage in anaerobic metabolism.

A thrombotic or embolic stroke causes ischemia. Some of the neurons served by the occluded vessel die from lack of oxygen and nutrients. This results in cerebral infarction, in which tissue injury triggers an inflammatory response that in turn increases intracranial pressure (ICP). Injury to the surrounding cells disrupts metabolism and leads to changes in ionic transport, localized acidosis, and free radical formation. Calcium, sodium, and water accumulate in the injured cells, and excitatory neurotransmitters are released. Consequent continued cellular injury and swelling set up a vicious cycle of further damage.

Types of stroke

Ischemic: Thrombotic
✦ Most common
✦ Commonly resulting from atherosclerosis

Ischemic: Embolic
✦ Second most common
✦ Embolus originates during atrial fibrillation

Ischemic: Lacunar
✦ Subtype of thrombotic stroke
✦ Hypertension creates cavities deep in white matter of the brain

Hemorrhagic
✦ Third most common type
✦ Caused by hypertension or rupture of aneurysm

How it happens

✦ Underlying event is deprivation of oxygen and nutrients
✦ Brain cells cease to function
✦ Thrombotic or embolic stroke causes ischemia
✦ Results in cerebral infarction
✦ Injury to surrounding cells disrupts metabolism
✦ Calcium, sodium, and water accumulate in injured cells, excitatory neurotransmitters released
✦ Hemorrhage impairs cerebral perfusion; causes infarction
✦ Blood exerts pressure on brain tissues
✦ Brain's regulatory mechanisms attempt to maintain equilibrium
✦ Increased ICP forces CSF out
✦ If bleeding is heavy, ICP increases rapidly and perfusion stops

TIAs
+ Episodes of neurologic deficit
+ Recurrent attacks may last from seconds to an hour
+ Considered warning sign for stroke
+ Features include transient focal deficits with complete return of function

Key signs and symptoms
+ Stroke in one hemisphere causes signs and symptoms on opposite side of body
+ Stroke damaging cranial nerves affects structures on same side as infarction
+ Unilateral limb weakness
+ Speech difficulties
+ Numbness on one side
+ Headache
+ Vision disturbances

Middle cerebral artery
+ Aphasia
+ Dysphasia
+ Hemiparesis of affected side

Cartoid artery
+ Paralysis
+ Bruits
+ Headaches
+ Ptosis

Understanding TIAs

A transient ischemic attack (TIA) is an episode of neurologic deficit resulting from cerebral ischemia. The recurrent attacks may last from seconds to an hour. It's usually considered a warning sign for stroke. In 14% of patients who experience a TIA, another TIA or a full stroke will occur within 1 year.

In a TIA, microemboli released from a thrombus may temporarily interrupt blood flow, especially in the small distal branches of the brain's arterial tree. Small spasms in those arterioles may impair blood flow and also precede a TIA.

The most distinctive features of TIAs are transient focal deficits with complete return of function. The deficits usually involve some degree of motor or sensory dysfunction. They may range to loss of consciousness and loss of motor or sensory function, but only for a brief time. Commonly, the patient experiences weakness in the lower part of the face and arms, hands, fingers, and legs on the side opposite the affected region. Other manifestations may include transient dysphagia, numbness or tingling of the face and lips, double vision, slurred speech, and dizziness.

When hemorrhage is the cause, impaired cerebral perfusion causes infarction, and the blood itself acts as a space-occupying mass, exerting pressure on the brain tissues. The brain's regulatory mechanisms attempt to maintain equilibrium by increasing blood pressure to maintain cerebral perfusion pressure. The increased ICP forces cerebrospinal fluid (CSF) out, thus restoring the balance. If the hemorrhage is small, this may be enough to keep the patient alive with only minimal neurologic deficits. However, if the bleeding is heavy, ICP increases rapidly and perfusion stops. Even if the pressure returns to normal, many brain cells die.

Initially, the ruptured cerebral blood vessels may constrict to limit the blood loss. This vasospasm further compromises blood flow, leading to more ischemia and cellular damage. If a clot forms in the vessel, decreased blood flow also promotes ischemia. If the blood enters the subarachnoid space, meningeal irritation occurs. The blood cells that pass through the vessel wall into the surrounding tissue also may break down and block the arachnoid villi, causing hydrocephalus.

SIGNS AND SYMPTOMS

The clinical features of stroke vary according to the affected artery and the region of the brain it supplies, the severity of the damage, and the extent of collateral circulation developed. A stroke in one hemisphere causes signs and symptoms on the opposite side of the body; a stroke that damages cranial nerves affects structures on the same side as the infarction.

General symptoms of a stroke include unilateral limb weakness, speech difficulties, numbness on one side, headache, vision disturbances (diplopia, hemianopsia, ptosis), dizziness, anxiety, and altered level of consciousness (LOC).

Additionally, symptoms are usually classified by the artery affected. Signs and symptoms associated with middle cerebral artery involvement include aphasia, dysphasia, visual field deficits, and hemiparesis of the affected side (more severe in the face and arm than in the leg).

Symptoms associated with carotid artery involvement include weakness, paralysis, numbness, sensory changes, vision disturbances on the affected side, altered LOC, bruits, headaches, aphasia, and ptosis.

Symptoms associated with vertebrobasilar artery involvement include weakness on the affected side, numbness around lips and mouth, visual field deficits, diplopia, poor coordination, dysphagia, slurred speech, dizziness, nystagmus, amnesia, and ataxia.

Signs and symptoms associated with anterior cerebral artery involvement include confusion, weakness, numbness, especially in the legs on the affected side, incontinence, loss of coordination, impaired motor and sensory functions, and personality changes.

Signs and symptoms associated with posterior cerebral artery involvement include visual field deficits (homonymous hemianopsia), sensory impairment, dyslexia, perseveration (abnormally persistent replies to questions), coma, cortical blindness, and absence of paralysis (usually).

COMPLICATIONS

Complications vary with the severity and type of stroke, but may include unstable blood pressure (from loss of vasomotor control), cerebral edema, fluid imbalances, sensory impairment, infections such as pneumonia, altered LOC, aspiration, contractures, pulmonary embolism, and death.

DIAGNOSIS

Computed tomography (CT) scan identifies an ischemic stroke within the first 72 hours of symptom onset and evidence of a hemorrhagic stroke (lesions larger than 1 cm) immediately.

Magnetic resonance imaging (MRI) assists in identifying areas of ischemia or infarction and cerebral swelling. Cerebral angiography reveals disruption or displacement of the cerebral circulation by occlusion, such as stenosis or acute thrombus, or hemorrhage. Digital subtraction angiography shows evidence of occlusion of cerebral vessels, lesions, or vascular abnormalities. Carotid duplex scan identifies the degree of stenosis.

Brain scan shows ischemic areas but may not be conclusive for up to 2 weeks after a stroke. Single photon emission CT and positron emission tomography scans identify areas of altered metabolism surrounding lesions not yet able to be detected by other diagnostic tests. Transesophageal echocardiogram reveals cardiac disorders, such as atrial thrombi, atrial septal defect, or patent foramen ovale, as causes of thrombotic stroke.

Lumbar puncture (performed if there are no signs of increased ICP) reveals bloody CSF when stroke is hemorrhagic. Ophthalmoscopy may identify signs of hypertension and atherosclerotic changes in retinal arteries. EEG helps identify damaged areas of the brain.

TREATMENT

Treatment is supportive to minimize and prevent further cerebral damage. Measures include ICP management with monitoring, hyperventilation (to decrease partial pressure of arterial carbon dioxide [$PaCO_2$] to lower ICP), osmotic diuretics (mannitol, to reduce cerebral edema), and corticosteroids (dexamethasone, to reduce inflammation and cerebral edema).

Medications useful in treating a stroke include stool softeners to prevent straining, which increases ICP, and anticonvulsants to treat or prevent seizures.

The patient may undergo surgery for large cerebellar infarction to remove infarcted tissue and decompress remaining live tissue. He may also have aneurysm repair to prevent further hemorrhage, or percutaneous transluminal angioplasty or stent insertion to open occluded vessels.

Key signs and symptoms

Vertebrobasilar artery
+ Poor coordination
+ Slurred speech

Anterior cerebral artery
+ Confusion
+ Weakness

Posterior cerebral artery
+ Dyslexia
+ Perseveration

Complications
+ Vary with the severity and type
+ Unstable blood pressure
+ Cerebral edema
+ Fluid imbalances
+ Sensory impairment
+ Infections

Diagnosis
+ CT scan identifies ischemic and hemorrhagic stroke
+ MRI helps identify areas of ischemia, infarction, cerebral swelling
+ Cerebral angiography reveals disruption or displacement of cerebral circulation
+ Lumbar puncture reveals bloody CSF
+ Ophthalmoscopy may show hypertension and atherosclerotic changes
+ EEG helps identify damaged areas of brain

Treatment
+ Hyperventilation
+ Osmotic diuretics
+ Corticosteroids
+ Stool softeners
+ Anticoagulant therapy
+ Antiplatelet agents

For ischemic stroke, thrombolytic therapy (tissue plasminogen activator, alteplase) is administered within the first 3 hours after the onset of symptoms to dissolve the clot, remove the occlusion, and restore blood flow, thus minimizing cerebral damage. (See *Treating ischemic stroke,* pages 344 and 345.)

Anticoagulant therapy (heparin, warfarin) maintains vessel patency and prevents further clot formation in cases of high-grade carotid stenosis or in newly diagnosed cardiovascular disease.

For TIAs, antiplatelet agents (aspirin, ticlopidine, dipyridamole and aspirin reduce the risk of platelet aggregation and subsequent clot formation. A carotid endarterectomy may be necessary to open partially (greater than 70%) occluded carotid arteries.

Analgesics such as acetaminophen relieve the headache associated with hemorrhagic stroke.

NURSING CONSIDERATIONS

During the acute phase, efforts focus on survival and the prevention of further complications. Effective care emphasizes continuing neurologic assessment, respiratory support, continuous monitoring of vital signs, careful positioning to prevent aspiration and contractures, management of GI problems, and careful monitoring of fluid, electrolyte, and nutritional status. Patient care must also include measures to prevent such complications as infection.

✦ Maintain patent airway and oxygenation. Loosen constrictive clothing. Watch for ballooning of the cheek with respiration. The side that balloons is the side affected by the stroke. If the patient is unconscious, he could aspirate saliva, so keep him in a lateral position to allow secretions to drain naturally or suction secretions, as needed. Insert an artificial airway, and start mechanical ventilation or supplemental oxygen, if necessary.

✦ Check vital signs and neurologic status, record observations, and report any significant changes to the physician. Monitor blood pressure, LOC, pupillary changes, motor function (voluntary and involuntary movements), sensory function, speech, skin color, temperature, signs of increased ICP, and nuchal rigidity or flaccidity. If a stroke is impending, blood pressure rises suddenly, pulse is rapid and bounding, and the patient may complain of a headache. Also, watch for signs of pulmonary emboli, such as chest pains, shortness of breath, dusky color, tachycardia, fever, and changed sensorium. If the patient is unresponsive, monitor blood gases often and alert the physician to increased $PaCO_2$ or decreased partial pressure of arterial oxygen.

Monitor status of fluid, electrolytes, and nutrition

✦ Maintain fluid and electrolyte balance. If the patient can take liquids orally, offer them as often as fluid limitations permit. Administer I.V. fluids as ordered; never give too much too fast because this can increase ICP. Offer the urinal or bedpan every 2 hours. If the patient is incontinent, he may need an indwelling urinary catheter, but this should be avoided, if possible, because of the risk of infection.

✦ Ensure adequate nutrition. Check for gag reflex before offering oral feedings of semisolid foods. Place the food tray within the patient's visual field; loss of peripheral vision is common. If oral feedings aren't possible, insert a nasogastric tube.

✦ Manage GI problems. Be alert for signs that the patient is straining at elimination because this increases ICP. Modify diet, administer stool softeners as ordered, and give laxatives if necessary. If the patient vomits (usually during the first few days), keep him positioned on his side to prevent aspiration.

✦ Provide careful mouth care. Clean and irrigate the patient's mouth to remove food particles. Care for his dentures, as needed.

Key nursing actions

✦ During the acute phase, efforts focus on survival and the prevention of further complications.

✦ Maintain patent airway and oxygenation. Loosen constrictive clothing. Watch for ballooning of the cheek with respiration.

✦ Check vital signs and neurologic status, record observations, and report any significant changes to the physician.

✦ Maintain fluid and electrolyte balance.

✦ Ensure adequate nutrition. Check for gag reflex before offering small oral feedings of semisolid foods.

✦ Manage GI problems. Be alert for signs that the patient is straining at elimination because this increases ICP.

✦ Provide meticulous eye care. Remove secretions with a cotton ball and sterile normal saline solution. Instill eyedrops, as ordered. Patch the patient's affected eye if he can't close the lid.

✦ Position the patient and align his extremities correctly. Use high-topped sneakers to prevent footdrop and contracture and convoluted foam, flotation, or pulsating mattress or sheepskin to prevent pressure ulcers. To prevent pneumonia, turn the patient at least every 2 hours. Elevate the affected hand to control dependent edema, and place it in a functional position.

✦ Assist the patient with exercise. Perform range-of-motion (ROM) exercises for both the affected and unaffected sides. Teach and encourage the patient to use his unaffected side to exercise his affected side.

✦ Give medications, as ordered, and watch for and report adverse effects.

✦ Establish and maintain communication with the patient. If he's aphasic, set up a simple method of communicating basic needs. Remember to phrase your questions so he can answer, using this system. Repeat yourself quietly and calmly (remember, he doesn't have hearing difficulty) and use gestures if necessary to help him understand. Even the unresponsive patient can hear, so don't say anything in his presence that you wouldn't want him to hear and remember.

✦ Provide psychological support. Set realistic short-term goals. Involve the patient's family in his care when possible, and explain his deficits and strengths.

Early rehabilitation

Begin your rehabilitation of the patient with a stroke on admission. The amount of teaching you'll have to do depends on the extent of neurologic deficit.

✦ Establish rapport with the patient. Spend time with him, and provide a means of communication. Simplify your language, asking "yes-or-no" questions whenever possible. Don't correct his speech or treat him like a child. Remember that building rapport may be difficult because of the mood changes that may result from brain damage or as a reaction to being dependent.

✦ If necessary, teach the patient to comb his hair, dress, and wash. With the aid of a physical therapist and an occupational therapist, obtain appliances, such as walking frames, hand bars by the toilet, and ramps, as needed. The patient may fail to recognize that he has a paralyzed side (called *unilateral neglect*) and must be taught to inspect that side of his body for injury and to protect it from harm. If speech therapy is indicated, encourage the patient to begin soon and follow through with the speech pathologist's suggestions. To reinforce teaching, involve the patient's family in all aspects of rehabilitation. With their cooperation and support, devise a realistic discharge plan, and let them help decide when the patient can return home.

✦ Before discharge, warn the patient and his family to report any premonitory signs of a stroke, such as severe headache, drowsiness, confusion, and dizziness. Emphasize the importance of regular follow-up visits.

✦ If aspirin has been prescribed, tell the patient to watch for GI bleeding. Make sure the patient and his family realize that acetaminophen isn't a substitute.

To help prevent stroke

✦ Stress the need to control such diseases as diabetes or hypertension.

✦ Teach all patients (especially those at high risk) the importance of following a low-cholesterol, low-salt diet; watching their weight; increasing activity; avoiding smoking and prolonged bed rest; and minimizing stress.

✦ If symptoms develop, go to the emergency department immediately.

Key nursing actions
(continued)

✦ Provide careful mouth care. Clean and irrigate the patient's mouth to remove food particles.

✦ Provide meticulous eye care. Remove secretions with a cotton ball and sterile normal saline solution.

✦ Position the patient and align his extremities correctly.

✦ Assist the patient with exercise. Perform ROM exercises for both the affected and unaffected sides.

✦ Give medications, as ordered, and watch for adverse effects.

✦ Establish and maintain communication with the patient.

✦ Provide psychological support. Set realistic short-term goals.

✦ Begin your rehabilitation of the patient with a stroke on admission.

✦ If necessary, teach the patient to comb his hair, dress, and wash.

✦ Before discharge, warn the patient and his family to report any premonitory signs of a stroke.

To help prevent stroke

✦ Stress the need to control such diseases as diabetes or hypertension.

✦ Teach all patients the importance of following a low-cholesterol, low-salt diet; watching their weight; increasing activity; avoiding smoking and prolonged bed rest; and minimizing stress.

✦ If symptoms develop, go to the emergency department immediately.

(Text continues on page 346.)

Treating ischemic stroke

In an ischemic stroke, a thrombus occludes a cerebral vessel or one of its branches and blocks blood flow to the brain. The thrombus may either have formed in that vessel or have lodged there after traveling through the circulation from another site such as the heart. Prompt treatment with thrombolytic agents or anticoagulants helps to minimize the effects of the occlusion. This flowchart shows how these drugs disrupt an ischemic stroke, thus minimizing the effects of cerebral ischemia and infarction. Keep in mind that thrombolytic agents should be used within 3 hours after onset of the patient's symptoms.

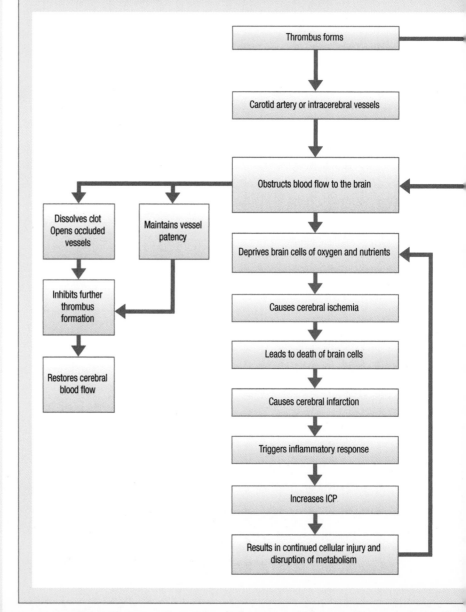

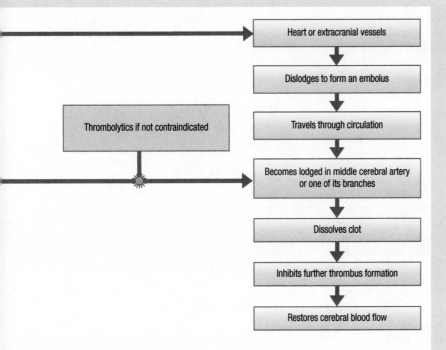

Heart or extracranial vessels

↓

Dislodges to form an embolus

↓

Travels through circulation

↓

Thrombolytics if not contraindicated

Becomes lodged in middle cerebral artery
or one of its branches

↓

Dissolves clot

↓

Inhibits further thrombus formation

↓

Restores cerebral blood flow

Key: ☀ = treatment

Characteristics of West Nile encephalitis

✦ Vector-borne disease causing inflammation of brain
✦ Risk of contracting is higher in those older than age 50 or those with compromised immune systems
✦ Occurs when mosquitoes are most active
✦ Mortality ranges from 3% to 15%

Causes

✦ WNV: found in humans, birds, other vertebrates in Africa, West Asia, Middle East

How it happens

✦ Mosquitoes feed on contaminated birds
✦ Transmitted to human by bite of infected mosquito
✦ Causes inflammation of brain

Key signs and symptoms

Moderate
✦ Fever
✦ Headache
✦ Body aches
✦ Swollen lymph glands

Severe
✦ Headache
✦ High fever
✦ Neck stiffness
✦ Stupor

Alert!

✦ Researchers estimate that 1 in 300 people who are bitten by a mosquito infected with WNV develops the disease.

WEST NILE ENCEPHALITIS

West Nile encephalitis, part of a family of vector-borne diseases that also includes malaria, yellow fever, and Lyme disease, is an infectious disease that primarily causes encephalitis (inflammation) of the brain. The first documented cases of West Nile virus (WNV) in the Western Hemisphere didn't occur until late in August 1999, when numerous dead birds in the New York, New Jersey, and Connecticut region tested positive for WNV after genetic sequencing. Scientists traced the Western Hemisphere origin of the disease to the vicinity of New York's Bronx Zoo and believe that mosquitoes feeding off diseased birds helped to spread the disease.

All people living in endemic areas carry a risk of contracting West Nile encephalitis, but those older than age 50 or those with compromised immune systems have the greatest risk. In temperate areas, West Nile encephalitis occurs mainly in the late summer or early autumn. In southern climates with milder temperatures, West Nile encephalitis can occur year-round.

Mortality of West Nile encephalitis is measured by case-fatality rates, which range from 3% to 15% (higher in the elderly population).

CAUSES

Etiology stems from WNV, a flavivirus commonly found in humans, birds, and other vertebrates in Africa, West Asia, and the Middle East.

PATHOPHYSIOLOGY

Mosquitoes become infected by feeding on birds contaminated with the virus. The virus is transmitted to a human by the bite of an infected mosquito (primarily the Culex species). Disease primarily causes inflammation or encephalitis of the brain. (See *Routes of transmission of West Nile virus.*)

Ticks infected with WNV have been found in Africa and Asia, but their role in transmission and maintenance of the virus is uncertain; they aren't considered vectors for WNV in the United States.

The Centers for Disease Control and Prevention has reported that there's no evidence that a person can contract the virus from handling live or dead infected birds. However, bare-handed contact when handling dead animals, including dead birds, should be avoided; if a dead animal must be handled, gloves or other protective measures should be used to place the carcass in a garbage can. A dead bird is a sign that there may be infected mosquitoes in the area; findings should be reported to the nearest Emergency Management Office.

SIGNS AND SYMPTOMS

Mild WNV infections are more common than severe infections and include symptoms such as fever, headache, and body aches, commonly accompanied by swollen lymph glands and a skin rash. Patients with severe infections present with such symptoms as headache, high fever, neck stiffness, stupor, disorientation, coma, tremors, occasional seizures, and paralysis. Rarely, death occurs before the infection is diagnosed.

The incubation period for West Nile encephalitis is anywhere from 5 to 15 days after exposure.

 CLINICAL ALERT Researchers estimate that only 1 in 300 people who are bitten by a mosquito infected with WNV develops the disease.

Routes of transmission of West Nile virus

Birds serve as the reservoir of the West Nile virus. They harbor the virus but are unable to spread it on their own. Mosquitoes serve as the vectors, spreading it from bird to bird and from birds to people. Humans are believed to be the "dead end hosts" — the virus lives in people and can make them ill; however, so far as is known, a feeding mosquito won't pick up the virus from biting an infected person.

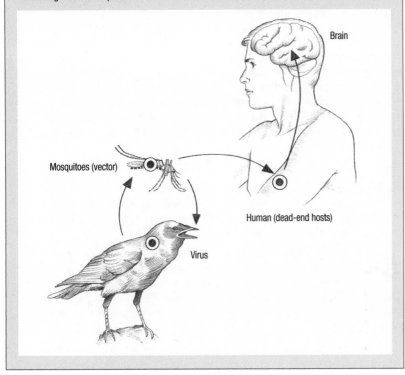

Brain

Mosquitoes (vector)

Human (dead-end hosts)

Virus

Complications
✦ Neurologic impairment
✦ Seizures
✦ Death

COMPLICATIONS

Complications may include neurologic impairment, seizures, and death.

DIAGNOSIS

The immunoglobulin M antibody capture–enzyme-linked immunosorbent assay (MAC-ELISA) is the test of choice for rapid definitive diagnosis. It has a high probability of accurate diagnosis of WNV infection when performed with acute serum or cerebrospinal fluid specimens obtained while the patient is hospitalized.

Encephalitis can also be caused by numerous viral and bacterial infections, so data must be carefully examined to determine a definitive diagnosis. St. Louis encephalitis, which produces symptoms similar to West Nile encephalitis, should be considered.

TREATMENT

There's no specific therapy utilized to treat West Nile encephalitis and no known cure. Treatment is generally aimed at controlling the specific symptoms. Supportive

Diagnosis
✦ Immunoglobulin M antibody capture–enzyme-linked immunosorbent assay
✦ Rule out other causes of encephalitis
✦ St. Louis encephalitis should be considered

Treatment
✦ No specific therapy or cure
✦ Supportive care: I.V. fluids, fever control, respiratory support

Key nursing actions

✦ Obtain an extensive history of the patient's whereabouts within the last 2 to 3 weeks.
✦ Perform a comprehensive physical assessment.
✦ Perform a complete neurologic examination.
✦ Maintain adequate hydration with I.V. fluids.
✦ Monitor strict intake and output.
✦ Utilize fever control methods.
✦ Provide respiratory support measures if necessary.
✦ Use standard precautions when handling body fluids and blood.
✦ Report suspected cases of West Nile encephalitis to the state's Department of Health.

Alert!

✦ An effective insect repellent will contain 20% to 30% DEET.
✦ Tell the patient to avoid products containing more than 30% DEET, because they may cause adverse effects, particularly in children.
✦ Because repellents may irritate the eyes and mouth, instruct parents to avoid applying repellent to children's hands.

care, such as I.V. fluids, fever control, and respiratory support, is rendered when necessary.

NURSING CONSIDERATIONS

✦ Obtain an extensive history of the patient's whereabouts within the last 2 to 3 weeks. Ask him if he has spent time near a body of water, such as a lake or pond, been in the presence of dead birds or other animals, or received a mosquito bite.
✦ Perform a comprehensive physical assessment. Report signs of fever, headache, lymphadenopathy, and maculopapular rash.
✦ Perform a complete neurologic examination. Report signs of confusion, lethargy, weakness, or slurred speech.
✦ Maintain adequate hydration with I.V. fluids.
✦ Monitor strict intake and output.
✦ Utilize fever control methods.
✦ Provide respiratory support measures if necessary.
✦ Use standard precautions when handling body fluids and blood.
✦ Report suspected cases of West Nile encephalitis to the state's Department of Health.

To reduce your patient's risk of becoming infected with West Nile encephalitis, instruct him to:
✦ stay indoors at dawn, dusk, and in the early evening
✦ wear long-sleeved shirts and long pants whenever outdoors
✦ apply insect repellent containing N, N-diethyl-meta-toluamide (DEET) sparingly to exposed skin and clothing.

 CLINICAL ALERT An effective insect repellent will contain 20% to 30% DEET. Tell the patient to avoid products containing more than 30% DEET, because they may cause adverse effects, particularly in children. Also tell the patient that whenever he uses an insecticide or insect repellent, he should read and follow the manufacturer's directions for use, as printed on the product.

 CLINICAL ALERT Because repellents may irritate the eyes and mouth, instruct parents to avoid applying repellent to children's hands. Insect repellents shouldn't be applied to children younger than age 3.

Gastrointestinal system

The GI system has the critical task of supplying essential nutrients to fuel the body's physiologic and pathophysiologic activities. Its functioning profoundly affects quality of life through its impact on overall health. The GI system has two major components: the alimentary canal, or GI tract, and the accessory organs. A malfunction anywhere in the system can produce far-reaching metabolic effects, eventually threatening life itself.

The alimentary canal is a hollow muscular tube that begins in the mouth and ends at the anus. It includes the oral cavity, pharynx, esophagus, stomach, small intestine, and large intestine. Peristalsis propels the ingested material along the tract; sphincters prevent its reflux. Accessory glands and organs include the salivary glands, liver, biliary duct system (gallbladder and bile ducts), and pancreas.

Together, the GI tract and accessory organs serve two major functions: digestion (breaking down food and fluids into simple chemicals that can be absorbed into the bloodstream and transported throughout the body) and elimination of waste products from the body through defecation.

PATHOPHYSIOLOGIC CHANGES

Disorders of the GI system typically manifest as vague, nonspecific complaints or problems that reflect disruption in one or more of the system's functions. For example, movement through the GI tract can be slowed, accelerated, or blocked; and secretion, absorption, or motility can be altered. As a result, one patient may present with several problems, the most common being anorexia, constipation, diarrhea, dysphagia, jaundice, nausea, and vomiting.

Anorexia

+ Loss of appetite or a lack of desire for food
+ May include nausea, abdominal pain, diarrhea
+ Can result from dysfunction in GI or other systems
+ Physiologic stimuli are present but person has no appetite or desire to eat
+ Can be result of slow gastric emptying or gastric stasis
+ High neurotransmitter, excess cortisol levels possible causes

Constipation

+ Hard stools
+ Difficult or infrequent defecation
+ Decrease in number of stools per week
+ Defined individually

Causes

+ Dehydration
+ Low-bulk diet
+ Sedentary lifestyle
+ Lack of regular exercise
+ Frequent repression of urge to defecate

Alert!

+ Elderly patients experience a decrease in intestinal motility.

Diarrhea

+ Increase in fluidity or volume of feces, frequency of defecation

Factors

+ Water content of colon and presence of unabsorbed food
+ Unabsorbable material
+ Intestinal secretions
+ Three major mechanism: osmotic, secretory, motility

ANOREXIA

Anorexia is a loss of appetite or a lack of desire for food. Nausea, abdominal pain, and diarrhea may accompany it. Anorexia can result from dysfunction in the GI system or other systems, such as cancer, heart disease, or renal disease.

Normally, a physiologic stimulus causes the sensation of hunger. Falling blood glucose levels stimulate the hunger center in the hypothalamus; rising blood fat and amino acid levels promote satiety. Hunger is also stimulated by contraction of an empty stomach and suppressed when the GI tract becomes distended, possibly as a result of stimulation of the vagus nerve. Sight, touch, and smell play subtle roles in controlling the appetite center.

In anorexia, the physiologic stimuli are present but the person has no appetite or desire to eat. Slow gastric emptying or gastric stasis can cause anorexia. High levels of neurotransmitters such as serotonin (may contribute to satiety) and excess cortisol levels (may suppress hypothalamic control of hunger) also have been implicated as causes of anorexia.

CONSTIPATION

Constipation is hard stools and difficult or infrequent defecation, as defined by a decrease in the number of stools per week. It's defined individually because normal bowel habits range from two to three episodes of stool passage per day to one per week. Causes of constipation include dehydration, consumption of a low-bulk diet, a sedentary lifestyle, lack of regular exercise, and frequent repression of the urge to defecate.

When a person is dehydrated or delays defecation, more fluid is absorbed from the intestine, the stool becomes harder, and constipation ensues. High-fiber diets cause water to be drawn into the stool by osmosis, thereby keeping stool soft and encouraging movement through the intestine. High-fiber diets also cause intestinal dilation, which stimulates peristalsis. Conversely, a low-fiber diet would contribute to constipation.

 CLINICAL ALERT Elderly patients typically experience a decrease in intestinal motility in addition to a slowing and dulling of neural impulses in the GI tract. Many older persons restrict fluid intake to prevent waking at night to use the bathroom or because of a fear of incontinence. This places them at risk for dehydration and constipation.

A sedentary lifestyle, lack of exercise, limitations in physical activity, or inability to engage in physical activity can cause constipation because exercise stimulates the GI tract and promotes defecation. Antacids, opiates, and other drugs that inhibit bowel motility also lead to constipation.

Stress stimulates the sympathetic nervous system, and GI motility slows. Absence or degeneration in the neural pathways of the large intestine also contributes to constipation. Other conditions, such as spinal cord trauma, multiple sclerosis, intestinal neoplasms, and hypothyroidism, can also cause constipation.

DIARRHEA

Diarrhea is an increase in the fluidity or volume of feces and the frequency of defecation. Factors that affect stool volume and consistency include water content of the colon and the presence of unabsorbed food, unabsorbable material, and intestinal secretions. Large-volume diarrhea is usually the result of an excessive amount of water, secretions, or both in the intestines. Small-volume diarrhea is usually caused by excessive intestinal motility. Diarrhea may also be caused by a parasympathetic stimulation of the intestine initiated by psychological factors, such as fear or stress.

There are three major mechanisms of diarrhea. *Osmotic diarrhea* occurs when a nonabsorbable substance such as synthetic sugar or increased numbers of osmotic particles in the intestine increases osmotic pressure and draws excess water into the intestine, thereby increasing the weight and volume of the stool. *Secretory diarrhea* is the result of a pathogen or tumor that irritates the muscle and mucosal layers of the intestine. The consequent increase in motility and secretions (water, electrolytes, and mucus) results in diarrhea. *Motility diarrhea* is due to inflammation, neuropathy, or obstruction that causes a reflex increase in intestinal motility that may expel the irritant or clear the obstruction.

DYSPHAGIA

Dysphagia — difficulty swallowing — can be caused by a mechanical obstruction of the esophagus or by impaired esophageal motility secondary to another disorder. Mechanical obstruction is characterized as intrinsic or extrinsic.

Intrinsic obstructions originate in the esophagus itself. Causes of intrinsic obstructions include tumors, strictures, and diverticular herniations. Extrinsic obstructions originate outside of the esophagus and narrow the lumen by exerting pressure on the esophageal wall. Most extrinsic obstructions result from a tumor.

Distention and spasm at the site of the obstruction during swallowing may cause pain. Upper esophageal obstruction causes pain 2 to 4 seconds after swallowing; lower esophageal obstructions, 10 to 15 seconds after swallowing. If a tumor is present, dysphagia begins with difficulty swallowing solids and eventually progresses to difficulty swallowing semisolids and liquids. Impaired motor function makes both liquids and solids difficult to swallow.

Neural or muscular disorders can also interfere with voluntary swallowing or peristalsis. This is known as functional dysphagia. Causes of functional dysphagia include dermatomyositis, stroke, Parkinson's disease, or achalasia. Malfunction of the upper esophageal striated muscles interferes with the voluntary phase of swallowing. (See *What happens in swallowing,* page 352.)

In achalasia, the esophageal ganglionic cells are thought to have degenerated, and the cardiac sphincter of the stomach can't relax. The lower end of the esophagus loses neuromuscular coordination and muscle tone, and food accumulates, causing hypertrophy and dilation. Eventually, accumulated food raises the hydrostatic pressure and forces the sphincter open, and small amounts of food slowly move into the stomach.

JAUNDICE

Jaundice — yellow pigmentation of the skin and sclera — is caused by an excess accumulation of bilirubin in the blood. Bilirubin, a product of red blood cell (RBC) breakdown, accumulates when production exceeds metabolism and excretion. This imbalance can result from excessive release of bilirubin precursors into the bloodstream or from impairment of its hepatic uptake, metabolism, or excretion. (See *Jaundice: Impaired bilirubin metabolism,* page 353.)

Jaundice occurs when bilirubin levels exceed 2.5 mg/dl, which is about twice the upper limit of the normal range. Lower levels of bilirubin may cause detectable jaundice in patients with fair skin, and jaundice may be difficult to detect in patients with dark skin.

Dysphagia

+ Difficulty swallowing from mechanical obstruction or impaired motility
+ Intrinsic obstructions in esophagus: tumors, strictures, diverticular herniations
+ Extrinsic obstruction outside esophagus: tumor
+ Distention and spasm may cause pain
+ Dysphagia with tumor begins with difficulty swallowing solids
+ Neural or muscular disorders — functional dysphagia

Jaundice

+ Yellow pigmentation of skin and sclera
+ Caused by excess accumulation of bilirubin
+ Imbalance results from impairment of hepatic uptake, metabolism, or excretion

CLOSER LOOK

What happens in swallowing

Before peristalsis can begin, the neural pattern to initiate swallowing (illustrated here) must occur:

✦ Food reaching the back of the mouth stimulates swallowing receptors that surround the pharyngeal opening.

✦ The receptors transmit impulses to the brain by way of the sensory portions of the trigeminal (V) and glossopharyngeal (IX) nerves.

✦ The brain's swallowing center relays motor impulses to the esophagus by way of the trigeminal (V), glossopharyngeal (IX), vagus (X), and hypoglossal (XII) nerves.

✦ Swallowing occurs.

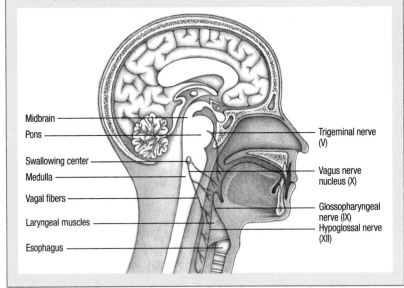

Alert!

✦ Jaundice in dark-skinned people may appear as yellow staining in the sclera, hard palate, and palmar or plantar surfaces.

3 types of jaundice

✦ Hemolytic
✦ Hepatocellular
✦ Obstructive

CLINICAL ALERT Jaundice in dark-skinned people may appear as yellow staining in the sclera, hard palate, and palmar or plantar surfaces.

There are three main types of jaundice. When RBC lysis exceeds the liver's capacity to conjugate bilirubin (binding bilirubin to a polar group makes it water-soluble and able to be excreted by the kidneys), *hemolytic jaundice* occurs. Causes include transfusion reactions, sickle cell anemia, thalassemia, and autoimmune disease.

Hepatocellular jaundice occurs as a result of hepatocyte dysfunction, which limits uptake and conjugation of bilirubin. Liver dysfunction can occur in hepatitis, cancer, cirrhosis, or congenital disorders, and can be caused by some drugs.

When the flow of bile out of the liver (through the hepatic duct) or through the bile duct is blocked, the liver can conjugate bilirubin, but the bilirubin can't reach the small intestine. This is called *obstructive jaundice*. Blockage of the hepatic duct by calculi or a tumor is considered an intrahepatic cause of obstructive jaundice. A blocked bile duct is an extrahepatic cause that may be attributed to gallstones or a tumor.

Jaundice: Impaired bilirubin metabolism

Jaundice occurs in three forms: prehepatic, hepatic, and posthepatic. In all three, bilirubin levels in the blood increase.

PREHEPATIC JAUNDICE

Certain conditions and disorders, such as transfusion reactions and sickle cell anemia, cause massive hemolysis.

✦ Red blood cells rupture faster than the liver can conjugate bilirubin.

✦ Large amounts of unconjugated bilirubin pass into the blood.

✦ Intestinal enzymes convert bilirubin to water-soluble urobilinogen for excretion in urine and stools. (Unconjugated bilirubin is insoluble in water, so it can't be directly secreted in urine.)

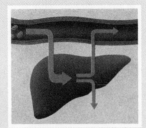

HEPATIC JAUNDICE

The liver becomes unable to conjugate or excrete bilirubin, leading to increased blood levels of conjugated and unconjugated bilirubin. This occurs in such disorders as hepatitis, cirrhosis, and metastatic cancer, and during prolonged use of drugs metabolized by the liver.

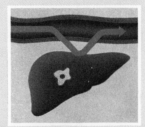

POSTHEPATIC JAUNDICE

In biliary and pancreatic disorders, bilirubin forms at its normal rate.

✦ Inflammation, scar tissue, tumor, or gallstones block the flow of bile into the intestines.

✦ Water-soluble conjugated bilirubin accumulates in the blood.

✦ The bilirubin is excreted in the urine.

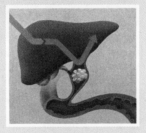

NAUSEA

Nausea is feeling the urge to vomit. It may occur independently of vomiting, or it may precede or accompany it. Specific neural pathways haven't been identified, but increased salivation, diminished functional activities of the stomach, and altered small intestinal motility have been associated with nausea. The same parts of the brain that control involuntary bodily functions are thought to control nausea.

VOMITING

Vomiting is the forceful oral expulsion of gastric contents. The gastric musculature provides the ejection force. The gastric fundus and gastroesophageal sphincter relax, and forceful contractions of the diaphragm and abdominal wall muscles increase intra-abdominal pressure, which combined with the annular contraction of

Jaundice

Prehepatic
✦ RBCs rupture faster than the liver can conjugate bilirubin

Hepatic
✦ Liver can't conjugate or excrete bilirubin

Posthepatic
✦ Bilirubin forms at normal rate and is excreted in urine

Nausea

✦ Feeling urge to vomit
✦ May occur independently or may precede vomiting
✦ Specific neural pathways not identified
✦ Probably controlled by parts of brain that control involuntary bodily functions

Vomiting

✦ Forceful oral expulsion of gastric contents
✦ Gastric musculature provides ejection force
✦ Increased intrathoracic pressure moves gastric content from esophagus to mouth

Vomiting
(continued)

+ Controlled by vomiting center and CTZ in medulla
+ Various stimuli activate CTZ
+ Nausea and vomiting manifestations of other disorders
+ May be psychogenic

Characteristics of appendicitis

+ Inflammation and obstruction of vermiform appendix
+ May occur at any age and affects both genders equally
+ Incidence and death rate have declined with anitbiotics
+ Fatal if untreated

Causes

+ Mucosal ulceration
+ Fecal mass
+ Stricture
+ Barium ingestion
+ Viral infection

How it happens

+ Mucosal ulceration triggers inflammation
+ Temporarily obstructs appendix, blocks mucus flow
+ Pressure increases, appendix contracts
+ Bacteria multiply, inflammation and pressure increase
+ Blood flow restricted — severe abdominal pain

Key signs and symptoms

+ Pain in epigastric region, shifting to right lower quadrant
+ Nausea
+ Vomiting

---

the gastric pylorus forces gastric contents into the esophagus. Increased intrathoracic pressure then moves the gastric content from the esophagus to the mouth.

Vomiting is controlled by two centers in the medulla: the vomiting center and the chemoreceptor trigger zone (CTZ). The vomiting center initiates the act of vomiting when it's stimulated by the GI tract, from higher brain stem and cortical centers, and from the CTZ. By itself the CTZ can't induce vomiting. Various stimuli or drugs, such as apomorphine, levodopa, cardiac glycosides, bacterial toxins, radiation, and metabolic abnormalities activate the zone. The activated zone sends impulses to the medullary vomiting center, and this sequence begins:

+ The abdominal muscles and diaphragm contract.
+ Reverse peristalsis begins, causing intestinal material to flow back into the stomach, distending it.
+ The stomach pushes the diaphragm into the thoracic cavity, raising the intrathoracic pressure.
+ The pressure forces the upper esophageal sphincter open, the glottis closes, and the soft palate blocks the nasopharynx.
+ The pressure also forces the material up through the sphincter and out through the mouth.

Nausea and vomiting are manifestations of other disorders, such as acute abdominal emergencies, infections of the intestinal tract, central nervous system disorders, myocardial infarction, heart failure, metabolic and endocrinologic disorders, or as the adverse effect of many drugs. Nausea and vomiting can also occur in pregnancy. Vomiting may also be psychogenic, resulting from emotional or psychological disturbance.

APPENDICITIS

The most common disease requiring emergency surgery, appendicitis is inflammation and obstruction of the vermiform appendix (a narrow tube of bowel which is closed at one end and attached to the cecum). Appendicitis may occur at any age and affects both genders equally; however, between puberty and age 25, it's more prevalent in men. Since the advent of antibiotics, the incidence and death rate of appendicitis have declined. If untreated, this disease is invariably fatal.

CAUSES

Causes of appendicitis include mucosal ulceration, fecal mass, stricture, barium ingestion, and viral infection.

PATHOPHYSIOLOGY

Mucosal ulceration triggers inflammation, which temporarily obstructs the appendix. The obstruction blocks mucus outflow. Pressure in the now distended appendix increases, and the appendix contracts. Bacteria multiply, and inflammation and pressure continue to increase, restricting blood flow to the pouch and causing severe abdominal pain.

SIGNS AND SYMPTOMS

Inflammation of the appendix and bowel obstruction and distention cause abdominal pain in appendicitis. The pain begins in the epigastric region, and then shifts to the right lower quadrant. The inflammation also causes nausea, vomiting, and tenderness. Anorexia follows the onset of pain. The patient may experience a low-grade fever from systemic manifestation of inflammation and leukocytosis.

COMPLICATIONS

Complications may include wound infection, intra-abdominal abscess, fecal fistula, intestinal obstruction, incisional hernia, peritonitis, and death.

DIAGNOSIS

White blood cell count is moderately high with an increased number of immature cells when appendicitis is present. In addition, an X-ray with radiographic contrast agent will reveal failure of the appendix to fill with contrast.

TREATMENT

Maintain a nothing-by-mouth status and GI intubation for decompression until appendectomy. To aid in pain relief, the patient should be placed in Fowler's position. Antibiotics are prescribed to treat infection if peritonitis occurs. To reverse possible dehydration resulting from surgery or nausea and vomiting, replace fluid and electrolytes parenterally.

NURSING CONSIDERATIONS

If appendicitis is suspected, or during preparation for appendectomy
◆ Administer I.V. fluids to prevent dehydration. Never administer cathartics or enemas, which may rupture the appendix. Maintain nothing-by-mouth status, and administer analgesics judiciously because they may mask symptoms.
◆ To lessen pain, place the patient in Fowler's position. Never apply heat to the right lower abdomen; this may cause the appendix to rupture. An ice bag may be used for pain relief.

After appendectomy
◆ Monitor vital signs and intake and output. Give analgesics as ordered.
◆ Encourage the patient to cough, breathe deeply, and turn frequently to prevent pulmonary complications.
◆ Document bowel sounds, passing of flatus, and bowel movements. If the patient's nausea and abdominal rigidity have subsided, it may indicate his readiness to resume oral fluids.
◆ Watch closely for possible surgical complications. Continuing pain and fever may signal an abscess. The complaint that "something gave way" may mean wound dehiscence. If an abscess or peritonitis develops, incision and drainage may be necessary. Frequently assess the dressing for wound drainage.
◆ Help the patient ambulate as soon as possible after surgery.
◆ In appendicitis complicated by peritonitis, a nasogastric (NG) tube may be needed to decompress the stomach and reduce nausea and vomiting. If so, record drainage and provide appropriate mouth and nose care.

CHOLECYSTITIS

Cholecystitis—acute or chronic inflammation causing painful distention of the gallbladder—is usually associated with a gallstone impacted in the cystic duct.

Complications
◆ Wound infection
◆ Intra-abdominal abscess
◆ Fecal fistula
◆ Intestinal obstruction

Diagnosis
◆ WBC count moderately high with increased immature cells
◆ X-ray with contrast agent will reveal failure to fill with agent

Treatment
◆ Nothing-by-mouth status
◆ GI intubation for decompression until appendectomy
◆ Place patient in Fowler's position
◆ Antibiotics
◆ Parenteral fluids and electrolytes

Key nursing actions

If appendicitis is suspected, or to prepare for appendectomy
◆ Administer I.V. fluids; maintain nothing by mouth status.
◆ Administer analgesics judiciously. Never apply heat to the right lower abdomen.

After appendectomy
◆ Document bowel sounds, passing of flatus, and bowel movements.
◆ Watch closely for possible surgical complications.

Characteristics of cholecystitis
◆ Acute or chronic inflammation causing painful distention of gallbladder
◆ Associated with gallstone impacted in cystic duct
◆ Acute form most common among middle-age women
◆ Prognosis good with treatment

Causes

+ Gallstones
+ Poor blood flow to gallbladder
+ Abnormal metabolism of cholesterol and bile salts

How it happens

+ Usually develops after gallstone lodges in cystic duct
+ Bile flow blocked, gallbladder inflamed and distended
+ Bacterial growth may contribute to inflammation
+ Edema of gallbladder obstructs bile flow, irritates gallbladder
+ Cells in gallbladder wall die as organ presses on vessels
+ Exudate covers ulcerated areas, causing gallbladder to adhere

Key signs and symptoms

+ Acute abdominal pain in right upper quadrant; may radiate to back, between shoulders, and in front of chest
+ Jaundice
+ Nausea, vomiting

Complications

+ Perforation and abscess
+ Fistula
+ Gangrene

Diagnosis

+ X-ray reveals gallstones, helps disclose other conditions
+ Ultrasonography detects gallstones, distinguishes between obstructive and nonobstructive jaundice
+ Technetium-labeled scan reveals cystic duct obstruction, acute or chronic cholecystitis

Cholecystitis accounts for 10% to 25% of all patients requiring gallbladder surgery. The acute form is most common among middle-age women; the chronic form, among elderly people. The prognosis is good with treatment.

CAUSES

Gallstones (most common), poor or absent blood flow to the gallbladder, and abnormal metabolism of cholesterol and bile salts are all causes of cholecystitis.

PATHOPHYSIOLOGY

In acute cholecystitis, inflammation of the gallbladder wall usually develops after a gallstone lodges in the cystic duct. (See *Understanding gallstone formation*.)

When bile flow is blocked, the gallbladder becomes inflamed and distended. Bacterial growth, usually *Escherichia coli*, may contribute to the inflammation. Edema of the gallbladder (and sometimes the cystic duct) obstructs bile flow, which chemically irritates the gallbladder. Cells in the gallbladder wall may become oxygen starved and die as the distended organ presses on vessels and impairs blood flow. The dead cells slough off, and an exudate covers ulcerated areas, causing the gallbladder to adhere to surrounding structures.

SIGNS AND SYMPTOMS

In cholecystitis, the patient complains of acute abdominal pain in the right upper quadrant that may radiate to the back, between the shoulders, or to the front of the chest secondary to inflammation and irritation of nerve fibers. Obstruction of the common bile duct by calculi results in jaundice, and passage of gallstones along the bile duct results in colic. Nausea, vomiting, and a low-grade fever are triggered by the inflammatory response, and chills are related to the fever.

COMPLICATIONS

Complications of cholecystitis include perforation and abscess formation, fistula formation, gangrene, empyema, cholangitis, hepatitis, pancreatitis, gallstone ileus, and carcinoma.

DIAGNOSIS

+ X-ray reveals gallstones if they contain enough calcium to be radiopaque; also helps disclose porcelain gallbladder (hard, brittle gallbladder due to calcium deposited in wall), limy bile, and gallstone ileus.
+ Ultrasonography detects gallstones as small as 2 mm and distinguishes between obstructive and nonobstructive jaundice.
+ Technetium-labeled scan reveals cystic duct obstruction and acute or chronic cholecystitis if ultrasound doesn't visualize the gallbladder.
+ Percutaneous transhepatic cholangiography supports the diagnosis of obstructive jaundice and reveals calculi in the ducts.
+ Levels of serum alkaline phosphate, lactate dehydrogenase, aspartate aminotransferase, and total bilirubin are high; serum amylase level slightly elevated; and icteric index elevated.
+ White blood cell (WBC) counts are slightly elevated during cholecystitis attack.

Understanding gallstone formation

Abnormal metabolism of cholesterol and bile salts plays an important role in gallstone formation. The liver makes bile continuously. The gall bladder concentrates and stores the bile until the duodenum signals that it needs it to help digest fat. Changes in the composition of bile may allow gallstones to form. Changes to the absorptive ability of the gallbladder lining may also contribute to gallstone formation.

TOO MUCH CHOLESTEROL

Certain conditions, such as age, obesity, and estrogen imbalance, cause the liver to secrete bile that's abnormally high in cholesterol or lacking the proper concentration of bile salts.

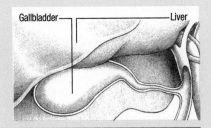

INSIDE THE GALLBLADDER

When the gallbladder concentrates this bile, inflammation may occur. Excessive reabsorption of water and bile salts makes the bile less soluble. Cholesterol, calcium, and bilirubin precipitate into gallstones.

Fat entering the duodenum causes the intestinal mucosa to secrete the hormone cholecystokinin, which stimulates the gallbladder to contract and empty. If a stone lodges in the cystic duct, the gallbladder contracts but can't empty.

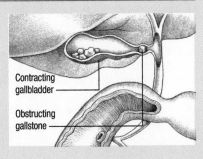

JAUNDICE, IRRITATION, INFLAMMATION

If a stone lodges in the common bile duct, the bile can't flow into the duodenum. Bilirubin is absorbed into the blood and causes jaundice.

Biliary narrowing and swelling of the tissue around the stone can also cause irritation and inflammation of the common bile duct.

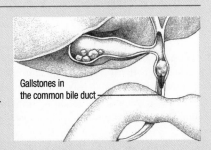

UP THE BILIARY TREE

Inflammation can progress up the biliary tree into any of the bile ducts. This causes scar tissue, fluid accumulation, cirrhosis, portal hypertension, and bleeding.

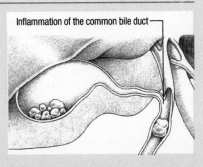

Understanding gallstone formation

+ Abnormal metabolism of cholesterol and bile salts plays role
+ Changes in bile composition may allow stone formation
+ Changes in gallbladder lining may allow stone formation
+ Composed of cholesterol, calcium, bilirubin precipitate
+ Can lodge in cystic ducts, blocking gallbladder drainage
+ Can lodge in bile duct, causing jaundice, inflammation
+ Can progress up bilary tree into ducts, causing scarring, cirrhosis, bleeding

Treatment

+ Cholecystectomy
+ Percutaneous transhepatic cholecystostomy
+ Choledochostomy
+ Endoscopic retrograde cholangiopancreatography
+ Lithotripsy
+ Oral chenodeoxycholic acid or ursodeoxycholic acids
+ Low-fat diet
+ Vitamin K relieves itching, jaundice, and bleeding tendencies
+ Antibiotics
+ Nasogastric tube inserted to decompress abdomen

Key nursing actions

+ Before surgery, teach the patient to deep breathe, cough, expectorate, and perform leg exercises as necessary after surgery.
+ After surgery, monitor vital signs for signs of bleeding, infection, or atelectasis.
+ Evaluate the incision site for bleeding.
+ Measure and record T-tube drainage daily.
+ Teach patients who will be discharged with a T-tube how to perform dressing changes and routine skin care.
+ If the patient doesn't void within 8 hours, percuss over the symphysis pubis for bladder distention.
+ At discharge, advise the patient against heavy lifting or straining for 6 weeks and urge him to walk daily.
+ Instruct patient to notify surgeon of postdischarge pain lasting longer than 24 hours, nausea, vomiting, fever, abdominal tenderness, or jaundice.

TREATMENT

Cholecystectomy may be performed to surgically remove the inflamed gallbladder. Percutaneous transhepatic cholecystostomy or choledochostomy may be performed to create an opening into the common bile duct for drainage. Gallstones may also be removed by endoscopic retrograde cholangiopancreatography. To break up gallstones and relieve obstruction, lithotripsy may be performed.

Oral chenodeoxycholic acid or ursodeoxycholic acids may be used to dissolve calculi, and a low-fat diet may help prevent attacks. Vitamin K relieves itching, jaundice, and bleeding tendencies due to vitamin K deficiencies. Antibiotics can treat infection during an acute attack. Additionally, a nasogastric tube is inserted into the patient to decompress the abdomen.

NURSING CONSIDERATIONS

Patient care for cholecystitis focuses on supportive care and close postoperative observation.

+ Before surgery, teach the patient to deep breathe, cough, expectorate, and perform leg exercises as necessary after surgery. Teach splinting, repositioning, and ambulation techniques. Explain the procedures that will be performed before, during, and after surgery to help ease the patient's anxiety and to help ensure his cooperation.
+ After surgery, monitor vital signs for signs of bleeding, infection, or atelectasis.
+ Evaluate the incision site for bleeding. Serosanguineous drainage is common during the first 24 to 48 hours if the patient has a wound drain. If, after a choledochostomy, a T-tube drain is placed in the duct and attached to a drainage bag, make sure the drainage tube has no kinks. Also check that the connecting tubing from the T-tube is well secured to the patient to prevent dislodgment.
+ Measure and record T-tube drainage daily (200 to 300 ml is normal).
+ Teach patients who will be discharged with a T-tube how to perform dressing changes and routine skin care.
+ Monitor intake and output. Allow the patient nothing by mouth for 24 to 48 hours or until bowel sounds return and nausea and vomiting cease (postoperative nausea may indicate a full bladder).
+ If the patient doesn't void within 8 hours (or if the amount voided is inadequate based on I.V. fluid intake), percuss over the symphysis pubis for bladder distention (especially in patients receiving anticholinergics). Patients who have had a laparoscopic cholecystectomy may be discharged the same day or within 24 hours after surgery. These patients should have minimal pain, be able to tolerate a regular diet within 24 hours after surgery, and be able to return to normal activity within 1 week.
+ Encourage deep breathing and leg exercises every hour. The patient should ambulate after surgery. Provide elastic stockings to support leg muscles and promote venous blood flow, thus preventing stasis and clot formation.
+ Evaluate the pain's location, duration, and character. Administer adequate medication to relieve pain, especially before such activities as deep breathing and ambulation, which increase pain.
+ At discharge, advise the patient against heavy lifting or straining for 6 weeks and urge him to walk daily. Tell him that food restrictions are unnecessary unless he has an intolerance to a specific food or some underlying condition (such as diabetes, atherosclerosis, or obesity) that requires such restriction.
+ Instruct the patient to notify the surgeon if he has pain for more than 24 hours, anorexia, nausea or vomiting, fever, tenderness in the abdominal area, or if he no-

tices any jaundice, as these may indicate a biliary tract injury from the cholestectomy, requiring immediate attention.

CIRRHOSIS

Cirrhosis is a chronic disease characterized by diffuse destruction and fibrotic regeneration of hepatic cells. As necrotic tissue yields to fibrosis, cirrhosis damages liver tissue and normal vasculature, impairs blood and lymph flow, and ultimately causes hepatic insufficiency. It's twice as common in men as in women, and is especially prevalent among malnourished persons older than age 50 with chronic alcoholism. Mortality is high; many patients die within 5 years of onset.

CAUSES

Cirrhosis may be a result of a wide range of diseases. These clinical types of cirrhosis reflect its diverse etiology:

Hepatocellular diseases
◆ Postnecrotic cirrhosis accounts for 10% to 30% of patients and stems from various types of hepatitis (such as types A, B, C, D viral hepatitis) or toxic exposures.
◆ Laënnec's cirrhosis, also called *portal, nutritional,* or *alcoholic cirrhosis,* is the most common type and is primarily caused by hepatitis C and alcoholism. Liver damage results from malnutrition (especially dietary protein) and chronic alcohol ingestion. Fibrous tissue forms in portal areas and around central veins.
◆ Autoimmune disease, such as sarcoidosis or chronic inflammatory bowel disease, may cause cirrhosis.

Cholestatic diseases
This group includes diseases of the biliary tree (biliary cirrhosis resulting from bile duct diseases suppressing bile flow) and sclerosing cholangitis.

Metabolic diseases
This group includes such disorders as Wilson's disease, alpha$_1$-antitrypsin, and hemochromatosis (pigment cirrhosis).

Other types of cirrhosis
Other types of cirrhosis include Budd-Chiari syndrome (epigastric pain, liver enlargement, and ascites due to hepatic vein obstruction), cardiac cirrhosis, and cryptogenic cirrhosis. Cardiac cirrhosis is rare; the liver damage results from right-sided heart failure. *Cryptogenic* refers to cirrhosis of unknown etiology.

PATHOPHYSIOLOGY

Cirrhosis begins with hepatic scarring or fibrosis. The scar begins as an increase in extracellular matrix components—fibril-forming collagens, proteoglycans, fibronectin, and hyaluronic acid. The site of collagen deposition varies with the cause. Hepatocyte function is eventually impaired as the matrix changes. Fat-storing cells are believed to be the source of the new matrix components. Contraction of these cells may also contribute to disruption of the lobular architecture and obstruction of the flow of blood or bile. Cellular changes producing bands of scar tissue also disrupt the lobular structure.

Characteristics of cirrhosis
◆ Chronic diffuse destruction and fibrotic regeneration of hepatic cells
◆ Damages liver tissue, normal vasculature, impairs blood and lymph flow, causes hepatic insufficiency
◆ Twice as common in men
◆ Prevalent among malnourished, chronic alcoholics older than age 50
◆ High mortality

Causes
Hepatocellular diseases
◆ Postnecrotic cirrhosis: hepatitis, toxic exposures
◆ Laënnec's cirrhosis: hepatitis C and alcoholism
◆ Autoimmune disease

Cholestatic diseases
◆ Diseases of biliary tree and sclerosing cholangitis

Metabolic diseases
◆ Wilson's disease
◆ Alpha$_1$-antitrypsin
◆ Hemochromatosis

Other types
◆ Budd-Chiari syndrome
◆ Cardiac cirrhosis
◆ Cryptogenic cirrhosis

How it happens
◆ Begins with hepatic scarring or fibrosis
◆ Scar begins as increase in extracellular matrix components
◆ Hepatocyte function impaired as matrix changes
◆ Fat-storing cells believed to be source of new matrix components
◆ Cellular changes produce bands of scar tissue

SIGNS AND SYMPTOMS

In the early stages of cirrhosis, anorexia may result from distaste for certain foods. Nausea and vomiting are due to the inflammatory response and systemic effects of liver inflammation. The patient may complain of a dull abdominal ache from liver inflammation. In addition, malabsorption causes diarrhea.

Late-stage signs and symptoms include:

+ *Respiratory* — pleural effusion, limited thoracic expansion due to abdominal ascites; interferes with efficient gas exchange, which causes hypoxia
+ *Central nervous system* — progressive signs or symptoms of hepatic encephalopathy, including lethargy, mental changes, slurred speech, asterixis, peripheral neuritis, paranoia, hallucinations, extreme obtundation, and coma — secondary to the loss of ammonia to urea conversion and consequent delivery of toxic ammonia to the brain
+ *Hematologic* — bleeding tendencies (nosebleeds, easy bruising, bleeding gums), splenomegaly, anemia resulting from thrombocytopenia (secondary to splenomegaly and decreased vitamin K absorption), and portal hypertension
+ *Endocrine* — testicular atrophy, menstrual irregularities, gynecomastia, and loss of chest and axillary hair from decreased hormone metabolism
+ *Skin* — abnormal pigmentation, spider angiomas, palmar erythema, and jaundice related to impaired hepatic function; severe pruritus secondary to jaundice from bilirubinemia; extreme dryness and poor tissue turgor related to malnutrition
+ *Hepatic* — jaundice from decreased bilirubin metabolism; hepatomegaly secondary to liver scarring and portal hypertension; ascites and edema of the legs from portal hypertension and decreased plasma proteins; hepatic encephalopathy from ammonia toxicity; and hepatorenal syndrome from advanced liver disease and subsequent renal failure.

Other signs and symptoms of late-stages cirrhosis include musty breath secondary to ammonia buildup; enlarged superficial abdominal veins due to portal hypertension; pain in the right upper abdominal quadrant that worsens when the patient sits up or leans forward, due to inflammation and irritation of area nerve fibers; palpable liver or spleen due to organomegaly; temperature of 101° to 103° F (38.3° to 39.4° C) due to inflammatory response; hemorrhage from esophageal varices resulting from portal hypertension. (See *What happens in portal hypertension.*)

COMPLICATIONS

Complications may include respiratory compromise, ascites, portal hypertension, jaundice, coagulopathy, hepatic encephalopathy, bleeding esophageal varices, acute GI bleeding, liver failure, and renal failure.

DIAGNOSIS

To diagnose cirrhosis, these tests results may be obtained:

+ Liver biopsy reveals tissue destruction and fibrosis.
+ Abdominal X-ray shows enlarged liver, cysts, or gas within the biliary tract or liver, liver calcification, and massive fluid accumulation (ascites).
+ Computed tomography and liver scans show liver size, abnormal masses, and hepatic blood flow and obstruction.
+ Esophagogastroduodenoscopy reveals bleeding esophageal varices, stomach irritation or ulceration, or duodenal bleeding and irritation.

CLOSER LOOK

What happens in portal hypertension

Portal hypertension (elevated pressure in the portal vein) occurs when blood flow meets increased resistance. This common result of cirrhosis may also stem from mechanical obstruction and occlusion of the hepatic veins (Budd-Chiari syndrome).

As the pressure in the portal vein rises, blood backs up into the spleen and flows through collateral channels to the venous system, bypassing the liver. Thus, portal hypertension causes:

✦ splenomegaly with thrombocytopenia

✦ dilated collateral veins (esophageal varices, hemorrhoids, or prominent abdominal veins)

✦ ascites.

In many patients, the first sign of portal hypertension is bleeding esophageal varices (dilated tortuous veins in the submucosa of the lower esophagus).

Esophageal varices commonly cause massive hematemesis, requiring emergency care to control hemorrhage and prevent hypovolemic shock.

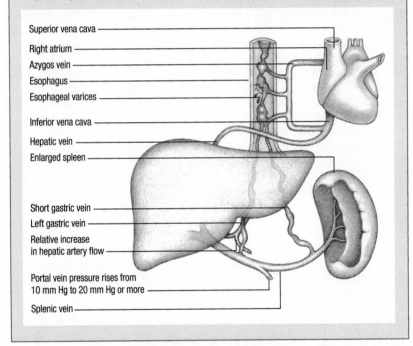

Superior vena cava
Right atrium
Azygos vein
Esophagus
Esophageal varices
Inferior vena cava
Hepatic vein
Enlarged spleen
Short gastric vein
Left gastric vein
Relative increase in hepatic artery flow
Portal vein pressure rises from 10 mm Hg to 20 mm Hg or more
Splenic vein

Portal hypertension
✦ Occurs when blood flow meets increased resistance
✦ Common result of cirrhosis
✦ Causes splenomegaly, dilated collateral veins, ascites
✦ First sign is bleeding esophageal varices

✦ Blood studies reveal elevated levels of liver enzymes, total serum bilirubin, and indirect bilirubin; decreased levels of total serum albumin and protein; prolonged prothrombin time; decreased hemoglobin level, hematocrit, and serum electrolytes; and deficiency of vitamins A, C, and K.

✦ Urine studies show increased bilirubin and urobilirubinogen level.

✦ Fecal studies show decreased fecal urobilirubinogen level.

TREATMENT

Treatment of cirrhosis may include vitamins and nutritional supplements, which help heal damaged liver cells and improve nutritional status. Antacids may reduce gastric distress and decrease the potential for GI bleeding. Potassium-sparing di-

Treatment
✦ Vitamins and nutritional supplements
✦ Antacids
✦ Potassium-sparing diuretics
✦ Paracentesis
✦ Surgical shunt placement
✦ Vasopressin
✦ Multilumen balloon
✦ Sclerosing agents
✦ Portosystemic shunt

uretics may be prescribed to reduce fluid accumulation; paracentesis may be performed to relieve abdominal pressure and remove ascitic fluid.

In addition, a surgical shunt placement may be used to help divert ascites into venous circulation, leading to weight loss, decreased abdominal girth, increased sodium excretion from the kidneys, and improved urine output.

Vasopressin may be used to treat bleeding esophageal varices and many options are available to control bleeding esophageal varices. A multilumen balloon can exert pressure on the bleeding sites, stopping blood loss from the vessel. Sclerosing agents may be injected into oozing vessels to cause clotting and sclerosis. Lastly, a portosystemic shunt may be inserted to control bleeding from esophageal varices and decrease portal hypertension (diverts a portion of the portal vein blood flow away from the liver; seldom performed).

NURSING CONSIDERATIONS

Patients with cirrhosis need close observation, intensive supportive care, and sound nutritional counseling.

✦ Check skin, gums, stools, and vomitus regularly for bleeding. Apply pressure to injection sites to prevent bleeding. Warn the patient against taking nonsteroidal anti-inflammatory drugs, straining at stool, and blowing his nose or sneezing too vigorously. Suggest using an electric razor and soft toothbrush.

✦ Observe closely for signs of behavioral or personality changes. Report increasing stupor, lethargy, hallucinations, or neuromuscular dysfunction. Awaken the patient periodically to determine level of consciousness. Watch for asterixis, a sign of developing hepatic encephalopathy.

✦ To assess fluid retention, weigh the patient and measure abdominal girth at least daily; inspect ankles and sacrum for dependent edema; and accurately record intake and output. Carefully evaluate the patient before, during, and after paracentesis; this drastic loss of fluid may induce shock.

✦ To prevent skin breakdown associated with edema and pruritus, avoid using soap when you bathe the patient; instead, use lubricating lotion or moisturizing agents. Handle the patient gently, and turn and reposition him often to keep his skin intact.

✦ Tell the patient that rest and good nutrition will conserve energy and decrease metabolic demands on the liver. Urge him to eat frequent small meals. Stress the need to avoid infections and abstain from alcohol. Refer the patient to Alcoholics Anonymous if necessary.

CROHN'S DISEASE

Crohn's disease, also known as *regional enteritis* or *granulomatous colitis,* is inflammation of any part of the GI tract (usually the proximal portion of the colon and less commonly the terminal ileum), extending through all layers of the intestinal wall. It may also involve regional lymph nodes and the mesentery. Crohn's disease is most prevalent in adults ages 20 to 40.

CAUSES

The exact cause of Crohn's disease is unknown but conditions that may contribute include lymphatic obstruction, allergies, immune disorders, infection, and genetic predisposition.

PATHOPHYSIOLOGY

Whatever the cause of Crohn's disease, inflammation spreads slowly and progressively. Enlarged lymph nodes block lymph flow in the submucosa. Lymphatic obstruction leads to edema, mucosal ulceration and fissures, abscesses, and sometimes granulomas. Mucosal ulcerations are called "skipping lesions" because they aren't continuous, as in ulcerative colitis.

Oval, elevated patches of closely packed lymph follicles, called *Peyer's patches,* develop in the lining of the small intestine. Subsequent fibrosis thickens the bowel wall and causes stenosis, or narrowing of the lumen. (See *Bowel changes in Crohn's disease,* page 364.)

The serous membrane becomes inflamed (serositis), inflamed bowel loops adhere to other diseased or normal loops, and diseased bowel segments become interspersed with healthy ones. Finally, diseased parts of the bowel become thicker, narrower, and shorter.

SIGNS AND SYMPTOMS

Signs and symptoms of Crohn's disease include steady, colicky pain in the right lower quadrant, cramping, and tenderness due to acute inflammation and nerve fiber irritation. A palpable mass may be present in the right lower quadrant.

Diarrhea occurs, due to bile salt malabsorption, loss of healthy intestinal surface area, and bacterial growth; steatorrhea occurs secondary to fat malabsorption; and bloody stools are secondary to bleeding from inflammation and ulceration. Weight loss occurs as a result of diarrhea and malabsorption.

COMPLICATIONS

Complications may include anal fistula; perineal abscess; fistulas to the bladder or vagina, or to the skin in an old scar area; intestinal obstruction; nutrient deficiencies from poor digestion and malabsorption of bile salts and vitamin B_{12}; and fluid imbalances.

DIAGNOSIS

These tests help to diagnose Crohn's disease:
+ Fecal occult blood test reveals minute amounts of blood in stools.
+ Small-bowel X-ray shows irregular mucosa, ulceration, and stiffening.
+ Barium enema reveals the string sign (segments of stricture separated by normal bowel) and possibly fissures and narrowing of the bowel.
+ Sigmoidoscopy and colonoscopy reveal patchy areas of inflammation (helps to rule out ulcerative colitis), with cobblestone-like mucosal surface. With colon involvement, ulcers may be seen.
+ Biopsy reveals granulomas in up to one-half of all specimens.
+ Blood tests reveal increased white blood cell count and erythrocyte sedimentation rate, and decreased potassium, calcium, magnesium, and hemoglobin levels.

TREATMENT

Various medications can treat Crohn's disease. Corticosteroids reduce the inflammation and, subsequently, diarrhea, pain, and bleeding; sulfasalazine also reduces inflammation. Immunosuppressants are prescribed to suppress the response to antigens. Antidiarrheals are used to combat diarrhea (not used with patients with significant bowel obstruction) and metronidazole treats perianal complications. In

How it happens
+ Inflammation spreads slowly and progressively
+ Enlarged lymph nodes block lymph flow in submucosa
+ Lymphatic obstruction leads to edema, mucosal ulceration and fissures, abscesses, granulomas
+ Peyer's patches develop in lining of small intestine
+ Subsequent fibrosis thickens bowel wall, causes stenosis
+ Serous membrane becomes inflamed
+ Inflamed bowel loops adhere to other loops
+ Diseased parts of the bowel become thicker, narrower, shorter

Key signs and symptoms
+ Steady, colicky pain
+ Cramping and tenderness
+ Diarrhea, steatorrhea, and bloody stool
+ Weight loss

Complications
+ Anal fistula
+ Perineal abscess
+ Nutrient deficiencies

Diagnosis
+ Minute amounts of blood in stool
+ Small-bowel X-ray — irregular mucosa, ulceration, stiffening
+ Barium enema shows string sign
+ Colonoscopy shows patchy areas of inflammation

Treatment
+ Corticosteroids
+ Sulfasalazine
+ Immunosuppressants
+ Antidiarrheals

Bowel changes in Crohn's disease

As Crohn's disease progresses, fibrosis thickens the bowel wall and narrows the lumen. Narrowing — or stenosis — can occur in any part of the intestine and cause varying degrees of intestinal obstruction. At first, the mucosa may appear normal, but as the disease progresses it takes on a "cobblestone" appearance as shown here.

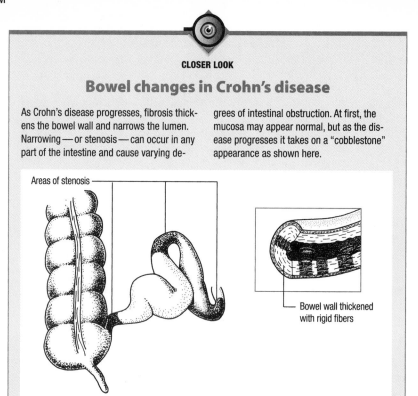

Areas of stenosis

Bowel wall thickened with rigid fibers

addition, opioid analgesics control diarrhea while also controlling pain. Vitamin supplements replace and compensate for the bowel's inability to absorb vitamins.

Lifestyle changes are also part of the treatment of Crohn's disease. Stress reduction and reduced physical activity rest the bowel and allow it to heal. Dietary changes are necessary to decrease bowel activity while still providing adequate nutrition. These changes include elimination of fruits, vegetables, high-fiber foods, dairy products, spicy and fatty foods, foods that irritate the mucosa, carbonated or caffeinated beverages, and other foods or liquids that stimulate excessive intestinal activity.

Surgery may be performed, if necessary, to repair bowel perforation and correct massive hemorrhage, fistulas, or acute intestinal obstruction. A colectomy with ileostomy may be indicated for patients with extensive disease of the large intestine and rectum.

NURSING CONSIDERATIONS

Although treatment is based largely on symptoms, you should monitor the patient's status carefully for signs of worsening condition.

✦ Record fluid intake and output (including the amount of stools), and weigh the patient daily. Watch for dehydration and maintain fluid and electrolyte balance. Be alert for signs of intestinal bleeding (bloody stools); check stools daily for occult blood.

✦ If the patient is receiving steroids, watch for adverse effects, such as GI bleeding and hyperglycemia. Remember that steroids can mask signs of infection.

Key nursing actions
✦ Monitor the patient's status carefully for signs of worsening condition.
✦ Record fluid intake and output, and weigh the patient daily. Watch for dehydration and maintain fluid and electrolyte balance. Be alert for signs of intestinal bleeding.
✦ If the patient is receiving steroids, watch for adverse effects, such as GI bleeding and hyperglycemia. Remember that steroids can mask signs of infection.

◆ Check hemoglobin levels and hematocrit regularly. Give iron supplements and blood transfusions, as ordered.

◆ Give analgesics as ordered.

◆ Provide good patient hygiene and meticulous mouth care if the patient is restricted to nothing-by-mouth status. After each bowel movement, give good skin care. Always keep a clean, covered bedpan within the patient's reach. Ventilate the room to eliminate odors.

◆ Observe the patient for fever and pain or pneumaturia, which may signal a bladder fistula. Abdominal pain and distention and fever may indicate intestinal obstruction. Watch for stools from the vagina and an enterovaginal fistula.

◆ Before ileostomy, arrange for a visit by an enterostomal therapist.

◆ After surgery, frequently check the patient's I.V. and nasogastric tube for proper functioning. Monitor vital signs and fluid intake and output. Watch for wound infection. Provide meticulous stoma care, and teach it to the patient and his family. Know that an ileostomy changes the patient's body image, so offer reassurance and emotional support.

◆ Stress the need for a severely restricted diet and bed rest, which may be demanding, particularly for the young patient. Encourage him to try to reduce tension. If stress is clearly an aggravating factor, refer him for counseling.

◆ Refer the patient to a support group such as the Crohn's and Colitis Foundation of America.

DIVERTICULAR DISEASE

In diverticular disease, bulging pouches (diverticula) in the GI wall push the mucosal lining through the surrounding muscle. Although the most common site for diverticula is in the sigmoid colon, they may develop anywhere, from the proximal end of the pharynx to the anus. Other typical sites include the duodenum, near the pancreatic border or the ampulla of Vater, and the jejunum.

 CLINICAL ALERT Diverticular disease is common in Western countries, suggesting that a low-fiber diet reduces stool bulk and leads to excessive colonic motility. The consequent increased intraluminal pressure causes herniation of the mucosa.

Diverticular disease of the stomach is rare and is usually a precursor of peptic or neoplastic disease. Diverticular disease of the ileum (Meckel's diverticulum) is the most common congenital anomaly of the GI tract.

Diverticular disease has two clinical forms. In *diverticulosis,* diverticula are present but don't cause symptoms. In *diverticulitis,* diverticula are inflamed and may cause potentially fatal obstruction, infection, or hemorrhage.

 CLINICAL ALERT Diverticular disease is most prevalent in men older than age 40 and in people who eat a low-fiber diet. More than 50% of all patients older than age 50 have colonic diverticula.

CAUSES

Causes of diverticular disease may include diminished colonic motility and increased intraluminal pressure, a low-fiber diet, and defects in colon wall strength.

How it happens

+ High intraluminal pressure on weakness in GI wall
+ Retained undigested food, bacteria accumulate in diverticular sac
+ Hard mass cuts off blood supply to thin walls of sac, making them susceptible to bacteria
+ Inflammation follows

Key signs and symptoms

+ Diverticulosis patients usually show no symptoms

Mild diverticulitis

+ Moderate left lower abdominal pain

Severe diverticulitis

+ Rupture of diverticula may cause abdominal rigidity
+ Subsequent inflammation produces left lower quadrant pain

Chronic diverticulitis

+ Constipation or diarrhea
+ Ribbonlike stools

Diagnosis

+ Upper GI series to confirm or rule out diverticulosis of esophagus, upper bowel
+ Barium enema reveals filling of diverticula
+ Blood studies show elevated erythrocyte sedimentation rate

Complications

+ Rectal bleeding
+ Peritonitis
+ Bowel perforation

Treatment

+ Liquid or bland diet
+ Stool softeners
+ Occasional doses of mineral oil

PATHOPHYSIOLOGY

Diverticula probably result from high intraluminal pressure on an area of weakness in the GI wall, where blood vessels enter. Diet may be a contributing factor because insufficient fiber reduces fecal residue, narrows the bowel lumen, and leads to high intra-abdominal pressure during defecation.

In diverticulitis, retained undigested food and bacteria accumulate in the diverticular sac. This hard mass cuts off the blood supply to the thin walls of the sac, making them more susceptible to attack by colonic bacteria. Inflammation follows and may lead to perforation, abscess, peritonitis, obstruction, or hemorrhage. Occasionally, the inflamed colon segment may adhere to the bladder or other organs and cause a fistula.

SIGNS AND SYMPTOMS

Typically, the patient with diverticulosis usually shows no symptoms unless diverticulitis develops. In mild diverticulitis, moderate left lower abdominal pain is secondary to inflammation of diverticula. The patient may experience a low-grade fever from trapping of bacteria-rich stools in the diverticula and may have leukocytosis from infection secondary to trapping of bacteria-rich stools in the diverticula.

In severe diverticulitis, rupture of the diverticula, abscesses, and peritonitis may cause abdominal rigidity. Rupture of the diverticula and subsequent inflammation and infection produce a left lower quadrant pain. Sepsis and shock from the release of fecal material from the rupture site cause high fever, chills, and hypotension. Microscopic or massive hemorrhage may result from rupture of diverticulum near a vessel.

Signs and symptoms of chronic diverticulitis include constipation, ribbonlike stools, intermittent diarrhea, and abdominal distention resulting from intestinal obstruction (possible when fibrosis and adhesions narrow the bowel's lumen). Abdominal rigidity and pain, diminishing or absent bowel sounds, nausea, and vomiting may occur secondary to intestinal obstruction.

DIAGNOSIS

To diagnose diverticular disease, many tests may be performed. An upper GI series can confirm or rule out diverticulosis of the esophagus and upper bowel. Diagnosis can be confirmed if a barium enema reveals filling of diverticula or if blood studies show an elevated erythrocyte sedimentation rate. Evidence of benign disease from a biopsy will rule out cancer.

COMPLICATIONS

Complications of diverticular disease generally result from diverticulitis. Small, fragile blood vessels in the diverticula can cause rectal bleeding. An infected diverticulum may progress to form an abscess. If the abscess doesn't respond to antibiotics, it can rupture and lead to peritonitis. An infected diverticulum can also cause bowel thickening and scarring, a condition that can lead to intestinal obstruction. When an inflamed diverticulum tears, bowel perforation results.

TREATMENT

Treatment of diverticular disease may include a liquid or bland diet, stool softeners, and occasional doses of mineral oil for symptomatic diverticulosis to relieve symptoms, minimize irritation, and lessen the risk of progression to diverticulitis.

After pain has subsided, a high-residue diet decreases intra-abdominal pressure during defecation. Exercise increases the rate of stool passage. Antibiotics are prescribed to treat infection of the diverticula. Analgesics, such as meperidine (Demerol) or morphine, help control pain and relax smooth muscle, and antispasmodics control muscle spasms.

Surgical interventions include colon resection with removal of the involved segment to correct cases refractory to medical treatment. Temporary colostomy may be necessary to drain abscesses and rest the colon in diverticulitis accompanied by perforation, peritonitis, obstruction, or fistula. Blood transfusions may be necessary to treat blood loss from hemorrhage, and fluid replacement should be provided as needed.

NURSING CONSIDERATIONS

Management of uncomplicated diverticulosis chiefly involves thorough patient education about fiber and dietary habits.
+ Explain what diverticula are and how they form.
+ Make sure the patient understands the importance of dietary fiber and the harmful effects of constipation and straining during defecation. Encourage increased intake of foods high in indigestible fiber, including fresh fruits and vegetables, whole grain bread, and wheat or bran cereals. Warn that a high-fiber diet may temporarily cause flatulence and discomfort. Advise the patient to relieve constipation with stool softeners or bulk-forming cathartics. Caution against taking bulk-forming cathartics without plenty of water; if swallowed dry, they may absorb enough moisture in the mouth and throat to swell and obstruct the esophagus or trachea.
+ If the patient with diverticulosis is hospitalized, administer medications as ordered. Observe his stools carefully for frequency, color, and consistency, and keep accurate pulse and temperature charts because they may signal developing inflammation or complications.

Management of diverticulitis depends on the severity of symptoms.
+ In mild disease, administer medications as ordered. Explain diagnostic tests and preparations for such tests; observe stools carefully; and maintain accurate records of temperature, pulse, respirations, and intake and output.
+ If diverticular bleeding occurs, the patient may require angiography and catheter placement for vasopressin infusion. If so, inspect the insertion site frequently for bleeding, check pedal pulses often, and keep him from flexing his legs at the groin.
+ Watch for vasopressin-induced fluid retention (apprehension, abdominal cramps, seizures, oliguria, or anuria) and severe hyponatremia (hypotension; rapid, thready pulse; cold, clammy skin; and cyanosis).

After surgery to resect the colon is performed
+ Watch for signs of infection.
+ Provide meticulous wound care because perforation may have infected the area.
+ Check drain sites frequently for signs of infection (purulent drainage or foul odor) or fecal drainage.
+ Change dressings as necessary.
+ Encourage coughing and deep breathing to prevent atelectasis.
+ Watch for signs of postoperative bleeding (hypotension and decreased hemoglobin levels and hematocrit).
+ Record intake and output accurately.
+ Keep the NG tube patent.
+ Teach ostomy care as needed.
+ Arrange for a visit by an enterostomal therapist.

Key nursing actions
+ Management of uncomplicated diverticulosis chiefly involves thorough patient education about fiber and dietary habits.
+ Explain what diverticula are and how they form.
+ Make sure the patient understands the importance of dietary fiber and the harmful effects of constipation and straining during defecation.
+ In mild disease, administer medications as ordered.
+ If diverticular bleeding occurs, the patient may require angiography and catheter placement for vasopressin infusion.
+ Watch for vasopressin-induced fluid retention and severe hyponatremia.

After surgery to resect the colon is performed
+ Watch for signs of infection.
+ Provide meticulous wound care because perforation may have infected the area.
+ Check drain sites frequently for signs of infection or fecal drainage.
+ Change dressings as necessary.
+ Watch for signs of postoperative bleeding.
+ Keep the NG tube patent.
+ Arrange for a visit by an enterostomal therapist.

Characteristics of GERD

+ Also known as *heartburn*
+ Backflow of gastric or duodenal contents past LES without associated belching or vomiting
+ Causes acute epigastric pain, usually after meals
+ Pain radiates to chest or arms
+ Commonly occurs in pregnant or obese people

Causes

+ Weakened esophageal sphincter
+ Hiatal hernia
+ Increased abdominal pressure
+ Medications

How it happens

+ LES doesn't remain closed
+ Pressure in stomach pushes contents into esophagus
+ High acidity of stomach contents causes pain

Key signs and symptoms

+ Burning pain in epigastric area
+ Feeling of fluid accumulation in throat

Complications

+ Reflux esophagitis
+ Esophageal stricture
+ Esophageal ulceration

Diagnosis

+ Esophageal acidity test evaluates LES
+ Acid perfusion test confirms esophagitis
+ Barium swallow identifies hiatal hernia
+ Esophagoscopy confirms pathologic changes in mucosa

GASTROESOPHAGEAL REFLUX DISEASE

Popularly known as *heartburn,* gastroesophageal reflux disease (GERD) refers to backflow of gastric or duodenal contents or both into the esophagus and past the lower esophageal sphincter (LES), without associated belching or vomiting. The reflux of gastric contents causes acute epigastric pain, usually after a meal. The pain may radiate to the chest or arms. It commonly occurs in pregnant or obese people. Lying down after a meal also contributes to reflux.

CAUSES

GERD may result from several conditions, including weakened esophageal sphincter, hiatal hernia, and increased abdominal pressure, such as with obesity or pregnancy. Medications such as morphine, diazepam, calcium channel blockers, meperidine, and anticholinergic agents have also been found to cause GERD. Food, alcohol, and cigarettes lower LES pressure, which causes GERD; nasogastric (NG) intubation for longer than 4 days causes the condition as well.

PATHOPHYSIOLOGY

Normally, the LES maintains enough pressure around the lower end of the esophagus to close it and prevent reflux. Typically the sphincter relaxes after each swallow to allow food into the stomach. In GERD, the sphincter doesn't remain closed (usually due to deficient LES pressure or pressure within the stomach exceeding LES pressure) and the pressure in the stomach pushes the stomach contents into the esophagus. The high acidity of the stomach contents causes pain and irritation when it enters the esophagus. (See *How heartburn occurs.*)

SIGNS AND SYMPTOMS

In GERD, a burning pain in the epigastric area, possibly radiating to the arms and chest, is a result of the reflux of gastric contents into the esophagus causing irritation and esophageal spasm.

Increased abdominal pressure causes reflux and pain, usually after a meal or when lying down. The patient may also report a feeling of fluid accumulation in the throat without a sour or bitter taste due to hypersecretion of saliva.

COMPLICATIONS

Complications include reflux esophagitis, esophageal stricture, esophageal ulceration, and chronic pulmonary disease from aspiration of gastric contents in the throat.

DIAGNOSIS

Diagnostic tests are aimed at determining the underlying cause of GERD:
+ Esophageal acidity test evaluates the competence of the LES and provides objective measure of reflux.
+ Acid perfusion test confirms esophagitis and distinguishes it from cardiac disorders.
+ Esophagoscopy allows visual examination of the lining of the esophagus to reveal the extent of the disease and confirm pathologic changes in mucosa.
+ Barium swallow identifies hiatal hernia as the cause.

CLOSER LOOK

How heartburn occurs

Hormonal fluctuations, mechanical stress, and the effects of certain foods and drugs can decrease lower esophageal sphincter (LES) pressure. When LES pressure falls and intra-abdominal or intragastric pressure rises, the normally contracted LES relaxes inappropriately and allows reflux of gastric acid or bile secretions into the lower esophagus. There, the reflux irritates and inflames the esophageal mucosa, causing pyrosis.

Persistent inflammation can cause LES pressure to decrease even more and may trigger a recurrent cycle of reflux and pyrosis.

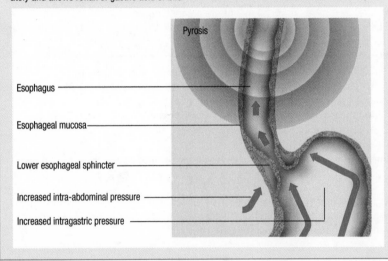

♦ Upper GI series detects hiatal hernia or motility problems.
♦ Esophageal manometry evaluates resting pressure of LES and determines sphincter competence.

TREATMENT

Treatment of GERD includes diet therapy with frequent, small meals and avoidance of eating before going to bed to reduce abdominal pressure and reduce the incidence of reflux. Positioning—sitting up during and after meals and sleeping with head of the bed elevated—helps by reducing abdominal pressure and preventing reflux. Increased fluid intake washes gastric contents out of the esophagus.

Medications such as antacids neutralize the stomach's acidic content and minimize irritation. Histamine-2 receptor antagonists inhibit gastric acid secretion. Proton pump inhibitors are prescribed to reduce gastric acidity. LES pressure is improved through the use of cholinergic agents and by smoking cessation (nicotine lowers LES pressure).

If hiatal hernia is the cause of GERD, or if the patient has refractory symptoms, surgical correction may be indicated.

Treatment
♦ Diet therapy
♦ Positioning
♦ H_2-receptor antagonists
♦ Proton pump inhibitors
♦ Cholinergic agents
♦ Smoking cessation
♦ Surgical correction

Key nursing actions

+ Teach the patient what causes reflux, how to avoid reflux with an antireflux regimen, and what symptoms to watch for.
+ Advise the patient to sit upright, particularly after meals, and to eat small, frequent meals.
+ After surgery, carefully watch and record chest tube drainage and respiratory status.

Characteristics of nonviral hepatitis

+ An inflammation of the liver that usually results from exposure to certain chemicals or drugs
+ Most patients recover; a few develop fulminating hepatitis or cirrhosis

Causes

+ Hepatotoxic chemicals and drugs

How it happens

+ Hepatotoxins cause hepatic cellular necrosis, scarring, Kupffer's cell hyperplasia
+ Infiltration by mononuclear phagocytes occur with varying severity
+ Alcohol, anoxia, and preexisting liver disease exacerbate effects of toxins
+ Idiosyncratic hepatitis may begin with a hypersensitivity reaction

Key signs and symptoms

+ Anorexia, nausea, vomiting
+ Hepatomegaly and possible abdominal pain
+ Jaundice and pruritus
+ Dark urine, clay-colored stool

NURSING CONSIDERATIONS

Teach the patient what causes reflux, how to avoid reflux with an antireflux regimen (medication, diet, and positional therapy), and what symptoms to watch for and report.

+ Instruct the patient to avoid circumstances that increase intra-abdominal pressure (such as bending, coughing, vigorous exercise, tight clothing, constipation, and obesity) as well as substances that reduce sphincter control (cigarettes, alcohol, fatty foods, and caffeine).

+ Advise the patient to sit upright, particularly after meals, and to eat small, frequent meals. Tell him to avoid highly seasoned food, acidic juices, alcoholic drinks, bedtime snacks, and foods high in fat or carbohydrates, which reduce LES pressure. He should eat meals at least 2 to 3 hours before lying down.

+ Tell the patient to take antacids as ordered (usually 1 and 3 hours after meals and at bedtime).

+ Teach the patient correct preparation for diagnostic testing. For example, he shouldn't eat for 6 to 8 hours before a barium swallow or endoscopy.

+ After surgery using a thoracic approach, carefully watch and record chest tube drainage and respiratory status. If needed, give chest physiotherapy and oxygen. Position the patient with an NG tube in semi-Fowler's position to help prevent reflux. Offer reassurance and emotional support.

HEPATITIS, NONVIRAL

Nonviral hepatitis is an inflammation of the liver that usually results from exposure to certain chemicals or drugs. Most patients recover from this illness, although a few develop fulminating hepatitis or cirrhosis.

CAUSES

Causes of nonviral hepatitis include hepatotoxic chemicals and hepatotoxic drugs.

PATHOPHYSIOLOGY

Various hepatotoxins, such as carbon tetrachloride, acetaminophen, trichloroethylene, poisonous mushrooms, and vinyl chloride, can cause hepatitis. After exposure to these agents, hepatic cellular necrosis, scarring, Kupffer's cell hyperplasia, and infiltration by mononuclear phagocytes occur with varying severity. Alcohol, anoxia, and preexisting liver disease exacerbate the effects of some toxins.

Drug-induced (idiosyncratic) hepatitis may begin with a hypersensitivity reaction unique to the individual, unlike toxic hepatitis, which appears to affect all exposed people indiscriminately. Among possible causes are niacin, halothane, sulfonamides, isoniazid, acetaminophen, methyldopa, and phenothiazines (cholestasis-induced hepatitis). Symptoms of hepatic dysfunction may appear at any time during or after exposure to these drugs, but the disorder usually manifests after 2 to 5 weeks of therapy.

SIGNS AND SYMPTOMS

In nonviral hepatitis, anorexia, nausea, and vomiting are due to the systemic effects of liver inflammation. Hepatomegaly and possible abdominal pain are results of liver inflammation. Jaundice results from decreased bilirubin metabolism, leading to hyperbilirubinemia. Dark urine is due to elevated urobilinogen. Decreased bile in the GI tract from liver necrosis causes the patient to have clay-colored stools. Jaundice and hyperbilirubinemia cause pruritus.

COMPLICATIONS

Complications of nonviral hepatitis include cirrhosis and hepatic failure.

DIAGNOSIS

Key tests can be performed to determine if the patient has nonviral hepatitis. If the condition is present, liver enzyme levels (such as serum aspartate aminotransferase and alanine aminotransferase levels), total and direct bilirubin levels, alkaline phosphatase levels, WBC count, and eosinophil count are all elevated.

Liver biopsy identifies underlying disorder, especially infiltration with WBCs and eosinophils.

TREATMENT

In order to treat nonviral hepatitis, treatments, such as lavage, catharsis, or hyperventilation, are used (depending on the route of exposure) to remove the causative agent.

For acetaminophen poisoning, acetylcysteine, the antidote to acetaminophen, is prescribed. Symptoms of drug-induced nonviral hepatitis are usually relieved by the use of corticosteroids.

NURSING CONSIDERATIONS

Preventive measures should include instructing the patient about the proper use of drugs and the proper handling of cleaning agents and solvents.

HEPATITIS, VIRAL

Viral hepatitis is a common infection of the liver, resulting in hepatic cell destruction, necrosis, and autolysis. In most patients, hepatic cells eventually regenerate with little or no residual damage. However, old age and serious underlying disorders make complications more likely. The prognosis is poor if edema and hepatic encephalopathy develop.

Five major forms of hepatitis are currently recognized:

✦ Type A (infectious or short-incubation hepatitis) is most common among male homosexuals and in people with human immunodeficiency virus (HIV) infection. It's commonly spread via the fecal-oral route by the ingestion of fecal contaminants.

✦ Type B (serum or long-incubation hepatitis) is also most common among HIV-positive individuals. Routine screening of donor blood for the hepatitis B surface antigen has reduced the incidence of posttransfusion cases, but transmission by needles shared by drug users remains a major problem.

✦ Type C (HCV) accounts for about 20% of all viral hepatitis cases and for most posttransfusion cases.

✦ Type D (delta hepatitis) causes about 50% of all cases of fulminant hepatitis, which has a high mortality. Developing in 1% of patients with viral hepatitis, fulminant hepatitis causes unremitting liver failure with encephalopathy. It progresses to coma and commonly leads to death within 2 weeks. In the United States, type D occurs only in people who are frequently exposed to blood and blood products,

Complications
✦ Cirrhosis
✦ Hepatic failure

Diagnosis
✦ Elevated liver enzyme, bilirubin, and alkaline phosphatase levels
✦ Elevated WBC and eosinophil count

Treatment
✦ Lavage
✦ Catharsis
✦ Hyperventilation
✦ Corticosteroids

Key nursing actions
✦ Instruct the patient about the proper use of drugs and handling of cleaning agents and solvents.

Characteristics of viral hepatitis
✦ Infection of liver causing hepatic cell destruction and necrosis
✦ Hepatic cells usually regenerate with little residual damage
✦ Prognosis poor with edema and hepatic encephalopathy

Five major forms
✦ Type A: infectious; spread by fecal-oral route
✦ Type B: serum; most common in HIV-positive, I.V. drug users
✦ Type C: 20% of all viral hepatitis and most posttransfusion cases
✦ Type D: in the United States, occurs in people frequently exposed to blood and blood products; high mortality
✦ Type E: occurs primarily among patients who have recently returned from an endemic area

Causes

+ Infection with causative viruses A, B, C, D, or E

How it happens

+ Hepatic damage is similar in all types
+ Varying degrees of cell injury, necrosis
+ Virus causes hepatocyte injury and death
+ Inflammatory and immune reactions injure hepatocytes
+ Direct antibody attack against antigens further destroys infected cells
+ Edema and swelling lead to collapse of capillaries, decreased blood flow, tissue hypoxia, scarring, fibrosis

Key signs and symptoms

Prodromal stage
+ Easy fatigue, malaise
+ Anorexia, nausea, and vomiting
+ Dark urine, clay-colored stool
+ Right upper quadrant tenderness

Clinical stage
+ Worsening of symptoms
+ Itching
+ Jaundice

Recovery stage
+ Symptoms subside
+ Appetite returns

Complications

+ Chronic persistent hepatitis
+ Chronic active hepatitis
+ Cirrhosis
+ Hepatic failure
+ Death

such as I.V. drug users and hemophilia patients. Type D hepatitis is found only in patients with an acute or chronic episode of hepatitis B and requires the presence of hepatitis B surface antigen. The type D virus depends on the double-shelled type B virus to replicate. (Therefore, type D infection can't outlast a type B infection.)
+ Type E (formerly grouped with types C and D under the name non-A, non-B hepatitis) occurs primarily among patients who have recently returned from an endemic area (such as India, Africa, Asia, or Central America). It's more common in young adults and is more severe in pregnant woman. (See *Viral hepatitis from A to E,* pages 374 and 375.)
+ Other types continue to be identified with growing patient populations and sophisticated laboratory identification techniques.

CAUSES

The five major forms of viral hepatitis result from infection with the causative viruses: A, B, C, D, or E.

PATHOPHYSIOLOGY

Hepatic damage is usually similar in all types of viral hepatitis. Varying degrees of cell injury and necrosis occur.

On entering the body, the virus causes hepatocyte injury and death, either by directly killing the cells or by activating inflammatory and immune reactions. The inflammatory and immune reactions, in turn, injure or destroy hepatocytes by lysing the infected or neighboring cells. Later, direct antibody attack against the viral antigens causes further destruction of the infected cells. Edema and swelling of the interstitium lead to collapse of capillaries and decreased blood flow, tissue hypoxia, and scarring and fibrosis.

SIGNS AND SYMPTOMS

Signs and symptoms reflect the stage of the disease. In the *prodromal stage,* easy fatigue, generalized malaise, anorexia, mild weight loss, arthralgia, and myalgia are all results of systemic effects of liver inflammation. Nausea and vomiting occur as a result of GI effects of liver inflammation. Changes in taste and smell senses are related to liver inflammation; fever occurs secondary to this inflammatory process. This liver inflammation and irritation of area nerve fibers cause right upper quadrant tenderness. Dark urine results from elevated urobilinogen; clay-colored stools result from decreased bile in the GI tract.

During the *clinical stage* the patient may experience worsening of all symptoms of the prodromal stage. As such, increased bilirubin in the blood results in itching and jaundice. The patient's abdominal pain or tenderness is a result of the continued liver inflammation. During the *recovery stage,* the patient's symptoms subside and appetite returns.

COMPLICATIONS

Complications may include chronic persistent hepatitis, which may prolong recovery up to 8 months, chronic active hepatitis, cirrhosis, hepatic failure, primary hepatocellular carcinoma, and death.

DIAGNOSIS

To diagnose hepatitis, a hepatitis profile study should be performed to identify antibodies specific to the causative virus, establishing the type of hepatitis. Serum aspartate aminotransferase levels and serum alanine aminotransferase levels are increased in the prodromal stage, whereas the serum alkaline phosphatase level is slightly increased. In addition, the serum bilirubin level may remain high into late disease, especially in severe cases.

Prothrombin time is prolonged—more than 3 seconds longer than normal indicates severe liver damage. Transient neutropenia and lymphopenia followed by lymphocytosis are revealed in white blood cell counts. To confirm suspicions of chronic hepatitis, a liver biopsy should be performed.

TREATMENT

Treatment of hepatitis includes rest, which helps to minimize energy demands. Small, high-calorie meals combat anorexia; parenteral nutrition should be used if the patient can't eat due to persistent vomiting. In addition, avoidance of alcohol and other drugs will help prevent further hepatic damage.

Immunity to hepatitis A and B before transmission occurs is accomplished through vaccination.

NURSING CONSIDERATIONS

Use enteric precautions when caring for patients with type A or E hepatitis. Practice standard precautions for all patients.
+ Inform visitors about isolation precautions.
+ Provide rest periods throughout the day. Schedule treatments and tests so that the patient can rest between bouts of activity.
+ Because inactivity may make the patient anxious, include diversionary activities as part of his care. Gradually add activities to his schedule as he begins to recover.
+ Encourage the patient to eat. Don't overload his meal tray or overmedicate him because this will diminish his appetite.
+ Encourage fluids (at least 135 oz [3,992 ml]/day). Encourage the anorectic patient to drink fruit juices. Also offer chipped ice and effervescent soft drinks to maintain hydration without inducing vomiting.
+ Administer supplemental vitamins and commercial feedings, as ordered. If symptoms are severe and the patient can't tolerate oral intake, provide I.V. therapy and parenteral nutrition, as ordered by the physician.
+ Record the patient's weight daily, and keep intake and output records. Observe stools for color, consistency, and amount, and record the frequency of bowel movements.
+ Watch for signs of fluid shift, such as weight gain and orthostasis.
+ Watch for signs of hepatic coma, dehydration, pneumonia, vascular problems, and pressure ulcers.
+ In fulminant hepatitis, maintain electrolyte balance and a patent airway, prevent infections, and control bleeding. Correct hypoglycemia and any other complications while awaiting liver regeneration and repair.
+ Before discharge, emphasize the importance of having regular medical checkups for at least 1 year. The patient will have an increased risk of developing hepatoma. Warn the patient against using any alcohol or over-the-counter drugs during this period. Teach him to recognize the signs of a recurrence.

Diagnosis
+ Hepatitis profile study to identify antibodies specific to the causative virus, establishing the type of hepatitis
+ Serum aspartate aminotransferase, serum alanine aminotransferase levels increased in prodromal stage
+ Serum alkaline phosphatase level slightly increased
+ Serum bilirubin level may remain high into late disease
+ Prothrombin time prolonged

Treatment
+ Rest
+ Small, high-calorie meals
+ Parenteral nutrition
+ Avoidance of alcohol and other drugs
+ Vaccination before transmission

Key nursing actions
+ Use enteric precautions when caring for patients with type A or E hepatitis.
+ Inform visitors about isolation precautions.
+ Provide rest periods throughout the day.
+ Encourage the patient to eat, and encourage fluids.
+ Watch for signs of hepatic coma, dehydration, pneumonia, vascular problems, and pressure ulcers.
+ Before discharge, emphasize the importance of having regular medical checkups for at least 1 year.

Viral hepatitis from A to E

This chart compares the features of each (characterized) type of viral hepatitis. Other types are emerging.

FEATURE	HEPATITIS A	HEPATITIS B
Incubation	15 to 45 days	30 to 180 days
Onset	Acute	Insidious
Age-group most affected	Children, young adults	Any age
Transmission	Fecal-oral, sexual (especially oral-anal contact), nonpercutaneous (sexual, maternal-neonatal), percutaneous (rare)	Blood-borne; parenteral route, sexual, maternal-neonatal; virus is shed in all body fluids
Severity	Mild	Usually severe
Prognosis	Generally good	Worsens with age and debility
Progression to chronicity	None	Occasional

Severity of hepatitis

- Hepatitis A: mild
- Hepatitis B: usually severe
- Hepatitis C: moderate
- Hepatitis D: can be severe and lead to fulminant hepatitis
- Hepatitis E: highly virulent with common progression to fulminant hepatitis and hepatic failure, especially in pregnant women

Characteristics of intestinal obstruction

- Partial or complete blockage of lumen in small or large bowel
- Small-bowel obstruction more common, more serious
- Complete obstruction can cause death within hours
- Most likely to occur after abdominal surgery or in persons with congenital bowel deformities

Causes

- Adhesions and strangulated hernias
- Carcinomas
- Foreign bodies
- Compression of the bowel wall
- Physiologic disturbances

INTESTINAL OBSTRUCTION

Intestinal obstruction is the partial or complete blockage of the lumen in the small or large bowel. Small-bowel obstruction is far more common (90% of patients) and usually more serious. Complete obstruction in any part of the bowel, if untreated, can cause death within hours due to shock and vascular collapse. Intestinal obstruction is most likely to occur after abdominal surgery or in persons with congenital bowel deformities.

CAUSES

Adhesions and strangulated hernias usually cause small-bowel obstruction; large-bowel obstruction is typically due to carcinomas. Mechanical intestinal obstruction results from foreign bodies (fruit pits, gallstones, or worms) or compression of the bowel wall due to stenosis, intussusception, volvulus of the sigmoid or cecum, tumors, or atresia. Nonmechanical obstruction results from physiologic disturbances, such as paralytic ileus, electrolyte imbalances, toxicity (uremia or generalized infection), neurogenic abnormalities (spinal cord lesions), and thrombosis or embolism of mesenteric vessels. (See *Paralytic ileus*, page 376.)

HEPATITIS C	HEPATITIS D	HEPATITIS E
15 to 160 days	14 to 64 days	14 to 60 days
Insidious	Acute and chronic	Acute
More common in adults	Any age	Ages 20 to 40
Blood-borne; parenteral route	Parenteral route; most people infected with hepatitis D are also infected with hepatitis B	Primarily fecal-oral
Moderate	Can be severe and lead to fulminant hepatitis	Highly virulent with common progression to fulminant hepatitis and hepatic failure, especially in pregnant women
Moderate	Fair, worsens in chronic cases; can lead to chronic hepatitis D and chronic liver disease	Good unless pregnant
10% to 50% of cases	Occasional	None

PATHOPHYSIOLOGY

Intestinal obstruction develops in three forms. In a *simple intestinal obstruction,* blockage prevents intestinal contents from passing, with no other complications. In a *strangulated intestinal obstruction,* blood supply to part or all of the obstructed section is cut off, in addition to blockage of the lumen. Lastly, both ends of a bowel section are occluded, isolating it from the rest of the intestine in a *closed-loop intestinal obstruction.*

The physiologic effects are similar in all three forms of obstruction: When intestinal obstruction occurs, fluid, air, and gas collect near the site. Peristalsis increases temporarily as the bowel tries to force its contents through the obstruction, injuring intestinal mucosa and causing distention at and above the site of the obstruction. Distention blocks the flow of venous blood and halts normal absorptive processes; as a result, the bowel begins to secrete water, sodium, and potassium into the fluid pooled in the lumen.

Obstruction in the small intestine results in metabolic alkalosis from dehydration and loss of gastric hydrochloric acid; lower bowel obstruction causes slower dehydration and loss of intestinal alkaline fluids, resulting in metabolic acidosis. Ultimately, intestinal obstruction may lead to ischemia, necrosis, and death. (See *Symptom progression in intestinal obstruction,* page 377.)

How it happens
+ Simple intestinal obstruction: blockage prevents intestinal contents from passing
+ Strangulated intestinal obstruction: blood supply to obstructed section cut off, in addition to blockage of lumen
+ Closed-loop intestinal obstruction: both ends of bowel section are occluded
+ When obstruction occurs, fluid, air, gas collect near site
+ Peristalsis increases temporarily, injuring intestinal mucosa, causing distention
+ Distention blocks flow of venous blood, halts normal absorptive processes
+ Bowel begins to secrete water, sodium, potassium into fluid pooled in lumen
+ Small intestine obstruction results in metabolic alkalosis
+ Lower bowel obstruction results in metabolic acidosis
+ Obstruction may lead to ischemia, necrosis, death

Paralytic ileus

Causes
- Trauma, toxemia, or peritonitis
- Electrolyte deficiencies
- Vascular causes

Treatment
- Intubation
- Intestinal tube
- Cholinergic agents

Alert!
- Watch for air-fluid lock syndrome in older adults who remain recumbent for extended periods.

Key signs and symptoms
- Colicky pain
- Nausea and vomiting
- Constipation
- Abdominal distention
- Drowsiness
- Intense thirst
- Malaise
- Aching
- Dry oral mucous membranes, tongue
- Bowel sounds, borborygmi, rushes
- Abdominal tenderness, moderate distention

Paralytic ileus

Paralytic ileus is a physiologic form of intestinal obstruction that usually develops in the small bowel after abdominal surgery. It causes decreased or absent intestinal motility that usually disappears spontaneously after 2 to 3 days. Clinical effects of paralytic ileus include severe abdominal distention, extreme distress and, possibly, vomiting. The patient may be severely constipated or may pass flatus and small liquid stools.

CAUSES
Paralytic ileus can develop as a response to trauma, toxemia, or peritonitis or as a result of electrolyte deficiencies (especially hypokalemia) and the use of certain drugs, such as ganglionic blocking agents and anticholinergics. It can also result from vascular causes, such as thrombosis and embolism. Excessive air swallowing may contribute to the condition, but paralytic ileus brought on by this factor alone seldom lasts more than 24 hours.

TREATMENT
Paralytic ileus lasting longer than 48 hours requires intubation for decompression and nasogastric suctioning. Because of the absence of peristaltic activity, a long, weighted intestinal tube—called a *Miller-Abbott tube*—may be necessary in the patient with extraordinary abdominal distention. However, such procedures must be used with extreme caution because any additional trauma to the bowel can aggravate ileus. When paralytic ileus results from surgical manipulation of the bowel, treatment may also include cholinergic agents, such as neostigmine or bethanechol.

When caring for patients with paralytic ileus, warn those receiving cholinergic agents to expect certain paradoxical adverse effects, such as intestinal cramps and diarrhea. Remember that neostigmine produces cardiovascular adverse effects, usually bradycardia and hypotension. Check frequently for returning bowel sounds.

 CLINICAL ALERT Watch for air-fluid lock syndrome in older adults who remain recumbent for extended periods. In this syndrome, fluid collects in the dependent bowel loops. Then, peristalsis is too weak to push fluid "uphill." The resulting obstruction primarily occurs in the large bowel.

SIGNS AND SYMPTOMS

Colicky pain, nausea, vomiting, constipation, and abdominal distention characterize small-bowel obstruction. The condition may also cause drowsiness, intense thirst, malaise, and aching and may dry up oral mucous membranes and the tongue.

Auscultation reveals bowel sounds, borborygmi, and rushes; occasionally, these are loud enough to be heard without a stethoscope. Palpation elicits abdominal tenderness, with moderate distention; rebound tenderness occurs when obstruction has caused strangulation with ischemia. In late stages, signs of hypovolemic shock result from progressive dehydration and plasma loss.

In complete small-bowel obstruction, vigorous peristaltic waves propel bowel contents toward the mouth instead of the rectum. Spasms may occur every 3 to 5 minutes and last about 1 minute each, with persistent epigastric or periumbilical pain. Passage of small amounts of mucus and blood may occur. The higher the obstruction, the earlier and more severe the vomiting will be. Vomitus initially contains gastric juice, then bile and, lastly, contents of the ileum.

Symptoms of large-bowel obstruction develop more slowly because the colon can absorb fluid from its contents and distend well beyond its normal size. Constipation may be the only clinical effect for days. Colicky abdominal pain may then appear suddenly, producing spasms that last less than 1 minute each and recur

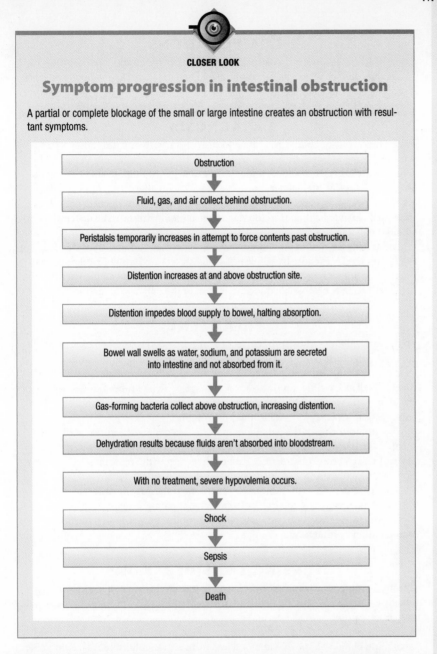

CLOSER LOOK

Symptom progression in intestinal obstruction

A partial or complete blockage of the small or large intestine creates an obstruction with resultant symptoms.

Obstruction

↓

Fluid, gas, and air collect behind obstruction.

↓

Peristalsis temporarily increases in attempt to force contents past obstruction.

↓

Distention increases at and above obstruction site.

↓

Distention impedes blood supply to bowel, halting absorption.

↓

Bowel wall swells as water, sodium, and potassium are secreted into intestine and not absorbed from it.

↓

Gas-forming bacteria collect above obstruction, increasing distention.

↓

Dehydration results because fluids aren't absorbed into bloodstream.

↓

With no treatment, severe hypovolemia occurs.

↓

Shock

↓

Sepsis

↓

Death

every few minutes. Continuous hypogastric pain and nausea may develop, but vomiting is usually absent at first. Large-bowel obstruction can cause dramatic abdominal distention; loops of the large bowel may become visible on the abdomen. Eventually, complete large-bowel obstruction may cause fecal vomiting, continuous pain, or localized peritonitis.

Patients with partial obstruction may display any of the aforementioned signs and symptoms in a milder form. However, leakage of liquid stools around the obstruction is common in partial obstruction.

Complications

+ Perforation
+ Peritonitis
+ Septicemia
+ Secondary infection
+ Metabolic alkalosis or acidosis

Diagnosis

+ Progressive, colicky, abdominal pain, distention, with or without nausea and vomiting
+ X-rays show presence and location of intestinal gas or fluid
+ "Stepladder" pattern emerges in small bowel on X-ray
+ Barium enema reveals distended, air-filled colon or closed loop of sigmoid with extreme distention

Treatment

+ Correction of fluid and electrolyte imbalances
+ Decompression of bowel
+ Treatment of shock, peritonitis
+ Blood replacement
+ I.V. fluid administration
+ Passage of NG tube
+ Miller-Abbott or Cantor tube
+ Surgical resection with anastomosis, colostomy, ileostomy

Key nursing actions

+ Monitor vital signs and observe for signs of shock.
+ Stay alert for signs and symptoms of metabolic alkalosis or acidosis.
+ Watch for signs and symptoms of secondary infection.
+ Monitor urine output carefully to assess renal function, circulating blood volume, and possible urine retention caused by bladder compression by the distended intestine.

COMPLICATIONS

Complications of intestinal obstruction may include perforation, peritonitis, septicemia, secondary infection, metabolic alkalosis or acidosis, hypovolemic or septic shock and, if untreated, death.

DIAGNOSIS

Progressive, colicky, abdominal pain and distention, with or without nausea and vomiting, suggest bowel obstruction. X-rays confirm the diagnosis. Abdominal films show the presence and location of intestinal gas or fluid. In small-bowel obstruction, a typical "stepladder" pattern emerges, with alternating fluid and gas levels apparent in 3 to 4 hours. In large-bowel obstruction, barium enema reveals a distended, air-filled colon or a closed loop of sigmoid with extreme distention (in sigmoid volvulus).

Laboratory results support this diagnosis. Decreased sodium, chloride, and potassium levels are cause by vomiting. A slightly elevated white blood cell count may be present with necrosis, peritonitis, or strangulation, and an increased serum amylase level may be possible due to irritation of the pancreas by a bowel loop.

TREATMENT

Preoperative therapy consists of correction of fluid and electrolyte imbalances, decompression of the bowel to relieve vomiting and distention, and treatment of shock and peritonitis. Strangulated obstruction usually necessitates blood replacement as well as I.V. fluid administration. Passage of an NG tube, followed by use of the longer and weighted Miller-Abbott or Cantor tube, usually accomplishes decompression, especially in small-bowel obstruction.

Close monitoring of the patient's condition determines the duration of treatment; if the patient fails to improve or if his condition deteriorates, surgery is necessary. In large-bowel obstruction, surgical resection with anastomosis, colostomy, or ileostomy commonly follows decompression with an NG tube.

Total parenteral nutrition may be appropriate if the patient suffers a protein deficit from chronic obstruction, postoperative or paralytic ileus, or infection. Drug therapy includes analgesics, sedatives, and antibiotics for peritonitis due to bowel strangulation or infarction.

NURSING CONSIDERATIONS

Effective management of intestinal obstruction, a life-threatening condition that usually causes overwhelming pain and distress, requires skillful supportive care and keen observation.

+ Monitor vital signs frequently. A drop in blood pressure may indicate reduced circulating blood volume due to blood loss from a strangulated hernia. Remember, as much as 10 qt (9.5 L) of fluid can collect in the small bowel, drastically reducing plasma volume. Observe the patient closely for signs of shock (pallor, rapid pulse, and hypotension).

+ Stay alert for signs and symptoms of metabolic alkalosis (changes in sensorium; slow, shallow respirations; hypertonic muscles; and tetany) or acidosis (shortness of breath on exertion; disorientation; and, later, deep, rapid breathing, weakness, and malaise).

+ Watch for signs and symptoms of secondary infection, such as fever and chills.

+ Monitor urine output carefully to assess renal function, circulating blood volume, and possible urine retention caused by bladder compression by the distended intestine. If you suspect bladder compression, catheterize the patient for residual urine immediately after he has voided. In addition, measure abdominal girth frequently to detect progressive distention.

✦ Provide fastidious mouth and nose care if the patient has vomited or undergone decompression by intubation. Look for signs of dehydration (thick, swollen tongue; dry, cracked lips; and dry oral mucous membranes).

✦ Record the amount and color of drainage from the decompression tube. Irrigate the tube with normal saline solution to maintain patency. If a weighted tube has been inserted, check periodically to make sure that it's advancing. Help the patient turn from side to side (or walk around, if he can) to facilitate passage of the tube.

✦ Keep the patient in Fowler's position as much as possible to promote pulmonary ventilation and ease respiratory distress from abdominal distention. Listen for bowel sounds, and watch for signs of returning peristalsis (passage of flatus and mucus through the rectum).

✦ Explain all diagnostic and therapeutic procedures to the patient, and answer any questions he may have. Make sure he understands that these procedures are necessary to relieve the obstruction and reduce pain. Tell him to lie on his left side for about a half hour before X-rays are taken.

✦ Prepare the patient and his family for the possibility of surgery, and provide emotional support and positive reinforcement afterward. Arrange for an enterostomal therapist to visit the patient who has had an ostomy.

IRRITABLE BOWEL SYNDROME

Also referred to as *spastic colon* or *spastic colitis,* irritable bowel syndrome (IBS) is marked by chronic symptoms of abdominal pain, alternating constipation and diarrhea, excess flatus, a sense of incomplete evacuation, and abdominal distention. IBS is a common, stress-related disorder. However, 20% of patients never seek medical attention. IBS is a benign condition that has no anatomical abnormality or inflammatory component. It's twice as common in women as in men.

CAUSES

Causes of IBS include psychological stress (most common), ingestion of irritants (drinks or foods high in caffeine or fat, beans, cabbage, and some fruits), lactose intolerance, abuse of laxatives, and hormonal changes (menstruation).

PATHOPHYSIOLOGY

IBS appears to reflect motor disturbances of the entire colon in response to stimuli. Some muscles of the small bowel are particularly sensitive to motor abnormalities and distention; others are particularly sensitive to certain foods and drugs. The patient may be hypersensitive to the hormones gastrin and cholecystokinin. The pain of IBS seems to be caused by abnormally strong contractions of the intestinal smooth muscle as it reacts to distention, irritants, or stress. (See *What happens in irritable bowel syndrome,* page 380.)

SIGNS AND SYMPTOMS

Lower abdominal pains characterized by cramping that usually occur during the day are secondary to muscle contractions; they're generally relieved by defecation

Key nursing actions
(continued)
✦ Look for signs of dehydration.
✦ Record the amount and color of drainage from the decompression tube.
✦ Keep the patient in Fowler's position as much as possible.

Characteristics of IBS
✦ Also referred to as *spastic colon* or *spastic colitis*
✦ Marked by chronic abdominal pain, alternating constipation and diarrhea, excess flatus and abdominal distention
✦ Stress-related
✦ Benign condition with no anatomical abnormality or inflammatory component

Causes
✦ Psychological stress
✦ Ingestion of irritants
✦ Lactose intolerance

How it happens
✦ May reflect motor disturbances of entire colon in response to stimuli
✦ Patient may be hypersensitive to gastrin and cholecystokinin
✦ Pain caused by abnormally strong contractions of intestinal smooth muscle

Key signs and symptoms
✦ Lower abdominal pains
✦ Pain that intensifies 1 to 2 hours after a meal
✦ Passage of mucus through the rectum
✦ Alternating constipation and diarrhea.

Occurrences in IBS

+ Autonomic nervous system doesn't cause alternating contractions and relaxations that propels stools smoothly toward rectum
+ Constipation or diarrhea, or a combination, may occur

Complications

+ Associated with a higher incidence of diverticulitis, colon cancer
+ May lead to chronic inflammatory bowel disease

Diagnosis

+ Physical examination reveals contributing psychological factors
+ Tests rule out infection, lactose intolerance, malignancy
+ Barium enema may reveal colon spasm, tubular appearance of descending colon
+ Sigmoidoscopy or colonoscopy may reveal spastic contractions

---

What happens in irritable bowel syndrome

Typically, the patient with irritable bowel syndrome (IBS) has a normal-appearing GI tract. However, careful examination of the colon may reveal functional irritability — an abnormality in colonic smooth-muscle function marked by excessive peristalsis and spasms, even during remission.

INTESTINAL FUNCTION

To understand what happens in IBS, consider how smooth muscle controls bowel function. Normally, segmental muscle contractions mix intestinal contents while peristalsis propels the contents through the GI tract. Motor activity is most propulsive in the proximal (stomach) and the distal (sigmoid) portions of the intestine. Activity in the rest of the intestines is slower, permitting nutrient and water absorption.

In IBS, the autonomic nervous system, which innervates the large intestine, doesn't cause the alternating contractions and relaxations that propel stools smoothly toward the rectum.

The result is constipation or diarrhea or both.

Constipation

Some patients have spasmodic intestinal contractions that set up a partial obstruction by trapping gas and stools. This causes distention, bloating, gas pain, and constipation.

Diarrhea

Other patients have dramatically increased intestinal motility. Eating or cholinergic stimulation triggers the small intestine's contents to rush into the large intestine, dumping watery stools and irritating the mucosa. The result is diarrhea.

Mixed symptoms

If further spasms trap liquid stools, the intestinal mucosa absorbs water from the stools, leaving them dry, hard, and difficult to pass. The result: a pattern of alternating diarrhea and constipation.

---

or passage of flatus. The patient may report a pain that intensifies 1 to 2 hours after a meal; it's caused by irritation of nerve fibers by causative stimulus.

Constipation may alternate with diarrhea, with one dominant (that is, occurring more than the other). These bowel patterns are due to motor disturbances from causative stimulus. Motor abnormalities cause altered mucus secretion in intestinal lumen. This results in the passage of mucus through the rectum. Flatus and constipation cause abdominal distention and bloating.

COMPLICATIONS

IBS is associated with a higher-than-normal incidence of diverticulitis and colon cancer. Although complications are usually few, the disorder may lead to chronic inflammatory bowel disease, although this progression is rare.

DIAGNOSIS

A physical examination of the patient with IBS reveals contributing psychological factors such as a recent stressful life change. Many tests conducted will rule out other disorders. Stool specimen tests for ova, parasites, bacteria, and blood rule out infection; lactose intolerance test rules out lactose intolerance; and rectal biopsy rules out malignancy.

A barium enema may reveal colon spasm and tubular appearance of descending colon without evidence of cancers and diverticulosis. In addition, a sigmoidoscopy or colonoscopy may reveal spastic contractions without evidence of colon cancer or inflammatory bowel disease.

TREATMENT

Treatment may include stress relief measures, including counseling or mild antianxiety agents. Investigation and avoidance of food irritants help by eliminating the stimulus causing the problem.

To reduce abdominal symptoms, application of heat may be used. Bulking agents can reduce episodes of diarrhea and minimize the effects of nonpropulsive colonic contractions. Additionally, antispasmodics (propantheline or diphenoxylate and atropine) may help alleviate pain, and loperamide may reduce urgency and fecal soiling in patients with persistent diarrhea.

Bowel training may be necessary to regain muscle control if chronic laxative use is the cause of the patient's IBS.

NURSING CONSIDERATIONS

Because the patient with IBS isn't hospitalized, focus your care on patient teaching.
✦ Tell the patient to avoid irritating foods, and encourage him to develop regular bowel habits.
✦ Help the patient deal with stress, and warn against dependence on sedatives or antispasmodics.
✦ Encourage regular checkups because IBS is associated with a higher-than-normal incidence of diverticulitis and colon cancer. For patients older than age 40, emphasize the need for an annual sigmoidoscopy and rectal examination.

▼ *LIFE-THREATENING DISORDER*

LIVER FAILURE

Liver failure can be the end result of any liver disease. The liver performs over 100 separate functions in the body. When it fails, a complex syndrome involving the impairment of many different organs and body functions ensues. (See *Functions of the liver,* page 382.)

Hepatic encephalopathy and hepatorenal syndrome are two conditions occurring in liver failure. The only cure for liver failure is a liver transplant.

CAUSES

Causes of liver failure include viral hepatitis, nonviral hepatitis, cirrhosis, and liver cancer.

PATHOPHYSIOLOGY

Manifestations of liver failure include hepatic encephalopathy and hepatorenal syndrome.

Hepatic encephalopathy, a set of central nervous system disorders, occurs when the liver can no longer detoxify the blood. Liver dysfunction and collateral vessels that shunt blood around the liver to the systemic circulation permit toxins absorbed from the GI tract to circulate freely to the brain. Ammonia, a by-product of protein metabolism, is one of the main toxins causing hepatic encephalopathy. The normal liver transforms ammonia to urea, which the kidneys excrete. When the liver fails and can no longer transform ammonia to urea, ammonia blood levels rise and the ammonia is delivered to the brain. Short-chain fatty acids, serotonin, tryptophan, and false neurotransmitters may also accumulate in the blood and contribute to hepatic encephalopathy.

Treatment
✦ Stress relief measures
✦ Investigation and avoidance of food irritants
✦ Application of heat
✦ Bulking agents
✦ Antispasmodics

Key nursing actions
✦ Focus your care on patient teaching.
✦ Tell the patient to avoid irritating foods, and encourage him to develop regular bowel habits.
✦ Help the patient deal with stress, and warn against dependence on sedatives or antispasmodics.

Characteristics of liver failure
✦ Life-threatening disorder
✦ Can be end result of any liver disease
✦ Complex syndrome involving impairment of many different organs and body functions
✦ Only cure is transplantation

Causes
✦ Viral hepatitis
✦ Nonviral hepatitis
✦ Cirrhosis
✦ Liver cancer

How it happens
Hepatic encephalopathy
✦ Liver dysfunction permits toxins from GI tract to circulate to brain
✦ Ammonia blood levels rise and ammonia delivered to brain
✦ Short-chain fatty acids, serotonin, tryptophan, false neurotransmitters may accumulate in blood

Key functions of the liver

+ Detoxified chemicals
+ Makes bile
+ Stores energy
+ Manufactures new proteins
+ Produces plasma

How it happens

Hepatorenal syndrome
+ Kidneys appear normal but abruptly cease functioning
+ Causes expanded blood volume, accumulation of hydrogen ions, electrolyte disturbances
+ Vasoconstriction may be compensatory response to portal hypertension, pooling of blood in splenic circulation

Key signs and symptoms

+ Jaundice
+ Pruritus
+ Abdominal pain or tenderness
+ Nausea
+ Anorexia
+ Fatigue and weight loss
+ Oliguria

Complications

+ Variceal bleeding
+ GI hemorrhage
+ Coma
+ Death

Diagnosis

+ Elevated levels of aspartate aminotransferase, alanine aminotransferase, alkaline phosphatase, bilirubin
+ Anemia
+ Impaired RBC production

Functions of the liver

The liver is one of the body's most essential organs. To understand how liver disease affects the body, it's best to understand its main functions:
+ detoxifies poisonous chemicals, including alcohol, beer, wine, and drugs (prescribed and over-the-counter as well as illegal substances)
+ makes bile to help digest food
+ stores energy by stockpiling sugar (carbohydrates, glucose, and fat) until needed
+ stores iron reserves as well as vitamins and minerals
+ manufactures new proteins
+ produces important plasma proteins necessary for blood coagulation, including prothrombin and fibrinogen
+ serves as a site for hematopoiesis during fetal development.

Hepatorenal syndrome is renal failure concurrent with liver disease; the kidneys appear to be normal but abruptly cease functioning. It causes expanded blood volume, accumulation of hydrogen ions, and electrolyte disturbances. It's most common in patients with alcoholic cirrhosis or fulminating hepatitis. The cause may be the accumulation of vasoactive substances that produce inappropriate constriction of renal arterioles, leading to decreased glomerular filtration and oliguria. The vasoconstriction may also be a compensatory response to portal hypertension and the pooling of blood in the splenic circulation.

SIGNS AND SYMPTOMS

Jaundice in liver failure occurs as a result of the liver's failure to conjugate bilirubin; pruritus results from the accumulation of bilirubin on the skin.

Liver inflammation causes abdominal pain or tenderness; the systemic effects of this inflammation result in nausea and anorexia. The patient may report fatigue and weight loss as a result of a failure of hepatic metabolism. He may also have oliguria from intrarenal vasoconstriction.

Ascites, splenomegaly, and varices of the esophagus, rectum, and abdominal wall occur secondary to portal hypertension. Decreased plasma proteins also contribute to the accumulation of ascites and peripheral edema. Thrombocytopenia causes bleeding tendencies and petechia. A prolonged prothrombin time from the impaired production of coagulation factors also result in bleeding tendencies.

Amenorrhea occurs as a result of altered steroid hormone production; metabolism and gynecomastia in males results because of estrogen buildup from failure of hepatic biotransformation functions.

COMPLICATIONS

Complications of liver failure include variceal bleeding, GI hemorrhage, coma, and death.

DIAGNOSIS

In diagnosing liver failure, liver function tests reveal elevated levels of aspartate aminotransferase, alanine aminotransferase, alkaline phosphatase, and bilirubin. In addition, blood studies reveal anemia, impaired RBC production, elevated bleeding and clotting times, low blood glucose levels, and increased serum ammonia levels. Urine osmolarity is increased as well.

TREATMENT

To cure liver failure, the patient must receive a liver transplantation.

Treatment of liver failure should include maintenance of a low-protein, high-carbohydrate diet to correct nutritional deficiencies and prevent overtaxing the liver. Oral lactulose or lactulose enemas reduce ammonia blood levels and help alleviate some symptoms of hepatic encephalopathy.

Ascites is treated with sodium restriction and potassium-sparing diuretics that increase water excretion as well as potassium supplements to reverse the effects of high aldosterone. Paracentesis is performed to remove ascitic fluid, alleviate abdominal discomfort, and obtain specimens for culture. Shunt placement may be necessary to aid in removal of ascitic fluid and alleviate abdominal discomfort.

To treat portal hypertension, shunt placement between the portal vein and another systemic vein may be performed to divert blood flow and relieve pressure. For variceal bleeding, vasoconstrictor drugs are prescribed. In addition, a balloon catheter may be inserted and inflated to exert pressure on the varicies and tamponade bleeding. The patient undergoes an embolization procedure to control bleeding from collaterals sprouting from the portal vein. Prothrombin time is decreased by the administration of vitamin K, which also helps control bleeding.

NURSING CONSIDERATIONS

Patient care for liver failure includes monitoring of symptoms and support.
✦ Frequently assess and record the patient's level of consciousness. Continually orient him to time, place, and person. Keep a daily record of the patient's handwriting to monitor progression of neurologic involvement.
✦ Monitor intake, output, and fluid and electrolyte balance. Check daily weight and measure abdominal girth. Watch for, and immediately report, signs of anemia (decreased hemoglobin levels), infection, alkalosis (increased serum bicarbonate), and GI bleeding (melena and hematemesis).
✦ Administer medications as ordered, and watch for adverse effects.
✦ Ask the dietary department to provide the specified low-protein diet, with carbohydrates supplying most of the calories. Provide good mouth care.
✦ Promote rest, comfort, and a quiet atmosphere. Discourage stressful exercise.
✦ Use restraints, if necessary, but avoid sedatives.
✦ Protect the comatose patient's eyes from corneal injury by using artificial tears or eye patches.
✦ Provide emotional support for the patient's family in the terminal stage of encephalopathy.

MALABSORPTION

Malabsorption is failure of the intestinal mucosa to absorb single or multiple nutrients efficiently. Absorption of amino acids, fat, sugar, or vitamins may be impaired, resulting in an inadequate movement of nutrients from the small intestine to the bloodstream or lymphatic system. Manifestations depend primarily on what isn't being absorbed.

CAUSES

A wide variety of disorders result in malabsorption. (See *Causes of malabsorption,* page 384.) Causes may include prior gastric surgery, pancreatic disorders, hepatobiliary disease, disease of the small intestine such as celiac disease, hereditary disorder, and drug toxicity.

Treatment
✦ Maintenance of a low-protein, high-carbohydrate diet
✦ Oral lactulose or lactulose enemas
✦ Sodium restriction; potassium-sparing diuretics
✦ Paracentesis
✦ Shunt placement
✦ Vasoconstrictor drugs
✦ Administration of vitamin K
✦ Liver transplantation

Key nursing actions
✦ Patient care for liver failure includes monitoring of symptoms and support.
✦ Frequently assess and record the patient's level of consciousness.
✦ Monitor intake, output, and fluid and electrolyte balance.
✦ Ask the dietary department to provide the specified low-protein diet, with carbohydrates supplying most of the calories. Provide good mouth care.
✦ Promote rest, comfort, and a quiet atmosphere. Discourage stressful exercise.
✦ Use restraints, if necessary, but avoid sedatives.
✦ Protect the comatose patient's eyes from corneal injury by using artificial tears or eye patches.

Characteristics of malabsorption
✦ Failure of intestinal mucosa to absorb nutrients efficiently

Causes of malabsorption

Many disorders — from systemic to organ-specific diseases — may give rise to malabsorption.

DISEASES OF THE SMALL INTESTINE

Primary small-bowel disease
+ Bacterial overgrowth due to stasis in afferent loop after Billroth II gastrectomy
+ Massive bowel resection
+ Nontropical sprue (celiac disease)
+ Regional enteritis
+ Tropical sprue

Ischemic small-bowel disease
+ Chronic heart failure
+ Mesenteric atherosclerosis

Small-bowel infections and infestations
+ Acute enteritis
+ Giardiasis

Systemic disease involving small bowel
+ Amyloidosis
+ Lymphoma
+ Sarcoidosis
+ Scleroderma
+ Whipple's disease

DRUG-INDUCED MALABSORPTION
+ Calcium carbonate
+ Neomycin

HEPATOBILIARY DISEASE
+ Biliary fistula
+ Biliary tract obstruction
+ Cirrhosis and hepatitis

HEREDITARY DISORDER
+ Primary lactase deficiency

PANCREATIC DISORDERS
+ Chronic pancreatitis
+ Cystic fibrosis
+ Pancreatic cancer
+ Pancreatic resection
+ Zollinger-Ellison syndrome

PREVIOUS GASTRIC SURGERY
+ Billroth II gastrectomy
+ Pyloroplasty
+ Total gastrectomy
+ Vagotomy

Causes of malabsorption
+ Diseases of the small intestine
+ Drug-induced malabsorption
+ Hepatobiliary disease
+ Hereditary disorder
+ Pancreatic disorders
+ Previous gastric surgery

How it happens
+ Mechanism depends on cause
+ Celiac disease
+ Lactase deficiency
+ Gastrectomy
+ Zollinger-Ellison syndrome
+ Bacterial overgrowth in duodenal stump

PATHOPHYSIOLOGY

The small intestine's inability to absorb nutrients efficiently may result from various disease processes. The mechanism of malabsorption depends on the cause. Some common causes of malabsorption syndrome include celiac disease, lactase deficiency, gastrectomy, Zollinger-Ellison syndrome, and bacterial overgrowth in the duodenal stump.

In celiac sprue, dietary gluten — a product of wheat, barley, rye, and oats — is toxic to the patient, causing injury to the mucosal villi. The mucosa appear flat and have lost absorptive surface. Symptoms generally disappear when gluten is removed from the diet.

Lactase deficiency is a disaccharide deficiency syndrome. Lactase is an intestinal enzyme that splits nonabsorbable lactose (a disaccharide) into the absorbable monosaccharides glucose and galactose. Production may be deficient, or another intestinal disease may inhibit the enzyme.

Malabsorption may occur after gastrectomy. Poor mixing of chyme with gastric secretions causes postsurgical malabsorption.

In Zollinger-Ellison syndrome, increased acidity in the duodenum inhibits release of cholecystokinin, which stimulates pancreatic enzyme secretion. Pancreatic enzyme deficiency leads to decreased breakdown of nutrients and malabsorption.

Bacterial overgrowth in the duodenal stump (loop created in the Billroth II procedure) causes malabsorption of vitamin B_{12}.

SIGNS AND SYMPTOMS

In malabsorption, weight loss and generalized malnutrition occur as a result of impaired absorption of carbohydrate, fat, and protein. Diarrhea occurs from a decreased absorption of fluids, electrolytes, bile acids, and fatty acids in the colon, and causes an electrolyte depletion, which in turn causes weakness and fatigue. Steatorrhea results from excess fat in the stool; flatulence and abdominal distention are secondary to fermentation of undigested lactose. In addition, delayed absorption of water causes the patient to experience nocturia.

Signs and symptoms may occur as a result of impaired absorption; for example, impaired absorption of amino acids results in protein depletion and hypoproteinemia and causes edema. Impaired absorption of iron, folic acid, and vitamin B_{12} causes anemia.

Other signs and symptoms result from vitamin deficiencies. A deficiency of iron, folic acid, vitamin B_{12}, and other vitamins cause glossitis and cheilosis. A deficiency of vitamin B_{12} and thiamine results in peripheral neuropathy. Osteoporosis occurs due to protein depletion.

Various other signs and symptoms occur because of malabsorption. Bone pain, skeletal deformities, and fractures result from calcium malabsorption that leads to hypocalcemia. Vitamin D malabsorption causes impaired calcium absorption. Additionally, tetany and paresthesia are due to calcium malabsorption (causing hypocalcemia) and magnesium malabsorption (leading to hypomagnesemia and hypokalemia).

COMPLICATIONS

Complications of malabsorption include fractures, anemia, bleeding disorders, tetany, and malnutrition.

DIAGNOSIS

These tests can help diagnose malabsorption:
+ Stool specimen for fat reveals excretion of greater than 6 g of fat per day.
+ D-xylose absorption test shows less than 20% of 25 g of D-xylose in the urine after 5 hours (reflects disorders of proximal bowel).
+ Schilling test reveals deficiency of vitamin B_{12} absorption.
+ Culture of duodenal and jejunal contents confirms bacterial overgrowth in the proximal bowel.
+ GI barium studies show characteristic features of the small intestine.
+ Small-intestine biopsy reveals the atrophy of mucosal villi.

TREATMENT

Treatment involves identifying the cause and correcting it appropriately. Dietary treatment includes a gluten-free diet to stop the progression of celiac disease and malabsorption, a lactose-free diet to treat lactase deficiency, and supplementation to replace nutrient deficiencies. Vitamin B_{12} injections may be necessary to treat vitamin B_{12} deficiency.

NURSING CONSIDERATIONS

+ Explain the necessity of a gluten-free diet to the patient (and to his parents, if the patient is a child). Advise him on the elimination of wheat, barley, rye, and oats, and foods made from them, such as breads and baked goods; suggest substitution

Key signs and symptoms
+ Weight loss, generalized malnutrition
+ Diarrhea
+ Steatorrhea
+ Edema
+ Anemia
+ Glossitis, cheilosis
+ Osteoporosis
+ Bone pain, skeletal deformities, fractures

Complications
+ Fractures
+ Anemia
+ Bleeding disorders
+ Tetany
+ Malnutrition

Diagnosis
+ Excretion > 6 g fat/day
+ < 20% of 25 g D-xylose in urine after 5 hours
+ Vitamin B_{12} absorption deficiency in Shilling test
+ Bacterial overgrowth in proximal bowel
+ Small-intestine biopsy reveals atrophy of mucosal villi

Treatment
+ Identifying cause and correcting appropriately
+ Gluten-free diet
+ Lactose-free diet
+ Dietary supplementation
+ Vitamin B_{12} injections

Key nursing actions

✦ Explain the necessity of a gluten-free diet to the patient.
✦ Check serum electrolyte levels. Watch for signs of hypokalemia and low calcium levels.
✦ Assess fluid status. Watch for dehydration.

Characteristics of pancreatitis

✦ Life-threatening
✦ Inflammation of pancreas
✦ Acute and chronic forms
✦ May be due to edema, necrosis, hemorrhage
✦ Commonly associated with alcoholism, trauma, peptic ulcer in men
✦ Associated with biliary tract disease in women
✦ Prognosis good when associated with biliary tract disease; poor when associated with alcoholism

Causes

✦ Biliary tract disease
✦ Alcoholism
✦ Abnormal organ structure
✦ Metabolic or endocrine disorders
✦ Pancreatic cysts or tumors

How it happens

✦ Edematous and necrotizing forms
✦ Edematous causes fluid accumulation and swelling
✦ Necrotizing causes cell death and tissue damage
✦ Inflammation with both caused by premature enzyme activation; causes tissue damage
✦ Enzymes back up, spill into pancreas, resulting in autodigestion of pancreas

---

of corn or rice. Advise the patient to consult a dietitian for a gluten-free diet that's high in protein but low in carbohydrates and fats. Depending on individual tolerance, the diet initially consists of proteins and gradually expands to include other foods. Assess the patient's acceptance and understanding of the disease, and encourage regular reevaluation.

✦ Observe nutritional status and progress by daily calorie counts and weight checks. Evaluate the patient's tolerance to new foods. In the early stages, offer small, frequent meals to counteract anorexia.

✦ Assess fluid status: record intake, urine output, and number of stools (may exceed 10 per day). Watch for signs of dehydration, such as dry skin and mucous membranes and poor skin turgor.

✦ Check serum electrolyte levels. Watch for signs of hypokalemia (weakness, lethargy, rapid pulse, nausea, and diarrhea) and low calcium levels (impaired blood clotting, muscle twitching, and tetany).

✦ Monitor prothrombin time, hemoglobin level, and hematocrit. Protect the patient from bleeding and bruising. Administer vitamin K, iron, folic acid, and vitamin B_{12}, as ordered. Early in treatment, give hematinic supplements I.M. using a separate syringe for each. Use the Z-track method to give iron I.M. If the patient can tolerate oral iron, give it between meals, when absorption is best. Dilute oral iron preparations, and give them through a straw to prevent staining teeth. Assess the patient's need for stool softeners because iron may cause constipation.

✦ Protect patients with osteomalacia from injury by keeping the side rails up and assisting with ambulation, as necessary.

✦ Give steroids as ordered, and assess regularly for cushingoid adverse effects, such as hirsutism and muscle weakness.

▼ *LIFE-THREATENING DISORDER*

PANCREATITIS

Pancreatitis, inflammation of the pancreas, occurs in acute and chronic forms and may be due to edema, necrosis, or hemorrhage. In men, this disease is commonly associated with alcoholism, trauma, or peptic ulcer; in women, it's associated with biliary tract disease. The prognosis in pancreatitis associated with biliary tract disease is good; however, the prognosis is poor when it's associated with alcoholism. Mortality is as high as 60% when pancreatitis is related to necrosis and hemorrhage.

CAUSES

Causes of pancreatitis include biliary tract disease, alcoholism, abnormal organ structure, metabolic or endocrine disorders (such as high cholesterol levels or overactive thyroid), pancreatic cysts or tumors, penetrating peptic ulcers, blunt or surgical trauma, drugs (such as glucocorticoids, sulfonamides, thiazides, hormonal contraceptives, and nonsteroidal anti-inflammatory drugs), kidney failure or transplantation, and endoscopic examination of the bile ducts and pancreas.

PATHOPHYSIOLOGY

Acute pancreatitis occurs in two forms: edematous (interstitial) and necrotizing (hemorrhagic). Edematous pancreatitis causes fluid accumulation and swelling. Necrotizing pancreatitis causes cell death and tissue damage. The inflammation that occurs with both types is caused by premature activation of enzymes, which causes tissue damage. Enzymes back up and spill out into the pancreatic tissue resulting in autodigestion of the pancreas.

Normally, the acini in the pancreas secrete enzymes in an inactive form. Two theories explain why enzymes become prematurely activated.

In one view, a toxic agent such as alcohol alters the way the pancreas secretes enzymes. Alcohol probably increases pancreatic secretion, alters the metabolism of the acinar cells, and encourages duct obstruction by causing pancreatic secretory proteins to precipitate.

Another theory suggests that a reflux of duodenal contents containing activated enzymes enters the pancreatic duct, activating other enzymes and setting up a cycle of more pancreatic damage.

In chronic pancreatitis, persistent inflammation produces irreversible changes in the structure and function of the pancreas. It sometimes follows an episode of acute pancreatitis. Protein precipitates block the pancreatic duct and eventually harden or calcify. Structural changes lead to fibrosis and atrophy of the glands. Growths called pseudocysts contain pancreatic enzymes and tissue debris. An abscess results if pseudocysts become infected.

If pancreatitis damages the islets of Langerhans, diabetes mellitus may result. Sudden severe pancreatitis causes massive hemorrhage and total destruction of the pancreas, manifested as diabetic acidosis, shock, or coma.

SIGNS AND SYMPTOMS

A patient with pancreatitis may complain of midepigastric abdominal pain, which can radiate to the back. This pain is caused by the escape of inflammatory exudates and enzymes into the back of the peritoneum, edema and distention of the pancreatic capsule, and obstruction of the biliary tract.

The patient may have mottled skin from hemorrhagic necrosis of the pancreas. He may report tachycardia that's secondary to dehydration and possible hypovolemia. A low-grade fever occurs as a result of the inflammatory response and cold, sweaty extremities are secondary to cardiovascular collapse. Restlessness is related to pain associated with acute pancreatitis and extreme malaise, in chronic pancreatitis, is related to malabsorption or diabetes.

In a severe attack, persistent vomiting from hypermotility or a paralytic ileus occurs secondary to pancreatitis or peritonitis. Abdominal distention is due to hypermotility also, as is the accumulation of fluids in the abdominal cavity. In addition, diminished bowel activity suggests altered motility secondary to peritonitis. Heart failure causes crackles at the lung bases; circulating pancreatic enzymes contribute to the development of a left pleural effusion.

COMPLICATIONS

Complications of pancreatitis include massive hemorrhage, shock, pseudocysts, biliary and duodenal obstruction, portal and splenic vein thrombosis, diabetes mellitus, and respiratory failure.

DIAGNOSIS

Certain tests can help diagnose pancreatitis. Elevated serum amylase and lipase levels confirm diagnosis. Furthermore, an endoscopic retrograde cholangiopancreatography identifies ductal system abnormalities, such as calcification or strictures and helps differentiate pancreatitis from other disorders such as pancreatic cancer. Blood and urine glucose tests reveal transient glucose in urine and hyperglycemia.

How it happens
(continued)
- Chronic pancreatitis: persistent inflammation, irreversible changes in pancreas
- Sometimes follows acute pancreatitis
- Protein precipitates block pancreatic duct, eventually harden or calcify
- Structural changes lead to fibrosis, atrophy of glands
- Pseudocysts contain pancreatic enzymes and tissue debris
- Abscess results if pseudocysts become infected
- Sudden severe pancreatitis causes massive hemorrhage, total destruction of the pancreas

Key signs and symptoms
- Midepigastric abdominal pain
- Mottled skin
- Tachycardia
- Low-grade fever
- Restlessness
- Persistent vomiting

Complications
- Massive hemorrhage
- Shock
- Pseudocysts
- Biliary and duodenal obstruction
- Portal and splenic vein thrombosis

Diagnosis
- Elevated serum amylase and lipase levels
- Ductal system abnormalities
- Transient glucose in urine and hyperglycemia
- Transiently elevated serum glucose levels
- Pleural effusions

In chronic pancreatitis, serum glucose levels may be transiently elevated. In addition, WBC count is elevated, as are serum bilirubin levels in both acute and chronic pancreatitis. Conversely, blood calcium levels may be decreased. Another test finding for chronic pancreatitis is elevated lipid and trypsin levels in stool analysis.

An enlarged pancreas with cysts and pseudocysts will be revealed in a computed tomography scan and ultrasonography. Abdominal and chest X-rays detect pleural effusions and differentiate pancreatitis from diseases that cause similar symptoms; they may also detect pancreatic calculi.

TREATMENT

Treatment of shock in pancreatitis includes I.V. replacement of fluids, protein, and electrolytes. Fluid volume replacement also helps correct metabolic acidosis. Blood loss from hemorrhage is replaced with blood transfusions.

Maintaining the patient on nothing-by-mouth status rests the pancreas and reduces pancreatic enzyme secretions. Maintaining an NG tube to suction decreases stomach distention and suppresses pancreatic secretions.

Pharmacologic treatment of pancreatitis includes antiemetics to alleviate nausea and vomiting and meperidine to relieve abdominal pain. Antacids neutralize gastric secretions and histamine-2 receptor antagonists decrease hydrochloric acid production. Antibiotics fight bacterial infections, and anticholinergics reduce vagal stimulation, decrease GI motility, and inhibit pancreatic enzyme secretion. Insulin corrects hyperglycemia.

Surgical treatment involves drainage of pancreatic abscesses or pseudocysts, surgery to reestablish drainage of the pancreas or a laparotomy (if a biliary tract obstruction causes acute pancreatitis) to remove the obstruction.

NURSING CONSIDERATIONS

Acute pancreatitis is a life-threatening emergency, requiring meticulous supportive care and continuous monitoring of vital systems.

◆ Monitor vital signs and pulmonary artery pressure closely. If the patient has a central venous pressure line instead of a pulmonary artery catheter, monitor it closely for volume expansion (it shouldn't rise above 10 cm H_2O). Give plasma or albumin, if ordered, to maintain blood pressure. Record fluid intake and output, check urine output hourly, and monitor electrolyte levels. Assess for crackles, rhonchi, or decreased breath sounds.

◆ For bowel decompression, maintain constant NG suctioning, and give nothing by mouth. Perform good mouth and nose care.

◆ Watch for signs and symptoms of calcium deficiency, such as tetany, cramps, carpopedal spasm, and seizures. If you suspect hypocalcemia, keep airway and suction apparatus handy and pad side rails.

◆ Administer analgesics as needed to relieve the patient's pain and anxiety. Remember that anticholinergics reduce salivary and sweat gland secretions. Warn the patient that he may experience dry mouth and facial flushing. *Caution:* Angle-closure glaucoma contraindicates the use of atropine or its derivatives.

◆ Watch for adverse reactions to antibiotics: nephrotoxicity with aminoglycosides, pseudomembranous enterocolitis with clindamycin, and blood dyscrasias with chloramphenicol.

◆ Don't confuse thirst resulting from hyperglycemia (indicated by serum glucose levels up to 350 mg/dl and sugar and acetone in urine) with dry mouth due to NG intubation and anticholinergics.

Treatment
◆ I.V. replacement of fluids, protein, electrolytes
◆ Fluid volume replacement
◆ Nothing-by-mouth status
◆ Maintaining NG tube
◆ Antiemetics
◆ Antacids
◆ Antibiotics
◆ Anticholinergics
◆ Insulin
◆ Surgical treatment

Key nursing actions
◆ Monitor vital signs and pulmonary artery pressure closely.
◆ For bowel decompression, maintain constant NG suctioning, and give nothing by mouth. Perform good mouth and nose care.
◆ Watch for signs and symptoms of calcium deficiency, such as tetany, cramps, carpopedal spasm, and seizures.
◆ Administer analgesics as needed to relieve the patient's pain and anxiety.
◆ Watch for adverse reactions to antibiotics.
◆ Don't confuse thirst resulting from hyperglycemia with dry mouth due to NG intubation and anticholinergics.
◆ Watch for complications due to TPN.

✦ Watch for complications due to total parenteral nutrition (TPN), such as sepsis, hypokalemia, overhydration, and metabolic acidosis. Watch for fever, cardiac irregularities, changes in arterial blood gas measurements, and deep respirations. Use strict sterile technique when caring for the catheter insertion site.

PEPTIC ULCERS

Peptic ulcers, circumscribed lesions in the mucosal membrane extending below the epithelium, can develop in the lower esophagus, stomach, pylorus, duodenum, or jejunum. Although erosions are commonly referred to as *ulcers*, erosions are breaks in the mucosal membranes that don't extend below the epithelium. Ulcers may be acute or chronic in nature. Chronic ulcers are identified by scar tissue at their base. (See *Peptic ulcers,* page 390.)

About 80% of peptic ulcers are duodenal ulcers, which affect the proximal part of the small intestine and occur most commonly in men between ages 20 and 50. Duodenal ulcers usually follow a chronic course with remissions and exacerbations; 5% to 10% of patients develop complications that necessitate surgery.

Gastric ulcers are most common in middle-age and elderly men, especially in chronic users of nonsteroidal anti-inflammatory drugs (NSAIDs), alcohol, or tobacco.

CAUSES

Causes of peptic ulcer include *Helicobacter pylori* infection, use of NSAIDs, and pathologic hypersecretory disorders.

PATHOPHYSIOLOGY

Although the stomach contains acidic secretions that can digest substances, intrinsic defenses protect the gastric mucosal membrane from injury. A thick, tenacious layer of gastric mucus protects the stomach from autodigestion, mechanical trauma, and chemical trauma. Prostaglandins provide another line of defense. Gastric ulcers may be a result of destruction of the mucosal barrier.

The duodenum is protected from ulceration by the function of Brunner's glands. These glands produce a viscid, mucoid, alkaline secretion that neutralizes the acid chyme. Duodenal ulcers appear to result from excessive acid production.

H. pylori releases a toxin that destroys the gastric and duodenal mucosa, reducing the epithelium's resistance to acid digestion and causing gastritis and ulcer disease.

Salicylates and other NSAIDs inhibit the secretion of prostaglandins (substances that block ulceration). Certain illnesses, such as pancreatitis, hepatic disease, Crohn's disease, preexisting gastritis, and Zollinger-Ellison syndrome also contribute to ulceration.

Besides peptic ulcer's main causes, several predisposing factors are acknowledged. They include blood type (gastric ulcers and type A; duodenal ulcers and type O) and other genetic factors. Exposure to irritants, such as alcohol, coffee, and tobacco, may contribute by accelerating gastric acid emptying and promoting mucosal breakdown. Emotional stress also contributes to ulcer formation because of the increased stimulation of acid and pepsin secretion and decreased mucosal defense. Physical trauma and normal aging are additional predisposing conditions.

Characteristics of peptic ulcers
✦ Circumscribed lesions in mucosal membrane extending below epithelium
✦ Can develop in lower esophagus, stomach, pylorus, duodenum, jejunum
✦ Erosions commonly called *ulcers* but don't extend below epithelium
✦ May be acute or chronic
✦ Chronic ulcers identified by scar tissue at base
✦ 80% of peptic ulcers: duodenal
✦ Most common in men between ages 20 and 50
✦ Usually follow chronic course with remissions, exacerbations
✦ 5% to 10% of patients need surgery
✦ Gastric ulcers most common in middle-age and elderly men, users of NSAIDs, alcohol, tobacco

Causes
✦ *H. pylori* infection
✦ Use of NSAIDs
✦ Pathologic hypersecretory disorders

How it happens
✦ May result from destruction of mucosal barrier
✦ Duodenal ulcers appear to result from excessive acid production
✦ *H. pylori* releases toxin that destroys gastric and duodenal mucosa
✦ Epithelium's resistance to acid digestion reduced
✦ Results in gastritis, ulcer disease
✦ Salicylates and NSAIDs inhibit secretion of prostaglandins

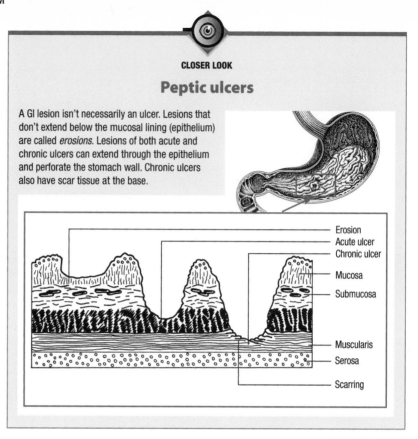

CLOSER LOOK

Peptic ulcers

A GI lesion isn't necessarily an ulcer. Lesions that don't extend below the mucosal lining (epithelium) are called *erosions*. Lesions of both acute and chronic ulcers can extend through the epithelium and perforate the stomach wall. Chronic ulcers also have scar tissue at the base.

- Erosion
- Acute ulcer
- Chronic ulcer
- Mucosa
- Submucosa
- Muscularis
- Serosa
- Scarring

Key signs and symptoms
- Vary by type of ulcer
- Gastric ulcer: pain, worsens with eating; nausea and anorexia
- Duodenal ulcer: gnawing, dull, aching, "hungerlike" epigastric pain; relieved by food or antacids; usually recurs 2 to 4 hours later

Complications
- Hemorrhage
- Shock
- Gastric perforation
- Gastric outlet obstruction

Diagnosis
- Barium swallow
- Upper GI and small bowel series
- Urea breath test results reflect activity of *H. pylori*

SIGNS AND SYMPTOMS

Symptoms vary by the type of ulcer. A patient with a gastric ulcer reports pain that worsens with eating due to stretching of the mucosa by food, and nausea and anorexia secondary to mucosal stretching.

A duodenal ulcer causes the patient to experience epigastric pain that's gnawing, dull, aching, or "hungerlike" due to excessive acid production and that's relieved by food or antacids. The pain usually recurs 2 to 4 hours later because the food acts as a buffer for acid.

COMPLICATIONS

Complications include hemorrhage, shock, gastric perforation, and gastric outlet obstruction.

DIAGNOSIS

Of the many diagnostic tests for peptic ulcers, the first tests that should be performed on a patient if his symptoms aren't severe are a barium swallow or upper GI and small-bowel series; these may reveal the presence of the ulcer. Esophagogastroduodenoscopy confirms the presence of an ulcer also and permits cytologic studies and biopsy to rule out *H. pylori* or cancer.

In addition, other tests may reveal abnormalities: upper GI tract X-rays reveal mucosal abnormalities; stool analysis may reveal occult blood; serologic testing may disclose clinical signs of infection such as elevated WBC count; gastric secretory studies show hyperchlorhydria; and urea breath test results reflect activity of *H. pylori*.

TREATMENT

Treatment may include the use of antimicrobial agents (bismuth subsalicylate, metronidazole, and tetracycline) to eradicate *H. pylori* infection. (See *Treating peptic ulcers*, pages 392 and 393.)

Medications may be used to aid in decreasing acid gastric contents. Misoprostol (a prostaglandin analog) may be used to inhibit gastric acid secretion and increase carbonate and mucus production, to protect the stomach lining. Antacids are prescribed to neutralize acid gastric contents by elevating the gastric pH, thus protecting the mucosa and relieving pain. In addition, anticholinergic drugs inhibit the effect of the vagal nerve on acid-secreting cells and histamine-2 (H_2) blockers reduce acid secretion. Sucralfate, a mucosal protectant forms an acid-impermeable membrane that adheres to the mucous membrane and accelerates mucus production. A proton gastric acid pump inhibitor (omeprazole) helps by decreasing gastric acid secretion.

Small infrequent meals and avoidance of eating before bedtime are dietary measures that neutralize gastric contents. To avoid stimulation of gastric acid, the patient should avoid caffeine and alcohol intake.

In instances where the patient experiences GI bleeding, an NG tube performs gastric decompression and rest, and permits iced saline lavage that may contain norepinephrine. Gastroscopy allows visualization of the bleeding site and coagulation by laser or cautery to control bleeding.

In order to repair perforation or to treat unresponsiveness to conservative treatment or suspected malignancy, surgery may be necessary.

NURSING CONSIDERATIONS

Management of peptic ulcers requires careful administration of medications, thorough patient teaching, and skillful postoperative care.
+ Administer prescribed medications.
+ Watch for adverse reactions to H_2-receptor antagonists and omeprazole (dizziness, fatigue, rash, and mild diarrhea).
+ Advise any patient who uses antacids, has a history of heart disease, or follows a sodium-restricted diet to take only those antacids that contain low amounts of sodium.
+ Warn the patient to avoid steroids and NSAIDs because they irritate the gastric mucosa. For the same reason, advise the patient to stop smoking and to avoid stressful situations, excessive intake of coffee, and any ingestion of alcoholic beverages during exacerbations of peptic ulcer disease.
+ Inform the patient about the potential adverse effects of antibiotic therapy, such as superinfection and diarrhea. Instruct him to notify the physician if these occur.
+ Describe follow-up testing that the physician will order to confirm eradication of *H. pylori* infection.
+ Tell the patient taking bismuth subsalicylate that this drug may cause constipation.

After gastric surgery
+ Keep the NG tube patent. If the tube isn't functioning, don't reposition it; you might damage the suture line or anastomosis. Notify the surgeon promptly.

(*Text continues on page 394.*)

Treatment
+ Antimicrobial agents
+ Misoprostol
+ Antacids
+ Anticholinergic drugs
+ Sucralfate
+ Proton gastric acid pump inhibitor
+ Dietary measures
+ NG tube
+ Gastroscopy
+ Surgery

Key nursing actions
+ Watch for adverse reactions to H_2-receptor antagonists and omeprazole.
+ Advise any patient who uses antacids, has a history of heart disease, or follows a sodium-restricted diet to take only those antacids that contain low amounts of sodium.
+ Warn the patient to avoid steroids and NSAIDs because they irritate the gastric mucosa.

After gastric surgery
+ Keep the NG tube patent.
+ Monitor intake and output, including NG tube drainage.
+ Replace fluids and electrolytes.
+ Monitor for possible complications.

FOCUS ON TREATMENT

Treating peptic ulcers

Peptic ulcers can result from factors that increase gastric acid production or from factors that impair mucosal barrier protection. This illustration highlights the actions of the major treatments used for peptic ulcer and where they interfere with the pathophysiologic chain of events.

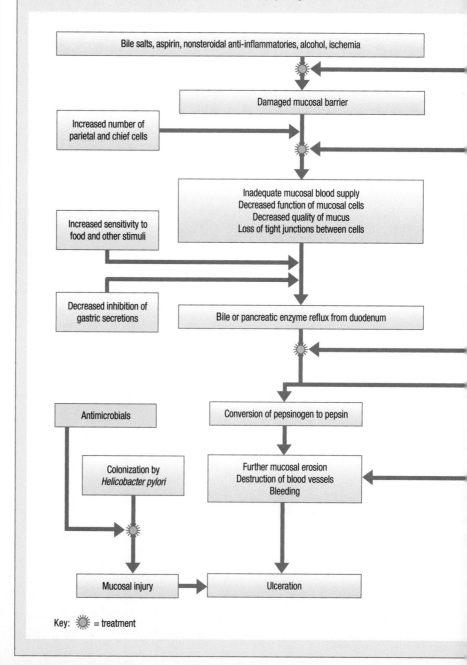

Key: ☀ = treatment

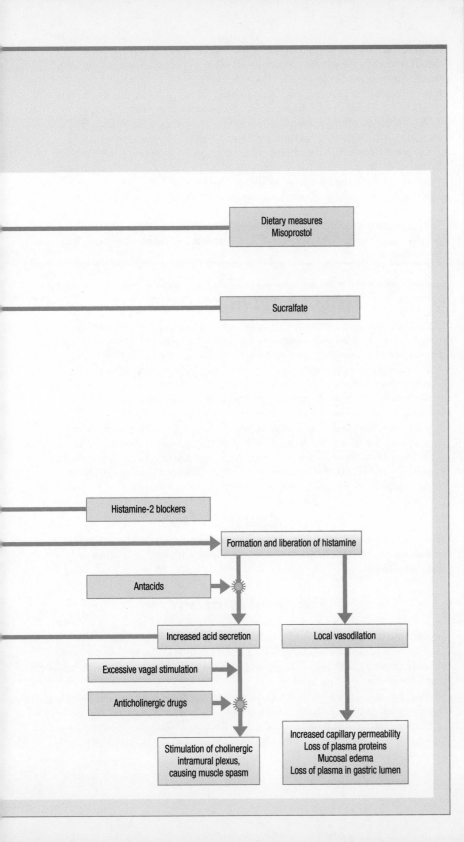

Characteristics of ulcerative colitis

- Inflammatory, usually chronic disease of mucosa of colon
- Begins in rectum and sigmoid colon, extends upward into entire colon, rarely affecting small intestine
- Produces edema, ulcerations
- Mild to fulminant
- May cause perforated colon, progressing to peritonitis, toxemia
- Occurs primarily in young adults, especially women
- Onset of symptoms peaks between ages 15 and 20 and 55 and 60

Causes

- Specific causes unknown
- May be related to abnormal immune response in GI tract
- Possibly associated with food or bacteria

How it happens

- Begins as inflammation in base of mucosal layer of large intestine
- Mucosal surface becomes dark, red, velvety
- Inflammation leads to erosions that form ulcers
- Mucosa becomes ulcerated, with hemorrhage, congestion, edema, exudative inflammation
- Abscesses in mucosa drain purulent exudate, become necrotic, ulcerate
- Scarring and thickening may appear in bowel's inner muscle layer
- Granulation tissue replaces muscle layer, colon loses haustral folds

- Monitor intake and output, including NG tube drainage. Check for bowel sounds, and allow the patient nothing by mouth until peristalsis resumes and the NG tube is removed or clamped.
- Replace fluids and electrolytes. Assess for signs of dehydration, sodium deficiency, and metabolic alkalosis, which may occur secondary to gastric suction.
- Monitor for possible complications including hemorrhage; shock; iron, folate, or vitamin B_{12} deficiency anemia from malabsorption (pernicious anemia) due to lack of intrinsic factor; and dumping syndrome (a rapid gastric emptying, causing distention of the duodenum or jejunum produced by a bolus of food). Signs and symptoms of dumping syndrome include diaphoresis, weakness, nausea, flatulence, explosive diarrhea, distention, and palpitations within 30 minutes after a meal.
- To avoid dumping syndrome, advise the patient to lie down after meals, to drink fluids between meals rather than with meals, to avoid eating large amounts of carbohydrates, and to eat four to six small, high-protein, low-carbohydrate meals during the day.

ULCERATIVE COLITIS

Ulcerative colitis is an inflammatory, usually chronic disease that affects the mucosa of the colon. It invariably begins in the rectum and sigmoid colon, and commonly extends upward into the entire colon, rarely affecting the small intestine. Ulcerative colitis produces edema (leading to mucosal friability) and ulcerations. Severity ranges from a mild, localized disorder to a fulminant disease that may cause a perforated colon, progressing to potentially fatal peritonitis and toxemia. The disease cycles between exacerbation and remission.

Ulcerative colitis occurs primarily in young adults, especially women. It's more prevalent among Ashkenazic Jews and in higher socioeconomic groups, and there seems to be a familial tendency. The prevalence is unknown; however, some studies suggest as many as 100 of 100,000 persons have the disease. Onset of symptoms seems to peak between ages 15 and 20 and between ages 55 and 60.

CAUSES

Specific causes of ulcerative colitis are unknown but may be related to abnormal immune response in the GI tract, possibly associated with food or bacteria such as *Escherichia coli*.

PATHOPHYSIOLOGY

Ulcerative colitis usually begins as inflammation in the base of the mucosal layer of the large intestine. The colon's mucosal surface becomes dark, red, and velvety. Inflammation leads to erosions that coalesce and form ulcers. The mucosa becomes diffusely ulcerated, with hemorrhage, congestion, edema, and exudative inflammation. Ulcerations are continuous.

Abscesses in the mucosa drain purulent exudate, become necrotic, and ulcerate. Sloughing causes bloody, mucus filled stools. As abscesses heal, scarring and thickening may appear in the bowel's inner muscle layer. As granulation tissue replaces the muscle layer, the colon narrows, shortens, and loses its characteristic pouches (haustral folds).

SIGNS AND SYMPTOMS

Signs and symptoms of ulcerative colitis include recurrent bloody diarrhea (as many as 10 to 20 stools per day), typically containing pus and mucus (hallmark sign) from accumulated blood and mucus in the bowel.

The accumulated blood and mucus also cause abdominal cramping and rectal urgency. Malabsorption causes weight loss, weakness, and anemia.

COMPLICATIONS

Complications may include perforation, toxic megacolon, liver disease, stricture formation, colon cancer, and anemia.

DIAGNOSIS

If the patient doesn't have active signs and symptoms a colonoscopy should be performed, which will reveal the extent of the disease, stricture areas, and pseudopolyps. A biopsy with a colonoscopy will confirm the diagnosis. Another test that can be performed when a patient is free from active symptoms is a barium enema, which will reveal the extent of the disease, detect complications, and identify cancer.

A sigmoidoscopy confirms rectal involvement; specifically, it confirms mucosal friability and flattening and thick, inflammatory exudate. A stool specimen analysis reveals blood, pus, and mucus but no disease-causing organisms.

In addition, a serologic test shows decreased serum potassium, magnesium, and albumin levels, decreased WBC count, decreased hemoglobin level, and prolonged prothrombin time. Elevated erythrocyte sedimentation rate correlates with severity of the attack.

TREATMENT

Treatment of ulcerative colitis includes corticotropin and adrenal corticosteroids to control inflammation, sulfasalazine for its anti-inflammatory and antimicrobial effects, antidiarrheals to relieve frequent, troublesome diarrhea in patients whose ulcerative colitis is otherwise under control, and iron supplements to correct anemia.

TPN and a nothing-by-mouth status is maintained for patients with severe disease to rest the intestinal tract, decrease stool volume, and restore nitrogen balance. Supplemental drinks supplement nutrition in patients with moderate symptoms, and I.V. hydration replaces fluid loss from diarrhea and prevents dehydration.

Patients with symptoms that are unbearable or unresponsive to drugs and supportive measures may require surgery to correct massive dilation of the colon. A proctocolectomy with ileostomy may be necessary to divert stools and to allow rectal anastomosis to heal. This procedure removes all the potentially malignant epithelia of the rectum and colon.

NURSING CONSIDERATIONS

Patient care includes close monitoring for changes in status.
✦ Accurately record intake and output, particularly the frequency and volume of stools. Watch for signs of dehydration and electrolyte imbalances, especially signs and symptoms of hypokalemia (muscle weakness and paresthesia) and hypernatremia (tachycardia, flushed skin, fever, and dry tongue). Monitor the patient's hemoglobin level and hematocrit, and give blood transfusions, as ordered. Provide good mouth care for the patient who's on nothing-by-mouth status.

Key signs and symptoms
✦ Recurrent bloody diarrhea containing pus and mucus
✦ Abdominal cramping
✦ Rectal urgency
✦ Weight loss
✦ Weakness
✦ Anemia

Complications
✦ Perforation
✦ Toxic megacolon
✦ Liver disease
✦ Stricture formation
✦ Colon cancer
✦ Anemia

Diagnosis
✦ Colonoscopy to reveal extent of disease, stricture areas, pseudopolyps
✦ Biopsy with colonoscopy will confirm diagnosis
✦ Barium enema
✦ Sigmoidoscopy confirms rectal involvement
✦ Blood, pus, mucus, no disease-causing organisms in stool
✦ Decreased serum potassium, magnesium, albumin levels

Treatment
✦ Corticotropin
✦ Adrenal corticosteroids
✦ Sulfasalazine
✦ Antidiarrheals
✦ Iron supplements
✦ I.V. hydration
✦ Surgery
✦ Proctocolectomy with ileostomy
✦ TPN and nothing-by-mouth status in severe disease

Key nursing actions

+ Accurately record intake and output, particularly the frequency and volume of stools. Watch for signs of dehydration and electrolyte imbalances.
+ After each bowel movement, thoroughly clean the skin around the rectum.
+ Watch for adverse effects of prolonged corticosteroid therapy.
+ Take precautionary measures if the patient is prone to bleeding.
+ Watch for signs of perforated colon, peritonitis, and toxic megacolon.

For patients requiring surgery

+ Carefully prepare the patient for surgery, and inform him about ileostomy.
+ After surgery, provide meticulous supportive care and continue teaching correct stoma care.
+ Keep the NG tube patent.
+ After a proctocolectomy and ileostomy, teach good stoma care.
+ After a pouch ileostomy, uncork the catheter every hour to allow contents to drain.

+ After each bowel movement, thoroughly clean the skin around the rectum. Provide an air mattress or sheepskin to help prevent skin breakdown.
+ Administer medications as ordered. Watch for adverse effects of prolonged corticosteroid therapy (moonface, hirsutism, edema, and gastric irritation). Be aware that corticosteroid therapy may mask infection.
+ If the patient needs TPN, change dressings as ordered, assess for inflammation at the insertion site, and check capillary blood glucose levels every 4 to 6 hours.
+ Take precautionary measures if the patient is prone to bleeding. Watch closely for signs of complications, such as a perforated colon and peritonitis (fever, severe abdominal pain, abdominal rigidity and tenderness, and cool, clammy skin), and toxic megacolon (abdominal distention and decreased bowel sounds).

For patients requiring surgery

+ Carefully prepare the patient for surgery, and inform him about ileostomy.
+ Do a bowel preparation as ordered.
+ After surgery, provide meticulous supportive care and continue teaching correct stoma care.
+ Keep the NG tube patent. After removal of the tube, provide a clear-liquid diet, and gradually advance to a low-residue diet, as tolerated.
+ After a proctocolectomy and ileostomy, teach good stoma care. Wash the skin around the stoma with soapy water and dry it thoroughly. Apply karaya gum around the stoma's base to avoid irritation, and make a watertight seal. Attach the pouch over the karaya ring. Cut an opening in the ring to fit over the stoma, and secure the pouch to the skin. Empty the pouch when it's one-third full.
+ After a pouch ileostomy, uncork the catheter every hour to allow contents to drain. After 10 to 14 days, gradually increase the length of time the catheter is left corked until it can be opened every 3 hours. Then remove the catheter and reinsert it every 3 to 4 hours for drainage. Teach the patient how to insert the catheter and how to take care of the stoma.
+ Encourage the patient to have regular physical examinations.
+ Provide the patient with information related to community resources and support groups. Encourage the patient to verbalize his feelings related to his body image.

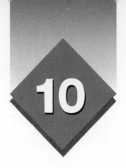

10

Musculoskeletal system

The musculoskeletal system is a complex system of bones, joints, muscles, ligaments, tendons, and other tissues that give the body form and shape. It also protects vital organs, makes movement possible, stores calcium and other minerals in the bony matrix for mobilization if deficiency occurs, and provides sites for hematopoiesis (blood cell production) in the marrow.

BONES

The human skeleton contains 206 bones, which are composed of inorganic salts (primarily calcium and phosphate) embedded in a framework of collagen fibers.

BONE SHAPE AND STRUCTURE

Bones are classified by shape as long, short, flat, or irregular. Long bones are found in the extremities and include the humerus, radius, and ulna of the arm; the femur, tibia, and fibula of the leg; and the phalanges, metacarpals, and metatarsals of the hands and feet. (See *Structure of long bones,* page 398.)

Short bones include the tarsal and carpal bones of the feet and hands, respectively. Flat bones include the frontal and parietal bones of the cranium, ribs, sternum, scapulae, ilium, and pubis. Irregular bones include the bones of the spine (vertebrae, sacrum, coccyx) and certain bones of the skull (the temporal, sphenoid, ethmoid, and mandible).

Classified according to structure, bone is either cortical (compact) or cancellous (spongy or trabecular). Adult cortical bone consists of networks of interconnecting canals, or canaliculi. Each of these networks, or *haversian systems,* runs parallel to the bone's long axis and consists of a central haversian canal surrounded by layers (lamellae) of bone. Between adjacent lamellae are small openings called *lacunae,* which contain bone cells or osteocytes. The canaliculi, each containing one capillary or more, provide a route for tissue fluids transport; they connect all the lacunae.

(See *Structure of long bones,* page 398.)

Bone shape and structure
(continued)

+ Irregular bones include spine, some of skull
+ Either cortical or cancellous
+ Cortical bone—consists of networks of canaliculi
+ Each haversian system runs parallel to bone's long axis, consists of central canal surrounded by lamellae
+ Lacunae between lamellae contain bone cells
+ Canaliculi capillaries provide tissue fluid transport; connect all lacunae
+ Cancellous bone consists of trabeculae that form interior meshwork
+ Trabeculae arranged to correspond with lines of maximum stress or pressure; gives bone added strength
+ Mature bone 70% inorganic salts; salts give bone elasticity, ability to withstand compression

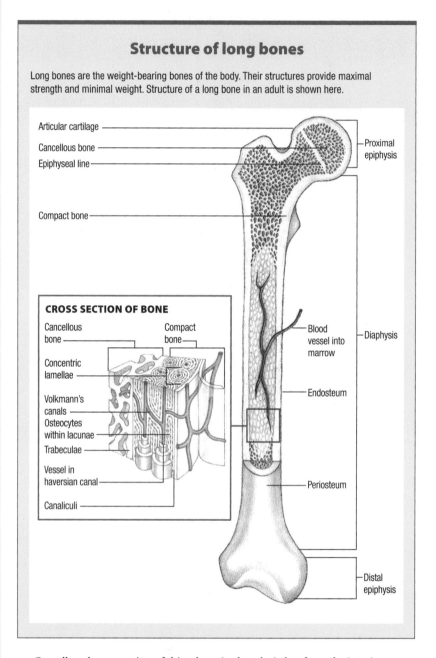

Structure of long bones

Long bones are the weight-bearing bones of the body. Their structures provide maximal strength and minimal weight. Structure of a long bone in an adult is shown here.

Cancellous bone consists of thin plates (trabeculae) that form the interior meshwork of bone. These trabeculae are arranged in various directions to correspond with the lines of maximum stress or pressure. This gives the bone added structural strength. Chemically, inorganic salts (calcium and phosphate, with small amounts of sodium, potassium carbonate, and magnesium ions) comprise 70% of the mature bone. The salts give bone its elasticity and ability to withstand compression.

BONE GROWTH

Bone formation is ongoing and is determined by hormonal stimulation, dietary factors, and the amount of stress put on the bone. It's accomplished by the continual actions of bone-forming *osteoblasts* and bone-reabsorbing cells called *osteoclasts*. Osteoblasts are present on the outer surface of and within bones. They respond to various stimuli to produce the bony matrix, or *osteoid*. As calcium salts precipitate on the organic matrix, the bone hardens. As the bone forms, a system of microscopic canals forms around the osteocytes (mature bone cells). Osteoclasts are phagocytic cells that digest old, weakened bone section by section. As they finish, osteoblasts simultaneously replace the cleared section with new, stronger bone.

Vitamin D supports bone calcification by stimulating osteoblast activity and calcium absorption from the gut to make it available for bone building. When serum calcium levels fall, the parathyroid gland releases parathyroid hormone, which then stimulates osteoclast activity and bone breakdown, freeing calcium into the blood. Parathyroid hormone also increases serum calcium by decreasing renal excretion of calcium and increasing renal excretion of phosphate ions.

Phosphates are essential to bone formation; about 85% of the body's phosphates are found in bone. The intestine absorbs many phosphates from dietary sources, but adequate levels of vitamin D are necessary for their absorption. Because calcium and phosphates interact in a reciprocal relationship, renal excretion of phosphates increases or decreases in inverse proportion to serum calcium levels. Alkaline phosphatase (ALP) influences bone calcification and lipid and metabolite transport. Osteoblasts contain an abundance of ALP. A rise in serum ALP levels can identify skeletal diseases, primarily those characterized by marked osteoblastic activity such as bone metastasis or Paget's disease. It can also identify biliary obstruction or hyperparathyroidism, or excessive ingestion of vitamin D.

In children and young adults, bone growth occurs in the epiphyseal plate, a layer of cartilage between the diaphysis and epiphysis of long bones.

Osteoblasts deposit new bone in the area just beneath the epiphysis, making the bone longer; osteoclasts model the new bone's shape by reabsorbing previously deposited bone. These remodeling activities promote longitudinal bone growth, which continues until the epiphyseal growth plates, located at both ends, close during adolescence. In adults, bone growth is complete, and this cartilage is replaced by bone, becoming the epiphyseal line.

JOINTS

The tendons, ligaments, cartilage, and other tissues that connect two bones constitute a joint. Depending on their structures, joints either predominantly permit motion or provide stability. Joints, like bones, are classified according to structure and function.

CLASSIFICATION OF JOINTS

There are three structures of joints: fibrous, cartilaginous, and synovial. Fibrous joints, or *synarthroses*, have only minute motion and provide stability when tight union is necessary as in the sutures that join the cranial bones. Cartilaginous joints, or *amphiarthroses*, allow limited motion, as between vertebrae. Synovial joints, or *diarthroses*, are the most common and permit the greatest degree of movement. These joints include the elbows and knees. (See *Structure of a synovial joint*, page 400.)

(See *Structure of a synovial joint*, page 400.)

Bone growth

+ Ongoing and determined by hormonal stimulation, diet, amount of stress on bone
+ Accomplished by osteoblasts and osteoclasts
+ Osteoblasts on outer surface of and within bones
+ Respond to various stimuli to produce bony matrix
+ Calcium salts precipitate on organic matrix; bone hardens
+ System of microscopic canals forms around osteocytes
+ Osteoclasts — phagocytic cells; digest old, weakened bone
+ Osteoblasts simultaneously replace with new, stronger bone
+ Vitamin D supports bone calcification
+ Parathyroid gland releases parathyroid hormone to stimulate osteoclast
+ Phosphates essential to bone formation
+ Bone growth occurs in epiphyseal plate

Key facts about joints

+ Tendons, ligaments, cartilage, other tissues that connect two bones
+ Permit motion, provide stability
+ Classified according to structure and function

Classification of joints

Three structures

+ Fibrous: only minute motion, provide stability when tight union is necessary
+ Cartilaginous: allow limited motion
+ Synovial: most common, permit greatest degree of movement

Structure of a synovial joint

The metacarpophalangeal joint depicted here permits angular motion between the finger and the hand. A synovial joint is characterized by a synovial pouch full of fluid that lubricates the two articulating bones.

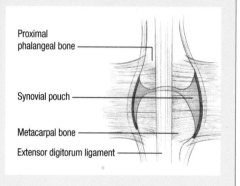

Proximal phalangeal bone

Synovial pouch

Metacarpal bone

Extensor digitorum ligament

Joint movement

Angular

+ Joints of knees, elbows, phalanges permit angular movement
+ Allow flexion, extension, and hyperextension
+ Other joints permit abduction and adduction

Circular

+ Include rotation, pronation, supination
+ Other kinds of movement: inversion, protraction, retraction

---

Key facts about muscles

+ Contractility makes movement of bones and joints possible
+ Normal skeletal muscles contract in response to neural impulses
+ Contraction usually applies force to tendons
+ Force pulls one bone toward, away from, or around a second bone
+ Permit and maintain body positions
+ Pump blood through body
+ Move food through intestines
+ Make breathing possible
+ Muscle activity produces heat
+ Muscle mass is 40% of average male weight

Synovial joints have distinguishing characteristics. The two articulating surfaces of the bones have a smooth hyaline covering (articular cartilage) that's resilient to pressure. Their opposing surfaces are congruous and glide smoothly on each other, while a fibrous (articular) capsule holds them together. Beneath the capsule, lining the joint cavity, is the synovial membrane, which secretes a clear viscous fluid called *synovial fluid*. This fluid lubricates the two opposing surfaces during motion and nourishes the articular cartilage. Surrounding a synovial joint are ligaments, muscles, and tendons, which strengthen and stabilize the joint but allow free movement.

JOINT MOVEMENT

The two types of synovial joint movement are angular and circular.

Angular movement

Joints of the knees, elbows, and phalanges permit angular movements. They allow flexion (closing of the joint angle), extension (opening of the joint angle), and hyperextension (extension of the angle beyond the usual arc).

Other joints, including the shoulders and hips, permit abduction (movement away from the body's midline) and adduction (movement toward the midline).

Circular movements

Circular movements include rotation (motion around a central axis), as in the ball and socket joints of the hips and shoulders, pronation (downward wrist or ankle motion), and supination (upward wrist motion).

Other kinds of movement are inversion (inward turning, as of foot), eversion (outward turning, as of foot), protraction (as in forward motion of the mandible), and retraction (returning protracted part into place).

MUSCLES

The most specialized feature of muscle tissue — contractility — makes the movement of bones and joints possible. Normal skeletal muscles contract in response to neural impulses. Appropriate contraction of muscle usually applies force to one or more tendons. The force pulls one bone toward, away from, or around a second bone, depending on the type of muscle contraction and the type of joint involved. Abnormal metabolism in the muscle may result in inappropriate contractility. For example, when stored glycogen or lipids can't be used because of the lack of an enzyme necessary to convert energy for contraction, the result may be cramps, fatigue, and exercise intolerance.

Muscles permit and maintain body positions, such as sitting and standing. Muscles also pump blood through the body (cardiac contraction and vessel compression), move food through the intestines (peristalsis), and make breathing possible. Skeletal muscular activity produces heat; it's an important component in temperature regulation. Deep body temperature regulators are found in the abdominal viscera, spinal cord, and great veins. These receptors detect changes in the body core temperature and stimulate the hypothalamus to institute appropriate temperature changing responses, such as shivering in response to cold. About 40% of the weight of an average man is muscle mass.

MUSCLE CLASSIFICATION

Muscles are classified according to structure, anatomic location, and function. Skeletal muscles are attached to bone and have striped (striated) appearances that reflect their cellular structures. Smooth (nonstriated) muscles that move contents through internal organs are visceral muscles. Cardiac muscles (smooth) constitute the heart wall.

When muscles are classified according to activity, they're called either *voluntary* or *involuntary*. (See chapter 8, Nervous system.) Voluntary muscles can be controlled at will and are under the influence of the somatic nervous system; these are the skeletal muscles. Involuntary muscles, controlled by the autonomic nervous system, include the cardiac and visceral muscles. Some organs contain voluntary and involuntary muscles.

MUSCLE CONTRACTION

Each skeletal muscle consists of many elongated muscle cells, called *muscle fibers*, through which run slender threads of protein, called *myofibrils*. Muscle fibers are held together in bundles by sheaths of fibrous tissues called *fascia*. Blood vessels and nerves pass into muscles through the fascia to reach the individual muscle fibers. Motor neurons synapse with the motor nerve fibers of voluntary muscles. These fibers reach the membranes of skeletal muscle cells at neuromuscular (myoneural) junctions. When an impulse reaches the myoneural junction, the junction releases the neurotransmitter, acetylcholine, which releases calcium from the sarcoplasmic reticulum, a membranous network in the muscle fiber, which, in turn, triggers muscle contraction. Muscle contraction is isometric or isotonic. Isometric contraction results in an increase in tension without change in length. Isotonic contraction occurs when the muscle shortens as weight is lifted. The energy source for this contraction is adenosine triphosphate (ATP). ATP release is also triggered by the impulse at the myoneural junction. Relaxation of a muscle is believed to take place by reversal of these mechanisms.

Muscle fatigue results when the sources of ATP in a muscle are depleted. If a muscle is deprived of oxygen, fatigue occurs rapidly. As the muscle fatigues, it switches to anaerobic metabolism of glycogen stores, in which the stored glycogen is split into glucose (glycolysis) without the use of oxygen. Lactic acid is a by-product of anaerobic glycolysis and may accumulate in the muscle and blood with intense or prolonged muscle contraction.

Muscle classification
+ Classified according to structure, anatomic location, function
+ Skeletal muscles — attached to bone
+ Visceral muscles — smooth, move content through organs
+ Cardiac muscles — smooth, constitute heart wall
+ Classified by activity: voluntary or involuntary

Muscle contraction
+ Skeletal muscle consists of muscle fibers
+ Myofibrils: protein running through muscle fibers
+ Fibers held in bundles by fascia
+ Vessels and nerves pass into muscles through fascia
+ Motor neurons synapse with motor nerve fibers of voluntary muscles
+ Fibers reach membranes of skeletal muscle cells at neuromuscular junctions
+ Impulse reaches the myoneural junction, triggers muscle contraction
+ Isometric contraction: increase in tension without change in length
+ Isotonic contraction: muscle shortens as weight is lifted
+ Relaxation of muscle believed to be reversal of these mechanisms
+ Muscle fatigue results when ATP in muscle depleted
+ Lactic acid: by-product of anaerobic glycolysis; may accumulate in muscle and blood

Tendons and ligaments
+ Tendons: fibrous cords connecting muscle to bone
+ Least movable end of muscle attachment is point of origin; most movable is point of insertion
+ Ligaments: fibrous connections that control joint movement between two bones or cartilages; support and strengthen joints

Alterations in bone
+ Most musculoskeletal disorders caused by or affect other body systems
+ Alterations of the normal functioning of bones and muscles may occur

Density
+ Resorption of bone cells exceeds formation

Growth
+ Lack of blood supply to femoral head leads to septic necrosis
+ Revascularization initiates new, malformed bone formation in femoral head or tibial tubercle

Bone strength
+ Any loss of the inorganic salts weaken bone
+ Tend to affect cancellous bone more quickly than cortical bone

Alert!
+ Bone density and structural integrity decrease after age 30 in women and after age 45 in men.
+ Age, race, and gender affect bone mass, structural integrity (ability to withstand stress), and bone loss.

TENDONS AND LIGAMENTS

Skeletal muscles are attached to bones—directly or indirectly—by fibrous cords known as *tendons*. The least movable end of the muscle attachment (generally proximal) is called the *point of origin;* the most movable end (generally distal) is called the *point of insertion.*

Ligaments are fibrous connections that control joint movement between two bones or cartilages. Their purpose is to support and strengthen joints.

PATHOPHYSIOLOGIC CHANGES

Most musculoskeletal disorders are caused by or profoundly affect other body systems; alterations of the normal functioning of bones and muscles may occur.

ALTERATIONS IN BONE
Disease may alter density, growth, or bone strength.

Density
In healthy young adults, the resorption and formation phases are tightly coupled to maintain bone mass in a steady state. Bone loss occurs when the two phases become uncoupled, and resorption exceeds formation. Estrogen not only regulates calcium uptake and release, it also regulates osteoblastic activity. Decreased estrogen levels may lead to diminished osteoblastic activity and loss of bone mass, called *osteoporosis.* In children, vitamin D deficiency prevents normal bone growth and leads to rickets.

 CLINICAL ALERT Bone density and structural integrity decrease after age 30 in women and after age 45 in men. The relatively steady loss of bone matrix can be partially offset by exercise and appropriate dietary calcium intake.

 CLINICAL ALERT Age, race, and gender affect bone mass, structural integrity (ability to withstand stress), and bone loss. For example, blacks commonly have denser bones than whites, and men typically have denser bones than women.

Growth
The osteochondroses are a group of disorders characterized by avascular necrosis of the epiphyseal growth plates in growing children and adolescents. In these disorders, a lack of blood supply to the femoral head leads to septic necrosis, with softening and resorption of bone. Revascularization then initiates new bone formation in the femoral head or tibial tubercle, which leads to a malformed femoral head.

Bone strength
Both cortical and trabecular bone contribute to skeletal strength. Any loss of the inorganic salts that constitute the chemical structure of bone will weaken bone. Cancellous bone is more sensitive to metabolic influences, so conditions that produce rapid bone loss tend to affect cancellous bone more quickly than cortical bone.

ALTERATIONS OF MUSCLE

Pathologic effects on muscle include atrophy, fatigue, weakness, myotonia, and spasticity.

Atrophy

Atrophy is a decrease in the size of a tissue or cell. In muscles, the myofibrils atrophy after prolonged inactivity from bed rest or trauma (casting), when local nerve damage makes movement impossible, or when illness removes needed nutrients from muscles. The effects of muscular deconditioning associated with lack of physical activity may be apparent in a matter of days. An individual on bed rest loses muscle strength and muscle mass from baseline levels at a rate of 3% per day. Conditioning and stretching exercises may help prevent atrophy. If reuse isn't restored within 1 year, regeneration of muscle fibers is unlikely.

 CLINICAL ALERT **Some degree of muscle atrophy is normal with aging.**

Fatigue

Pathologic muscle fatigue may be the result of impaired neural stimulation of muscle or energy metabolism or disruption of calcium flux. See chapter 5, Fluid and electrolytes, for a detailed discussion of these events.

Weakness

 CLINICAL ALERT **Muscle mass and muscle strength decrease in the elderly, usually as a result of disuse. This can be reversed with moderate, regular, weight-bearing exercise.**

Periodic paralysis is a disorder that can be triggered by exercise or a process or chemical that increases serum potassium levels. This hyperkalemic periodic paralysis may be caused by a high-carbohydrate diet, emotional stress, prolonged bed rest, or hyperthyroidism. During an attack of periodic paralysis, the muscle membrane is unresponsive to neural stimuli, and the electrical charge needed to initiate the impulse (resting membrane potential) is reduced from –90 to –45 millivolts.

Myotonia and spasticity

Myotonia is delayed relaxation after a voluntary muscle contraction—such as grip, eye closure, or muscle percussion—accompanied by prolonged depolarization of the muscle membrane. Depolarization is the reversal of the resting potential in stimulated cell membranes. It's the process by which the cell membrane "resets" its positive charge with respect to the negative charge outside the cell. Myotonia occurs in myotonic muscular dystrophy and some forms of periodic paralysis.

Stress-induced muscle tension, or spasticity, is presumably caused by increased activity in the reticular activating system and gamma loop in the muscle fiber. The reticular activating system consists of multiple diffuse pathways in the brain that control wakefulness and response to stimuli. A pathologic contracture is permanent muscle shortening caused by muscle spasticity, seen in central nervous system injury or severe muscle weakness.

 CLINICAL ALERT **Patients with musculoskeletal disorders are commonly elderly, have other concurrent medical conditions, or are victims of trauma. Generally, they face prolonged immobilization.** (See *Managing musculoskeletal pain,* page 404.)

Alterations in muscle

Atrophy
- Decrease in size of a tissue or cell
- Myofibrils atrophy after prolonged inactivity
- May be apparent in matter of days
- If reuse not restored within 1 year, regeneration of muscle fibers unlikely

Fatigue
- Result of impaired neural stimulation of muscle or energy metabolism, disruption of calcium flux

Weakness
- Periodic paralysis
- Can be triggered by exercise, process, chemical
- Muscle membrane unresponsive to neural stimuli
- Electrical charge needed to initiate the impulse reduced

Myotonia and spasticity
- Myotonia: delayed relaxation after voluntary muscle contraction; accompanied by prolonged depolarization of muscle membrane; occurs in myotonic muscular dystrophy and some forms of periodic paralysis
- Spasticity: stress-induced muscle tension

Alert!
- Some degree of muscle atrophy is normal with aging.
- Muscle mass and muscle strength decrease in the elderly, usually as a result of disuse.
- Patients with musculoskeletal disorders are commonly elderly, have other concurrent medical conditions, or are trauma victims.

Characteristics of carpal tunnel syndrome

◆ Repetitive stress injury
◆ Most common nerve entrapment syndrome
◆ Usually occurs in women between ages 30 and 60
◆ Strenuous use of hands aggravates condition

Causes

◆ Repetitive stress injury
◆ Rheumatoid arthritis
◆ Flexor tenosynovitis
◆ Nerve compression
◆ Pregnancy
◆ Multiple myeloma
◆ Diabetes mellitus

How it happens

◆ Sheaths passing through carpal tunnel cause edema, compression of median nerve
◆ Sensory, motor changes occur in median distribution of hands

Key signs and symptoms

◆ Weakness
◆ Pain, burning, numbness
◆ Tingling hands
◆ Paresthesia affects thumb, forefinger, middle finger, one-half of fourth finger
◆ Patient can't make fist
◆ Nails may be atrophic, skin dry and shiny

Managing musculoskeletal pain

A patient with a musculoskeletal disorder that causes chronic, nonmalignant pain should be assessed and treated in a stepped approach. Measures include:
◆ nonpharmacologic methods, such as heat, ice, elevation, and rest
◆ acetaminophen (Tylenol)
◆ nonsteroidal anti-inflammatory drugs such as ibuprofen (Motrin)
◆ other nonopioid analgesics, such as tramadol (Ultram) or topical capsaicin (Zostrix)
◆ tricyclic antidepressants such as amitriptyline (Elavil), which may decrease the pain signal at the neurosynaptic junctions
◆ opioid analgesics alone or with a tricyclic antidepressant.

CARPAL TUNNEL SYNDROME

Carpal tunnel syndrome, a form of repetitive stress injury, is the most common nerve entrapment syndrome. Carpal tunnel syndrome usually occurs in women between ages 30 and 60 (posing a serious occupational health problem). However, people who are employed as assembly-line workers and packers and who repeatedly use poorly designed tools are just as likely to develop this disorder. Any strenuous use of the hands—sustained grasping, twisting, or flexing—aggravates this condition.

CAUSES

Carpal tunnel syndrome is mostly idiopathic. It may result from repetitive stress injury, rheumatoid arthritis, flexor tenosynovitis (commonly associated with rheumatic disease), nerve compression, pregnancy, multiple myeloma, diabetes mellitus, acromegaly, hypothyroidism, amyloidosis, obesity, benign tumor, other conditions that increase fluid pressure in the wrist (including alterations in the endocrine or immune systems), and wrist dislocation or sprain (including Colles' fracture followed by edema).

PATHOPHYSIOLOGY

The carpal bones and the transverse carpal ligament form the carpal tunnel. (See *The carpal tunnel.*) Inflammation or fibrosis of the tendon sheaths that pass through the carpal tunnel usually causes edema and compression of the median nerve. This compression neuropathy causes sensory and motor changes in the median distribution of the hands, initially impairing sensory transmission to the thumb, index finger, second finger, and inner aspect of the third finger.

SIGNS AND SYMPTOMS

The patient with carpal tunnel syndrome usually complains of weakness, pain, burning, numbness, or tingling in one or both hands. This paresthesia affects the thumb, forefinger, middle finger, and one-half of the fourth finger. The patient can't clench his hand into a fist; the nails may be atrophic, the skin dry and shiny.

Because of vasodilation and venous stasis, symptoms are typically worse at night and in the morning. The pain may spread to the forearm and, in severe cases, as far as the shoulder. The patient can usually relieve such pain by shaking or rubbing his hands vigorously or dangling his arms at his side.

The carpal tunnel

The carpal tunnel is clearly visible in this palmar view and cross section of a right hand. Note the blood vessels and median nerve flexor tendons of the fingers passing through the tunnel on their way from the forearm to the hand.

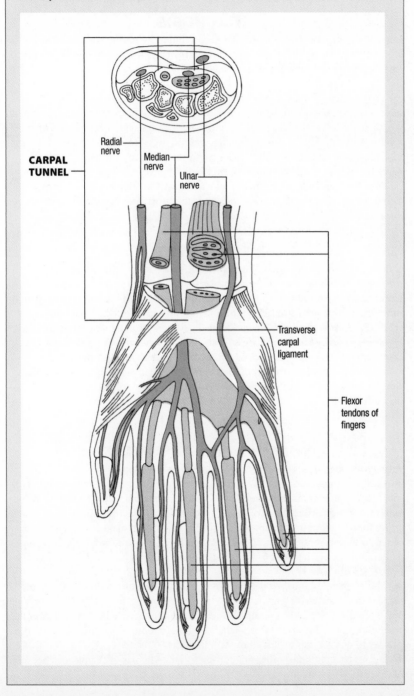

CARPAL TUNNEL

Radial nerve

Median nerve

Ulnar nerve

Transverse carpal ligament

Flexor tendons of fingers

Complications

+ Decrease in wrist function
+ Permanent nerve damage
+ Loss of movement and sensation

Diagnosis

+ Decreased sensation to light touch in affected fingers
+ Thenar muscle atrophy
+ Tinel's sign
+ Phalen's maneuver

Treatment

+ Splinting wrist in neutral extension 1 to 2 weeks
+ NSAIDs
+ Hydrocortisone and lidocaine injections
+ Resection of transverse carpal tunnel ligament
+ Neurolysis

Key nursing actions

+ Administer mild analgesics as needed. Encourage the patient to use his hands as much as possible.
+ Teach the patient how to apply a splint. Show him how to remove the splint to perform gentle ROM exercises.
+ After surgery, monitor vital signs and regularly check the color, sensation, and motion of the affected hand.
+ Advise the patient who's about to be discharged to exercise his hands occasionally in warm water.

COMPLICATIONS

Continued use of the affected wrist may increase tendon inflammation, compression, and neural ischemia, causing a decrease in wrist function. Untreated carpal tunnel syndrome can produce permanent nerve damage with loss of movement and sensation.

DIAGNOSIS

Physical examination reveals decreased sensation to light touch or pinpricks in the affected fingers. Thenar muscle atrophy occurs in about one-half of all cases of carpal tunnel syndrome but is usually a late sign.

Three tests provide rapid diagnosis of carpal tunnel syndrome. Tingling over the median nerve on light percussion is known as *Tinel's sign.* Performing *Phalen's maneuver,* holding the forearms vertically and allowing both hands to drop into complete flexion at the wrists for 1 minute, reproduces symptoms of carpal tunnel syndrome. To perform a *compression test* a blood pressure cuff is inflated above systolic pressure on the forearm for 1 to 2 minutes. Doing this provokes pain and paresthesia along the distribution of the median nerve.

Other tests include electromyography to detect a median nerve motor conduction delay of more than 5 milliseconds and laboratory tests to identify underlying disease.

TREATMENT

Conservative treatment, including resting the hands by splinting the wrist in neutral extension for 1 to 2 weeks, should be tried first. Nonsteroidal anti-inflammatory drugs usually provide symptomatic relief. Injection of the carpal tunnel with hydrocortisone and lidocaine may provide significant but temporary relief. If a definite link has been established between the patient's occupation and the development of repetitive stress injury, he may have to seek other work. Effective treatment may also require correction of an underlying disorder.

When conservative treatment fails, the only alternative is surgical decompression of the nerve by resecting the entire transverse carpal tunnel ligament or by using endoscopic surgical techniques. Neurolysis (freeing of the nerve fibers) may also be necessary.

NURSING CONSIDERATIONS

Patient care for carpal tunnel syndrome includes these steps:
+ Administer mild analgesics as needed. Encourage the patient to use his hands as much as possible. If his dominant hand has been impaired, you may have to help with eating and bathing.
+ Teach the patient how to apply a splint. Tell him not to make it too tight. Show him how to remove the splint to perform gentle range-of-motion (ROM) exercises, which should be done daily. Make sure the patient knows how to do these exercises before he's discharged.
+ After surgery, monitor vital signs and regularly check the color, sensation, and motion of the affected hand.
+ Advise the patient who's about to be discharged to exercise his hands occasionally in warm water. If the arm is in a sling, tell him to remove the sling several times per day to do exercises for his elbow and shoulder.
+ Suggest occupational counseling for the patient who has to change jobs because of repetitive stress injury.

GOUT

Gout, also called *gouty arthritis,* is a metabolic disease marked by urate deposits that cause painful arthritic joints. It's found mostly in the foot, especially the great toe, ankle, and midfoot, but may affect any joint. Gout follows an intermittent course, and patients may be totally free from symptoms for years between attacks. With treatment, the prognosis is good.

 CLINICAL ALERT Primary gout usually occurs in men older than age 30 and in postmenopausal women; secondary gout occurs in elderly people.

CAUSES

Although the exact cause of primary gout remains unknown, it may be caused by a genetic defect in purine metabolism, causing overproduction of uric acid (hyperuricemia), retention of uric acid, or both.

In secondary gout, which develops during the course of another disease (such as obesity, diabetes mellitus, hypertension, sickle cell anemia, and renal disease), the cause may be a breakdown of nucleic acid causing hyperuricemia or it may be the result of drug therapy, especially after the use of hydrochlorothiazide or pyrazinamide, which decrease urate excretion (ionic form of uric acid).

PATHOPHYSIOLOGY

When uric acid becomes supersaturated in blood and other body fluids, it crystallizes and forms a precipitate of urate salts that accumulate in connective tissue throughout the body; these deposits are called *tophi.* The presence of the crystals triggers an acute inflammatory response when neutrophils begin to ingest the crystals. Tissue damage begins when the neutrophils release their lysosomes (see chapter 12, Immune system). The lysosomes not only damage the tissues, but also perpetuate the inflammation.

In cases of gout that produce no symptoms, serum urate levels increase but don't crystallize or produce symptoms. As the disease progresses, it may cause hypertension or the formation of urate renal calculi.

The first acute attack strikes suddenly and peaks quickly. Although it generally involves only one or a few joints, this initial attack is extremely painful. Affected joints appear hot, tender, inflamed, dusky red, or cyanotic. The metatarsophalangeal joint of the great toe usually becomes inflamed first (podagra), then the instep, ankle, heel, knee, or wrist joints. Sometimes a low-grade fever is present. Mild acute attacks commonly subside quickly but tend to recur at irregular intervals. Severe attacks may persist for days or weeks.

Intercritical periods are the symptom-free intervals between gout attacks. Most patients have a second attack within 6 months to 2 years, but some attacks, common in those who are untreated, tend to be longer and more severe than initial attacks. Such attacks are also polyarticular, invariably affecting joints in the feet and legs, and sometimes accompanied by fever. A migratory attack sequentially strikes various joints and the Achilles tendon and is associated with either subdeltoid or olecranon bursitis.

Eventually, chronic polyarticular gout sets in. This final, unremitting stage of the disease is marked by persistent painful polyarthritis, with large tophi in cartilage, synovial membranes, tendons, and soft tissue. Tophi form in fingers, hands, knees, feet, ulnar sides of the forearms, helices of the ears, Achilles tendons and, rarely, in internal organs, such as the kidneys and myocardium. The skin over the tophus

Characteristics of gout
+ Also called *gouty arthritis*
+ Marked by urate deposits that cause painful arthritic joints
+ Found mostly in the foot
+ Follows intermittent course
+ Prognosis good with treatment

Alert!
+ Primary gout usually occurs in men older than age 30 and in postmenopausal women.
+ Secondary gout occurs in elderly people.

Causes
+ Exact cause unknown
+ May be genetic defect in purine metabolism
+ Secondary gout cause may be breakdown of nucleic acid or result of drug therapy

How it happens
+ Uric acid becomes supersaturated in blood, body fluids
+ Crystallizes into precipitate of urate salts, accumulates in connective tissue
+ Crystals trigger acute inflammatory response
+ Lysosomes damage tissues, perpetuate inflammation
+ First acute attack strikes suddenly, peaks quickly
+ Symptom-free intervals between gout attacks
+ Second attack within 6 months to 2 years
+ Chronic polyarticular gout sets in, marked by persistent painful polyarthritis
+ Skin over tophus may ulcerate and release white exudate

Key signs and symptoms

+ Joint pain
+ Tophi in great toe, ankle, pinna of ear
+ Elevated skin temperature
+ Red, swollen joints

Complications

+ Erosions
+ Deformity
+ Disability
+ Hypertension

Diagnosis

+ Needlelike monosodium urate crystals in synovial fluid
+ Tissue sections of tophaceous deposits
+ Hyperuricemia
+ Elevated 24-hour urine uric acid

Treatment

Acute
+ Immobilization and protection of joints
+ Local application of heat or cold
+ Fluid intake up to 3 qt/day
+ Concomitant colchicine
+ NSAIDs

Chronic
+ Maintenance allopurinol
+ Colchicine
+ Uricosuric agents
+ Dietary restrictions

Alert!

+ Older patients are at risk for GI bleeding associated with the use of NSAIDs.

---

may ulcerate and release a chalky, white exudate that's composed primarily of uric acid crystals.

SIGNS AND SYMPTOMS

Joint pain occurs due to uric acid deposits and inflammation, whereas tophi in the great toe, ankle, and pinna of the ear occur as a result of urate deposits. Elevated skin temperature and red, swollen joints are due to uric acid deposits and irritation from inflammation.

COMPLICATIONS

Gout may cause eventual erosions, deformity, and disability due to chronic inflammation and tophi that cause secondary joint degeneration. Gout may lead to hypertension and albuminuria in some patients. Other patients may experience kidney involvement, with tubular damage from aggregates of urate crystals. The patient will eventually experience progressively poorer excretion of uric acid and chronic renal dysfunction.

DIAGNOSIS

These are test results that help diagnose gout.
+ Needlelike monosodium urate crystals in synovial fluid (shown by needle aspiration) or tissue sections of tophaceous deposits
+ Hyperuricemia (uric acid greater than 420 μmol/mmol of creatinine)
+ Elevated 24-hour urine uric acid (usually higher in secondary than in primary gout)
+ X-rays initially normal; in chronic gout, damage of articular cartilage and subchondral bone. Outward displacement of the overhanging margin from the bone contour characterizes gout.

TREATMENT

The goals of treatment are to end the acute attack as quickly as possible, to prevent recurrent attacks, and to prevent or reverse complications.

Acute gout is treated with immobilization and protection of the inflamed, painful joints and local application of heat or cold. A fluid intake of up to 3 qt (3 L)/day (if not contraindicated by other conditions) will prevent renal calculus formation. In acute inflammation, concomitant treatment with colchicine (oral or I.V.) every hour for 8 hours will inhibit phagocytosis of uric acid crystals by neutrophils, until the pain subsides or nausea, vomiting, cramping, or diarrhea develops. Nonsteroidal anti-inflammatory drugs (NSAIDs) are prescribed for pain and inflammation.

 CLINICAL ALERT Older patients are at risk for GI bleeding associated with the use of NSAIDs. Encourage the patient to take these drugs with meals, and monitor the patient's stools for occult blood.

Chronic gout treatment aims to decrease serum uric acid levels. A maintenance dosage of allopurinol (Zyloprim) suppresses uric acid formation or controls uric acid levels. This prevents further attacks but must be used cautiously in patients with renal failure. Colchicine prevents recurrent acute attacks until uric acid returns to its normal level, yet doesn't affect the uric acid level. Uricosuric agents (probenecid [Benemid] and sulfinpyrazone [Anturane]) promote uric acid excretion and inhibit uric acid accumulation. These agents are of limited value in patients with renal impairment. Alcohol and purine-rich foods (shellfish, liver, sardines, anchovies, and kidneys) increase urate levels. The necessary dietary restrictions must be made.

NURSING CONSIDERATIONS

Patient care for gout includes these steps:
✦ Encourage bed rest, but use a bed cradle to keep bedcovers off extremely sensitive, inflamed joints.
✦ Administer pain medication as needed, especially during acute attacks. Apply hot or cold packs to inflamed joints according to what the patient finds effective. Administer anti-inflammatory medication and other drugs as ordered. Watch for adverse effects. Be alert for GI disturbances with colchicine.
✦ Urge the patient to drink plenty of fluids (up to 2 qt [2 L] per day) to prevent formation of renal calculi. When encouraging fluids, record intake and output accurately. Be sure to monitor serum uric acid levels regularly. Alkalinize urine with sodium bicarbonate or other agent if ordered.
✦ Watch for acute gout attacks 24 to 96 hours after surgery. Even minor surgery can precipitate an attack. Before and after surgery, administer colchicine, as ordered, to help prevent attacks of gout.
✦ Make sure the patient understands the importance of checking serum uric acid levels periodically. Tell him to avoid high-purine foods, such as anchovies, liver, sardines, kidneys, sweetbreads, lentils, and alcoholic beverages—especially beer and wine—which raise the urate level. Explain the principles of a gradual weight reduction diet to obese patients. Such a diet features foods containing moderate amounts of protein and very little fat.
✦ Advise the patient receiving allopurinol, probenecid, and other drugs to immediately report any adverse effects, such as drowsiness, dizziness, nausea, vomiting, urinary frequency, or dermatitis. Warn the patient taking probenecid or sulfinpyrazone to avoid aspirin or any other salicylate. Their combined effect causes urate retention.
✦ Inform the patient that long-term colchicine therapy is essential during the first 3 to 6 months of treatment with uricosuric drugs or allopurinol.

HERNIATED DISK

Herniated disk, also called *ruptured* or *slipped disk* and *herniated nucleus pulposus,* occurs when all or part of the nucleus pulposus—the soft, gelatinous, central portion of an intervertebral disk—is forced through the disk's weakened or torn outer ring (anulus fibrosus).

Herniated disk usually occurs in adults (mostly men) under age 45. About 90% of herniated disks are lumbar or lumbosacral, 8% are cervical, and 1% to 2% are thoracic. Patients with a congenitally small lumbar spinal canal or with osteophyte formation along the vertebrae may be more susceptible to nerve root compression and more likely to have neurologic symptoms.

CAUSES

Causes of herniated disk may include severe trauma or strain and intervertebral joint degeneration.

Key nursing actions
✦ Encourage bed rest.
✦ Administer pain medication and apply hot and cold packs as needed, especially during acute attacks.
✦ Urge the patient to drink plenty of fluids.
✦ Before and after surgery, administer colchicine, as ordered, to help prevent attacks of gout.
✦ Make sure the patient understands the importance of checking serum uric acid levels periodically.
✦ Advise the patient receiving allopurinol, probenecid, and other drugs to immediately report any adverse effects.

Characteristics of herniated disk
✦ Also called *ruptured* or *slipped disk* and *herniated nucleus*
✦ All or part of nucleus pulposus forced through disk's outer ring
✦ Usually occurs in adults younger than age 45
✦ 90% lumbar or lumbosacral; 8% cervical; 1% to 2% thoracic
✦ Patients with small lumbar spinal canal or osteophyte formation along vertebrae more likely to have neurologic symptoms

Causes
✦ Severe trauma or strain
✦ Intervertebral joint degeneration

Alert!

+ In older patients whose disks have begun to degenerate, even minor trauma may cause herniation.

How it happens

+ Physical stress tears anulus fibrosus so nucleus pulposus herniates into spinal canal
+ Extruded disk may impinge on spinal nerve roots
+ Vertebrae move closer together, exert pressure on nerve roots
+ Pain, sensory, and motor loss
+ Three steps: protrusion, extrusion, sequestration

Key signs and symptoms

+ Severe low back pain radiating to buttocks, legs, feet
+ Pain may begin suddenly, subside, then recur at shorter intervals
+ Valsalva's maneuver, coughing, sneezing, or bending intensifies pain
+ Sensory and motor loss in area innervated by compressed spinal nerve root

Complications

+ Neurologic deficits
+ Bowel and bladder problems

Diagnosis

+ Obtain detailed patient history
+ Straight-leg-raising test and variants; test is positive if patient complains of sciatic pain
+ X-rays of spine

CLINICAL ALERT In older patients whose disks have begun to degenerate, even minor trauma may cause herniation.

PATHOPHYSIOLOGY

An intervertebral disk has two parts: the soft center called the *nucleus pulposus* and the tough, fibrous surrounding ring called the *anulus fibrosus.* The nucleus pulposus acts as a shock absorber, distributing the mechanical stress applied to the spine when the body moves.

Physical stress, usually a twisting motion, can tear or rupture the anulus fibrosus so that the nucleus pulposus herniates into the spinal canal. When this happens, the extruded disk may impinge on spinal nerve roots as they exit from the spinal canal or on the spinal cord itself, resulting in back pain and other signs of nerve root irritation. The vertebrae move closer together and in turn exert pressure on the nerve roots as they exit between the vertebrae. Pain and possibly sensory and motor loss follow. A herniated disk can also follow intervertebral joint degeneration; minor trauma may cause herniation.

Herniation occurs in three steps. During the first step, *protrusion,* the nucleus pulposus presses against the anulus fibrosus. Next, the nucleus pulposus bulges forcibly through the anulus fibrosus, pushing against the nerve root. This is called *extrusion.* In the last step, *sequestration,* the anulus fibrosis gives way as the disk's core bursts and presses against the nerve root. (See *How a herniated disk develops.*)

SIGNS AND SYMPTOMS

The overriding symptom of lumbar herniated disk is severe low back pain that radiates to the buttocks, legs, and feet, usually unilaterally. When herniation follows trauma, the pain may begin suddenly, subside in a few days, and then recur at shorter intervals and with progressive intensity. Sciatic pain follows, beginning as a dull pain in the buttocks. Valsalva's maneuver, coughing, sneezing, or bending intensifies the pain, which is typically accompanied by muscle spasms.

Herniated disk may also cause sensory and motor loss in the area innervated by the compressed spinal nerve root and, in later stages, weakness and atrophy of leg muscles.

COMPLICATIONS

Complications of herniated disk may include neurologic deficits (most common) and bowel and bladder problems (with lumbar herniations).

DIAGNOSIS

Obtaining a detailed patient history is vital because the events that intensify disk pain are diagnostically significant.

The straight-leg-raising test and its variants are perhaps the best tests for herniated disk. For the straight-leg-raising test, the patient lies in a supine position while the examiner places one hand on the patient's ilium to stabilize the pelvis and the other hand under the ankle, and slowly raises the patient's leg. The test is positive only if the patient complains of posterior leg (sciatic) pain, not back pain. In Lasègue's sign, the patient lies flat while the thigh and knee are flexed to a 90-degree angle. Resistance and pain as well as loss of ankle or knee-jerk reflex indicate spinal root compression.

X-rays of the spine are essential to rule out other abnormalities but may not diagnose herniated disk because marked disk prolapse can be present despite a nor-

CLOSER LOOK

How a herniated disk develops

These illustrations show how herniation of an intervertebral disk develops.

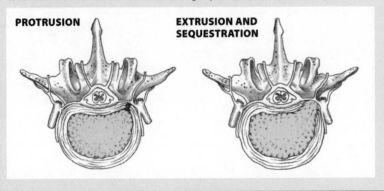

NORMAL VERTEBRA AND INTERVERTEBRAL DISK

Spinal canal

Nerve root

Nucleus pulposus

Anulus fibrosus

Physical stress from severe trauma or strain or from intervertebral joint degeneration may cause herniation. Herniation occurs in three stages: protrusion, extrusion, and sequestration.

PROTRUSION

EXTRUSION AND SEQUESTRATION

mal X-ray. A thorough check of the patient's peripheral vascular status — including posterior tibial and dorsalis pedis pulses and skin temperature of extremities — helps rule out ischemic disease, another cause of leg pain or numbness. After physical examination and X-rays, myelography, computed tomography scans, and magnetic resonance imaging (MRI) provide the most specific diagnostic information, showing spinal canal compression by herniated disk material. MRI is the method of choice to confirm the diagnosis and determine the exact level of herniation.

TREATMENT

Unless neurologic impairment progresses rapidly, treatment is initially conservative and may consist of several weeks of bed rest (possibly with pelvic traction), administration of nonsteroidal anti-inflammatory drugs, heat applications, and an exercise program. Epidural corticosteroids, short-term oral corticosteroids, nerve root blocks, or physical therapy may be used to decrease pain. Muscle relaxants, such as

Treatment
+ Several weeks bed rest (possibly with pelvic traction)
+ NSAIDs
+ Heat applications
+ Exercise
+ Corticosteroids
+ Nerve root blocks
+ Physical therapy
+ Muscle relaxants
+ Surgery
+ Injection of chymopapain

diazepam (Valium), methocarbamol (Robaxin), or cyclobenzaprine (Flexeril) may relieve associated muscle spasms.

A herniated disk that fails to respond to conservative treatment may need surgery. The most common procedure, laminectomy, involves excision of a portion of the lamina and removal of the nucleus pulposus of the protruding disk. If laminectomy doesn't alleviate pain and disability, a spinal fusion may be necessary to overcome segmental instability. Laminectomy and spinal fusion are sometimes performed concurrently to stabilize the spine. Microdiskectomy can also be used to remove fragments of nucleus pulposus.

Injection of chymopapain (Chymodiactin) into the herniated disk produces a loss of water and proteoglycans from the disk, thereby reducing both the disk's size and the pressure in the nerve root. Chymopapain is most commonly used for herniations in the lumbar region.

NURSING CONSIDERATIONS

Herniated disk requires supportive care, careful patient teaching, and strong emotional support to help the patient cope with the discomfort and frustration of chronic low back discomfort.

✦ If the patient requires myelography, question him carefully about allergies to iodides, iodine-containing substances, or seafood because such allergies may indicate sensitivity to the test's radiopaque dye. Reinforce previous explanations of the need for this test, and tell the patient to expect some discomfort. Assure him that he'll receive a sedative before the test, if needed, to keep him as calm and comfortable as possible. After the test, urge the patient to remain in bed with his head elevated (especially if metrizamide was used) and to drink plenty of fluids. Monitor intake and output. Watch for seizures and allergic reaction.

✦ During conservative treatment, watch for any deterioration in the patient's neurologic status (especially during the first 24 hours after admission), which may indicate an urgent need for surgery. Use antiembolism stockings as prescribed, and encourage the patient to move his legs as allowed. Provide high-topped sneakers to prevent footdrop. Work closely with the physical therapy department to ensure a consistent regimen of leg- and back-strengthening exercises. Give plenty of fluids to prevent renal stasis, and remind the patient to deep-breathe, and use blow bottles or an incentive spirometer to preclude pulmonary complications. Provide good skin care. Assess for bowel function. Use a fracture bedpan for the patient on complete bed rest.

✦ After laminectomy, microdiskectomy, or spinal fusion, enforce bed rest as ordered. If a blood drainage system (closed drainage system or Jackson Pratt drain) is in use, check the tubing frequently for kinks and a secure vacuum. Empty the closed drainage system at the end of each shift, and record the amount and color of drainage. Report colorless moisture on dressings (possible cerebrospinal fluid leakage) or excessive drainage immediately. Observe neurovascular status of legs (color, motion, temperature, and sensation).

✦ Monitor vital signs and check for bowel sounds and abdominal distention. Use logrolling technique to turn the patient. Administer analgesics, as ordered, especially 30 minutes before initial attempts at sitting or walking. Give the patient assistance during his first attempt to walk. Provide a straight-backed chair for limited sitting.

✦ Teach the patient who has undergone spinal fusion how to wear a brace. Assist with straight-leg-raising and toe-pointing exercises as ordered. Before discharge, teach proper body mechanics: bending at the knees and hips (never at the waist), standing straight, and carrying objects close to the body. Advise the patient to lie

Key nursing actions

✦ If the patient requires myelography, question him carefully about allergies to iodides, iodine-containing substances, or seafood.

✦ During conservative treatment, watch for any deterioration in the patient's neurologic status.

✦ After laminectomy, microdiskectomy, or spinal fusion, enforce bed rest as ordered.

✦ Monitor vital signs and check for bowel sounds and abdominal distention. Use logrolling technique to turn the patient.

✦ Report colorless moisure on dressings (possible cerebrospinal fluid leakage) or excessive drainage immediately.

✦ Observe neurovascular status of legs.

✦ Teach the patient who has undergone spinal fusion how to wear a brace.

✦ If the patient requires chemonucleolysis, make sure he isn't allergic to meat tenderizers.

✦ Provide emotional support.

down when tired and to sleep on his side (never on his abdomen) on an extra-firm mattress or a bed board. Urge maintenance of proper weight to prevent lordosis caused by obesity.

✦ If the patient requires chemonucleolysis, make sure he isn't allergic to meat tenderizers (chymopapain is a similar substance). Such an allergy contraindicates the use of this enzyme, which can produce severe anaphylaxis in a sensitive patient. After chemonucleolysis, enforce bed rest as ordered. Administer analgesics and apply heat as needed. Urge the patient to cough and deep-breathe. Assist with special exercises, and tell the patient to continue these exercises after discharge.

✦ Tell the patient who must receive a muscle relaxant of possible adverse effects, especially drowsiness. Warn him to avoid activities that require alertness until he has built up a tolerance to the drug's sedative effects.

✦ Provide emotional support. Try to cheer the patient during periods of frustration and depression. Assure him of his progress, and offer encouragement.

LEGG-CALVÉ-PERTHES DISEASE

Legg-Calvé-Perthes disease (also called *coxa plana*) is ischemic necrosis leading to eventual flattening of the head of the femur due to vascular interruption. This typically unilateral condition occurs most commonly in boys ages 4 to 10 and tends to occur in families. It occurs bilaterally in 20% of patients.

Although this disease usually runs its course in 3 to 4 years, it may lead to premature osteoarthritis later in life from misalignment of the acetabulum and flattening of the femoral head.

CAUSES

The exact vascular obstructive changes that initiate Legg-Calvé-Perthes disease are unknown. Current etiologic theories include venous obstruction with secondary intraepiphyseal thrombosis, trauma to retinacular vessels, vascular irregularities (congenital or developmental), vascular occlusion secondary to increased intracapsular pressure from acute transient synovitis, and increased blood viscosity resulting in stasis and decreased blood flow.

PATHOPHYSIOLOGY

Legg-Calvé-Perthes disease occurs in four stages. The first stage, *synovitis,* is characterized by synovial inflammation and increased joint fluid, and typically lasts 1 to 3 weeks. In the second *(avascular)* stage, vascular interruption causes necrosis of the ossification center of the femoral head (usually in several months to 1 year). In the third stage, *revascularization,* a new blood supply causes bone resorption and deposition of immature bone cells. New bone replaces necrotic bone and the femoral head gradually reforms. The final, or *residual* stage, involves healing and regeneration. Normal bone cells replace immature bone cells, thereby fixing the shape of the joint. There may be residual deformity, based on the degree of necrosis that occurred in stage two.

SIGNS AND SYMPTOMS

The first indication of Legg-Calvé-Perthes disease is usually a persistent thigh pain or limp that becomes progressively severe. This symptom appears when bone resorption and deformity begin. The patient may also report a mild pain in the hip,

Characteristics of Legg-Calvé-Perthes disease
✦ Also called *coxa plana*
✦ Ischemic necrosis leading to flattening of head of femur
✦ Mostly occurs in boys ages 4 to 10
✦ Tends to occur in families
✦ Typically unilateral, occurs bilaterally in 20% of patients
✦ Runs its course in 3 to 4 years

Causes
✦ Vascular changes unknown
✦ Theories: venous obstruction, trauma to retinacular vessels, vascular irregularities, and vascular occlusion

How it happens
✦ Synovitis: synovial inflammation and increased joint fluid; typically lasts 1 to 3 weeks
✦ Avascular: interruption causes necrosis of ossification center of femoral head
✦ Revascularization: new blood supply causes bone resorption, deposition of immature bone cells; femoral head gradually reforms
✦ Residual: normal bone cells replace immature bone cells, fix shape of joint

Key signs and symptoms
✦ Persistent thigh pain or limp that becomes progressively severe
✦ Mild pain in hip, thigh, knee aggravated by activity, relieved by rest

thigh, or knee that's aggravated by activity and relieved by rest or a muscle spasm. Upon observation, atrophy of muscles in the upper thigh, slight shortening of the leg, and severely restricted abduction and internal rotation of the hip may be noted.

COMPLICATIONS

Complications result from misalignment of the acetabulum and the flattened femoral head. These complications can lead to permanent disability and premature osteoarthritis.

DIAGNOSIS

A thorough physical examination and clinical history suggest Legg-Calvé-Perthes disease. Hip X-rays taken every 3 to 4 months confirm the diagnosis, with findings that vary according to the stage of the disease. Anterior-posterior X-rays and magnetic resonance imaging enhance early diagnosis of necrosis and visualization of articular surface.

Diagnostic evaluation must also differentiate between Legg-Calvé-Perthes disease (restriction of only the abduction and rotation of the hip) and infection or arthritis (restriction of all motion). Aspiration and culture of synovial fluid rule out joint sepsis.

TREATMENT

The goal of treatment is to protect the femoral head from further stress and damage by containing it within the acetabulum. After 1 to 2 weeks of bed rest, therapy may include reduced weight bearing by means of bed rest in bilateral split counterpoised traction, then application of hip abduction splint or cast, or weight bearing while a splint, cast, or brace holds the leg in abduction. Braces may remain in place for 6 to 18 months. Analgesics help relieve pain. Physical therapy with passive and active ROM exercises after cast removal helps restore motion.

For a young child in the early stages of the disease, osteotomy and subtrochanteric derotation provide maximum confinement of the epiphysis within the acetabulum to allow return of the femoral head to normal shape and full ROM. Proper placement of the epiphysis thus allows remolding with ambulation. Postoperatively, the patient requires a hip-spica cast for about 2 months.

NURSING CONSIDERATIONS

When caring for the hospitalized child
✦ Monitor the intake and output of fluid. Maintain sufficient fluid balance. Provide a diet sufficient for growth without causing excessive weight gain, which might necessitate cast change and loss of the corrective position.
✦ Provide good cast care. Turn the child every 2 to 3 hours to expose the cast to air. When the cast is still wet, turn the child with your palms because depressions in the plaster may lead to pressure ulcers. After the cast dries, petal it with pieces of adhesive tape or moleskin, changing them as they become soiled. Protect the cast with a plastic covering during toileting.
✦ Watch for complications. Check toes for color, temperature, swelling, sensation, and motion; report dusky, cool, numb toes immediately. Check the skin under the cast with a flashlight every 4 hours while the patient is awake. Follow a consistent plan of skin care to prevent skin breakdown. Never use oils or powders under the cast because they increase skin breakdown and soften the cast. Check under the cast

Complications
✦ Permanent disability
✦ Premature osteoarthritis

Diagnosis
✦ Physical examination and clinical history
✦ Hip X-rays every 3 to 4 months confirm diagnosis
✦ X-rays and MRI enhance early diagnosis of necrosis
✦ Rules out infection or arthritis
✦ Aspiration, culture of synovial fluid rule out joint sepsis

Treatment
✦ Protect femoral head from further stress and damage
✦ 1 to 2 weeks of bed rest
✦ Bilateral split counterpoised traction
✦ Hip abduction splint or cast
✦ Braces
✦ Analgesics
✦ Physical therapy
✦ Hip-spica cast for a young child

Key nursing actions
When caring for the hospitalized child
✦ Monitor fluid intake and output. Maintain sufficient fluid balance.
✦ Provide a diet sufficient for growth without causing excessive weight gain.
✦ Provide good cast care.
✦ Watch for complications.

daily for odors, particularly after surgery, to detect skin breakdown or wound problems. Report persistent soreness.

✦ Administer analgesics as ordered.

✦ Relieve itching by using a hair dryer (set on cool) at the cast edges; this also decreases dampness from perspiration. If itching becomes excessive, get an order for an antipruritic. Never insert an object under the cast to scratch.

✦ Provide continuous emotional support. Explain all procedures and the need for bed rest, cast, or braces to the child; encourage him to verbalize his fears and anxiety. Encourage parents to participate in their child's care. Teach them proper cast care and how to recognize signs of skin breakdown. Offer tips for making home management of the bedridden child easier. Tell them what special supplies are needed: pajamas and trousers a size larger (open the side seam, and attach Velcro fasteners to close it), bedpan, adhesive tape, moleskin and, possibly, a hospital bed.

✦ When the cast is removed, debride dry, scaly skin gradually by applying lotion after bathing.

✦ Stress the need for follow-up care to monitor rehabilitation. Also stress home tutoring and socialization to promote normal mental and emotional growth and development.

MUSCULAR DYSTROPHY

Muscular dystrophy is a group of congenital disorders characterized by progressive symmetric wasting of skeletal muscles without neural or sensory defects. Paradoxically, some wasted muscles tend to enlarge (pseudohypertrophy) because connective tissue and fat replace muscle tissue, giving a false impression of increased muscle strength.

The four main types of muscular dystrophy include Duchenne's (pseudohypertrophic), which represents 50% of all cases; Becker's (benign pseudohypertrophic); Landouzy-Dejerine (facioscapulohumeral); and limb-girdle.

The prognosis varies with the form of disease. Duchenne's muscular dystrophy strikes during early childhood and is usually fatal during the second decade of life. It mostly affects males — 13 to 33 per 100,000 people. Patients with Becker's muscular dystrophy can live into their 40s. It primarily affects males — 1 to 3 per 100,000 people. Facioscapulohumeral and limb-girdle muscular dystrophies usually don't shorten life expectancy; they affect both genders equally.

CAUSES

Muscular dystrophy can be caused by various genetic mechanisms typically involving an enzymatic or metabolic defect.

X-linked recessive disorders, such as Duchenne's and Becker's muscular dystrophies, cause an error in the Xp21 locus. This affects the muscle protein dystrophin, which is essential for maintaining the muscle cell membrane. In fact, muscle cells deteriorate or die without it.

Landouzy-Dejerine (facioscapulohumeral) muscular dystrophy is an autosomal dominant disorder, whereas limb-girdle muscular dystrophy is an autosomal recessive disorder.

PATHOPHYSIOLOGY

Abnormally permeable cell membranes allow leakage of various muscle enzymes, particularly creatine kinase. This metabolic defect that causes the muscle cells to die

Key signs and symptoms

Duchenne's
+ Insidious onset between ages 3 and 5
+ Waddling gait, toe walking, lumbar lordosis
+ Difficulty climbing stairs
+ Enlarged, firm calf muscles

Becker's
+ Similar to Duchenne's with slower progression

Landouzy-Dejerine
+ Weakened face, shoulder, upper arm muscles
+ Pendulous lip, absent nasolabial fold, inability to pucker

Limb-girdle
+ Weakness in upper arms and pelvis
+ Lumbar lordosis
+ Waddling gait

Complications

+ Tachycardia
+ Electrocardiographic abnormalities
+ Pulmonary complications
+ Facial and shoulder deformities
+ Hearing loss
+ Contractures

Diagnosis

+ Family history
+ Electromyography shows abnormal impulses
+ Muscle biopsy shows muscle cell abnormalities
+ Immunologic and molecular biological techniques

is present from fetal life onward. The absence of progressive muscle wasting at birth suggests that other factors compound the effect of dystrophin deficiency. The specific trigger is unknown, but phagocytosis of the muscle cells by inflammatory cells causes scarring and loss of muscle function.

As the disease progresses, skeletal muscle becomes almost totally replaced by fat and connective tissue. The skeleton eventually becomes deformed, causing progressive immobility. Cardiac and smooth muscle of the GI tract typically become fibrotic. No consistent structural abnormalities are seen in the brain.

SIGNS AND SYMPTOMS

Duchenne's muscular dystrophy generally has an insidious onset between ages 3 and 5 with an initial effect on the legs, pelvis, and shoulders. A waddling gait, toe walking, and lumbar lordosis are observed due to muscle weakness. The child may have difficulty climbing stairs and may fall frequently. He also may have enlarged, firm calf muscles. By ages 9 to 12, the child is usually confined to wheelchair.

Signs and symptoms of Becker's (benign pseudohypertrophic) muscular dystrophy are similar to those of Duchenne's muscular dystrophy but with slower progression.

Patients with Landouzy-Dejerine (facioscapulohumeral) muscular dystrophy initially exhibit a weakened face, shoulder, and upper arm muscles. They may have a pendulous lip, an absent nasolabial fold, and an inability to pucker their mouth or whistle. Their abnormal facial movements—an absence of facial movements when laughing or crying and diffuse facial flattening leading to a masklike expression—are also signs of this disorder. The patient will also be unable to raise his arms above his head.

The first signs and symptoms of limb-girdle muscular dystrophy are weakness in the upper arms and the pelvis. Others include lumbar lordosis with abdominal protrusion, winging of the scapulae, waddling gait, poor balance, and an inability to raise the arms.

COMPLICATIONS

Possible complications of Duchenne's and Becker's muscular dystrophy are weakened cardiac and respiratory muscles leading to tachycardia, electrocardiographic abnormalities, pulmonary complications, and death commonly due to sudden heart failure, respiratory failure, or infection. Complications of Landouzy-Dejerine muscular dystrophy include facial and shoulder deformities, hearing loss and, rarely, vision loss. Limb-girdle muscular dystrophy may result in contractures and abnormal cardiac rhythms.

DIAGNOSIS

Diagnosis depends on typical clinical findings, family history, and diagnostic test findings. If another family member has muscular dystrophy, its clinical characteristics can suggest the type of dystrophy the patient has and how he may be affected.

Certain tests may help in the diagnosis. Electromyography shows short, weak bursts of electrical activity in the affected muscles. Muscle biopsy shows a combination of muscle cell degeneration and regeneration and in the later stages, fat and connective tissue deposits. In addition, immunologic and molecular biological techniques (now available in specialized medical centers) facilitate accurate prenatal and postnatal diagnosis of Duchenne's and Becker's muscular dystrophies (replacing muscle biopsy and elevated serum creatine kinase levels in diagnosis).

TREATMENT

No treatment can stop the progressive muscle impairment. Supportive treatments can be employed to prevent complications and maximize the patient's functional abilities. The patient should perform coughing and deep-breathing exercises as well as diaphragmatic breathing. Parents should be taught to recognize the early signs of respiratory complications.

To help preserve mobility and independence, a combination of orthopedic appliances, exercise, physical therapy, and surgery to correct contractures may be used. Inactivity may cause constipation. Adequate fluid intake, increased dietary bulk, and stool softeners may help combat the problem. Inactivity also predisposes the patient to obesity. A low-calorie, high-protein, high-fiber diet will help prevent it.

Surgery, such as tendon releases for contractures and spinal fusions for scoliosis, may be performed to promote or maintain motility.

The family should be referred for genetic counseling to assess the risk of transmitting the disease.

NURSING CONSIDERATIONS

Comprehensive long-term care and follow-up, patient and family teaching, and psychological support can help the patient and his family deal with this disorder.

✦ When respiratory involvement occurs in Duchenne's muscular dystrophy, encourage coughing, deep-breathing exercises, and diaphragmatic breathing. Teach parents how to recognize early signs of respiratory complications.

✦ Encourage and assist with active and passive ROM exercises to preserve joint mobility and prevent muscle atrophy.

✦ Advise the patient to avoid long periods of bed rest and inactivity. If necessary, limit television viewing and other sedentary activities.

✦ Refer the patient for physical therapy. Splints, braces, and surgery to correct contractures; trapeze bars; overhead slings; and a wheelchair can help preserve mobility. A footboard or high-topped sneakers and a foot cradle increase comfort and prevent footdrop.

✦ Because inactivity may cause constipation, encourage adequate fluid intake, increase dietary bulk, and obtain an order for a stool softener. The patient is prone to obesity due to reduced physical activity; with him, help his family plan a low-calorie, high-protein, high-fiber diet.

✦ Always allow the patient plenty of time to perform even simple physical tasks because he's likely to be slow and awkward.

✦ Encourage communication between family members to help them deal with the emotional strain this disorder produces. Provide emotional support to help the patient cope with continual changes in body image.

✦ Help the child with Duchenne's muscular dystrophy maintain peer relationships and realize his intellectual potential by encouraging his parents to keep him in a regular school as long as possible.

✦ If necessary, refer adult patients for sexual counseling. Refer those who must acquire new job skills for vocational rehabilitation. (Contact the Department of Labor and Industry in your state for more information.) For information on social services and financial assistance, refer these patients and their families to the Muscular Dystrophy Association.

✦ Refer family members for genetic counseling.

Treatment

✦ No treatment stops progressive impairment
✦ Perform coughing, deep-breathing exercises, diaphragmatic breathing
✦ Orthopedic appliances, exercise, physical therapy
✦ Surgery to promote motility
✦ Adequate fluid intake, increased dietary bulk, stool
✦ Low-calorie, high-protein, high-fiber diet

Key nursing actions

✦ With respiratory involvement in Duchenne's muscular dystrophy, encourage coughing, deep-breathing exercises, and diaphragmatic breathing.
✦ Encourage and assist with active and passive ROM.
✦ Advise the patient to avoid long periods of bed rest and inactivity.
✦ Refer the patient for physical therapy.
✦ Help the child with Duchenne's muscular dystrophy maintain peer relationships and realize his intellectual potential by encouraging his parents to keep him in a regular school as long as possible.
✦ If necessary, refer adult patients for sexual counseling.
✦ Refer family members for genetic counseling.

Characteristics of osteoarthritis

+ Also called *degenerative joint disease*
+ Most common form of arthritis
+ Chronic, causing deterioration of joint cartilage, formation of reactive new bone
+ Can affect weight-bearing joints
+ Symptoms manifest in middle age and progress
+ Disability depends on site and severity

Causes

+ Primary defect is loss of articular cartilage

Idiopathic osteoarthritis
+ Process of aging
+ Metabolic, chemical, and mechanical factors

Secondary osteoarthritis
+ Trauma
+ Congenital deformity
+ Obesity

How it happens

+ Occurs in synovial joints
+ Joint cartilage deteriorates, reactive new bone forms
+ Cartilage flakes irritate synovial lining
+ Synovial lining becomes fibrotic, limits joint movement
+ Synovial fluid forced into defects in bone, causing cysts
+ Bone spur forms at joint margins as articular cartilage erodes

Key signs and symptoms

+ Increase with poor posture, obesity, occupational stress
+ Deep, aching joint pain
+ Stiffness
+ Crepitus during motion

OSTEOARTHRITIS

Osteoarthritis (commonly referred to as *degenerative joint disease*), the most common form of arthritis, is a chronic condition causing the deterioration of joint cartilage and the formation of reactive new bone at the margins and subchondral areas of the joints. It usually affects weight-bearing joints (knees, feet, hips, lumbar vertebrae). Osteoarthritis is widespread (affecting more than 60 million people in the United States) and is most common in women. Typically, its earliest symptoms manifest in middle age and progress from there.

Disability depends on the site and severity of involvement and can range from minor limitation of finger movement to severe disability in persons with hip or knee involvement. The rate of progression varies, and joints may remain stable for years in an early stage of deterioration.

CAUSES

The primary defect in both idiopathic and secondary osteoarthritis is loss of articular cartilage due to functional changes in chondrocytes (cells responsible for the formation of the proteoglycans, glycoproteins that act as cementing material in the cartilage, and collagen).

Idiopathic osteoarthritis, a normal part of aging, results from many factors, including metabolic factors (endocrine disorders such as hyperparathyroidism) and genetic factors (decreased collagen synthesis), chemical factors (drugs that stimulate the collagen-digesting enzymes in the synovial membrane such as steroids), and mechanical factors (repeated stress on the joint).

Secondary osteoarthritis usually follows an identifiable predisposing event that leads to degenerative changes, such as trauma (most common cause), congenital deformity, and obesity.

PATHOPHYSIOLOGY

Osteoarthritis occurs in synovial joints. The joint cartilage deteriorates, and reactive new bone forms at the margins and subchondral areas of the joints. The degeneration results from damage to the chondrocytes. Cartilage softens with age, narrowing the joint space. Mechanical injury erodes articular cartilage, leaving the underlying bone unprotected. This causes sclerosis, or thickening and hardening of the bone underneath the cartilage.

Cartilage flakes irritate the synovial lining, which becomes fibrotic and limits joint movement. Synovial fluid may be forced into defects in the bone, causing cysts. New bone, called *osteophyte* (bone spur), forms at joint margins as the articular cartilage erodes, causing gross alteration of the bony contours and enlargement of the joint.

SIGNS AND SYMPTOMS

Symptoms increase with poor posture, obesity, and occupational stress. Deep, aching joint pain is due to degradation of the cartilage, inflammation, and bone stress, particularly after exercise or weight bearing (the most common symptom, usually relieved by rest). Stiffness generally occurs in the morning and after exercise (relieved by rest). Crepitus, or "grating" of the joint occurs during motion due to cartilage damage. Heberden's nodes on physical examination (bony enlargements of the distal interphalangeal joints) may be present due to repeated inflammation.

Contractures due to overcompensation of the muscles supporting the joint result in altered gait. Pain and stiffness result in decreased range of motion (ROM). Stress on the bone and disordered bone growth cause notable joint enlargement. Lastly, cervical spine arthritis causes localized headaches.

COMPLICATIONS

Complications of osteoarthritis include irreversible joint changes and node formation (nodes eventually becoming red, swollen, and tender, causing numbness and loss of finger dexterity), subluxation of the joint, decreased joint ROM, joint contractures, pain (can be debilitating in later stages), and loss of independence in activities of daily living.

DIAGNOSIS

Findings that help diagnose osteoarthritis include absence of systemic symptoms (ruling out inflammatory joint disorder), arthroscopy showing bone spurs, narrowing of joint space, and increased erythrocyte sedimentation rate (with extensive synovitis).

X-rays of the affected joint help confirm the diagnosis but may be normal in the early stages. X-rays may require many views and typically show narrowing of joint space or margin, cystlike bony deposits in joint space and margins, sclerosis of the subchondral space, joint deformity due to degeneration or articular damage, bony growths at weight-bearing areas, and joint fusion.

TREATMENT

The goal of treatment is to relieve pain, maintain or improve mobility, and minimize disability. Weight loss can help reduce stress on the joint. Balance of rest and exercise is imperative.

Medications, including aspirin, fenoprofen (Nalfon), ibuprofen (Motrin), indomethacin (Indocin), phenylbutazone, and other nonsteroidal anti-inflammatory drugs; propoxyphene (Darvon), and celecoxib (Celebrex) (see *Specific care for arthritic joints*, page 420) are prescribed to relieve the symptoms of arthritis. Nutritional supplements, such as glucosamine sulfate and chondroitin, have recently gained popularity in the treatment of pain associated with osteoarthritis.

Support or stabilization of the joint may be achieved by using crutches, braces, a cane, walker, cervical collar, or traction to reduce stress. Intra-articular injections of corticosteroids (every 4 to 6 months) are given because they may delay node development in the hands. However, if used too frequently, they may accelerate arthritic progression by depleting the normal ground substance of the cartilage.

Surgical treatment is reserved for patients with severe disability or uncontrollable pain. Arthroplasty is partial or total replacement of a deteriorated part of the joint with a prosthetic appliance). Arthrodesis, which is primarily used to treat spinal arthritis, is a surgical fusion of bones. When performed on the spine, the procedure is called *laminectomy*.

Deteriorated bone may be scraped or lavaged from a joint during an osteoplasty. During an osteotomy, a change in the alignment of bones is made. This procedure relieves stress by excising a wedge of bone or by cutting bone.

Complications
+ Irreversible joint changes
+ Node formation
+ Subluxation of joint
+ Decreased joint ROM
+ Contractures
+ Debilitating pain
+ Loss of independence

Diagnosis
+ Absence of systemic symptoms
+ Arthroscopy showing bone spurs, narrowing of joint space, increased erythrocyte sedimentation rate
+ X-rays help confirm diagnosis

Treatment
+ Weight loss
+ Aspirin
+ NSAIDs
+ Propoxyphene
+ Celecoxib
+ Nutritional supplements
+ Support or stabilization of joint
+ Intra-articular corticosteroids
+ Surgery

Arthritic joint care

✦ Apply hot soaks to hands
✦ Check cervical spine collar for constriction
✦ Use moist heat pads to reduce hip pain
✦ Assist with ROM exercises for knees

Key nursing actions

✦ Promote adequate rest, particularly after activity.
✦ Assist with physical therapy.
✦ If the patient needs surgery, provide appropriate preoperative and postoperative care.
✦ Provide emotional support and reassurance to help the patient cope with limited mobility. Explain that osteoarthritis isn't a systemic disease.

Characteristics of osteogenesis imperfecta

✦ Also called *little bone disease*
✦ Genetic disease
✦ Bones thin, poorly developed, fracture easily
✦ Expression varies
✦ If autosomal dominant, heterozygote may eventually express disease
✦ If autosomal recessive, homozygous child likely to die at birth

---

Specific care for arthritic joints

Specific care depends on the affected joint.
✦ Hand: Apply hot soaks and paraffin dips to relieve pain as ordered.
✦ Lumbar and sacral spine: Recommend a firm mattress or bed board to decrease morning pain.
✦ Cervical spine: Check cervical collar for constriction; watch for redness with prolonged use.
✦ Hip: Use moist heat pads to relieve pain, and administer antispasmodic drugs as ordered. Assist with range-of-motion (ROM) and strengthening exercises, always making sure the patient gets the proper rest afterward. Check crutches, cane, braces, and walker for proper fit, and teach the patient to use them correctly. For example, a patient with unilateral joint involvement should use an orthopedic appliance (such as a cane or walker) on the unaffected side. Advise use of cushions when sitting and use of an elevated toilet seat.
✦ Knee: Assist with prescribed ROM exercises, muscle tone maintenance exercises,

and progressive resistance exercises to increase muscle strength. Provide elastic supports or braces if needed.

To minimize the long-term effects of osteoarthritis, teach the patient to:
✦ plan for adequate rest during the day, after exertion, and at night
✦ take medication exactly as prescribed and report adverse effects immediately
✦ avoid overexertion, take care to stand and walk correctly, minimize weight-bearing activities, and be especially careful when stooping or picking up objects
✦ always wear well-fitting supportive shoes and not let the heels become too worn down
✦ install safety devices at home such as guard rails in the bathroom
✦ perform ROM exercises as gently as possible
✦ maintain proper body weight to lessen strain on joints
✦ avoid percussive activities.

NURSING CONSIDERATIONS

Patient care for osteoarthritis includes the following:
✦ Promote adequate rest, particularly after activity. Plan rest periods during the day, and provide for adequate sleep at night. Moderation is the key; teach the patient to pace daily activities.
✦ Assist with physical therapy, and encourage the patient to perform gentle, isometric ROM exercises.
✦ If the patient needs surgery, provide appropriate preoperative and postoperative care.
✦ Provide emotional support and reassurance to help the patient cope with limited mobility. Explain that osteoarthritis isn't a systemic disease.

OSTEOGENESIS IMPERFECTA

Osteogenesis imperfecta (also called *little bone disease*) is a genetic disease in which bones are thin, poorly developed, and fracture easily.

The expression of the disease varies, depending on whether the defect is carried as a trait or is clinically obvious. (See chapter 5, Genetics.) If it's inherited as an autosomal dominant disorder, a heterozygote may eventually express the disease, which occurs in about 1 in 30,000 people. If inheritance is as an autosomal recessive disorder, the homozygous child will likely die before, during, or soon after birth from multiple fractures sustained *in utero* or during delivery.

CAUSES

One cause of osteogenesis perfecta is genetic disease, which is typically an autosomal dominant disease (characterized by a defect in the synthesis of connective tissue). The disease can also be an autosomal recessive gene defect that produces osteogenesis imperfecta in homozygotes and osteoporosis in some children.

PATHOPHYSIOLOGY

Most forms of the disease appear to be caused by mutations in the genes that determine the structure of collagen. Possible mutations in other genes may cause variations in the assembly and maintenance of bone and other connective tissues. Collectively or alone, these mutated genes lead to pathologic fractures and impaired healing.

SIGNS AND SYMPTOMS

In the autosomal dominant disorder, some symptoms may not be apparent until the child's mobility increases. For example, a child sustains frequent fractures and experiences poor healing due to falls as he begins to walk.

Short stature in autosomal dominant osteogenesis imperfecta is due to multiple fractures caused by minor physical stress. Multiple fractures cause deformed cranial structures and deformed limbs.

The child may have thin skin, bluish sclera of the eyes, and thin collagen fibers of the sclera that allow the choroid layer to be seen. Improper deposition of dentin results in abnormal tooth and enamel development. The child may have middle ear deafness.

COMPLICATIONS

Deafness is a complication of osteogenesis imperfecta. It results from bone deformity and scarring of the middle and inner ear. Stillbirth or death within the first year of life is a complication of the autosomal recessive disorder.

DIAGNOSIS

Fractures early in life, hearing loss, and blue sclera show that mutation is expressed in more than one connective tissue. These symptoms aid in proper diagnosis. During periods of rapid bone formation and cellular injury, the child will have elevated serum alkaline phosphatase levels. A skin culture shows reduced quantity of fibroblasts. An echocardiography may show mitral insufficiency or floppy mitral valves.

TREATMENT

Possible treatment options are prevention of fractures and internal fixation of fractures to ensure stabilization and prevent deformities.

NURSING CONSIDERATIONS

✦ Educate the family about the disorder. Teach the parents and their child how to recognize fractures and how to correctly splint them. Also teach the parents how to protect the child during diapering, dressing, and other activities of daily living.

Causes
✦ Genetic disease

How it happens
✦ Mutations in genes that determine structure of collagen
✦ Mutated genes lead to pathologic fractures, impaired healing

Key signs and symptoms
✦ Frequent fractures
✦ Poor healing
✦ Short stature
✦ Deformed cranial structures, limbs
✦ Thin skin, bluish sclera of eyes, thin collagen fibers of sclera
✦ Abnormal tooth, enamel development
✦ Middle ear deafness

Complications
✦ Deafness
✦ Stillbirth or death within first year of life

Diagnosis
✦ Fractures early in life
✦ Hearing loss
✦ Blue sclera
✦ Elevated serum alkaline phosphatase levels

Treatment
✦ Prevention of fractures
✦ Internal fixation of fractures

Key nursing actions

+ Advise the parents to encourage their child to develop interests that don't require strenuous physical activity and to develop his fine motor skills.
+ Teach the child to assume some responsibility for precautions during physical activity to help foster his independence.
+ Discuss alternatives for birth control and family planning.
+ Administer analgesics, as ordered, to relieve pain from frequent fractures, a hallmark of this disease.
+ Instruct the parents to provide a medical identification bracelet for the child.

Characteristics of osteomalacia and rickets

+ Vitamin D deficiency
+ Bone can't calcify normally
+ Called *rickets* in infants and young children, *osteomalacia* in adults
+ Occurs in areas where smog limits sunlight penetration
+ Prognosis good with treatment

Alert!

+ Incidence of rickets is highest in children with black or dark brown skin.

Causes

+ Inadequate dietary intake of preformed vitamin D
+ Malabsorption of vitamin D
+ Inadequate exposure to sunlight
+ Inherited impairment of renal tubular reabsorption of phosphate from vitamin D insensitivity

---

+ Advise the parents to encourage their child to develop interests that don't require strenuous physical activity and to develop his fine motor skills. These actions will promote the child's self-esteem.
+ Teach the child to assume some responsibility for precautions during physical activity to help foster his independence.
+ Stress the importance of good nutrition to heal bones.
+ Refer the parents and their child for genetic counseling to assess the recurrence risk.
+ Discuss alternatives for birth control and family planning if appropriate.
+ Administer analgesics, as ordered, to relieve pain from frequent fractures, a hallmark of this disease.
+ Monitor dental and hearing needs. Stress the need for regular dental care and immunizations.
+ Instruct the parents to provide a medical identification bracelet for the child.

OSTEOMALACIA AND RICKETS

In vitamin D deficiency, bone can't calcify normally; the result is called *rickets* in infants and young children and *osteomalacia* in adults.

Once a common childhood disease, rickets is now rare in the United States. It appears occasionally in breast-fed infants who don't receive a vitamin D supplement or in infants fed a formula with a nonfortified milk base. Rickets also occurs in overcrowded, urban areas where smog limits sunlight penetration.

 CLINICAL ALERT Incidence of rickets is highest in children with black or dark brown skin, who, because of their pigmentation, absorb less sunlight.

With treatment, the prognosis is good. In osteomalacia, bone deformities may disappear; however, they usually persist in children with rickets.

CAUSES

There are many causes of osteomalacia and rickets. An inadequate dietary intake of preformed vitamin D and malabsorption of vitamin D can cause the disease. Solar ultraviolet rays irradiate 7-dehydrocholesterol, a precursor of vitamin D, to form calciferol. Therefore, an inadequate exposure to sunlight is also a cause. In vitamin D-resistant rickets (refractory rickets, familial hypophosphatemia), inherited impairment of renal tubular reabsorption of phosphate from vitamin D insensitivity causes the disorder.

Conditions that reduce the absorption of fat-soluble vitamin D (such as chronic pancreatitis, celiac disease, Crohn's disease, cystic fibrosis, gastric or small-bowel resections, fistulas, colitis, and biliary obstruction), hepatic or renal diseases that interfere with hydroxylated calciferol formation (needed to form a calcium-binding protein in intestinal absorption sites), and a malfunctioning parathyroid gland (decreased secretion of parathyroid hormone), contribute to calcium deficiency (normally, vitamin D controls absorption of calcium and phosphorus through the intestine) and interfere with activation of vitamin D in the kidneys.

PATHOPHYSIOLOGY

Vitamin D regulates the absorption of calcium ions from the intestine. When vitamin D is lacking, falling serum calcium concentration stimulates synthesis and secretion of parathyroid hormone, causing release of calcium from bone, decreasing renal calcium excretion, and increasing renal phosphate excretion. When the concentration of phosphate in the bone decreases, osteoid may be produced, but mineralization can't proceed normally. Large quantities of osteoid accumulate, coating the trabeculae and linings of the haversian canals and areas beneath the periosteum.

When mineralization of bone matrix is delayed or inadequate, bone is disorganized in structure and lacks density. The result is gross deformity of both spongy and compact bone.

SIGNS AND SYMPTOMS

Osteomalacia may not produce symptoms until a fracture occurs. Chronic vitamin D deficiency induces numerous bone malformations due to bone softening. Possible signs and symptoms include pain in the legs and lower back due to vertebral collapse, bow legs, knock knees, rachitic rosary (beading of ends of ribs), enlarged wrists and ankles, pigeon breast (protruding ribs and sternum), delayed closing of fontanels, softening skull, bulging forehead, poorly developed muscles (pot belly), difficulty walking and climbing stairs, and kyphoscoliosis.

COMPLICATIONS

Complications of osteomalacia and rickets may include spontaneous multiple fractures, tetany in infants, and bone deformities.

DIAGNOSIS

Physical examination, dietary history, and laboratory tests establish the diagnosis. In addition, a serum calcium concentration less than 7.5 mg/dl, a serum inorganic phosphorus concentration less than 3 mg/dl, a serum citrate level less than 2.5 mg/dl, and alkaline phosphatase level less than 4 Bodansky units/dl all suggest vitamin D deficiency.

X-rays showing characteristic bone deformities and abnormalities such as Looser's transformation zones (radiolucent bands perpendicular to the surface of the bones indicating reduced bone ossification) confirm the diagnosis.

TREATMENT

Massive oral doses of vitamin D or cod liver oil are given for osteomalacia and rickets, except when caused by malabsorption. For rickets refractory to vitamin D or rickets accompanied by hepatic or renal disease, 25-hydroxycholecalciferol, 1,25-dihydroxycholecalciferol, or a synthetic analogue of active vitamin is the most effective treatment.

A diet consisting of foods high in vitamin D (fortified milk, fish liver oils, herring, liver, and egg yolks) and sufficient sun exposure are an important part of treatment. Supplemental aqueous preparations of vitamin D are given for chronic fat malabsorption, hydroxylated cholecalciferol is given for refractory rickets, and supplemental vitamin D is given to breast-fed infants to prevent rickets.

Surgical intervention may be necessary in the cases of intestinal disease.

NURSING CONSIDERATIONS

Here are important nursing steps for the patient with osteomalacia and rickets:
+ Obtain a dietary history to assess the patient's current vitamin D intake.

How it happens
+ Low vitamin D causes falling serum calcium concentration
+ Stimulates synthesis and secretion of parathyroid hormone
+ Calcium released from bone, renal calcium excretion decreased, renal phosphate excretion increased
+ Large quantities of osteoid accumulate
+ Mineralization of bone matrix delayed or inadequate

Key signs and symptoms
+ May not produce symptoms until fracture occurs
+ Bone malformations
+ Pain in legs and lower back
+ Bow legs

Complications
+ Spontaneous multiple fractures
+ Tetany in infants
+ Bone deformities

Diagnosis
+ Physical examination, dietary history, laboratory tests
+ Serum calcium concentration < 7.5 mg/dl
+ Serum inorganic phosphorus concentration < 3 mg/dl

Treatment
+ Massive oral doses of vitamin D or cod liver oil unless caused by malabsorption
+ 25-hydroxycholecalciferol, 1,25-dihydroxycholecalciferol, synthetic analogue of active vitamin
+ Sufficient sun exposure

Key nursing actions

+ If the patient must take vitamin D for a prolonged period, tell him to watch for vitamin D toxicity.
+ If the patient's vitamin D deficiency is linked to adverse socioeconomic conditions, refer him to an appropriate agency.

Characteristics of osteomyelitis

+ Bone infection
+ Progressive inflammatory destruction after new bone forms
+ Chronic or acute
+ Results from local trauma and acute infection
+ Localized; can spread through bone to marrow, cortex, periosteum
+ Chronic osteomyelitis characterized by draining sinus tracts, widespread lesions

Alert!

+ Osteomyelitis occurs more commonly in children than in adults.

Causes

+ *Staphylococcus aureus*
+ *Streptococcus pyogenes*
+ Pneumococcus

How it happens

+ Organisms find culture site in hematoma from recent trauma or weakened area; travel through bloodstream to metaphysis

Key signs and symptoms

+ Rapid onset of acute osteomyelitis
+ Pain, heat, swelling, and erythema

+ If the patient must take vitamin D for a prolonged period, tell him to watch for symptoms of vitamin D toxicity (headache, nausea, constipation and, after prolonged use, renal calculi).
+ If the patient's vitamin D deficiency appears to be linked to adverse socioeconomic conditions, refer the patient to an appropriate community agency.

OSTEOMYELITIS

Osteomyelitis is a bone infection characterized by progressive inflammatory destruction after formation of new bone. It may be chronic or acute. It commonly results from a combination of local trauma — usually trivial but causing a hematoma — and an acute infection originating elsewhere in the body. Although osteomyelitis usually remains localized, it can spread through the bone to the marrow, cortex, and periosteum. Acute osteomyelitis is usually a blood-borne disease and most commonly affects rapidly growing children. Chronic osteomyelitis, which is rare, is characterized by draining sinus tracts and widespread lesions.

 CLINICAL ALERT Osteomyelitis occurs more commonly in children (especially boys) than in adults — usually as a complication of an acute localized infection. Typical sites in children are the lower end of the femur and the upper ends of the tibia, humerus, and radius. The most common sites in adults are the pelvis and vertebrae, generally after surgery or trauma.

The incidence of both chronic and acute osteomyelitis is declining, except in drug abusers. With prompt treatment, the prognosis for acute osteomyelitis is very good; for chronic osteomyelitis, prognosis remains poor.

CAUSES

The most common pyogenic organism in osteomyelitis is *Staphylococcus aureus.* Other organisms include *Streptococcus pyogenes,* pneumococcus, *Pseudomonas aeruginosa, Escherichia coli, Proteus vulgaris,* and *Pasteurella multocida* (part of the normal mouth flora of cats and dogs).

PATHOPHYSIOLOGY

Typically, these organisms find a culture site in a hematoma from recent trauma or in a weakened area, such as the site of local infection (for example, furunculosis), and travel through the bloodstream to the metaphysis, the section of a long bone that's continuous with the epiphysis plates, where the blood flows into sinusoids. (See *Avoiding chronic osteomyelitis.*)

SIGNS AND SYMPTOMS

Clinical features of chronic and acute osteomyelitis are generally the same. The patient experiences rapid onset of acute osteomyelitis, with sudden pain in the affected bone, tenderness, heat, swelling, erythema, guarding of the affected region of the limb, and restricted movement. He also has a chronic infection persisting intermittently for years, flaring after minor trauma or persisting as drainage of pus from an old pocket in a sinus tract. The patient may also have fever and tachycardia. Young patients experience dehydration; infants are irritable and don't eat well.

FOCUS ON TREATMENT

Avoiding chronic osteomyelitis

Bones are essentially isolated from the body's natural defense system after an organism gets through the periosteum. Bones are limited in their ability to replace necrotic tissue caused by infection, which may lead to chronic osteomyelitis.

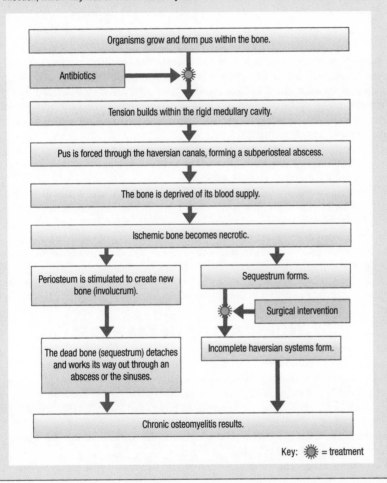

Organisms grow and form pus within the bone.

Antibiotics ────► ☀

Tension builds within the rigid medullary cavity.

Pus is forced through the haversian canals, forming a subperiosteal abscess.

The bone is deprived of its blood supply.

Ischemic bone becomes necrotic.

Periosteum is stimulated to create new bone (involucrum).

Sequestrum forms.

☀ ◄──── Surgical intervention

The dead bone (sequestrum) detaches and works its way out through an abscess or the sinuses.

Incomplete haversian systems form.

Chronic osteomyelitis results.

Key: ☀ = treatment

COMPLICATIONS

A possible complication of osteomyelitis includes the need for amputation of an arm or leg when resistant chronic osteomyelitis causes severe, unrelenting pain and decreases function. Other complications include weakened bone cortex that predisposes the bone to pathologic fracture, and arrested growth of an extremity in children with severe disease.

DIAGNOSIS

Diagnosis must rule out septicemia, foreign bodies, poliomyelitis (rare), rheumatic fever, myositis (inflammation of voluntary muscle), and bone fracture. History that

Complications

+ Need for amputation
+ Weakened bone cortex
+ Arrested growth of extremity

Diagnosis

+ Rule out other disease and bone fracture
+ History of urinary tract, respiratory tract, ear, skin infection
+ Human or animal bite
+ Penetrating trauma
+ WBC count showing leukocytosis

helps confirm osteomyelitis may include history of a urinary tract, respiratory tract, ear, or skin infection; human or animal bite; or other penetrating trauma. Laboratory tests supporting the diagnosis include a white blood cell count showing leukocytosis, an elevated erythrocyte sedimentation rate, and blood cultures showing the causative organism.

Magnetic resonance imaging facilitates diagnosis by delineating bone marrow from soft tissue. X-rays are helpful but they may not show bone involvement until the disease has been active for 2 to 3 weeks, and bone scans can detect early infection.

TREATMENT

Treatment of acute osteomyelitis should begin before definitive diagnosis. Large doses of antibiotics (usually a penicillinase-resistant penicillin, such as nafcillin [Nafcil] or oxacillin [Bactocill]) are administered after blood cultures are taken. Immobilization of the affected body part by cast, traction, or bed rest prevents failure to heal or recurrence. Early surgical drainage relieves pressure and reduces the likelihood of abscess formation.

Supportive measures include analgesics to control pain and I.V. fluids to maintain hydration. If an abscess or sinus tract forms, incision and drainage, followed by a culture of the drainage are performed.

Antibiotic therapy to control infection may include systemic antibiotics, intracavitary instillation of antibiotics through closed-system continuous irrigation with low intermittent suction, limited irrigation with blood drainage system with suction (closed drainage system), and packed, wet, antibiotic-soaked dressings.

In chronic osteomyelitis, surgery is usually required to remove dead bone and promote drainage. The prognosis remains poor even after surgery.

Hyperbaric oxygen is used to stimulate normal immune mechanisms, and skin, bone, and muscle grafts fill in dead space and increase blood supply.

NURSING CONSIDERATIONS

Major concerns in osteomalacia and rickets are to control infection, protect the bone from injury, and offer meticulous supportive care.

✦ Use strict sterile technique when changing dressings and irrigating wounds. If the patient is in skeletal traction for compound fractures, cover insertion points of pin tracks with small, dry dressings, and tell him not to touch the skin around the pins and wires.

✦ Administer I.V. fluids to maintain adequate hydration as necessary. Provide a diet high in protein and vitamin C.

✦ Assess vital signs, the wound appearance, and new pain and drainage, which may indicate secondary infection.

✦ Carefully monitor suctioning equipment. Monitor the amount of solution instilled and suctioned.

✦ Support the affected limb with firm pillows. Keep the limb level with the body; don't let it sag. Provide good skin care. Turn the patient gently every 2 hours and watch for signs of developing pressure ulcers. Report any signs of pressure ulcer formation immediately.

✦ Provide good cast care. Support the cast with firm pillows, and smooth rough edges by covering with pieces of adhesive tape or moleskin. Check circulation and drainage; if a wet spot appears on the cast, circle it with a marking pen and note the time of appearance (on the cast). Be aware of how much drainage is expected. Check the circled spot at least every 4 hours. Report any enlargement immediately.

Treatment

✦ Large doses of antibiotics
✦ Immobilization of affected body part
✦ Early surgical drainage
✦ Analgesics
✦ I.V. fluids
✦ Antibiotics
✦ Surgery
✦ Hyperbaric oxygen

Key nursing actions

✦ Use strict sterile technique when changing dressings and irrigating wounds. Tell the patient not to touch the skin around the pins and wires.
✦ Administer I.V. fluids to maintain adequate hydration as necessary.
✦ Support the affected limb with firm pillows.
✦ Provide good cast care. Check circulation and drainage.
✦ Provide emotional support and appropriate diversions.

✦ Protect the patient from mishaps, such as jerky movements and falls, which may threaten bone integrity. Report sudden pain, crepitus, or deformity immediately. Watch for any sudden malposition of the limb, which may indicate fracture.

✦ Provide emotional support and appropriate diversions. Before discharge, teach the patient how to protect and clean the wound and how to recognize signs of recurring infection (increased temperature, redness, localized heat, and swelling). Stress the need for follow-up examinations. Instruct the patient to seek prompt treatment for possible sources of recurrence, such as blisters, boils, sties, and impetigo.

OSTEOPOROSIS

Osteoporosis is a metabolic bone disorder in which the rate of bone resorption accelerates while the rate of bone formation slows, causing a loss of bone mass. Bones affected by this disease lose calcium and phosphate salts and become porous, brittle, and abnormally vulnerable to fractures. Osteoporosis may be primary or secondary to an underlying disease, such as Cushing's syndrome or hyperthyroidism. It primarily affects the weight-bearing vertebrae. Only when the condition is advanced or severe, as in secondary disease, do similar changes occur in the skull, ribs, and long bones. Usually, the femoral heads and pelvic acetabula are selectively affected.

Primary osteoporosis is commonly called *postmenopausal osteoporosis* because it most commonly develops in postmenopausal women.

CAUSES

The cause of primary osteoporosis is unknown, but contributing factors have been identified. A mild but prolonged negative calcium balance due to inadequate dietary intake of calcium may be an important contributing factor. Other factors include declining gonadal and adrenal function, a sedentary lifestyle, and faulty protein metabolism caused by relative or progressive estrogen deficiency. Estrogen stimulates osteoblastic activity and limits the osteoclastic-stimulating effects of parathyroid hormones.

Alcoholism, malnutrition, malabsorption, scurvy, lactose intolerance, osteogenesis imperfecta, Sudeck's atrophy (localized to hands and feet, with recurring attacks), medications (aluminum-containing antacids, corticosteroids, anticonvulsants, heparin [prolonged therapy]), endocrine disorders (hyperthyroidism, hyperparathyroidism, Cushing's syndrome, diabetes mellitus), and total immobilization or disuse of a bone are all causes of secondary osteoporosis.

PATHOPHYSIOLOGY

In normal bone, the rates of bone formation and resorption are constant; replacement follows resorption immediately, and the amount of bone replaced equals the amount of bone resorbed. Osteoporosis develops when the remodeling cycle is interrupted, and new bone formation falls behind resorption.

When bone is resorbed faster than it forms, the bone becomes less dense. Men have approximately 30% greater bone mass than women, which may explain why osteoporosis develops later in men.

Characteristics of osteoporosis

✦ Metabolic bone disorder
✦ Bone resorption accelerates and formation slows, causing loss of bone mass
✦ Bones become porous, brittle, abnormally vulnerable to fractures
✦ Primary or secondary to underlying disease
✦ Primarily affects weight-bearing vertebrae.
✦ Advanced disease causes changes in skull, ribs, long bones
✦ Primary osteoporosis commonly called *postmenopausal osteoporosis*

Causes

✦ Cause of primary condition unknown
✦ Mild but prolonged negative calcium balance
✦ Declining gonadal and adrenal function
✦ Sedentary lifestyle
✦ Faulty protein metabolism
✦ Alcoholism
✦ Malnutrition
✦ Malabsorption
✦ Scurvy

How it happens

✦ Remodeling cycle interrupted
✦ New bone formation falls behind resorption

SIGNS AND SYMPTOMS

Osteoporosis is typically discovered suddenly. A common scenario is a postmenopausal woman who bends to lift something, hears a snapping sound, and then feels a sudden pain in her lower back. Another is a vertebral collapse that causes back pain that radiates around the trunk (most common presenting feature) and is aggravated by movement or jarring.

In another common pattern, osteoporosis can develop insidiously, showing increasing deformity, kyphosis, loss of height, decreased exercise tolerance, a markedly aged appearance, spontaneous wedge fractures, pathologic fractures of the neck and femur, Colles' fractures of the distal radius after a minor fall, and hip fractures (common as bone is lost from the femoral neck).

COMPLICATIONS

Spontaneous fractures are possible complications of osteoporosis. As the bones lose volume and become brittle and weak, they're susceptible to spontaneous fracture. Shock, hemorrhage, and fat embolism are fatal complications of fractures.

DIAGNOSIS

Differential diagnosis must exclude other causes of bone loss, especially those affecting the spine, such as metastatic cancer or advanced multiple myeloma. History is the key to identifying the specific cause of osteoporosis.

Dual- or single-photon absorptiometry measures the bone mass of the extremities, hips, and spine, and computed tomography scans assess spinal bone loss. X-rays show typical degeneration in the lower thoracic and lumbar vertebrae. This degeneration causes vertebral bodies to appear flattened and denser than normal; bone mineral loss is evident in only later stages of osteoporosis.

Serum calcium, phosphorus, and alkaline phosphatase levels are normal but the level of parathyroid hormone may be elevated. Bone biopsy shows thin, porous, but otherwise normal-looking bone.

TREATMENT

Treatment is aimed at controlling bone loss, preventing fractures, and controlling pain. Because the mechanical stress of exercise stimulates bone formation, physical therapy emphasizes gentle exercise and activity and regular, moderate weight-bearing exercise to slow bone loss and possibly reverse demineralization.

Surgery may be indicated for treatment of pathologic fractures. Hormone replacement therapy with estrogen and progesterone may help slow the loss of bone and prevent occurrence of fractures. Analgesics and local heat to relieve pain and supportive devices such as a back brace help prevent fractures and control pain.

Calcium and vitamin D supplements support normal bone metabolism, calcitonin-salmon (Calcimar) reduces bone resorption and slows the decline in bone mass, bisphosphonates (such as etidronate [Didronel] increase bone density and restore lost bone, and fluoride (such as alendronate [Fosamax]) stimulates bone formation, requires strict dosage precautions, and can cause gastric distress. A balanced diet rich in vitamin C, calcium, and protein nutrients helps provide adequate support to skeletal metabolism.

Other treatment measures include early mobilization after surgery or trauma, decreased alcohol and tobacco consumption, and careful observation for signs of malabsorption (fatty stools, chronic diarrhea). Prompt, effective treatment of the underlying disorder may prevent secondary osteoporosis.

NURSING CONSIDERATIONS

Your care plan should focus on the patient's fragility, stressing careful positioning, ambulation, and prescribed exercises.

✦ Check the patient's skin daily for redness, warmth, and new sites of pain, which may indicate new fractures. Encourage activity; help the patient walk several times daily. As appropriate, perform passive ROM exercises or encourage the patient to perform active exercises. Make sure the patient regularly attends scheduled physical therapy sessions.

✦ Impose safety precautions. Keep the side rails of the patient's bed in raised position. Move the patient gently and carefully at all times. Explain to the patient's family and ancillary health care personnel how easily an osteoporotic patient's bones can fracture.

✦ Make sure the patient and her family clearly understand the prescribed drug regimen. Tell them how to recognize significant adverse effects and to report them immediately. The patient should also report any new pain sites immediately, especially after trauma, no matter how slight. Advise the patient to sleep on a firm mattress and avoid excessive bed rest. Make sure she knows how to wear her back brace.

✦ Thoroughly explain osteoporosis to the patient and her family. If the patient and her family don't understand the nature of this disease, they may feel the fractures could have been prevented if they had been more careful.

✦ Teach the patient good body mechanics: to stoop before lifting anything and to avoid twisting movements and prolonged bending.

✦ Instruct the female patient taking estrogen about the proper technique for breast self-examination. Tell her to perform this examination at least once per month and to report any lumps immediately. Emphasize the need for regular gynecologic exams. Tell her to report abnormal bleeding promptly.

PAGET'S DISEASE

Paget's disease, also called *osteitis deformans,* is a slowly progressive metabolic bone disease characterized by accelerated patterns of bone remodeling. An initial phase of excessive bone resorption (osteoclastic phase) is followed by a reactive phase of excessive abnormal bone formation (osteoblastic phase). Chronic accelerated remodeling eventually enlarges and softens the affected bones. The new bone structure, which is chaotic, fragile, and weak, causes painful deformities of both external contour and internal structure. Paget's disease usually localizes in one or several areas of the skeleton (most commonly the lumbosacral spine, skull, pelvis, femur, and tibia are affected), but occasionally skeletal deformity is widely distributed.

In the United States, Paget's disease affects about 2.5 million people older than age 40 (mostly men). It can be fatal, particularly when it's associated with heart failure (widespread disease creates a continuous need for high cardiac output), bone sarcoma, or giant-cell tumors.

CAUSES

Although the exact cause of Paget's disease is unknown, one theory is that early viral infection causes a dormant skeletal infection that erupts many years later as Paget's disease.

Other possible causes include benign or malignant bone tumors, vitamin D deficiency during the bone-developing years of childhood, autoimmune disease, and estrogen deficiency.

How it happens

+ Repeated episodes of accelerated resorption of spongy bone
+ Trabeculae diminish, vascular fibrous tissue replaces marrow
+ Short periods of rapid, abnormal bone formation
+ Collagen fibers disorganized, glycoprotein levels in matrix decrease
+ Partially resorbed trabeculae thicken, enlarge

Key signs and symptoms

+ Severe and persistent pain intensifying with weight bearing
+ Impaired movement
+ Cranial enlargement over frontal and occipital areas
+ Headaches, sensory abnormalities, impaired motor function
+ Kyphosis
+ Barrel chest

Complications

+ Blindness and hearing loss with tinnitus and vertigo
+ Heart failure
+ Respiratory failure
+ Malignant changes in involved bones

Diagnosis

+ Diagnosis may include X-rays, CT scan, MRI show increased bone expansion and density
+ Radionuclide bone scan shows early lesions
+ Bone biopsy shows mosaic pattern

PATHOPHYSIOLOGY

Repeated episodes of accelerated osteoclastic resorption of spongy bone occur. The trabeculae diminish, and vascular fibrous tissue replaces marrow. This is followed by short periods of rapid, abnormal bone formation. The collagen fibers in this new bone are disorganized, and glycoprotein levels in the matrix decrease. The partially resorbed trabeculae thicken and enlarge because of excessive bone formation, and the bone becomes soft and weak.

SIGNS AND SYMPTOMS

Clinical effects of Paget's disease vary. Early stages may produce no symptoms. Later, the patient may complain of severe and persistent pain intensifying with weight bearing. He may also have impaired movement due to impingement of abnormal bone on the spinal cord or sensory nerve root. The pain may also result from the constant inflammation accompanying cell breakdown.

Characteristic cranial enlargement over frontal and occipital areas (hat size may increase), headaches, sensory abnormalities, and impaired motor function (with skull involvement) are other later signs and symptoms.

A physical examination may reveal kyphosis (spinal curvature due to compression fractures of vertebrae), barrel chest, asymmetric bowing of the tibia and femur (commonly reduces height), and waddling gait (from softening of pelvic bones). Warm and tender disease sites are susceptible to pathologic fractures, which are usually slow to heal and don't heal completely after minor trauma.

COMPLICATIONS

Blindness and hearing loss with tinnitus and vertigo are complication of Paget's disease. They're due to bony impingement on the cranial nerves. Heart failure as a complication of Paget's is due to the high blood flow demands of remodeling bones. Deformed thoracic bones may result in respiratory failure and 1% of patients have malignant changes in involved bones. Other complications include pathologic fractures, hypertension, renal calculi, hypercalcemia, and gout.

DIAGNOSIS

Diagnosis of Paget's disease may include X-rays, computed tomography scan, and magnetic resonance imaging. These tests are done before overt symptoms develop and show increased bone expansion and density. A radionuclide bone scan (more sensitive than X-rays) clearly shows early Paget's lesions (radioisotope concentrates in areas of active disease) and bone biopsy shows a characteristic mosaic pattern.

Other laboratory findings include anemia, elevated serum alkaline phosphatase level (an index of osteoblastic activity and bone formation), elevated 24-hour urine levels for hydroxyproline (amino acid excreted by kidneys and an index of osteoclastic hyperactivity), and normal or elevated serum calcium level.

TREATMENT

Primary treatment consists of drug therapy. Bisphosphonates (alendronate [Fosamax], and etidronate [Didronel]) inhibit osteoclast-mediated bone resorption. Calcitonin-salmon (Calcimar), a hormone, and etidronate retard bone resorption and reduce serum alkaline phosphate and urinary hydroxyproline secretion. Calcitonin requires long-term maintenance therapy, but improvement is noticeable after the first few weeks of treatment; etidronate produces improvement after 1 to 3 months. Plicamycin (Mithracin), a cytotoxic antibiotic, decreases serum calcium, urinary hydroxyproline, and serum alkaline phosphatase level. This produces remission of symptoms within 2 weeks and biochemical improvement in 1 to 2 months, but may destroy platelets or compromise renal function.

Surgery may be performed to reduce or prevent pathologic fractures, correct secondary deformities, and relieve neurologic impairment. Drug therapy with calcitonin and etidronate or plicamycin must precede surgery to decrease the risk of excessive bleeding from hypervascular bone. Joint replacement may be helpful but is difficult because bonding material [methyl methacrylate] doesn't set properly on pagetic bone.

Aspirin, indomethacin (Indocin), or ibuprofen (Motrin) is used to control pain.

Nursing considerations

Incorporate the following considerations into your care of the patient with Paget's disease:

✦ To evaluate the effectiveness of analgesics, assess pain level daily. Watch for new areas of pain or restricted movements, which may indicate new fracture sites, and sensory or motor disturbances, such as difficulty in hearing, seeing, or walking.

✦ Monitor serum calcium and alkaline phosphatase levels.

✦ If the patient is confined to prolonged bed rest, prevent pressure ulcers by providing good skin care. Reposition the patient frequently, and use a flotation mattress. Provide high-topped sneakers to prevent footdrop.

✦ Monitor intake and output. Encourage adequate fluid intake to minimize renal calculi formation.

✦ Demonstrate how to inject calcitonin properly and rotate injection sites or how to perform nasal inhalation if that's the form prescribed. Warn the patient that adverse effects may occur (nausea, vomiting, local inflammatory reaction at injection site, facial flushing, itching of hands, and fever). Give reassurance that these adverse effects are usually mild and infrequent.

✦ If the patient is prescribed the nasal inhalation form of calcitonin, explain proper administration to the patient.

✦ To help the patient adjust to the changes in lifestyle imposed by this disease, teach him how to pace activities and, if necessary, how to use assistive devices. Encourage him to follow a recommended exercise program, avoiding both immobilization and excessive activity. Suggest a firm mattress or a bed board to minimize spinal deformities. Warn against imprudent use of analgesics because diminished sensitivity to pain resulting from analgesic use may make the patient unaware of new fractures. To prevent falls at home, advise removal of throw rugs and other obstacles.

✦ Emphasize the importance of regular checkups, including the eyes and ears.

✦ Tell the patient who's receiving etidronate to take this medication with fruit juice 2 hours before or after meals (milk or other high-calcium fluids impair absorption), to divide daily dosage to minimize adverse effects, and to watch for and report stomach cramps, diarrhea, fractures, and new or increased bone pain.

✦ Tell the patient receiving plicamycin to watch for signs of infection, easy bruising, bleeding, and temperature elevation and to report for regular follow-up laboratory tests.

✦ Help the patient and his family make use of community support resources, such as a visiting nurse or home health agency. For more information, refer them to the Paget Foundation.

Treatment

✦ Bisphosphonates
✦ Calcitonin-salmon
✦ Etidronate
✦ Plicamycin
✦ Surgery
✦ Aspirin and NSAIDs

Key nursing actions

✦ Monitor serum calcium and alkaline phosphatase levels.
✦ Demonstrate how to inject calcitonin properly and rotate injection sites or how to perform nasal inhalation if that's the form prescribed.
✦ Teach the patient how to pace activities and, if necessary, how to use assistive devices.
✦ Emphasize the importance of regular checkups, including the eyes and ears.
✦ Tell the patient who's receiving etidronate to take this medication with fruit juice 2 hours before or after meals, to divide daily dosage to minimize adverse effects, and to watch for and report stomach cramps, diarrhea, fractures, and new or increased bone pain.
✦ Help the patient and his family make use of community support resources. For more information, refer them to the Paget Foundation.

Characteristics of rhabdomyolysis

+ Life-threatening disorder
+ Breakdown of muscle tissue
+ Usually follows muscle trauma
+ Can cause renal failure

Causes

+ Familial tendency
+ Strenuous exertion
+ Heat stroke

How it happens

+ Muscle trauma compresses tissue, causes ischemia, necrosis
+ Local edema further increases compartment pressure and tamponade
+ Blood vessels collapse, tissue hypoxia, muscle infarction, neural damage in area of fracture
+ Release of myoglobin from necrotic muscle fibers into circulation

Key signs and symptoms

+ Tenderness
+ Swelling and muscle weakness
+ Dark, reddish brown urine

Complications

+ Renal failure
+ Amputation if necrosis substantial

Diagnosis

+ Urine myoglobin level > 0.5 mg/dl
+ Elevated creatinine kinase level

Treatment

+ Treat underlying disorder
+ Prevent renal failure
+ Bed rest

RHABDOMYOLYSIS

Rhabdomyolysis, the breakdown of muscle tissue, may cause myoglobinuria, in which varying amounts of muscle protein (myoglobin) appear in the urine. Rhabdomyolysis usually follows major muscle trauma, especially a muscle crush injury. Long-distance running, certain severe infections, and exposure to electric shock can cause extensive muscle damage and excessive release of myoglobin. The prognosis is good if contributing causes are stopped or disease is checked before damage has progressed to an irreversible stage. Unchecked, it can cause renal failure.

CAUSES

Possible causes of rhabdomyolysis include familial tendency, strenuous exertion, infection, anesthetic agents (halothane) causing intraoperative rigidity, heat stroke, electrolyte disturbances, cardiac arrhythmias, and excessive muscular activity associated with status epilepticus, electroconvulsive therapy, or high-voltage electric shock.

PATHOPHYSIOLOGY

Muscle trauma that compresses tissue causes ischemia and necrosis. The ensuing local edema further increases compartment pressure and tamponade. Pressure from severe swelling causes blood vessels to collapse, leading to tissue hypoxia, muscle infarction, neural damage in the area of the fracture, and release of myoglobin from the necrotic muscle fibers into the circulation.

SIGNS AND SYMPTOMS

Signs and symptoms of rhabdomyolysis include tenderness, swelling, muscle weakness due to muscle trauma and pressure, and dark, reddish-brown urine from myoglobin.

COMPLICATIONS

Possible complications of rhabdomyolysis include renal failure as myoglobin is trapped in renal capillaries or tubules, and amputation if muscle necrosis is substantial.

DIAGNOSIS

Laboratory values that support the diagnosis include a urine myoglobin level greater than 0.5 mg/dl (evident with only 200 g of muscle damage); an elevated creatinine kinase level (0.5 to 0.95 mg/dl) due to muscle damage; elevated serum potassium, phosphate, creatinine, and creatine levels; hypocalcemia in early stages; and hypercalcemia in later stages.

Computed tomography scans, magnetic resonance imaging, and bone scintigraphy detect muscle necrosis. Intracompartmental venous pressure measurements are obtained by inserting a wick catheter, needle, or slit catheter into the muscle.

TREATMENT

Treatment of rhabdomyolysis may include treating the underlying disorder, preventing renal failure, bed rest, anti-inflammatory agents, corticosteroids (in extreme cases), analgesics for pain, and immediate fasciotomy and debridement (if compartment venous pressure is greater than 25 mm Hg).

NURSING CONSIDERATIONS

✦ Administer I.V. fluids and diuretics as ordered to reduce nephrotoxicity.
✦ To prevent rhabdomyolysis due to physical exertion, such as long-distance running, recommend prolonged, low-intensity training as opposed to short bursts of intense exercise.

SCOLIOSIS

Scoliosis is a lateral curvature of the thoracic, lumbar, or thoracolumbar spine. The curve may be convex to the right (more common in thoracic curves) or to the left (more common in lumbar curves). Rotation of the vertebral column around its axis may cause rib cage deformity. Scoliosis is commonly associated with kyphosis (humpback) and lordosis (swayback).

About 2% to 3% of adolescents have scoliosis. In general, the greater the magnitude of the curve and the younger the child is at the time of diagnosis, the greater the risk of progression of the spinal abnormality. Favorable outcomes are usually achieved with optimal treatment.

There are three categories of structural scoliosis. The first is *congenital,* which includes wedge vertebrae, fused ribs or vertebrae, or hemivertebrae. The second is *paralytic* or *musculoskeletal* scoliosis. This type develops several months after asymmetric paralysis of the trunk muscles due to polio, cerebral palsy, or muscular dystrophy. The third category is *idiopathic* scoliosis, which is the most common. It may be transmitted as an autosomal dominant or multifactorial trait and appears in a previously straight spine during the growing years.

Idiopathic scoliosis can be further classified according to age at onset. *Infantile* idiopathic scoliosis affects mostly male infants between birth and 3 years and causes left thoracic and right lumbar curves. *Juvenile* idiopathic scoliosis affects both genders between ages 4 and 10 and causes varying types of curvature. Lastly, *adolescent* idiopathic scoliosis generally affects girls from age 10 until skeletal maturity and causes varying types of curvature.

CAUSES

Functional causes of scoliosis include poor posture, a discrepancy in leg lengths, and a deformity of the spinal column that wasn't fixed (postural scoliosis). There's also a structural cause: A deformity of the vertebral bodies leads to the curvature.

PATHOPHYSIOLOGY

Differential stress on vertebral bone causes an imbalance of osteoblastic activity; thus the curve progresses rapidly during the adolescent growth spurt. Without treatment, the imbalance continues into adulthood.

SIGNS AND SYMPTOMS

Scoliosis rarely produces subjective symptoms until it's well established. When symptoms occur, they include backache, fatigue, and dyspnea.

The most common curve in functional or structural scoliosis arises in the thoracic segment, with convexity to the right and compensatory curves (S curves) in

Key nursing actions
✦ Administer I.V. fluids and diuretics as ordered.
✦ To prevent rhabdomyolysis due to physical exertion recommend prolonged, low-intensity training.

Characteristics of scoliosis
✦ Lateral curvature of thoracic, lumbar, or thoracolumbar spine
✦ Curve may be convex to right or left
✦ Rotation of vertebral column around axis may cause rib cage deformity
✦ Commonly associated with kyphosis, lordosis
✦ Three categories: congenital, paralytic, idiopathic
✦ Idiopathic further classified according to age at onset: infantile, juvenile, adolescent

Causes
✦ Poor posture
✦ Discrepancy in leg lengths
✦ Deformity of spinal column or vertebral bodies

How it happens
✦ Stress on vertebral bone causes imbalance of osteoblastic activity
✦ Curve progresses rapidly during adolescent growth spurt

Key signs and symptoms
✦ Rarely produces subjective symptoms until well established
✦ Backache, fatigue, and dyspnea
✦ Unequal shoulder heights, elbow levels, heights of iliac crests
✦ Asymmetric thoracic cage

the cervical and lumbar segments, both with convexity to the left. As the spine curves laterally, compensatory curves develop to maintain body balance. Subtle signs include uneven hemlines or pant legs that appear unequal in length and one hip that appears higher than the other.

Physical examination shows unequal shoulder heights, elbow levels, and heights of iliac crests; asymmetric thoracic cage and misalignment of the spinal vertebrae when the patient bends over; asymmetric paraspinal muscles, rounded on the convex side of the curve and flattened on the concave side; and asymmetric gait.

COMPLICATIONS

Without treatment, curves greater than 40 degrees progress. Untreated scoliosis may result in pulmonary insufficiency (curvature may decrease lung capacity), back pain, degenerative arthritis of the spine, vertebral disk disease, and sciatica.

DIAGNOSIS

Diagnosis of scoliosis includes anterior, posterior, and lateral spinal X-rays, taken with the patient standing upright and bending. These confirm scoliosis and determine the degree of curvature (Cobb method) and flexibility of the spine. A scoliometer is used to measure the angle of trunk rotation.

TREATMENT

The severity of the deformity and potential spine growth determine appropriate treatment, which may include close observation, exercise, brace, surgery, or a combination of these treatments.

To be most effective, treatment should begin early, when spinal deformity is still subtle. For a curve less than 25 degrees, or mild scoliosis, treatment includes X-rays to monitor curve, an examination every 3 months, and an exercise program to strengthen torso muscles and prevent curve progression.

For a curve of 30 to 50 degrees, spinal exercises, transcutaneous electrical stimulation (alternative therapy), and a brace (may halt progression but doesn't reverse the established curvature) can be used. Braces can be adjusted as the patient grows and worn until bone growth is complete.

A lateral curve continues to progress at the rate of 1 degree per year even after skeletal maturity. For a curve of 40 degrees or more, treatment includes surgery (supportive instrumentation, with spinal fusion in severe cases) and periodic postoperative checkups for several months to monitor the stability of the correction.

NURSING CONSIDERATIONS

Scoliosis commonly affects adolescent girls, who are likely to be distressed by limitations on their activities and treatment with orthopedic appliances. Therefore, it's important to provide emotional support in addition to meticulous skin and cast care and patient teaching.

If the patient needs a brace
✦ Enlist the help of a physical therapist, a social worker, and an orthotist. Before the patient goes home, explain what the brace does and how to care for it (how to check the screws for tightness and pad the uprights to prevent excessive wear on clothing). Suggest that loose-fitting, oversized clothes be worn for greater comfort.
✦ Tell the patient to wear the brace 23 hours per day and to remove it only for bathing and exercise. While she's still adjusting to the brace, tell her to lie down and rest several times per day.

Complications
✦ Pulmonary insufficiency
✦ Back pain
✦ Degenerative arthritis of spine
✦ Vertebral disk disease
✦ Sciatica

Diagnosis
✦ Anterior, posterior, lateral spinal X-rays with patient standing upright and bending
✦ Scoliometer used to measure angle of trunk rotation

Treatment
✦ Close observation
✦ Exercise
✦ Brace
✦ Surgery
✦ Combination of treatments

◆ Suggest a soft mattress if a firm one is uncomfortable.

◆ To prevent skin breakdown, advise the patient not to use lotions, ointments, or powders on areas where the brace contacts the skin. Tell her to keep the skin dry and clean and to wear a snug T-shirt under the brace.

◆ Advise the patient to increase activities gradually and avoid vigorous sports. Emphasize the importance of conscientiously performing prescribed exercises. Recommend swimming during the 1 hour out of the brace but strongly warn against diving.

◆ Instruct the patient to turn her whole body, instead of just her head, when looking to the side. To make reading easier, tell her to hold the book so she can look straight ahead at it instead of down. If she finds this difficult, help her to obtain prism glasses.

If the patient needs traction or a cast before surgery

◆ Explain these procedures to the patient and her family. Remember that application of a body cast can be traumatic because it's placed on a special frame and the patient's head and face are covered throughout the procedure.

◆ Check the skin around the cast edge daily. Keep the cast clean and dry and the edges of the cast petaled. Warn the patient not to insert or let anything get under the cast and to immediately report cracks in the cast, pain, burning, skin breakdown, numbness, or odor.

◆ Before surgery, assure the patient and family that she'll have adequate pain control postoperatively.

After corrective surgery

◆ Check sensation, movement, color, and blood supply in all extremities every 2 to 4 hours for the first 48 hours and then several times per day for signs of neurovascular deficit, a serious complication after spinal surgery. Logroll the patient often.

◆ Measure intake, output, and urine specific gravity to monitor effects of blood loss, which is usually substantial.

◆ Monitor abdominal distention and bowel sounds.

◆ Encourage deep-breathing exercises to avoid pulmonary complications.

◆ Medicate for pain, especially before activity.

◆ Promote active ROM arm exercises to help maintain muscle strength. Remember that any exercise, even brushing the hair or teeth, is helpful. Encourage the patient to perform quadriceps-setting, calf-pumping, and active ROM exercises of ankles and feet.

◆ Watch for skin breakdown and signs of cast syndrome, such as nausea, abdominal pressure, and vague abdominal pain.

◆ Remove antiembolism stockings for at least 30 minutes daily.

◆ Offer emotional support to help prevent depression that may result from altered body image and immobility. Encourage the patient to wear her own clothes, wash her hair, and use makeup.

◆ If the patient is being discharged with a Harrington rod and cast and must have bed rest, arrange for a social worker and a visiting nurse to provide home care. Before discharge, check with the surgeon about activity limitations, and make sure the patient understands them.

◆ If you work in a school, screen children routinely for scoliosis during physical examinations.

Key nursing actions

If the patient needs a brace

◆ Enlist the help of a physical therapist, a social worker, and an orthotist.

◆ Tell the patient to wear the brace 23 hours per day and to remove it only for bathing and exercise.

◆ To prevent skin breakdown, advise the patient not to use lotions, ointments, or powders on areas where the brace contacts the skin.

◆ Advise the patient to increase activities gradually and avoid vigorous sports.

If the patient needs traction or a cast before surgery

◆ Explain these procedures to the patient and her family.

◆ Check the skin around the cast edge daily.

After corrective surgery

◆ Check sensation, movement, color, and blood supply in all extremities every 2 to 4 hours for the first 48 hours and then several times per day.

◆ Measure intake, output, and urine specific gravity to monitor effects of blood loss.

◆ Offer emotional support to help prevent depression that may result from altered body image and immobility.

◆ If the patient is being discharged with a Harrington rod and cast and must have bed rest, arrange for a social worker and a visiting nurse to provide home care.

Hematologic system

Key facts about the hematologic system
+ Blood is a major body tissue
+ Plasma factors and platelets control clotting
+ Erythrocytes carry oxygen; remove carbon dioxide
+ Leukocytes act in inflammatory and immune responses
+ Plasma carries antibodies and nutrients to tissues and carries away waste
+ Hematopoiesis occurs primarily in marrow
+ Average person has 5 to 6 L of circulating blood

Blood, although a fluid, is one of the body's major tissues. It continuously circulates through the heart and blood vessels, carrying vital elements to every part of the body.

Blood performs several vital functions through its special components: the liquid protein (plasma) and the formed constituents (erythrocytes, leukocytes, and thrombocytes) suspended in it. Erythrocytes (red blood cells [RBCs]) carry oxygen to the tissues and remove carbon dioxide. Leukocytes (white blood cells [WBCs]) act in inflammatory and immune responses. Plasma (a clear, straw-colored fluid) carries antibodies and nutrients to tissues and carries away waste. Plasma coagulation factors and thrombocytes (platelets) control clotting.

Hematopoiesis, the process of blood formation, occurs primarily in the marrow. There, primitive blood cells (stem cells) differentiate into the precursors of erythrocytes (normoblasts), leukocytes, and thrombocytes.

The average person has 5 to 6 L of circulating blood, which constitutes 5% to 7% of body weight (as much as 10% in premature neonates). Blood is three to five times more viscous than water, has an arterial pH of 7.35 to 7.45, and is either bright red (arterial blood) or dark red (venous blood), depending on the degree of oxygen saturation and the hemoglobin level.

Pathophysiologic changes
+ Bone marrow cells particularly vulnerable to physiologic changes
+ Disease can affect structure or concentration of any hematologic cell

PATHOPHYSIOLOGIC CHANGES

Bone marrow cells reproduce rapidly and have a short life span, and the storage of circulating cells in the marrow is minimal. Thus, bone marrow cells and their precursors are particularly vulnerable to physiologic changes that affect cell production. Disease can affect the structure or concentration of any hematologic cell.

Erythropoiesis

The tissues' demand for oxygen and the blood cells' ability to deliver it regulate red blood cell (RBC) production. Lack of oxygen in the tissues (hypoxia) stimulates RBC production, which triggers the formation and release of the hormone erythropoietin. In turn, erythropoietin, 90% of which is produced by the kidneys and 10% by the liver, activates bone marrow to produce RBCs. Androgens may also stimulate erythropoiesis, which accounts for higher RBC counts in men.

The formation of an erythrocyte (RBC) begins with an uncommitted stem cell that may eventually develop into an RBC or white blood cell. Such formation requires certain vitamins — B_{12} and folic acid — and minerals — copper, cobalt, and especially iron, which is vital to hemoglobin's oxygen-carrying capacity. Iron is obtained from various foods and is absorbed in the duodenum and jejunum. An excess of iron is temporarily stored in reticuloendothelial cells, especially those in the liver, as ferritin and hemosiderin until it's released for use in the bone marrow to form new RBCs.

HEMOGLOBIN

The protein hemoglobin is the major component of the RBC. Hemoglobin consists of an iron-containing molecule (heme) bound to the protein globulin. Oxygen binds to the heme component and is transported throughout the body and released to the cells. The hemoglobin picks up carbon dioxide and hydrogen ions from the cells and delivers them to the lungs, where they're released.

Various mutations or abnormalities in the hemoglobin protein can cause abnormal oxygen transport.

RED BLOOD CELLS

RBC disorders may be quantitative or qualitative. A deficiency of RBCs (anemia) can follow a condition that destroys or inhibits the formation of these cells. (See *Erythropoiesis.*)

Common factors leading to anemia include drugs, toxins, ionizing radiation, congenital or acquired defects that cause bone marrow to stop producing new RBCs (aplasia) and generally suppress production of all blood cells (hematopoiesis, aplastic anemia). Other factors include metabolic abnormalities (sideroblastic anemia); deficiency of vitamins (vitamin B_{12} deficiency, or pernicious anemia) or minerals (iron, folic acid, copper, and cobalt deficiency anemias) leading to inadequate erythropoiesis; excessive chronic or acute blood loss (posthemorrhagic anemia); chronic illnesses, such as renal disease, cancer, and chronic infections; and intrinsically (sickle cell anemia) or extrinsically (hemolytic transfusion reaction) defective RBCs.

Decreased plasma volume can cause a relative excess of RBCs. The few conditions characterized by excessive production of RBCs include abnormal proliferation of all bone marrow cells (polycythemia vera) and an abnormality of a single element (such as erythropoietin excess caused by hypoxemia or pulmonary disease).

LEUKOCYTOSIS

Leukocytosis is an elevation in the number of WBCs. All types of WBCs — or only one type — may be increased. (See *WBC types and functions,* page 438.)

Erythropoiesis

✦ Low oxygen stimulates RBC production
✦ RBC production triggers release of erythropoietin
✦ Erythropoietin activates bone marrow to produce RBCs

Hemoglobin

✦ Mutations or abnormalities can cause abnormal oxygen transport

RBCs

✦ Disorders may be quantitative or qualitative
✦ Anemia caused by drugs, toxins, ionizing radiation, congenital or acquired defects, metabolic abnormalities, vitamin or mineral deficiency, excessive blood loss, chronic illnesses, defective RBCs
✦ Decreased plasma volume can cause relative excess of RBCs

Leukocytosis

✦ Elevation in number of WBCs
✦ Normal response to infection or inflammation
✦ WBCs also increased by temperature, emotional disturbances, anesthesia, surgery, strenuous exercise, pregnancy, drugs, hormones, toxins
✦ Occurs in malignancies and bone marrow disorders

WBC types and functions

- Protect body against harmful bacteria or infection
- Classified as granular or non-granular leukocytes
- Neutrophils: predominant form of granulocyte; devour invading organisms
- Eosinophils: minor granulocytes; defend against parasites, lung and skin infections, act in allergic reactions
- Basophils: minor granulocytes; release heparin and histamine
- Monocytes: help devour invaders; process antigens for lymphocytes, form microphages in tissues
- Lymphocytes: occur as B cells and T cells; produce humoral antibodies; reject foreign cells, cell products
- Plasma cells: develop from lymphoblasts, reside in tissues, produce antibodies

Leukopenia

- Deficiency of WBCs
- Caused by disease, prolonged stress, radiation or chemotherapy
- Increases risk of infectious illness

Thrombocytosis

- Excess of circulating platelets to greater than 400,000/µl

Primary thrombocytosis
- Number of megakaryocytes increased and platelet count is > 1 million/µl
- May result from abnormality of platelet function and increased platelet mass
- May accompany polycythemia vera or chronic granulocytic leukemia

WBC types and functions

White blood cells (WBCs), or leukocytes, protect the body against harmful bacteria and infection. WBCs are classified as granular leukocytes (basophils, neutrophils, and eosinophils) or nongranular leukocytes (lymphocytes, monocytes, and plasma cells). WBCs are usually produced in bone marrow; lymphocytes and plasma cells are produced in lymphoid tissue as well. Neutrophils have a circulating half-life of less than 6 hours, while some lymphocytes may survive for weeks or months. Normally, WBCs number between 5,000 and 10,000 µl. There are six types of WBCs:

- Neutrophils—The predominant form of granulocyte, they make up about 60% of WBCs and help devour invading organisms by phagocytosis.
- Eosinophils—Minor granulocytes, they may defend against parasites and lung and skin infections and act in allergic reactions. They account for 1% to 5% of the total WBC count.

- Basophils—Minor granulocytes, they may release heparin and histamine into the blood and participate in delayed hypersensitivity reactions. They account for 0% to 1% of the total WBC count.
- Monocytes—Along with neutrophils, they help devour invading organisms by phagocytosis. Monocytes help process antigens for lymphocytes and form macrophages in the tissues. They account for 1% to 6% of the total WBC count.
- Lymphocytes—They occur as B cells and T cells. B cells form lymphoid follicles, produce humoral antibodies, and help T-cell mediated delayed hypersensitivity reactions and the rejection of foreign cells or cell products. Lymphocytes account for 20% to 40% of the total WBC count.
- Plasma cells—They develop from lymphoblasts, reside in the tissue, and produce antibodies.

Leukocytosis is a normal physiologic response to infection or inflammation. Other factors, such as temperature changes, emotional disturbances, anesthesia, surgery, strenuous exercise, pregnancy, and some drugs, hormones, and toxins, can also cause leukocytosis. Abnormal leukocytosis occurs in malignancies and bone marrow disorders.

LEUKOPENIA

Leukopenia is a deficiency of WBCs—all types or only one type. It can be caused by several conditions or diseases, such as human immunodeficiency virus (HIV) infection, prolonged stress, bone marrow disease or destruction, radiation or chemotherapy, lupus erythematosus, leukemia, thyroid disease, or Cushing's syndrome. Because WBCs fight infection, leukopenia increases the risk of infectious illness.

THROMBOCYTOSIS

Thrombocytosis is an excess of circulating platelets to greater than 400,000/µl and may be primary or secondary.

Primary thrombocytosis

In primary thrombocytosis, the number of platelet precursor cells, called *megakaryocytes*, is increased and the platelet count is greater than 1 million/µl. The condition may result from an intrinsic abnormality of platelet function and increased platelet mass. It may accompany polycythemia vera or chronic granulocytic leukemia.

Stroke

WHAT IS STROKE?

Stroke, or cerebrovascular accident, is the sudden death of brain tissue caused by a lack of oxygen resulting from an interrupted blood supply. An *infarct* is the area of the brain that has died because of this lack of oxygen.

There are two ways that brain tissue death can occur:

◆ Ischemic stroke, the most common cause of infarct, is a blockage or reduction of blood flow in an artery that feeds that area of the brain.

◆ Hemorrhagic stroke results from bleeding within and around the brain that causes compression and tissue injury.

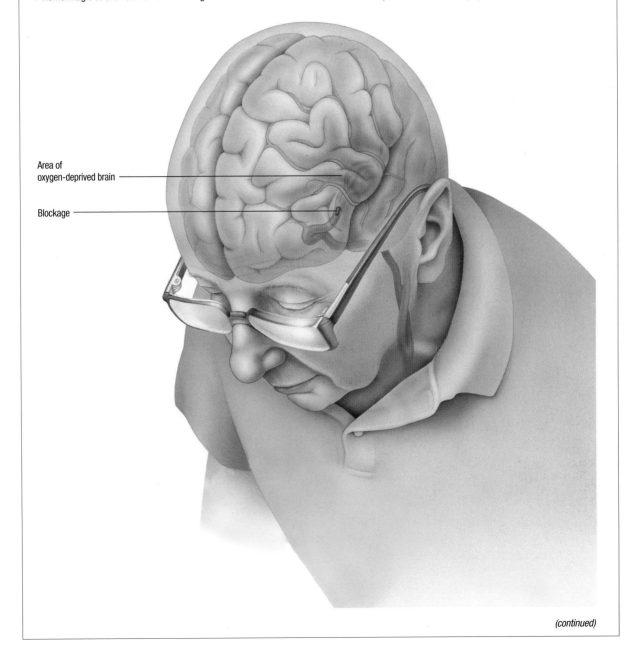

Area of
oxygen-deprived brain

Blockage

(continued)

Stroke *(continued)*

ISCHEMIC STROKE

Ischemic stroke results from a blockage or reduction of blood flow to an area of the brain. This blockage may result from atherosclerosis or blood clot formation.

Atherosclerosis is the deposit of cholesterol and plaque within the walls of the arteries. These deposits may become large enough to narrow the lumen and reduce the flow of blood while also causing the artery to lose its ability to stretch.

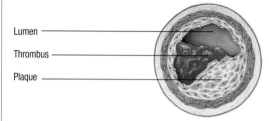

Lumen
Thrombus
Plaque

A **thrombus,** or blood clot, forms on the roughened surface of atherosclerotic plaques that develop in the wall of the artery. The thrombus can enlarge and eventually block the artery lumen.

Part of a thrombus may break off and become an **embolus**. An embolus travels through the bloodstream and may block smaller arteries. Emboli commonly come from the heart, where different conditions can cause thrombus formation.

COMMON SITES OF PLAQUE FORMATION

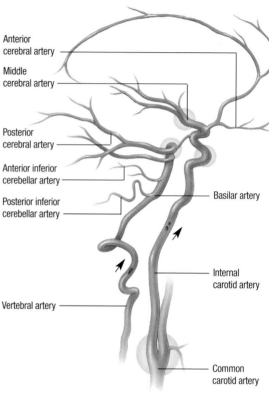

Anterior cerebral artery

Middle cerebral artery

Posterior cerebral artery

Anterior inferior cerebellar artery

Posterior inferior cerebellar artery

Basilar artery

Internal carotid artery

Vertebral artery

Common carotid artery

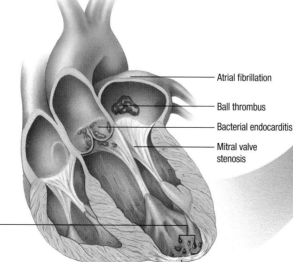

Atrial fibrillation

Ball thrombus

Bacterial endocarditis

Mitral valve stenosis

Embolus

Mural thrombi

Myocardial infarction

HEMORRHAGIC STROKE

Hemorrhagic stroke is caused by bleeding within and around the brain. Bleeding that fills the spaces between the brain and the skull is called a *subarachnoid hemorrhage* and is caused by ruptured aneurysms, arteriovenous malformation (AVM), and head trauma. Bleeding within the brain tissue itself is known as *intracerebral hemorrhage* and is primarily caused by hypertension.

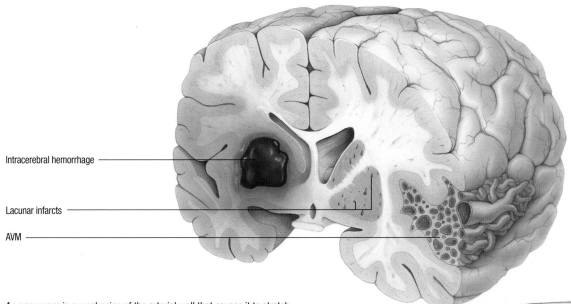

An **aneurysm** is a weakening of the arterial wall that causes it to stretch and balloon. It usually occurs where the artery branches.

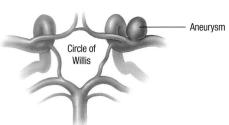

Hypertension is an elevation of blood pressure that may cause tiny arterioles to burst in the brain. Blood released inside brain tissue puts pressure on adjacent arterioles, causing them to burst and leading to more bleeding. Hypertension may also cause lacunar infarcts. These are miniature infarcts similar to complete strokes, but on a much smaller scale. They occur within the nuclei and spinal tracts of the brain and resemble little lakes or pits.

An **AVM** is an abnormality of the brain's blood vessels in which arteries lead directly into veins without first going through a capillary bed. The pressure of the blood coming through the arteries is too high for the veins, causing them to dilate in order to transport the higher volume of blood. This dilation can cause them to rupture.

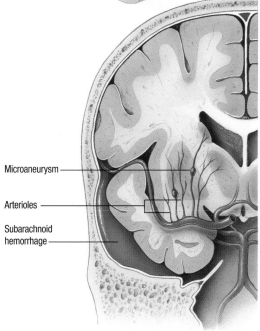

(continued)

Stroke (continued)

NORMAL FUNCTIONAL AREAS OF THE BRAIN

The brain has two sides: a right hemisphere that controls the left side of the body and a left hemisphere that controls the right side of the body. Each hemisphere has four lobes and a cerebellum that control our daily functions. Depending on what part of the brain has been affected, stroke victims experience many neurologic deficits. Rehabilitation is crucial to recovery. Physical therapists and speech therapists help patients relearn their lost functions and devise ways to cope with the loss of those they can't regain.

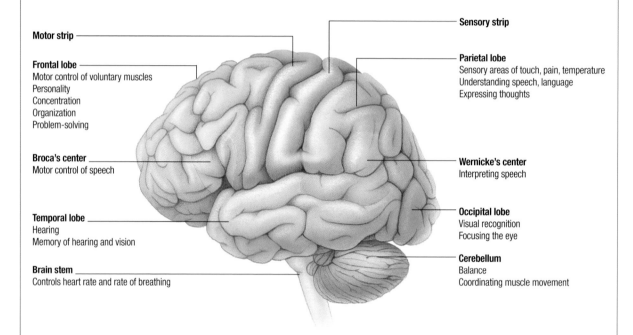

Motor strip

Frontal lobe
Motor control of voluntary muscles
Personality
Concentration
Organization
Problem-solving

Broca's center
Motor control of speech

Temporal lobe
Hearing
Memory of hearing and vision

Brain stem
Controls heart rate and rate of breathing

Sensory strip

Parietal lobe
Sensory areas of touch, pain, temperature
Understanding speech, language
Expressing thoughts

Wernicke's center
Interpreting speech

Occipital lobe
Visual recognition
Focusing the eye

Cerebellum
Balance
Coordinating muscle movement

COMMON NEUROLOGIC DEFICITS AFTER STROKE

Left-sided stroke	Right-sided stroke	Related terms
■ Right-sided paralysis	■ Left-sided paralysis	**Paralysis**
■ Speech and language deficits	■ Spatial and perceptual deficits	Loss of muscle function and sensation
■ Slow, cautious behavior	■ Quick, impulsive behavior	**Hemiparesis**
■ Hemianopsia of right visual field	■ Hemianopsia of left visual field	Weakness of muscles on one side of body
■ Memory loss in language	■ Memory loss in performance	**Hemianopsia**
■ Right-sided dysarthria	■ Left-sided dysarthria	Loss of sight in one-half of visual field
■ Aphasia		**Aphasia**
■ Apraxia		Inability to understand or produce language
		Apraxia
		Inability to control muscles; uncoordinated, jerky movements
		Dysarthria
		Slurring of speech and mouth droop on one side of the face due to muscle weakness

Acquired immunodeficiency syndrome

Human immunodeficiency virus (HIV) infection may cause acquired immunodeficiency syndrome (AIDS). The resulting immunodeficiency makes the patient susceptible to opportunistic infection, cancers, and other abnormalities that define AIDS.

MANIFESTATIONS OF HIV INFECTION AND AIDS

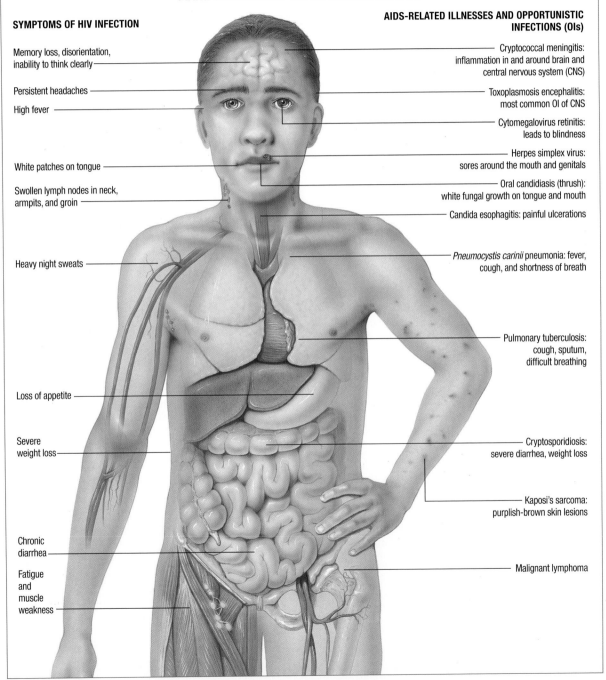

SYMPTOMS OF HIV INFECTION

Memory loss, disorientation, inability to think clearly

Persistent headaches

High fever

White patches on tongue

Swollen lymph nodes in neck, armpits, and groin

Heavy night sweats

Loss of appetite

Severe weight loss

Chronic diarrhea

Fatigue and muscle weakness

AIDS-RELATED ILLNESSES AND OPPORTUNISTIC INFECTIONS (OIs)

Cryptococcal meningitis: inflammation in and around brain and central nervous system (CNS)

Toxoplasmosis encephalitis: most common OI of CNS

Cytomegalovirus retinitis: leads to blindness

Herpes simplex virus: sores around the mouth and genitals

Oral candidiasis (thrush): white fungal growth on tongue and mouth

Candida esophagitis: painful ulcerations

Pneumocystis carinii pneumonia: fever, cough, and shortness of breath

Pulmonary tuberculosis: cough, sputum, difficult breathing

Cryptosporidiosis: severe diarrhea, weight loss

Kaposi's sarcoma: purplish-brown skin lesions

Malignant lymphoma

Anaphylaxis

An anaphylactic reaction requires previous sensitization or exposure to the specific antigen. The pathophysiology of anaphylaxis is described here.

1. RESPONSE TO ANTIGEN
Immunoglobulins (Ig) M and G recognize and bind to the antigen.

Complement cascade =

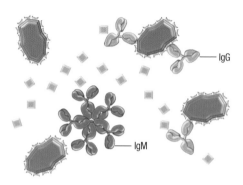

2. RELEASE OF CHEMICAL MEDIATORS
Activated IgE on basophils promotes the release of mediators: histamine, serotonin, and leukotrienes.

Histamine   = **H**
Serotonin   = ◆
Leukotrienes = ❖

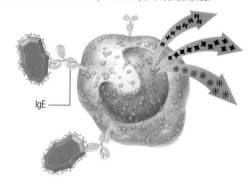

3. INTENSIFIED RESPONSE
Mast cells release more histamine and eosinophil chemotactic factor of anaphylaxis (ECF-A), which create venule-weakening lesions.

ECF-A   = ◗
Histamine = **H**

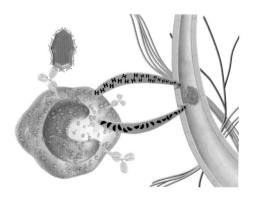

4. RESPIRATORY DISTRESS

In the lungs, histamine causes endothelial cell destruction and fluid leak into alveoli.

Leukotrienes = ✷
Histamine   = **H**

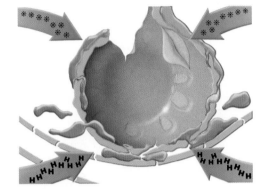

5. DETERIORATION

Meanwhile, mediators increase vascular permeability, causing fluid leak from the vessels.

Bradykinin   = ●
Histamine   = **H**
Prostaglandins = ✚
Serotonin   = ◆

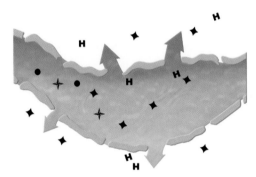

6. FAILURE OF COMPENSATORY MECHANISMS

Endothelial cell damage causes basophils and mast cells to release heparin and mediator-neutralizing substances. However, anaphylaxis is now irreversible.

Heparin   = ▲
Leukotrienes = ✷

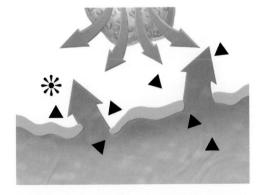

Rheumatoid arthritis

Rheumatoid arthritis is a chronic, systemic inflammatory disease that primarily attacks peripheral joints and the surrounding muscles, tendons, ligaments, and blood vessels.

JOINTS TYPICALLY AFFECTED BY RHEUMATOID ARTHRITIS

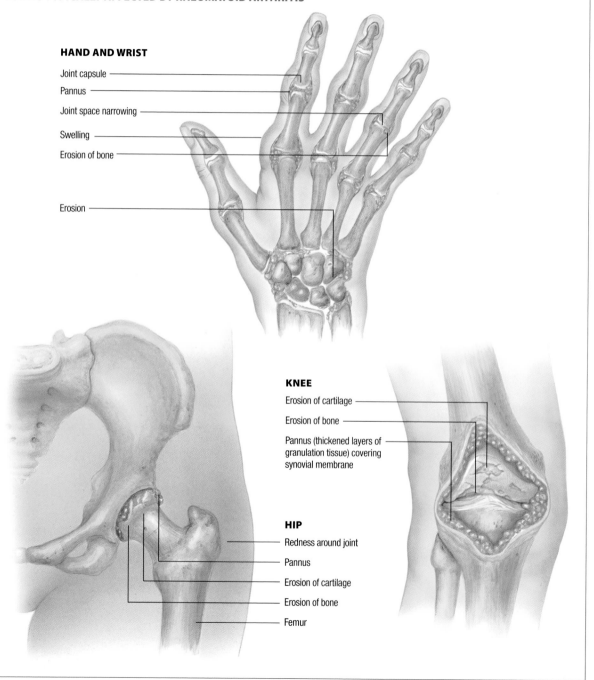

HAND AND WRIST

Joint capsule
Pannus
Joint space narrowing
Swelling
Erosion of bone

Erosion

KNEE

Erosion of cartilage
Erosion of bone
Pannus (thickened layers of granulation tissue) covering synovial membrane

HIP

Redness around joint
Pannus
Erosion of cartilage
Erosion of bone
Femur

In the presence of thrombocytosis, both hemorrhage and thrombosis may occur. This paradox occurs because accelerated clotting results in a generalized activation of prothrombin and a consequent excess of thrombin clots in the microcirculation. This process consumes exorbitant amounts of coagulation factors and thereby increases the risk of hemorrhage.

Secondary thrombocytosis

Secondary thrombocytosis is a result of an underlying cause, such as stress, exercise, hemorrhage, or hemolytic anemia. Stress and exercise release stored platelets from the spleen. Hemorrhage or hemolytic anemia signals the bone marrow to produce more megakaryocytes.

Thrombocytosis may also occur after a splenectomy. Because the spleen is the primary site of platelet storage and destruction, platelet count may rise after its removal until the bone marrow begins producing fewer platelets.

▼ *LIFE-THREATENING DISORDER*

ANEMIA, APLASTIC

Aplastic, or hypoplastic, anemia results from injury to or destruction of stem cells in bone marrow or the bone marrow matrix, causing pancytopenia (anemia, leukopenia, and thrombocytopenia) and bone marrow hypoplasia. Although used interchangeably with other terms for bone marrow failure, aplastic anemia properly refers to pancytopenia resulting from the decreased functional capacity of a hypoplastic, fatty bone marrow.

These disorders generally produce fatal bleeding or infection, especially when they're idiopathic or if they're caused by chloramphenicol (Chloromycetin) use or infectious hepatitis. The death rate for severe aplastic anemia is 80% to 90%.

CAUSES

About one-half of aplastic anemias result from drugs (antibiotics and anticonvulsants), toxic agents (such as benzene and chloramphenicol), or radiation. The rest may result from immunologic factors (unconfirmed), severe disease (especially hepatitis), or preleukemic and neoplastic infiltration of bone marrow.

Idiopathic anemias may be congenital. Two such forms of aplastic anemia have been identified: congenital hypoplastic anemia (Blackfan-Diamond anemia) develops between ages 2 and 3 months; Fanconi's syndrome develops between birth and age 10.

PATHOPHYSIOLOGY

Aplastic anemia usually develops when damaged or destroyed stem cells inhibit blood cell production. Less commonly, it develops when damaged bone marrow microvasculature creates an unfavorable environment for cell growth and maturation.

SIGNS AND SYMPTOMS

Signs and symptoms of aplastic anemia vary with the severity of pancytopenia but develop insidiously in many cases. They may include progressive weakness and fatigue, shortness of breath, headache, pallor, and ultimately tachycardia and heart failure due to hypoxia and increased venous return.

Thrombocytosis
Secondary thrombocytosis
+ Result of underlying cause, such as stress, exercise, hemorrhage, or hemolytic anemia

Characteristics of aplastic anemia
+ Life-threatening disorder
+ Results from injury to or destruction of stem cells in bone marrow or matrix
+ Pancytopenia resulting from decreased functional capacity of hypoplastic, fatty bone marrow
+ Generally produces fatal bleeding or infection
+ Death rate for severe cases: 80% to 90%

Causes
+ One-half result from drugs, toxic agents, radiation
+ Rest may result from immunologic factors, severe disease, preleukemic and neoplastic infiltration of bone marrow
+ Two congenital forms: congenital hypoplastic anemia, Fanconi's syndrome

How it happens
+ Damaged or destroyed stem cells inhibit blood cell production
+ Damaged bone marrow creates poor environment for cell growth and maturation

Key signs and symptoms
+ Vary with severity
+ Weakness and fatigue
+ Shortness of breath
+ Headache
+ Pallor

Thrombocytopenia leads to ecchymosis, petechiae, and hemorrhage, especially from the mucous membranes (nose, gums, rectum, vagina) or into the retina or central nervous system.

Neutropenia (neutrophil deficiency) may lead to infection (fever, oral and rectal ulcers, sore throat) without characteristic inflammation.

COMPLICATIONS

Life-threatening hemorrhage from the mucous membranes is the most common complication of aplastic or hypoplastic anemias because affected patients develop autoimmunization, which can make platelet transfusions ineffective. Immunosuppression can lead to secondary opportunistic infections.

DIAGNOSIS

Confirmation requires a series of laboratory tests. A total count of 1 million/µl or fewer RBCs of normal color and size (normochromic and normocytic) is seen. RBCs may be macrocytic (larger than normal) and anisocytotic (excessive variation in size). Absolute reticulocyte count is very low. An elevated serum iron level (unless bleeding occurs), normal or slightly reduced total iron-binding capacity, presence of hemosiderin (a derivative of hemoglobin), and microscopically visible tissue iron storage are present. Platelet, neutrophil, and lymphocyte counts fall.

Coagulation test results (bleeding time), reflecting decreased platelet count, are abnormal. Bone marrow aspiration at several sites may yield a "dry tap" (no cells) and biopsy will show severely hypocellular or aplastic marrow, with varied amounts of fat, fibrous tissue, or gelatinous replacement; absence of tagged iron (because iron is deposited in the liver rather than bone marrow) and megakaryocytes (platelet precursors); and depression of RBCs and precursors (erythroid elements).

Differential diagnosis must rule out paroxysmal nocturnal hemoglobinuria and other diseases in which pancytopenia is common.

TREATMENT

Effective treatment must eliminate an identifiable cause and provide vigorous supportive measures, including packed RBC or platelet transfusion, and experimental histocompatibility locus antigen-matched leukocyte transfusions. Bone marrow transplantation is the treatment of choice for anemia due to severe aplasia and for patients who need constant RBC transfusions.

For patients with leukopenia, special measures are needed to prevent infection, such as avoidance of exposure to communicable diseases and diligent hand washing. The patient may receive specific antibiotics for infection; however, these aren't given prophylactically because they encourage resistant strains of organisms.

Respiratory support with oxygen in addition to blood transfusions may be given to patients with low hemoglobin levels. Other appropriate treatments include corticosteroids to stimulate erythropoiesis; marrow-stimulating agents such as androgens (controversial); antilymphocyte globulin (experimental); immunosuppressive agents (if the patient doesn't respond to other therapy); and colony-stimulating factors to encourage growth of specific cellular components.

NURSING CONSIDERATIONS

♦ If the platelet count is low (less than 20,000/µl), prevent bleeding by avoiding I.M. injections, suggesting the use of an electric razor and a soft toothbrush, humidifying oxygen to prevent drying of mucous membranes, avoiding enemas and

Complications
♦ Life-threatening hemorrhage from mucous membranes
♦ Secondary opportunistic infections

Diagnosis
♦ RBCs < 1 million/µl
♦ Absolute reticulocyte count very low
♦ Elevated serum iron level
♦ Low platelet, neutrophil, and lymphocyte counts
♦ Coagulation test results abnormal (decreased platelet count)
♦ Bone marrow aspiration yields no cells
♦ Severely hypocellular or aplastic marrow

Treatment
♦ Eliminate identifiable cause
♦ Packed RBC or platelet transfusion
♦ Experimental histocompatibility locus antigen-matched leukocyte transfusions
♦ Bone marrow transplantation
♦ Infection prevention
♦ Respiratory support
♦ Corticosteroids

rectal temperatures, and promoting regular bowel movements through the use of a stool softener and a proper diet to prevent constipation. Also, apply pressure to venipuncture sites until bleeding stops. Detect bleeding early by checking for blood in urine and stools and assessing skin for petechiae.

✦ Take safety precautions to prevent falls, which could lead to prolonged bleeding or hemorrhage.

✦ Help prevent infection by washing your hands thoroughly before entering the patient's room, by making sure the patient is receiving a nutritious diet (high in vitamins and proteins) to improve his resistance, and by encouraging meticulous mouth and perianal care.

✦ Watch for life-threatening hemorrhage, infection, adverse effects of drug therapy, or blood transfusion reaction. Make sure routine throat, urine, nose, rectal, and blood cultures are done regularly and correctly to check for infection. Teach the patient to recognize signs of infection, and tell him to report them immediately.

✦ If the patient has a low hemoglobin level that causes fatigue, schedule frequent rest periods. Administer oxygen therapy as needed. If blood transfusions are necessary, assess for a transfusion reaction by checking the patient's temperature and watching for the development of other signs and symptoms, such as rash, hives, itching, back pain, restlessness, and shaking chills.

✦ Reassure and support the patient and his family by explaining the disease and its treatment, particularly if the patient has recurring acute episodes. Explain the purpose of all prescribed drugs and discuss possible adverse effects, including which ones he should report promptly. Encourage the patient who doesn't require hospitalization to continue his normal lifestyle, with appropriate restrictions (such as regular rest periods), until remission occurs.

✦ To prevent aplastic anemia, monitor blood studies carefully in the patient receiving anemia-inducing drugs.

✦ Support efforts to educate the public about the hazards of toxic agents. Tell parents to keep toxic agents out of the reach of children. Encourage people who work with radiation to wear protective clothing and a radiation-detecting badge and to observe plant safety precautions. Those who work with benzene (solvent) should know that 10 parts per million is the highest safe environmental level and that a delayed reaction to benzene may develop.

ANEMIA, IRON DEFICIENCY

Iron deficiency anemia is a disorder of oxygen transport in which hemoglobin synthesis is deficient. A common disease worldwide, iron deficiency anemia affects 10% to 30% of the adult population in the United States. Iron deficiency anemia occurs most commonly in premenopausal women, infants (particularly premature or low-birth-weight infants), children, and adolescents (especially girls). The prognosis after replacement therapy is favorable.

CAUSES

Possible causes of iron deficiency anemia include inadequate dietary intake of iron (less than 1 to 2 mg/day), as in prolonged nonsupplemented breast-feeding or bottle-feeding of infants or during periods of stress, such as rapid growth in children and adolescents; iron malabsorption, as in chronic diarrhea, partial or total gastrectomy, and malabsorption syndromes, such as celiac disease and pernicious anemia; and blood loss due to drug-induced GI bleeding (from anticoagulants, aspirin, steroids) or heavy menses, hemorrhage from trauma, peptic ulcers, cancer, in-

Key nursing actions

✦ If the platelet count is low, prevent bleeding.

✦ Check for blood in urine and stool.

✦ Take safety precautions to prevent falls.

✦ Help prevent infection.

✦ Watch for life-threatening hemorrhage, infection, adverse effects of drug therapy, or blood transfusion reaction.

✦ Reassure and support the patient and his family by explaining the disease and its treatment, particularly if the patient has recurring acute episodes.

✦ As a preventive measure, monitor blood studies carefully in the patient receiving anemia-inducing drugs.

Characteristics of iron deficiency anemia

✦ Disorder of oxygen transport — hemoglobin synthesis deficient

✦ Most common in premenopausal women, infants, children, adolescents

✦ Prognosis favorable after replacement therapy

Causes

✦ Inadequate dietary intake of iron

✦ Iron malabsorption

✦ Blood loss

✦ Pregnancy

✦ Intravascular hemolysis-induced hemoglobinuria

✦ Mechanical trauma to RBCs

How it happens

+ Supply of iron inadequate for optimal formation of RBCs
+ Body stores of iron become depleted
+ Concentration of serum transferrin decreases
+ Depleted RBC mass with subnormal hemoglobin concentration
+ Subnormal oxygen-carrying capacity of the blood

Key signs and symptoms

+ Progresses gradually
+ Dyspnea on exertion
+ Fatigue
+ Listlessness
+ Pallor
+ Inability to concentrate
+ Irritability
+ Headache

Complications

+ Infection and pneumonia
+ Pica
+ Bleeding
+ Overdosage of oral or I.M. iron supplements

Diagnosis

+ Blood studies and iron stores in bone marrow confirm iron deficiency
+ Some results can be misleading because of complicating factors
+ Low hemoglobin level
+ Low hematocrit
+ Depleted or absent iron stores
+ Low serum iron and ferritin

creased laboratory blood samples in chronically ill patients, sequestration in patients on dialysis, or varices.

Other possible causes include pregnancy, which diverts maternal iron to the fetus for erythropoiesis, intravascular hemolysis-induced hemoglobinuria or paroxysmal nocturnal hemoglobinuria, and mechanical trauma to RBCs caused by a prosthetic heart valve or vena cava filters.

PATHOPHYSIOLOGY

Iron deficiency anemia occurs when the supply of iron is inadequate for optimal formation of RBCs, resulting in smaller (microcytic) cells with less color (hypochromic) on staining. Body stores of iron, including plasma iron, become depleted, and the concentration of serum transferrin, which binds with and transports iron, decreases. Insufficient iron stores lead to a depleted RBC mass with subnormal hemoglobin concentration and, in turn, subnormal oxygen-carrying capacity of the blood.

SIGNS AND SYMPTOMS

Because iron deficiency anemia progresses gradually, many patients exhibit only symptoms of an underlying condition and tend not to seek medical treatment until anemia is severe.

At advanced stages, signs and symptoms include dyspnea on exertion, fatigue, listlessness, pallor, inability to concentrate, irritability, headache, and a susceptibility to infection due to decreased oxygen-carrying capacity of the blood caused by decreased hemoglobin levels.

Increased cardiac output and tachycardia are a result of decreased oxygen perfusion. Inspection reveals coarsely ridged, spoon-shaped (koilonychia), brittle, and thin nails due to decreased capillary circulation; a sore, red, and burning tongue due to papillae atrophy; and sore, dry skin in the corners of the mouth due to epithelial changes.

COMPLICATIONS

Possible complications include infection and pneumonia, pica (compulsive eating of nonfood materials, such as starch or dirt), bleeding, and overdosage of oral or I.M. iron supplements.

DIAGNOSIS

Blood studies (serum iron, total iron-binding capacity, ferritin levels) and iron stores in bone marrow may confirm iron deficiency anemia. However, the results of these tests can be misleading because of complicating factors, such as infection, pneumonia, blood transfusion, or iron supplements. Characteristic blood test results include low hemoglobin level (males, less than 12 g/dl; females, less than 10 g/dl), low hematocrit (males, less than 47; females, less than 42), low serum iron with high binding capacity level, low serum ferritin level, low RBC count with microcytic and hypochromic cells (in early stages, RBC count possibly normal, except in infants and children), decreased mean corpuscular hemoglobin level in severe anemia, depleted or absent iron stores (by specific staining), and hyperplasia of normal precursor cells (by bone marrow studies).

Diagnosis must also include exclusion of other causes of anemia, such as thalassemia minor, cancer, and chronic inflammatory, hepatic, or renal disease.

TREATMENT

The first priority of treatment is to determine the underlying cause of anemia. Only then can iron replacement therapy begin.

The treatment of choice is an oral preparation of iron or a combination of iron and ascorbic acid (enhances iron absorption). Iron may have to be administered parenterally if the patient is noncompliant with oral dose, needs more iron than can be given orally, has malabsorption preventing adequate iron absorption, or needs a maximum rate of hemoglobin regeneration.

Because total-dose I.V. infusion of supplemental iron is painless and requires fewer injections, it's usually preferred to I.M. administration. Pregnant patients and geriatric patients with severe anemia should receive a total-dose infusion of iron dextran (INFeD) in normal saline solution given over 8 hours. An I.V. test dose of 0.5 ml should be given first to minimize the risk of an allergic reaction.

NURSING CONSIDERATIONS

✦ Monitor the patient's compliance with the prescribed iron supplement therapy. Advise the patient not to stop therapy even if he feels better because replacement of iron stores takes time.

✦ Tell the patient he may take iron supplements with a meal to decrease gastric irritation. Advise him to avoid milk, milk products, and antacids because they interfere with iron absorption; however, vitamin C can increase absorption.

✦ Warn the patient that iron supplements may result in dark green or black stools and can cause constipation.

✦ Instruct the patient to drink liquid supplemental iron through a straw to prevent staining his teeth.

✦ Tell the patient to report reactions, such as nausea, vomiting, diarrhea, constipation, fever, or severe stomach pain, which may require a dosage adjustment.

✦ If the patient receives I.V. iron, monitor the infusion rate carefully, and observe for an allergic reaction. Stop the infusion and begin supportive treatment immediately if the patient shows signs of an adverse reaction. Also, watch for dizziness and headache and for thrombophlebitis around the I.V. site.

✦ Use the Z-track injection method when administering iron I.M. to prevent skin discoloration, scarring, and irritating iron deposits in the skin.

✦ Because an iron deficiency may recur, advise regular checkups and blood studies.

▼ *LIFE-THREATENING DISORDER*

DISSEMINATED INTRAVASCULAR COAGULATION

Disseminated intravascular coagulation (DIC) occurs as a complication of diseases and conditions that accelerate clotting, causing small blood vessel occlusion, organ necrosis, depletion of circulating clotting factors and platelets, activation of the fibrinolytic system, and consequent severe hemorrhage. Clotting in the microcirculation usually affects the kidneys and extremities but may occur in the brain, lungs, pituitary and adrenal glands, and GI mucosa. DIC, also called *consumption coagulopathy* or *defibrination syndrome,* is generally an acute condition but may be chronic in cancer patients. Prognosis depends on early detection and treatment, the severity of the hemorrhage, and treatment of the underlying disease. (See *Understanding disseminated intravascular coagulation and its treatment,* page 444.)

Treatment

✦ Determine underlying cause
✦ Oral preparation of iron or a combination of iron and ascorbic acid
✦ Parenteral iron; I.V. infusion preferred

Key nursing actions

✦ Monitor the patient's compliance with the prescribed iron supplement therapy.
✦ Tell the patient he may take iron supplements with a meal to decrease gastric irritation.
✦ Tell him to avoid milk, milk products, and antacids.
✦ Instruct the patient to drink liquid supplemental iron through a straw.
✦ Use the Z-track injection method when administering iron I.M.
✦ Advise regular checkups and blood studies.

Characteristics of DIC

✦ Life-threatening disorder
✦ Occurs as a complication of diseases and conditions that accelerate clotting
✦ Clotting in the microcirculation affects kidneys, extremities, brain, lungs, pituitary and adrenal glands, GI mucosa
✦ Also called *consumption coagulopathy* or *defibrination syndrome*
✦ Generally acute but may be chronic in cancer patients
✦ Prognosis depends on early detection and treatment, severity of hemorrhage, treatment of underlying disease

FOCUS ON TREATMENT

Understanding disseminated intravascular coagulation and its treatment

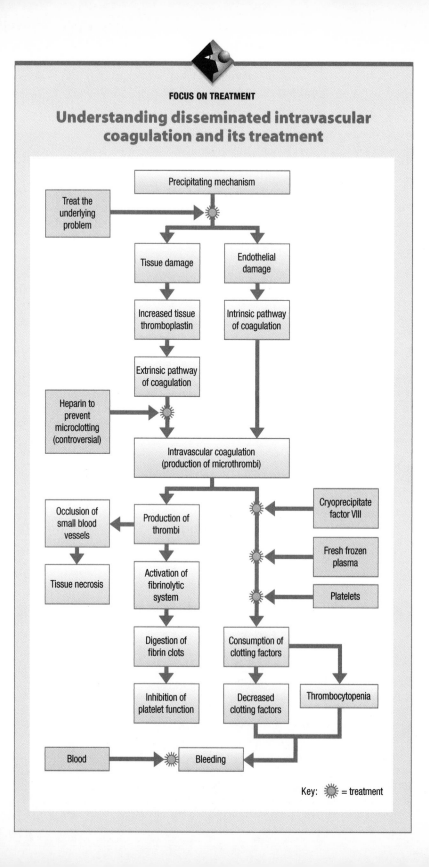

Key: ☀ = treatment

CAUSES

Causes of DIC include an infection, such as gram-negative or gram-positive septicemia, and viral, fungal, rickettsial, or protozoal infection. Obstetric complications include abruptio placentae, amniotic fluid embolism, retained dead fetus, septic abortion, and eclampsia.

Neoplastic disease includes acute leukemia, metastatic carcinoma, and aplastic anemia. Disorders that produce necrosis include extensive burns and trauma, brain tissue destruction, transplant rejection, and hepatic necrosis.

Other conditions include heatstroke, shock, poisonous snakebite, cirrhosis, fat embolism, incompatible blood transfusion, cardiac arrest, surgery requiring cardiopulmonary bypass, giant hemangioma, severe venous thrombosis, and purpura fulminans.

PATHOPHYSIOLOGY

It isn't clear why certain disorders lead to DIC or whether they use a common mechanism. In many patients, the triggering mechanisms may be the entrance of foreign protein into the circulation and vascular endothelial injury.

Regardless of how DIC begins, the typical accelerated clotting results in generalized activation of prothrombin and a consequent excess of thrombin. The thrombin converts fibrinogen to fibrin, producing fibrin clots in the microcirculation. This process uses huge amounts of coagulation factors (especially fibrinogen, prothrombin, platelets, and factors V and VIII), causing hypofibrinogenemia, hypoprothrombinemia, thrombocytopenia, and deficiencies in factors V and VIII. Circulating thrombin also activates the fibrinolytic system, which dissolves fibrin clots into fibrin degradation products. Hemorrhage may be mostly the result of the anticoagulant activity of fibrin degradation products as well as depletion of plasma coagulation factors.

SIGNS AND SYMPTOMS

Signs and symptoms of DIC caused by the anticoagulant activity of fibrin degradation products and depletion of plasma coagulation factors include abnormal bleeding, cutaneous oozing of serum, petechiae, or blood blisters, bleeding from surgical or I.V. sites, bleeding from the GI tract, epistaxis, and hemoptysis.

Other signs and symptoms include cyanotic, cold, mottled fingers and toes due to fibrin clots in the microcirculation resulting in tissue ischemia; severe muscle, back, abdominal, and chest pain from tissue hypoxia; nausea and vomiting (may be a manifestation of GI bleeding); shock due to hemorrhage; confusion, possibly due to cerebral thrombus and decreased cerebral perfusion; dyspnea due to poor tissue perfusion and oxygenation; and oliguria due to decreased renal perfusion.

COMPLICATIONS

Complications of DIC include acute tubular necrosis, shock, and multiple organ failure.

DIAGNOSIS

Diagnosis of DIC is based on a decreased platelet count (usually less than 100,000/μl, because platelets are consumed during thrombosis) and a fibrinogen level less than 150 mg/dl because fibrinogen is consumed in clot formation (levels

Causes

+ Infection
+ Obstetric complications
+ Neoplastic disease

How it happens

+ Foreign protein enters circulation or vascular endothelial injury occurs
+ Accelerated clotting, activation of prothrombin, excess of thrombin
+ Thrombin converts fibrinogen to fibrin
+ Fibrin clots in microcirculation
+ Hypofibrinogenemia, hypoprothrombinemia, thrombocytopenia, deficiencies in factors V and VIII
+ Fibrinolytic system activates, dissolves fibrin clots
+ Hemorrhage is result of fibrin degradation products, depletion of plasma coagulation factors

Key signs and symptoms

+ Abnormal bleeding
+ Cutaneous oozing of serum
+ Petechiae
+ Bleeding

Complications

+ Acute tubular necrosis
+ Shock
+ Multiple organ failure

Diagnosis

+ Based on decreased platelet count and low fibrinogen level
+ Prothrombin time > 15 seconds
+ Partial thromboplastin time > 60 seconds
+ Increased fibrin degradation products

may be normal if elevated by hepatitis or pregnancy). As the excessive clot breaks down, hemorrhagic diathesis occurs and tests reveal a prothrombin time greater than 15 seconds, partial thromboplastin time greater than 60 seconds, and increased fibrin degradation products (typically greater than 45 mcg/ml) due to excess fibrinolysis by plasmin.

D-dimer test (presence of an asymmetrical carbon compound fragment formed in the presence of fibrin split products) is positive at less than 1:8 dilution. Other supportive data include positive fibrin monomers, diminished levels of factors V and VIII, fragmentation of RBCs, and hemoglobin level less than 10 g/dl.

Assessment of renal status demonstrates a reduced urine output (less than 30 ml/hour), elevated blood urea nitrogen (greater than 25 mg/dl), and elevated serum creatinine (greater than 1.3 mg/dl).

Treatment

+ Treatment of underlying disorder
+ Administration of blood
+ Fresh frozen plasma, platelet, packed RBCs
+ Heparin therapy (controversial)

Key nursing actions

+ Patient care must focus on early recognition of abnormal bleeding, prompt treatment of the underlying disorders, and prevention of further bleeding.
+ Don't scrub bleeding areas.
+ Use pressure, cold compresses, and topical hemostatic agents to control bleeding.
+ Enforce complete bed rest during bleeding episodes.
+ Check all I.V. and venipuncture sites frequently for bleeding.
+ Monitor intake and output hourly in acute DIC.
+ Weigh dressings and linen to measure blood loss.
+ Watch for transfusion reactions and signs of fluid overload.
+ Weigh the patient daily.
+ Watch for bleeding from the GI and genitourinary tracts.

TREATMENT

Successful management requires prompt recognition and treatment of the underlying disorder. Active bleeding may require administration of blood, fresh frozen plasma, platelet, or packed RBC transfusions to support hemostasis.

Heparin therapy is controversial. It may be used in early stages to prevent microclotting and as a last resort in hemorrhage. (See *Understanding disseminated intravascular coagulation and its treatment,* page 444.)

NURSING CONSIDERATIONS

Patient care must focus on early recognition of abnormal bleeding, prompt treatment of the underlying disorders, and prevention of further bleeding.
+ To avoid dislodging clots and causing fresh bleeding, don't scrub bleeding areas. Use pressure, cold compresses, and topical hemostatic agents to control bleeding.
+ To prevent injury, enforce complete bed rest during bleeding episodes. If the patient is agitated, pad the side rails.
+ Check all I.V. and venipuncture sites frequently for bleeding. Apply pressure to injection sites for at least 20 minutes. Alert other personnel to the patient's tendency to hemorrhage.
+ Monitor intake and output hourly in acute DIC, especially when administering blood products. Watch for transfusion reactions and signs of fluid overload. To measure the amount of blood lost, weigh dressings and linen and record drainage. Weigh the patient daily, particularly if there's renal involvement.
+ Watch for bleeding from the GI and genitourinary tracts. If you suspect intra-abdominal bleeding, measure the patient's abdominal girth at least every 4 hours, and monitor closely for signs of shock.
+ Monitor the results of serial blood studies (particularly hematocrit, hemoglobin levels, and coagulation times).
+ Explain all diagnostic tests and procedures. Allow time for questions.
+ Inform the family of the patient's progress. Prepare them for his appearance (I.V. lines, nasogastric tubes, bruises, and dried blood). Provide emotional support for the patient and family. As needed, enlist the aid of a social worker, chaplain, and other members of the health care team in providing such support.

IDIOPATHIC THROMBOCYTOPENIC PURPURA

Idiopathic thrombocytopenic purpura (ITP) is a deficiency of platelets that occurs when the immune system destroys the body's own platelets. ITP may be acute, as in postviral thrombocytopenia, or chronic, as in essential thrombocytopenia or autoimmune thrombocytopenia.

 CLINICAL ALERT Acute ITP usually affects children between ages 2 and 6; chronic ITP mainly affects adults younger than age 50, especially women between ages 20 and 40.

The prognosis for acute ITP is excellent; nearly four of five patients recover without treatment. The prognosis for chronic ITP is good; remissions lasting weeks or years are common, especially among women.

CAUSES

ITP may be an autoimmune disorder because antibodies that reduce platelet life span have been found in nearly all patients. The spleen may help remove platelets modified by the antibody. Acute ITP usually follows a viral infection, such as rubella or chickenpox, and can follow immunization with a live virus vaccine. Chronic ITP seldom follows infection and is commonly linked to immunologic disorders such as systemic lupus erythematosus as well as to drug reactions. ITP commonly occurs in patients who have abused alcohol, heroin, or morphine, and in patients with acquired immunodeficiency syndrome who are exposed to the rubella virus.

PATHOPHYSIOLOGY

ITP occurs when circulating immunoglobulin (Ig) G molecules react with host platelets, which are then destroyed in the spleen and, to a lesser degree, in the liver. Normally, the life span of platelets in circulation is 7 to 10 days. In ITP, platelets survive 1 to 3 days or less.

SIGNS AND SYMPTOMS

Signs and symptoms of ITP are caused by decreased levels of platelets and may include nosebleeds; oral bleeding; hemorrhages into the skin, mucous membranes, and other tissues causing red discoloration of skin (purpura); small purplish hemorrhagic spots on skin (petechiae); and excessive menstrual bleeding.

COMPLICATIONS

Possible complications of ITP include hemorrhage, cerebral hemorrhage, and purpuric lesions of vital organs (such as the brain and kidney).

DIAGNOSIS

Platelet count of less than 20,000/µl and prolonged bleeding time suggest ITP. Platelet size and morphologic appearance may be abnormal; anemia may be present if bleeding has occurred. As in thrombocytopenia, bone marrow studies show an abundance of megakaryocytes and a shortened circulating platelet survival time (hours or days). Humoral tests that measure platelet-associated IgG may help establish the diagnosis; one-half of patients with ITP have an elevated IgG level.

Characteristics of ITP
+ Deficiency of platelets
+ Immune system destroys body's own platelets
+ Acute or chronic

Alert!
+ Acute ITP usually affects children between ages 2 and 6.
+ Chronic ITP mainly affects adults younger than age 50.

Causes
+ Antibodies that reduce life span of platelets found in patients
+ Spleen probably helps to remove platelets modified by antibodies
+ Acute form follows viral infection
+ Chronic form linked to immunologic disorders; drug reactions

How it happens
+ Circulating IgG molecules react with host platelets
+ Platelets then destroyed in spleen and liver

Key signs and symptoms
+ Nosebleeds
+ Oral bleeding
+ Hemorrhages into skin, mucous membranes, other tissues

Complications
+ Hemorrhage
+ Purpuric lesions of vital organs

Diagnosis
+ Platelet count < 20,000/µl
+ Prolonged bleeding time
+ Elevated IgG level

Treatment
+ Glucocorticoids
+ Immunoglobulin
+ Corticosteroids
+ Blood transfusions

Key nursing actions
+ Teach the patient to observe for petechiae, ecchymoses, and other signs of recurrence.
+ Monitor patients receiving immunosuppressants for signs of bone marrow depression, infection, mucositis, GI ulcers, and severe diarrhea or vomiting.

Characteristics of polycythemia vera
+ Chronic disorder characterized by increased RBC mass, erythrocytosis, leukocytosis, thrombocytosis, and increased hemoglobin level, with normal or increased plasma volume
+ Usually occurs between ages 40 and 60 among Jewish males of European ancestry
+ Mortality high if untreated or associated with leukemia, myeloid metaplasia

Causes
+ Unknown
+ Probably related to multipotential stem cell defect

How it happens
+ Uncontrolled, rapid cellular reproduction and maturation
+ Proliferation or hyperplasia of all bone marrow cells
+ Blood abnormally viscous
+ Blood flow to microcirculation inhibited
+ Intravascular thrombosis results

TREATMENT

Treatment for acute ITP includes glucocorticoids to prevent further platelet destruction, immunoglobulin to prevent platelet destruction, plasmapheresis, and platelet pheresis.

Treatment for chronic ITP includes corticosteroids to suppress phagocytic activity and enhance platelet production, splenectomy (when splenomegaly accompanies the initial thrombocytopenia), and blood and blood component transfusions and vitamin K to correct anemia and coagulation defects.

Alternative treatments include immunosuppressants to help stop platelet destruction, high-dose I.V. immunoglobulin, and immunoabsorption apheresis using staphylococcal protein A columns.

NURSING CONSIDERATIONS

Patient care for ITP is essentially the same as for other types of thrombocytopenia, with emphasis on teaching the patient to observe for petechiae, ecchymoses, and other signs of recurrence. Monitor patients receiving immunosuppressants for signs of bone marrow depression, infection, mucositis, GI ulcers, and severe diarrhea or vomiting. Tell the patient to avoid aspirin and ibuprofen.

POLYCYTHEMIA VERA

Polycythemia vera is a chronic disorder characterized by increased RBC mass, erythrocytosis, leukocytosis, thrombocytosis, and increased hemoglobin level, with normal or increased plasma volume. This disease is also known as *primary polycythemia, erythremia, polycythemia rubra vera, splenomegalic polycythemia,* or *Vaquez-Osler disease.* It usually occurs between ages 40 and 60, most commonly among Jewish males of European ancestry. It seldom affects children and doesn't appear to be familial.

The prognosis depends on age at diagnosis, the type of treatment used, and complications. Mortality is high if polycythemia is untreated, associated with leukemia, or associated with myeloid metaplasia (presence of marrow-like tissue and ectopic hematopoiesis in extramedullary sites, such as liver and spleen, and nucleated erythrocytes in blood).

CAUSES

The cause of polycythemia vera is unknown, but is probably related to a multipotential stem cell defect.

PATHOPHYSIOLOGY

In polycythemia vera, uncontrolled and rapid cellular reproduction and maturation cause proliferation or hyperplasia of all bone marrow cells (panmyelosis).

Increased RBC mass makes the blood abnormally viscous and inhibits blood flow to microcirculation. Diminished blood flow and thrombocytosis set the stage for intravascular thrombosis.

SIGNS AND SYMPTOMS

In its early stages, polycythemia vera may produce no signs or symptoms. As altered circulation (secondary to increased RBC mass) produces hypervolemia and hyperviscosity, the patient may report a vague feeling of fullness in the head; rushing in the ears; tinnitus; headache; dizziness; vertigo; epistaxis; night sweats; epigastric and joint pain; and visual alterations, such as scotomas, double vision, and blurred vision. He may also report a decrease in urine output, possibly due to increased uric acid production.

Late in the disease, the patient may report pruritus (which worsens after bathing and may be disabling), a sense of abdominal fullness, and pain, such as pleuritic chest pain or left upper quadrant pain.

COMPLICATIONS

Hyperviscosity may lead to thrombosis of smaller vessels with ruddy cyanosis of the nose and clubbing of the digits. Paradoxically, hemorrhage is a complication of polycythemia vera. It may occur as a result of defective platelet function or of hyperviscosity and the local effects from excess RBCs exerting pressure on distended venous and capillary walls. Uric acid stones are another possible complication.

DIAGNOSIS

Laboratory studies confirm polycythemia vera by showing increased RBC mass and normal arterial oxygen saturation in association with splenomegaly. Another common finding is increased uric acid level, leading to hyperuricemia and hyperuricuria. Other laboratory results include increased blood histamine levels, decreased serum iron concentration, and decreased or absent urinary erythropoietin. Bone marrow biopsy reveals excess production of myeloid stem cells.

TREATMENT

Treatment may include phlebotomy to reduce RBC mass. For severe symptoms, myelosuppressive therapy with radioactive phosphorus (^{32}P) may be used to suppress erythropoiesis (may increase the risk of leukemia) or hydroxyurea.

NURSING CONSIDERATIONS

If the patient requires phlebotomy, explain the procedure and reassure the patient that the procedure will relieve distressing symptoms. Check blood pressure, pulse rate, and respiratory rate. During phlebotomy, make sure the patient is lying down comfortably to prevent vertigo and syncope. Stay alert for tachycardia, clamminess, or complaints of vertigo. If these effects occur, the procedure should be stopped.
✦ Immediately after phlebotomy, check blood pressure and pulse rate. Have the patient sit up for about 5 minutes before allowing him to walk; this prevents vasovagal attack or orthostatic hypotension. Also, have the patient drink 24 oz (710 ml) of juice or water.
✦ Tell the patient to watch for and report any signs or symptoms of iron deficiency (pallor, weight loss, asthenia [weakness], and glossitis).
✦ Keep the patient active and ambulatory to prevent thrombosis. If bed rest is absolutely necessary, prescribe a daily program of both active and passive range-of-motion exercises.
✦ Watch for complications: hypervolemia, thrombocytosis, and signs or symptoms of an impending stroke (decreased sensation, numbness, transitory paralysis, fleeting blindness, headache, and epistaxis).
✦ Regularly examine the patient closely for bleeding. Tell him which are the most common bleeding sites (such as the nose, gingiva, and skin) so he can check for bleeding. Advise him to report any abnormal bleeding promptly.

Key signs and symptoms
✦ Vague feeling of fullness in head
✦ Rushing in ears, tinnitus
✦ Headache
✦ Dizziness, vertigo
✦ Epistaxis
✦ Night sweats
✦ Epigastric and joint pain

Complications
✦ Thrombosis of smaller vessels
✦ Ruddy cyanosis of nose, clubbing of digits
✦ Hemorrhage

Diagnosis
✦ Increased RBC mass, normal arterial oxygen saturation in association with splenomegaly
✦ Increased uric acid and blood histamine
✦ Decreased serum iron concentration and urinary erythropoietin

Treatment
✦ Phlebotomy
✦ Myelosuppressive therapy

Key nursing actions
✦ If the patient requires phlebotomy, explain the procedure and reassure the patient.
✦ Check blood pressure, pulse rate, and respiratory rate.
✦ Stay alert for tachycardia, clamminess, or complaints of vertigo.
✦ Immediately after phlebotomy, check blood pressure and pulse rate.
✦ Have the patient drink 24 oz (710 ml) of juice or water.
✦ Regularly examine the patient closely for bleeding.

Key nursing actions

During myelosuppressive treatment

✦ Monitor CBC and platelet count before and during therapy.

✦ Tell the patient to report signs of bleeding, infection, or reactions.

During treatment with ³²P

✦ Take a blood sample for CBC and platelet count before beginning treatment.

✦ Have the patient lie down during I.V. administration and for 15 to 20 minutes afterward.

Characteristics of thalassemia

✦ Hereditary group of hemolytic anemias

✦ Defective synthesis in polypeptide chains of protein component of hemoglobin

✦ In β-thalassemia, synthesis of beta polypeptide chain is defective

✦ Thalassemia major: patients seldom survive to adulthood; also known as *Cooley's anemia*

✦ Thalassemia intermedia: children develop normally into adulthood

✦ Thalassemia minor: normal lifespan

Alert!

✦ Thalassemia is most common in people of Mediterranean ancestry.

Causes

✦ Homozygous or heterozygous inheritance

✦ To compensate for increased uric acid production, give additional fluids, administer allopurinol, and alkalinize the urine to prevent uric acid calculi.

✦ If the patient has symptomatic splenomegaly, suggest or provide small, frequent meals, followed by a rest period, to prevent nausea and vomiting.

✦ Report acute abdominal pain immediately; it may signal splenic infarction, renal calculi, or abdominal organ thrombosis.

During myelosuppressive treatment

✦ Monitor complete blood count (CBC) and platelet count before and during therapy. Warn the outpatient who develops leukopenia that his resistance to infection is low; advise him to avoid crowds and watch for the symptoms of infection. If leukopenia develops in a hospitalized patient who needs reverse isolation, follow hospital guidelines. If thrombocytopenia develops, tell the patient to watch for signs of bleeding (blood in urine, nosebleeds, and black stools).

✦ Tell the patient about possible reactions (nausea, vomiting, and risk of infection) to alkylating agents. Alopecia may follow the use of busulfan, cyclophosphamide, and uracil mustard; sterile hemorrhagic cystitis may follow the use of cyclophosphamide (forcing fluids can prevent it). Watch for and report all reactions. If nausea and vomiting occur, begin antiemetic therapy and adjust the patient's diet.

During treatment with ³²P

✦ Explain the procedure to relieve anxiety. Tell the patient he may require repeated phlebotomies until ³²P takes effect. Take a blood sample for CBC and platelet count before beginning treatment. (*Note:* Use of ³²P requires radiation precautions to prevent contamination.)

✦ Have the patient lie down during I.V. administration (to facilitate the procedure and prevent extravasation) and for 15 to 20 minutes afterward.

THALASSEMIA

Thalassemia, a hereditary group of hemolytic anemias, is characterized by defective synthesis in the polypeptide chains of the protein component of hemoglobin. Consequently, RBC synthesis is also impaired.

 CLINICAL ALERT Thalassemia is most common in people of Mediterranean ancestry (especially Italian and Greek) but also occurs in people whose ancestors originated in Africa, southern China, Southeast Asia, and India.

In β-*thalassemia*, the most common form of this disorder, synthesis of the beta polypeptide chain is defective. It occurs in three clinical forms: major, intermedia, and minor. The severity of the resulting anemia depends on whether the patient is homozygous or heterozygous for the thalassemic trait and the prognosis varies. In *thalassemia major*, patients seldom survive to adulthood. In *thalassemia intermedia*, children develop normally into adulthood, although puberty is usually delayed. Patients have a normal life span in *thalassemia minor*.

CAUSES

Causes of thalassemia are homozygous inheritance of the partially dominant autosomal gene (thalassemia major or thalassemia intermedia) or heterozygous inheritance of the same gene (thalassemia minor).

PATHOPHYSIOLOGY

Total or partial deficiency of beta polypeptide chain production impairs hemoglobin synthesis and results in continual production of fetal hemoglobin, lasting even past the neonatal period. Normally, immunoglobulin synthesis switches from gamma- to beta-polypeptides at the time of birth. This conversion doesn't happen in thalassemic infants. Their red cells are hypochromic and microcytic.

SIGNS AND SYMPTOMS

Possible signs and symptoms of thalassemia major (also known as *Cooley's anemia, Mediterranean disease,* and *erythroblastic anemia*) include a healthy neonate at birth, but during the second 6 months of life developing severe anemia, bone abnormalities, failure to thrive, and life-threatening complications.

The first signs are pallor, yellow skin and sclera in infants ages 3 to 6 months. Later signs and symptoms include splenomegaly or hepatomegaly, with abdominal enlargement; frequent infections; bleeding tendencies (especially nosebleeds); and anorexia. Most children with thalassemia major have a small body, a large head (characteristic features), and possible mental retardation. Infants may have features similar to Down syndrome, because of thickened bone at the base of the nose from bone marrow hyperactivity.

Signs and symptoms of thalassemia intermedia include some degree of anemia, jaundice, and splenomegaly, and possibly signs of hemosiderosis due to increased intestinal absorption of iron.

Thalassemia minor may cause mild anemia but usually produces no symptoms and is commonly overlooked; it should be differentiated from iron deficiency anemia.

COMPLICATIONS

Possible complications of thalassemia include pathologic fractures due to expansion of the marrow cavities with thinning of the long bones, cardiac arrhythmias, and heart failure.

DIAGNOSIS

Diagnosis of thalassemia major includes low RBC and hemoglobin levels, microcytosis, and high reticulocyte count. Laboratory tests also reveal elevated bilirubin and urinary and fecal urobilinogen levels.

A low serum folate level reflects increased folate use by hypertrophied bone marrow. A peripheral blood smear reveals target cells, microcytes, pale nucleated RBCs, and marked anisocytosis. Thinning and widening of the marrow space is seen on skull and long bone X-rays due to overactive bone marrow. There's also a granular appearance of bones, of skull and vertebrae, areas of osteoporosis in long bones, and deformed (rectangular or biconvex) phalanges. Significantly increased fetal hemoglobin level and a slightly increased hemoglobin A_2 level on quantitative hemoglobin studies is revealed. Additionally, diagnosis must rule out iron deficiency anemia, which also produces hypochromic microcytic RBCs.

Diagnosis of thalassemia intermedia includes hypochromic microcytic RBCs (less severe than in thalassemia major).

Diagnosis of thalassemia minor includes hypochromic microcytic RBCs, significantly increased hemoglobin A_2 level, and moderately increased fetal hemoglobin level on quantitative hemoglobin studies.

How it happens

+ Hemoglobin synthesis impaired
+ Results in continual production of fetal hemoglobin
+ Red cells are hypochromic and microcytic

Key signs and symptoms

Thalassemia major

+ Severe anemia second 6 months of life
+ Bone abnormalities
+ Failure to thrive
+ Life-threatening complications
+ Pallor, yellow skin and sclera in infants ages 3 to 6 months
+ Splenomegaly or hepatomegaly

Thalassemia intermedia

+ Some degree of anemia, jaundice, splenomegaly
+ Signs of hemosiderosis

Thalassemia minor

+ Mild anemia

Complications

+ Pathologic fractures
+ Cardiac arrhythmias
+ Heart failure

Diagnosis

Thalassemia major

+ Low RBC and hemoglobin levels
+ Microcytosis
+ High reticulocyte count

Thalassemia intermedia

+ Hypochromic microcytic RBCs

Thalassemia minor

+ Increased hemoglobin A_2
+ Increased fetal hemoglobin level

Treatment

- ✦ Folic acid supplements
- ✦ Transfusions of packed RBCs
- ✦ Splenectomy and bone marrow transplantation

Key nursing actions

- ✦ During and after RBC transfusions for thalassemia major, watch for adverse reactions.
- ✦ Stress the importance of good nutrition, meticulous wound care, and periodic dental checkups to prevent infection.
- ✦ Refer parents and adult patients with thalassemia minor and thalassemia intermedia for genetic counseling.
- ✦ Be sure to tell people with thalassemia minor that their condition is benign.

Characteristics of thrombocytopenia

- ✦ Most common cause of hemorrhagic disorders
- ✦ Deficiency of circulating platelets
- ✦ Congenital or acquired
- ✦ Poses threat to hemostasis
- ✦ Prognosis excellent in drug-induced form if offending drug is withdrawn

Causes

- ✦ Decreased or defective platelet production in bone marrow or increased platelet destruction
- ✦ Sequestration or blood loss

TREATMENT

Treatment of thalassemia major is essentially supportive. Infections require prompt treatment with appropriate antibiotics. Folic acid supplements help maintain folic acid levels despite increased requirements.

Transfusions of packed RBCs are administered to increase hemoglobin levels but must be used judiciously to minimize iron overload. Splenectomy and bone marrow transplantation have been tried, but their effectiveness hasn't been confirmed.

Thalassemia intermedia and thalassemia minor generally don't require treatment. Iron supplements are contraindicated in all forms of thalassemia.

NURSING CONSIDERATIONS

- ✦ During and after RBC transfusions for thalassemia major, watch for adverse reactions — shaking chills, fever, rash, itching, and hives.
- ✦ Stress the importance of good nutrition, meticulous wound care, periodic dental checkups, and other measures to prevent infection.
- ✦ For young patients, discuss with parents various options for healthy physical and creative outlets. Such a child must avoid strenuous athletic activity because of increased oxygen demand and the tendency toward pathologic fractures, but he may participate in less stressful activities.
- ✦ Teach parents to watch for signs of hepatitis and iron overload — always possible with frequent transfusions.
- ✦ Because parents may have questions about the vulnerability of future offspring, refer them for genetic counseling. Also, refer adult patients with thalassemia minor and thalassemia intermedia for genetic counseling; they need to recognize the risk of transmitting thalassemia major to their children if they marry another person with thalassemia. If such people choose to marry and have children, all their children should be evaluated for thalassemia by age 1. Be sure to tell people with thalassemia minor that their condition is benign.

THROMBOCYTOPENIA

Thrombocytopenia, the most common cause of hemorrhagic disorders, is a deficiency of circulating platelets. It may be congenital or acquired; the acquired form is more common. Because platelets are needed for coagulation, this disease poses a serious threat to hemostasis. The prognosis is excellent in drug-induced thrombocytopenia if the offending drug — usually carbamazepine (Tegretol) or heparin — is withdrawn; in such cases, recovery may be immediate. In other types, the prognosis depends on the patient's response to treatment of the underlying cause.

CAUSES

Thrombocytopenia may be congenital or acquired. In either case, it usually results from decreased or defective platelet production in the bone marrow (as in leukemia, aplastic anemia, or drug toxicity) or from increased platelet destruction outside the marrow due to an underlying disorder (such as cirrhosis of the liver, disseminated intravascular coagulation, or severe infection). Less commonly, thrombocytopenia results from sequestration (increased amount of blood in a limited vascular area such as the spleen) or blood loss.

PATHOPHYSIOLOGY

In thrombocytopenia, lack of platelets can cause inadequate hemostasis. Four mechanisms are responsible: decreased platelet production, decreased platelet survival, pooling of blood in the spleen, and intravascular dilution of circulating platelets. Megakaryocytes, giant cells in the bone marrow, produce platelets. Platelet production decreases when the number of megakaryocytes is reduced or when platelet production becomes dysfunctional. (See *What happens in thrombocytopenia,* page 454.)

SIGNS AND SYMPTOMS

Thrombocytopenia typically produces a sudden onset of petechiae or blood blisters caused by bleeding into the skin or bleeding into the mucous membrane. Some patients may complain of malaise, fatigue, and general weakness. Large blood-filled blisters characteristically appear in the mouths of adults.

COMPLICATIONS

Complications of thrombocytopenia are usually related to bleeding. Severe thrombocytopenia can cause acute hemorrhage, which may be fatal without immediate therapy. The most common sites of severe bleeding include the brain and GI tract, although intrapulmonary bleeding and cardiac tamponade may also occur.

DIAGNOSIS

Coagulation tests reveal a platelet count usually less than 100,000 µl in adults and a prolonged bleeding time.

Platelet antibody studies can help determine why the platelet count is low and are also used to select treatment. Platelet survival studies help to differentiate between ineffective platelet production and platelet destruction as causes of thrombocytopenia.

Bone marrow studies determine the number, size, and maturity of megakaryocytes in severe disease, helping identify ineffective platelet production as the cause and ruling out malignant disease.

TREATMENT

Treatment of thrombocytopenia must include withdrawing the offending drug or treating the underlying cause, when possible. Corticosteroids may be used to increase platelet production. In addition, lithium (Eskalith) or folate is administered to stimulate bone marrow production and I.V. gamma globulin is administered to increase platelet production. Platelet transfusions are given to treat complications of severe hemorrhage.

Splenectomy may be necessary to correct disease caused by platelet destruction because the spleen is the primary site of platelet removal and antibody production.

NURSING CONSIDERATIONS

When caring for the patient with thrombocytopenia, take every possible precaution against bleeding.

✦ Protect the patient from trauma. Keep the side rails up and pad them, if possible. Promote the use of an electric razor and a soft toothbrush. Avoid invasive procedures, such as venipuncture or urinary catheterization, if possible. When venipunc-

How it happens

✦ Decreased platelet production
✦ Decreased platelet survival
✦ Pooling of blood in spleen
✦ Intravascular dilution of circulating platelets

Key signs and symptoms

✦ Sudden onset of petechiae
✦ Malaise, fatigue, general weakness
✦ Large blood-filled blisters in mouths of adults

Complications

✦ Acute hemorrhage in brain and GI tract
✦ Intrapulmonary bleeding
✦ Cardiac tamponade

Diagnosis

✦ Platelet count < 100,000 µl
✦ Prolonged bleeding time

Treatment

✦ Withdraw offending drug or treat underlying cause
✦ Corticosteroids
✦ Lithium or folate
✦ I.V. gamma globulin

Key nursing actions

✦ Take every possible precaution against bleeding.
✦ Protect the patient from trauma.
✦ Exert pressure on the venipuncture site for at least 20 minutes or until the bleeding stops.

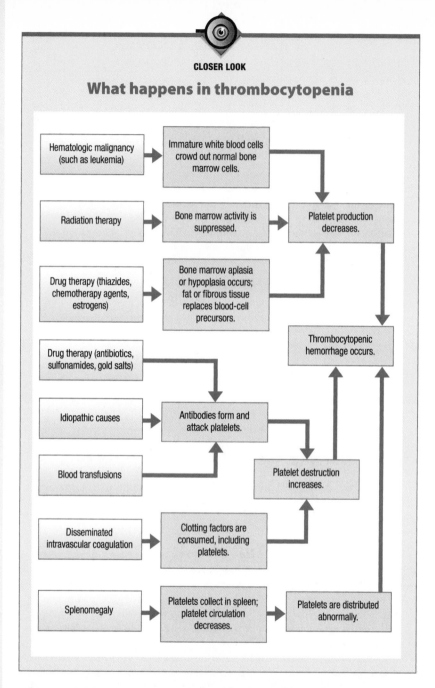

CLOSER LOOK

What happens in thrombocytopenia

Hematologic malignancy (such as leukemia)	Immature white blood cells crowd out normal bone marrow cells.	
Radiation therapy	Bone marrow activity is suppressed.	Platelet production decreases.
Drug therapy (thiazides, chemotherapy agents, estrogens)	Bone marrow aplasia or hypoplasia occurs; fat or fibrous tissue replaces blood-cell precursors.	

Thrombocytopenic hemorrhage occurs.

Drug therapy (antibiotics, sulfonamides, gold salts)	Antibodies form and attack platelets.	
Idiopathic causes		
Blood transfusions		Platelet destruction increases.
Disseminated intravascular coagulation	Clotting factors are consumed, including platelets.	
Splenomegaly	Platelets collect in spleen; platelet circulation decreases.	Platelets are distributed abnormally.

ture is unavoidable, be sure to exert pressure on the puncture site for at least 20 minutes or until the bleeding stops.

✦ Monitor platelet count daily.

✦ Test stool for guaiac; test urine and vomitus for traces of blood.

✦ Watch for bleeding (petechiae, ecchymoses, surgical or GI bleeding, and menor-rhagia).

✦ Warn the patient to avoid aspirin in any form and other drugs that impair coagulation. Teach him how to recognize aspirin or ibuprofen compounds on labels of over-the-counter remedies.

✦ Advise the patient to avoid straining at defecation or coughing as both can lead to increased intracranial pressure, possibly causing cerebral hemorrhage in the patient with thrombocytopenia. Provide a stool softener to avoid constipation.

✦ During periods of active bleeding, keep the patient on strict bed rest, if necessary.

✦ When administering platelet concentrate, remember that platelets are extremely fragile, so infuse them quickly. Don't give platelets to a patient with a fever.

✦ During platelet transfusion, monitor for febrile reaction (flushing, chills, fever, headache, tachycardia, and hypertension). Histocompatibility locus antigen-typed platelets may be ordered to prevent febrile reaction. A patient with a history of minor reactions may benefit from acetaminophen and diphenhydramine before transfusion.

✦ If thrombocytopenia is drug-induced, stress the importance of avoiding the offending drug.

✦ If the patient must receive long-term steroid therapy, teach him to watch for and report cushingoid signs (acne, moon face, hirsutism, buffalo hump, hypertension, girdle obesity, thinning arms and legs, glycosuria, and edema). Emphasize that steroid doses must be discontinued gradually. During steroid therapy, monitor fluid and electrolyte balance, and watch for infection, pathologic fractures, and mood changes.

✦ A 1- to 2-hour postplatelet count will aid assessment of response.

VON WILLEBRAND'S DISEASE

Von Willebrand's disease is a hereditary bleeding disorder, occurring more commonly in females. It's characterized by prolonged bleeding time, moderate deficiency of clotting factor VIII (antihemophilic factor), and impaired platelet function. This disease commonly causes bleeding from the skin or mucosal surfaces and, in females, excessive uterine bleeding. Bleeding may range from mild and producing no symptoms to severe, potentially fatal, hemorrhage. The prognosis is usually good.

CAUSES

Von Willebrand's disease is caused by an inherited autosomal dominant trait. Recently, an acquired form has been identified in patients with cancer and immune disorders.

PATHOPHYSIOLOGY

A possible mechanism of the disease is that mild to moderate deficiency of factor VIII and defective platelet adhesion prolong coagulation time. Specifically, this results from a deficiency of von Willebrand's factor (vWF), which stabilizes the factor VIII molecule and is needed for proper platelet function.

Defective platelet function is characterized in vivo by decreased agglutination and adhesion at the bleeding site and in vitro by reduced platelet retention when blood is filtered through a column of packed glass beads, and diminished ristocetin-induced platelet aggregation.

Key nursing actions
✦ Monitor platelet count daily.
✦ Test stools for guaiac; test urine and vomitus for traces of blood.
✦ Warn the patient to avoid aspirin in any form and other drugs that impair coagulation.
✦ Advise the patient to avoid straining at defecation or coughing.
✦ Provide a stool softener to avoid constipation.
✦ During platelet transfusion, monitor for febrile reaction.

Characteristics of von Willebrand's disease
✦ Hereditary bleeding disorder
✦ Occurs more commonly in females
✦ Prolonged bleeding time, deficiency of clotting factor VIII, impaired platelet function
✦ Causes bleeding from skin or mucosal surfaces, excessive uterine bleeding
✦ Mild and producing no symptoms to severe, potentially fatal, hemorrhage

Causes
✦ Inherited autosomal dominant trait
✦ Acquired form in patients with cancer and immune disorders

How it happens
✦ Mild to moderate deficiency of factor VIII and defective platelet adhesion prolong coagulation time

SIGNS AND SYMPTOMS

Prolonged coagulation time may cause easy bruising, epistaxis (nosebleed), and bleeding from the gums. Petechiae are rarely seen. Severe forms of this disease may cause hemorrhage after laceration or surgery, menorrhagia, and GI bleeding.

Excessive postpartum bleeding is uncommon because factor VIII levels and bleeding time abnormalities become less pronounced during pregnancy. Massive soft tissue hemorrhage and bleeding into joints seldom occur.

COMPLICATIONS

A complication of von Willebrand's disease is hemorrhage.

DIAGNOSIS

Typical laboratory findings include prolonged bleeding time (greater than 6 minutes), slightly prolonged partial thromboplastin time (greater than 45 seconds), absent or low factor VIII, absent or low factor VIII–related antigens, low factor VIII activity, ristocetin coagulation factor assay showing defective in vitro platelet aggregation, and normal platelet count and clot retraction.

TREATMENT

The aims of treatment are to shorten bleeding time and to replace factor VIII by infusion of cryoprecipitate or blood fractions rich in factor VIII. Parenteral or intranasal desmopressin is administered to increase serum levels of vWF.

NURSING CONSIDERATIONS

The care plan should include local measures to control bleeding and patient teaching to prevent bleeding, unnecessary trauma, and complications.
+ After surgery, monitor bleeding time for 24 to 48 hours, and watch for signs of new bleeding.
+ During a bleeding episode, elevate and apply cold compresses and gentle pressure to the bleeding site.
+ Refer parents of affected children for genetic counseling.
+ Advise the patient to consult the physician after even minor trauma and before all surgery to determine if replacement of blood components is necessary.
+ Tell the patient to watch for signs of hepatitis within 6 weeks to 6 months after transfusion.
+ Warn against using aspirin and other drugs that impair platelet function.
+ Advise the patient who has a severe form to avoid contact sports.

Immune system

The immune system is responsible for safeguarding the body from disease-causing microorganisms. It's part of a complex system of host defenses.

Host defenses may be innate or acquired. Innate defenses include physical and chemical barriers, the complement complex, and cells such as phagocytes (cells programmed to destroy foreign cells such as bacteria) and natural killer lymphocytes.

Physical barriers, such as the skin and mucous membranes, prevent invasion by most organisms. Chemical barriers include lysozymes (found in such body secretions as tears, mucus, and saliva) and hydrochloric acid in the stomach. Lysozymes destroy bacteria by removing cell walls. Hydrochloric acid breaks down foods and destroys pathogens carried by food or swallowed mucus.

Organisms that penetrate this first line of defense simultaneously trigger the inflammatory and immune responses, some innate and others acquired.

Acquired immunity comes into play when the body encounters a cell or cell product that it recognizes as foreign, such as a bacterium or a virus. The two kinds of immunity provided by cells are humoral (provided by B-lymphocytes) and cell-mediated (provided by T-lymphocytes). All cells involved in the inflammatory and immune responses arrive from a single type of stem cell in the bone marrow. B cells mature in the marrow and T cells migrate to the thymus, where they mature.

The inflammatory response is the immediate local response to tissue injury, whether from trauma or infection. It involves the action of polymorphonuclear leukocytes, basophils and mast cells, platelets and, to some extent, monocytes and macrophages.

IMMUNE RESPONSE

The immune response primarily involves the interaction of antigens (foreign proteins), B-lymphocytes, T-lymphocytes, macrophages, cytokines, complement, and polymorphonuclear leukocytes. Some immunoactive cells circulate constantly;

Key facts about the immune system

+ Responsible for protecting the body from disease-causing microorganisms
+ Innate defenses include physical and chemical barriers, complement complex, phagocytes, lymphocytes
+ Acquired immunity occurs when body encounters foreign cell or cell product
+ Inflammatory response — immediate local response to tissue injury

Immune response

+ Involves interaction of antigens, B-lymphocytes, T-lymphocytes, macrophages, cytokines, complement, and polymorphonuclear leukocytes
+ Immunoactive cells circulate constantly or remain in tissues, organs

457

others remain in the tissues and organs of the immune system, such as the thymus, lymph nodes, bone marrow, spleen, and tonsils. In the thymus, the T-lymphocytes, which are involved in cell-mediated immunity, become able to differentiate self (host) from nonself (foreign) substances (antigens). In contrast, B-lymphocytes, which are involved in humoral immunity, mature in the bone marrow. The key mechanism in humoral immunity is the production of immunoglobulin by B cells and the subsequent activation of the complement cascade. The lymph nodes, spleen, liver, and intestinal lymphoid tissue help remove and destroy circulating antigens in the blood and lymph.

ANTIGENS

An antigen is a substance that can induce an immune response. T- and B-lymphocytes have specific receptors that respond to specific antigen molecular shapes, called *epitopes*. In B cells, this receptor is an immunoglobulin, also called an *antibody*.

Major histocompatibility complex

The T-cell antigen receptor recognizes antigens only in association with specific cell-surface molecules known as the *major histocompatibility complex* (MHC).

The MHC, also known as the *human leukocyte antigen* (HLA) *locus,* is a cluster of genes on human chromosome 6 that has a pivotal role in the immune response. Every person receives one set of MHC genes from each parent, and both sets of genes are expressed on the individual's cells. These genes produce MHC molecules, which participate in the recognition of self versus nonself and the interaction of immunologically active cells by coding for cell-surface proteins.

MHC molecules differ among individuals. Slightly different antigen receptors can recognize a large number of distinct antigens, coded by distinct, variable region genes.

Groups or clones of lymphocytes exist that have identical receptors for a specific antigen. The clone of a lymphocyte rapidly proliferates when it's exposed to the specific antigen. Some lymphocytes further differentiate, while others become memory cells, which allow for a more rapid response—the memory or anamnestic response—to subsequent challenge by the antigen.

Haptens

Most antigens are large molecules, such as proteins or polysaccharides. Smaller molecules, such as drugs, that aren't antigenic by themselves are known as *haptens*. They can bind with larger molecules, or carriers, and become antigenic or immunogenic.

Antigenicity

Many factors influence the intensity of a foreign substance's interaction with the host's immune system (antigenicity). Among them are the physical and chemical characteristics of the antigen, the host's genetic makeup (especially the MHC molecules), and the antigen's relative foreignness. For example, little or no immune response may follow the transfusion of serum proteins between humans, but a vigorous immune response (serum sickness) commonly follows transfusion of horse serum proteins to a human.

HUMORAL IMMUNITY

The humoral immune response is one of two types of immune responses that can occur when foreign substances invade the body. The other is the cell-mediated response. The humoral response is also called an *antibody-mediated response.*

B-lymphocytes

B-lymphocytes and their products, immunoglobulins, are the basis of humoral immunity. A soluble antigen binds with the B-cell antigen receptor, initiating the humoral immune response. The activated B cells differentiate into plasma cells, which secrete immunoglobulins, also called *antibodies.* This response is regulated by T-lymphocytes and their products—lymphokines, such as interleukin-2 (IL-2), IL-4, IL-5, and interferon-8—determine which class of immunoglobulins a B cell will manufacture.

Immunoglobulins

The immunoglobulins secreted by plasma cells are four-chain molecules with two heavy and two light chains. Each chain has a variable (V) region and one or more constant (C) regions, which are coded by separate genes. The V regions of both light and heavy chains participate in antigen binding. The C regions of the heavy chain provide a binding site for crystallizable fragment (Fc) receptors on cells and govern other mechanisms. (See *Structure of the immunoglobulin molecule,* page 460.)

There are five known classes of immunoglobulins: IgG, IgM, IgA, IgE, and IgD. These classes are distinguished by the constant portions of their heavy chains. However, each class has a kappa or lambda light chain, which gives rise to many subtypes and provides almost limitless combinations of light and heavy chains that give immunoglobulins their specificity. (See *Classification of immunoglobulins,* page 461.)

A clone of B cells is specific for only one antigen, and the V regions of its Ig light chains determine that specificity. However, the class of immunoglobulin can change if the association between the cell's V region genes and heavy chain C region genes changes through a process known as *isotype switching.* For example, a clone of B cells genetically programmed to recognize tetanus toxoid will first make an IgM antibody against tetanus toxoid and later an IgG or other antibody against it.

CELL-MEDIATED IMMUNITY

The cell-mediated immune response protects the body against bacterial, viral, and fungal infections and defends against transplanted cells and tumor cells. T-lymphocytes and macrophages are the chief participants in the cell-mediated immune response. A macrophage processes the antigen and then presents it to T-lymphocytes.

Macrophages

Macrophages influence both immune and inflammatory responses. Macrophage precursors circulate in the blood. When the precursors collect in various tissues and organs, they differentiate into different types of macrophages. Unlike B- and T-lymphocytes, macrophages lack surface receptors for specific antigens. Instead, they have receptors for the C region of the heavy chain (Fc region) of immunoglobulin, for fragments of the third component of complement (C3), and for nonimmunologic substances such as carbohydrate molecules.

One of the most important functions of macrophages is presentation of antigen to T-lymphocytes. Macrophages ingest and process the antigen, then deposit it on

Humoral immunity
◆ One of two types of immune responses to foreign substances
◆ Also called an *antibody-mediated response*

B-lymphocytes
◆ Basis of humoral immunity
◆ Soluble antigen binds with B-cell antigen receptor
◆ Plasma cells secrete immunoglobulins
◆ Response regulated by T-lymphocytes and their products

Immunoglobulins
◆ Secreted by plasma cells
◆ Four-chain molecules with two heavy and two light chains
◆ Each chain has one variable, one or more constant regions
◆ Five known classes: IgG, IgM, IgA, IgE, IgD
◆ Clone of B cells specific for only one antigen
◆ Class of immunoglobulin can change (isotype switching)

Cell-mediated immunity
◆ Protects body against bacterial, viral, fungal infections
◆ Defends against transplanted and tumor cells

Macrophages
◆ Influence immune and inflammatory responses
◆ Macrophage precursors circulate in blood
◆ Collect in various tissues, organs, differentiate into different types of macrophages
◆ Produce IL-1, generating fever

Structure of the immunoglobulin molecule

The immunoglobulin molecule consists of four polypeptide chains: two heavy (H) and two light (L) chains held together by disulfide bonds. The H chain has one variable (V) and at least three constant (C) regions. The L chain has one V and one C region. Together, the V regions form a pocket known as the *antigen-binding site.* This site is located within the antigen-binding fragment (Fab) region of the molecule. Part of the C region of the H chains forms the crystallizable fragment (Fc) region of the molecule. This region mediates effector mechanisms, such as complement activation, and is the portion of the immunoglobulin molecule bound by Fc receptors on phagocytic cells, mast cells, and basophils. Each immunoglobulin molecule also has two antibody-combining sites (except for the immunoglobulin [Ig] M molecule, which has 10, and IgA, which may have 2 or more).

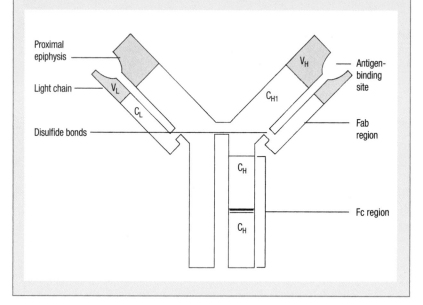

T-lymphocytes

+ Derived from bone marrow and migrate to thymus
+ Products of MHC genes "teach" T cells to distinguish between self and nonself
+ Five types of T cells: memory cells, lymphokine-producing cells, cytotoxic T cells, helper T cells, suppressor T cells
+ Markers and T-cell antigen receptor promote activation of each type
+ Requires presentation of antigens in context of specific HLA antigen

their own surfaces in association with HLA antigen. T-lymphocytes become activated when they recognize the antigen-HLA complex. Macrophages also function in the inflammatory response by producing IL-1, which generates fever, and by synthesizing complement proteins and other mediators that have phagocytic, microbicidal, and tumoricidal effects.

T-lymphocytes

Immature T-lymphocytes are derived from the bone marrow and migrate to the thymus, where they mature. In maturation, the products of the MHC genes "teach" T cells to distinguish between self and nonself.

Five types of T cells exist with specific functions. Memory cells are sensitized cells that remain dormant until the second exposure to the antigen and are also known as *secondary immune response.* Lymphokine-producing cells produce delayed hypersensitivity reactions. Cytotoxic T cells produce direct destruction of the antigen or the cells carrying the antigen. Helper T cells, also known as *T4 cells,* facilitate the humoral and cell-mediated responses. Suppressor T cells, also known as *T8 cells,* inhibit humoral and cell-mediated responses.

Classification of immunoglobulins

This chart shows the five classifications of immunoglobulins (Igs).

CLASSIFICATION	DESCRIPTION
IgA	✦ Secretory immunoglobulin (monomer in serum, dimer in secretory form) ✦ Found in colostrum, saliva, tears, nasal fluids, and respiratory, GI, and genitourinary secretions ✦ Accounts for 20% of total serum immunoglobulins ✦ Important role in preventing antigenic agents from attaching to epithelial surfaces
IgD	✦ Minute amounts found in serum (monomer) ✦ Predominant on surface of B-lymphocytes ✦ Primarily an antigen receptor ✦ Possible function in controlling lymphocyte activation or suppression
IgE	✦ Found only in trace amounts ✦ Involved in release of vasoactive amines stored in basophils and tissue mast cell granules that cause the allergic effects
IgG	✦ Smallest immunoglobulin (monomer) ✦ Found in all body fluids ✦ Can cross membranes as a single structural unit ✦ Accounts for 75% of total serum immunoglobulins ✦ Produced mainly in secondary immune response ✦ Classic antibody reactions, including precipitation, agglutination, neutralization, and complement fixation ✦ Major antibacterial and antiviral antibody
IgM	✦ Largest immunoglobulin (pentamer) ✦ Usually found only in the vascular system ✦ Can't readily cross membrane barriers because of its size ✦ Accounts for 5% of total serum immunoglobulins ✦ Dominant activity in primary or initial immune response ✦ Classic antibody reactions, including precipitation, agglutination, neutralization, and complement fixation

Classification of Igs

IgA
✦ Secretory
✦ Found in mucus, tears, other secretions
✦ Important in antigen rejection

IgD
✦ Monomer
✦ Predominant on B-lymphocyte surface
✦ Antigen receptor
✦ May activate or suppress lymphocytes

IgE
✦ Found in trace amounts
✦ Involved in release of vasoactive amines

IgG
✦ Monomer
✦ In all body fluids
✦ Crosses membranes as single unit
✦ Secondary immune response
✦ Antibacterial and antiviral property

IgM
✦ Largest Ig
✦ Found in vascular system
✦ Can't cross membranes easily
✦ Initial immune response
✦ Classic antibody reactions

T cells acquire specific surface molecules (markers) that identify their potential role when needed in the immune response. These markers and the T-cell antigen receptor together promote the particular activation of each type of T cell. T-cell activation requires presentation of antigens in the context of a specific HLA antigen: class II HLA for helper T cells; class I for cytotoxic T cells. T-cell activation also requires IL-1, produced by macrophages, and IL-2, produced by T cells.

Natural killer cells

This is a discrete population of large lymphocytes, some of which resemble T cells. Natural killer cells recognize surface changes on body cells infected with a virus. They bind to and, in many cases, kill the infected cells.

Natural killer cells

✦ Discrete population of large lymphocytes
✦ Recognize surface changes on body cells
✦ Bind to and usually kill infected cells

Cytokines
+ Low-molecular-weight proteins
+ Involved in communication among macrophages and lymphocytes
+ Induce or regulate immune or inflammatory responses
+ Include colony-stimulating factors, interferons, interleukins, tumor necrosis factors, transforming growth factor

Complement system
+ Chief humoral effector of inflammatory response
+ Includes more than 20 serum proteins

Classic pathway
+ IgM or IgG binds with antigen to form antigen-antibody complexes
+ Complexes activate C1
+ C1 activates C4, C2, C3

Alternate pathway
+ Activating surfaces amplify spontaneous cleavage of C3
+ C3 activates C5 to C9
+ Major biological effects include chemotaxis, phagocyte activation, and histamine release
+ Inflammation mediators interact with complement system

Polymorphonuclear leukocytes

Neutrophils
+ Derived from bone marrow
+ Increase in response to infection, inflammation
+ First to respond in infection
+ Main constituent of pus

Eosinophils
+ Derived from bone marrow
+ Multiply in allergic and parasitic disorders

Cytokines

Cytokines are low-molecular-weight proteins involved in the communication among macrophages and the lymphocytes. They induce or regulate various immune or inflammatory responses. Cytokines include colony-stimulating factors, interferons, interleukins, tumor necrosis factors, and transforming growth factor.

COMPLEMENT SYSTEM

The chief humoral effector of the inflammatory response, the complement system includes more than 20 serum proteins. When activated, these proteins interact in a cascade-like process that has profound biological effects. Complement activation takes place through one of two pathways.

Classic pathway

In the classic pathway, IgM or IgG binds with the antigen to form antigen-antibody complexes that activate the first complement component, C1. This in turn activates C4, C2, and C3.

Alternate pathway

In the alternate pathway, activating surfaces such as bacterial cell membranes directly amplify spontaneous cleavage of C3. After C3 is activated in either pathway, activation of the terminal components, C5 to C9, follows.

The major biological effects of complement activation include chemotaxis (phagocyte attraction), phagocyte activation, histamine release, viral neutralization, promotion of phagocytosis by opsonization (making the bacteria susceptible to phagocytosis), and lysis of cells and bacteria. Kinins (peptides that cause vasodilation and enhance vascular permeability and smooth muscle contraction) and other mediators of inflammation derived from the kinin and coagulation pathways interact with the complement system.

POLYMORPHONUCLEAR LEUKOCYTES

Other key factors in the inflammatory response are the polymorphonuclear leukocytes: neutrophils, eosinophils, basophils, and mast cells.

Neutrophils

Neutrophils, the most numerous of these leukocytes, derive from bone marrow and increase dramatically in number in response to infection and inflammation. They're the first to respond in acute infection. Neutrophils are highly mobile cells attracted to areas of inflammation and are the main constituent of pus.

Neutrophils have surface receptors for immunoglobulins and complement fragments, and they avidly ingest bacteria or other particles that are coated with target-identifying antibodies (opsonins). Toxic oxygen metabolites and enzymes such as lysozyme promptly kill the ingested organisms. Unfortunately, in addition to killing invading organisms, neutrophils also damage host tissues.

Eosinophils

Eosinophils, also derived from bone marrow, multiply in allergic and parasitic disorders. Although their phagocytic function isn't clearly understood, evidence suggests that they participate in host defense against parasites. Their products may also diminish inflammatory response in allergic disorders.

Basophils and mast cells

Basophils and mast cells also function in immune disorders. Mast cells, unlike basophils, aren't blood cells. Basophils circulate in peripheral blood, whereas mast cells accumulate in connective tissue, particularly in the lungs, intestines, and skin. Both types of cells have surface receptors for IgE. When their receptors are cross-linked by an IgE antigen complex, they release mediators characteristic of the allergic response.

PATHOPHYSIOLOGIC CHANGES

The host defense system and the immune response are highly complex processes, subject to malfunction at any point along the sequence of events. This malfunction may involve exaggeration, misdirection, or an absence or depression of activity leading to an immune disorder.

IMMUNE RESPONSE MALFUNCTION

When the immune system responds inappropriately, three basic categories of reactions may occur: hypersensitivity, autoimmune response, and alloimmune response. The type of reaction is determined by the source of the antigen, such as environmental, self, or other person, to which the immune system is responding.

Hypersensitivity

Hypersensitivity is an exaggerated or inappropriate response that occurs on second exposure to an antigen. The result is inflammation and the destruction of healthy tissue. *Allergy* refers to the harmful effects resulting from a hypersensitivity to antigens, also called *allergens*.

Hypersensitivity reactions may be *immediate*, occurring within minutes to hours of reexposure, or *delayed*, occurring several hours after reexposure. A delayed hypersensitivity reaction typically is most severe days after the reexposure.

Generally, hypersensitivity reactions are classified as one of four types: type I (mediated by IgE), type II (tissue-specific), type III (immune complex-mediated), type IV (cell-mediated). (See *Classification of hypersensitivity reactions*, pages 464 and 465.)

Type I hypersensitivity

Allergens activate T cells, which induce B-cell production of IgE, which binds to the Fc receptors on the surface of mast cells. Repeated exposure to relatively large doses of the allergen is usually necessary to cause this response. When enough IgE has been produced, the person is *sensitized* to the allergen. At the next exposure to the same antigen, the antigen binds with the surface IgE, cross-links the Fc receptors, and causes mast cells to degranulate and release various mediators. Degranulation may also be triggered by complement-driven anaphylatoxins — C3a and C5a — or by certain drugs such as morphine.

Some of the mediators released are preformed, whereas others are newly synthesized on activation of the mast cells. Preformed mediators include heparin, histamine, proteolytic (protein-splitting) and other enzymes, and chemotactic factors for eosinophils and neutrophils. Newly synthesized mediators include prostaglandins and leukotrienes. Mast cells also produce various cytokines, which initiate smooth-muscle contraction, vasodilation, bronchospasm, edema, increased vascular permeability, mucus secretion, and cellular infiltration by eosinophils and neu-

(*Text continues on page 466.*)

Polymorphonuclear leukocytes

Basophils and mast cells

✦ Mast cells are not blood cells and they accumulate in connective tissue
✦ Basophils circulate in peripheral blood
✦ Both have surface receptors for IgE
✦ Receptors cross-linked by IgE antigen complex release

Pathophysiologic changes

✦ Exaggeration
✦ Misdirection
✦ Absence or depression of activity

Immune response malfunction

✦ Immune system responds inappropriately
✦ Three basic categories of reactions

Hypersensitivity

✦ Exaggerated or inappropriate response on second exposure to antigen
✦ Results in inflammation and destruction of healthy tissue
✦ Allergy: harmful effects from hypersensitivity to antigens
✦ Reactions may be immediate or delayed
✦ Delayed hypersensitivity reaction most severe days after reexposure

Type I

✦ Response to repeated exposure to large doses of allergen

Classification of hypersensitivity reactions

Clinical examples of hypersensitivity

Type I
✦ Extrinsic asthma
✦ Seasonal allergic rhinitis
✦ Systemic anaphylaxis

Type II
✦ Goodpasture's syndrome
✦ Pernicious anemia
✦ Autoimmune hemolytic anemia

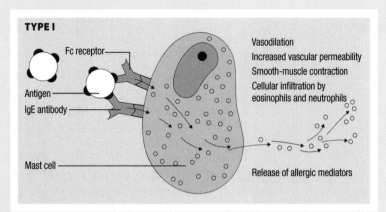

TYPE I

Fc receptor

Antigen

IgE antibody

Mast cell

Vasodilation
Increased vascular permeability
Smooth-muscle contraction
Cellular infiltration by
eosinophils and neutrophils

Release of allergic mediators

REACTIONS	PATHOPHYSIOLOGY	CLINICAL EXAMPLES
Anaphylactic (immediate, atopic, mediated by immunoglobulin [Ig] E)	Binding of antigens to IgE antibodies on mast cell surfaces releases allergic mediators, causing vasodilation, increased capillary permeability, smooth-muscle contraction, and eosinophilia.	Extrinsic asthma, seasonal allergic rhinitis, systemic anaphylaxis, reactions to insect stings, some food and drug reactions, some cases of urticaria, infantile eczema

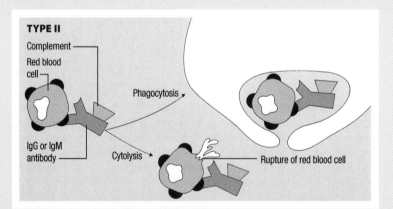

TYPE II

Complement

Red blood cell

Phagocytosis

IgG or IgM antibody

Cytolysis

Rupture of red blood cell

REACTIONS	PATHOPHYSIOLOGY	CLINICAL EXAMPLES
Cytotoxic (cytolytic, complement-dependent)	Binding of IgG or IgM antibodies to cellular or exogenous antigens activates the complement cascade, resulting in phagocytosis or cytolysis.	Goodpasture's syndrome, pernicious anemia, autoimmune hemolytic anemia, thrombocytopenia, some drug reactions, hyperacute renal allograft rejection, and hemolytic disease of the neonate

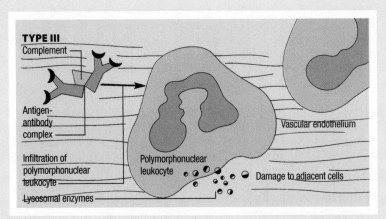

REACTIONS
Immune complex disease

PATHOPHYSIOLOGY
Activation of complement by immune complexes causes infiltration of polymorphonuclear leukocytes and release of lysosomal enzymes and permeability factors, producing an inflammatory response.

CLINICAL EXAMPLES
Serum sickness, systemic lupus erythematosus, rheumatoid arthritis, and polyarteritis

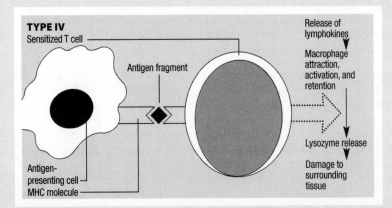

REACTIONS
Delayed (cell-mediated)

PATHOPHYSIOLOGY
Antigen-presenting cells present antigen to T cells in association with major histocompatibility complex (MHC). The sensitized T cells release lymphokines that stimulate macrophages. Lysozymes are released, and surrounding tissue is damaged.

CLINICAL EXAMPLES
Contact dermatitis, graft-versus-host disease, allograft rejection, some drug sensitivities, Hashimoto's thyroiditis, and sarcoidosis

Clinical examples of hypersensitivity

Type III
✦ Serum sickness
✦ Systemic lupus erythematosus
✦ Rheumatoid arthritis

Type IV
✦ Contact dermatitis
✦ Graft-versus-host disease
✦ Allograft rejection

Hypersensitivity

Type II
+ Tissue-specific reaction
+ Involves destruction of target cell by antibody directed against cell-surface antigens
+ Tissue damage occurs

Type III
+ Circulating antigen-antibody complexes accumulate, deposit in tissues
+ Deposited immune complexes cause local inflammation
+ Tissue damage occurs

Type IV
+ Involve processing of antigen by macrophages
+ Activated cytotoxic T cells attack and destroy target cells
+ Coagulation, kinin, complement cascades contribute to tissue damage

Autoimmune reactions
+ Body's normal defenses become self-destructive
+ Recognize self-antigens as foreign
+ Mechanism for misdirection is unclear
+ Genetic, hormonal, environmental influences
+ B-cell hyperactivity possibly related to T-cell abnormalities

trophils. These effects result in some of the classic associated signs and symptoms, such as hypotension, wheezing, swelling, urticaria, and rhinorrhea.

Type II hypersensitivity

Type II hypersensitivity, a tissue-specific reaction, generally involves the destruction of a target cell by an antibody directed against cell-surface antigens. Alternatively, the antibody may be directed against small molecules absorbed to cells or against cell-surface receptors, rather than against the cell constituents themselves. Tissue damage occurs through several mechanisms. Binding of antigen and antibody activates complement, which ultimately disrupts cellular membranes — complement-mediated lysis. Various phagocytic cells mediate another mechanism with receptors for immunoglobulin (Fc region) and complement fragments. These cells envelop and destroy opsonized targets, such as red blood cells (RBCs), leukocytes, and platelets. Cytotoxic T cells and natural killer cells, although not antigen specific, also contribute to tissue damage by releasing toxic substances that destroy the cells. Antibody binding causes the target cell to malfunction rather than causing its destruction.

Type III hypersensitivity

Circulating antigen-antibody complexes (immune complexes) accumulate and are deposited in the tissues. The most common tissues involved are the kidneys, joints, skin, and blood vessels. Normally, they clear excess immune complexes from the circulation. However, immune complexes deposited in the tissues activate the complement cascade, causing local inflammation, and trigger platelet release of vasoactive amines that increase vascular permeability, so that more immune complexes accumulate in the vessel walls.

Probably the most harmful effects result from the generation of complement fragments that attract neutrophils. The neutrophils attempt to ingest the immune complexes. They're generally unsuccessful, but in the attempt, the neutrophils release lysosomal enzymes, which exacerbate the tissue damage.

The formation of immune complexes is dynamic and always changing. The complexes that form in children may be totally different from those formed in later years. Also, more than one type of immune complex may be present at one time.

Type IV hypersensitivity

These cell-mediated reactions involve the processing of the antigen by the macrophages. Once processed, the antigen is presented to the T cells. Cytotoxic T cells, if activated, attack and destroy the target cells directly. When lymphokine T cells are activated, they release lymphokines, which recruit and activate other lymphocytes, monocytes, macrophages, and polymorphonuclear leukocytes. The coagulation, kinin, and complement cascades also contribute to tissue damage in this type of reaction.

Autoimmune reactions

In autoimmune reactions, the body's normal defenses become self-destructive, recognizing self-antigens as foreign. What causes this misdirected response isn't clearly understood. For example, drugs or viruses have been implicated as causing some autoimmune reactions, but in diseases such as rheumatoid arthritis and systemic lupus erythematosus, the mechanism for misdirection is unclear.

Autoimmune reactions are believed to result from a combination of factors, including genetic, hormonal, and environmental influences. Many are characterized by B-cell hyperactivity and by hypergammaglobulinemia. B-cell hyperactivity may be related to T-cell abnormalities. Hormonal and genetic factors strongly influence the onset of some autoimmune disorders.

 CLINICAL ALERT Immune function starts declining at sexual maturity and continues declining with age. During this decline, the immune system begins losing its ability to differentiate between self and nonself, leading to an increase in the incidence of autoimmune disorders.

Alloimmune reactions

Alloimmune reactions are directed at antigens from the tissues of others of the same species. Alloimmune reactions commonly occur in transplant and transfusion reactions, in which the recipient reacts to antigens, primarily HLA, on the donor cells. This immune response is also seen in infants with erythroblastosis fetalis. (See chapter 11, Hematologic system.) This type of response is commonly associated with a type II hypersensitivity reaction.

Immunodeficiency

An absent or depressed immune response increases susceptibility to infection. Immunodeficiency may be primary, reflecting a defect involving T cells, B cells, or lymphoid tissues, or secondary, resulting from an underlying disease or factor that depresses or blocks the immune response. The most common forms of immunodeficiency are caused by viral infection or are iatrogenic reactions to therapeutic drugs.

ACQUIRED IMMUNODEFICIENCY SYNDROME

Human immunodeficiency virus (HIV) infection may cause acquired immunodeficiency syndrome (AIDS). Although it's characterized by gradual destruction of cell-mediated (T cell) immunity, it also affects humoral immunity and even autoimmunity because of the central role of the CD4+ (helper) T-lymphocyte in immune reactions. The resulting immunodeficiency makes the patient susceptible to opportunistic infections, cancers, and other abnormalities that define AIDS.

This syndrome was first described by the Centers for Disease Control and Prevention (CDC) in 1981. Because transmission is similar, AIDS shares epidemiologic patterns with hepatitis B and sexually transmitted diseases.

Depending on individual variations and the presence of cofactors that influence disease progression, the time from acute HIV infection to the appearance of symptoms (mild to severe) to the diagnosis of AIDS and, eventually, to death varies greatly. Current combination drug therapy in conjunction with treatment and prophylaxis of common opportunistic infections can delay the natural progression and prolong survival.

CAUSES

The HIV-I retrovirus is the primary etiologic agent. Transmission occurs by contact with infected blood or body fluids and is associated with identifiable high-risk behaviors. It's disproportionately represented in homosexual and bisexual men, I.V. drug users, neonates born to infected women, recipients of contaminated blood or blood products (dramatically decreased since mid-1985), and heterosexual partners of persons in the former groups.

How it happens

+ Infection by HIV retrovirus through transmission of blood or body fluids
+ HIV strikes helper T cells bearing the CD4+ antigen
+ Genetic material is copied
+ Leads to profound structural and functional changes
+ Infectious process takes three forms: immunodeficiency, autoimmunity, neurologic dysfunction

Key signs and symptoms

+ Mononucleosis-like syndrome soon after infection
+ Laboratory evidence of seroconversion
+ Persistent generalized lymphadenopathy
+ Weight loss, fatigue, night sweats, fevers
+ HIV encephalopathy
+ Opportunistic infection or cancer

PATHOPHYSIOLOGY

AIDS begins with infection by the HIV retrovirus, which is detectable only by laboratory tests, and ends with death. Twenty years of data suggests that casual household or social contact doesn't transmit HIV. The HIV virus may enter the body by any of several routes involving the transmission of blood or body fluids, for example: direct inoculation during intimate sexual contact, especially associated with the mucosal trauma of receptive rectal intercourse, transfusion of contaminated blood or blood products (a risk diminished by routine testing of blood products), sharing contaminated needles, and transplacental or postpartum transmission from infected mother to fetus (by cervical or blood contact at delivery and in breast milk).

HIV strikes helper T cells bearing the CD4+ antigen. Normally a receptor for major histocompatibility complex molecules, the antigen serves as a receptor for the retrovirus and allows it to enter the cell. Viral binding also requires a coreceptor (believed to be the chemokine receptor CCR5) on the cell surface. The virus may also infect CD4+ antigen-bearing cells of the GI tract, cervix, and neuroglia.

Like other retroviruses, HIV copies its genetic material in a reverse manner compared with other viruses and cells. Through the action of reverse transcriptase, HIV produces deoxyribonucleic acid (DNA) from its viral ribonucleic acid (RNA). Transcription is typically poor, leading to mutations, some of which make HIV resistant to antiviral drugs. The viral DNA enters the nucleus of the cell and is incorporated into the host cell's DNA, where it's transcribed into more viral RNA. If the host cell reproduces, it duplicates the HIV DNA along with its own and passes it on to the daughter cells. Thus, if activated, the host cell carries this information and, if activated, replicates the virus. Viral enzymes, proteases, arrange the structural components and RNA into viral particles that move out to the periphery of the host cell, where the virus buds and emerges from the host cell. The virus is now free to travel and infect other cells.

HIV replication may lead to cell death or it may become latent. HIV infection leads to profound structural and functional changes, either directly through destruction of CD4+ cells, other immune cells, and neuroglial cells, or indirectly through the secondary effects of CD4+ T-cell dysfunction and resulting immunosuppression.

The HIV infectious process takes three forms: immunodeficiency (opportunistic infections and unusual cancers), autoimmunity (lymphoid interstitial pneumonitis, arthritis, hypergammaglobulinemia, and production of autoimmune antibodies), and neurologic dysfunction (AIDS dementia complex, HIV encephalopathy, and peripheral neuropathies).

SIGNS AND SYMPTOMS

HIV infection manifests in many ways. After a high-risk exposure and inoculation, the infected person usually experiences a mononucleosis-like syndrome, which may be attributed to flu or another virus and then may not produce symtoms for years. In this latent stage, the only sign of HIV infection is laboratory evidence of seroconversion.

When symptoms appear, they may take many forms, including persistent generalized lymphadenopathy secondary to impaired function of CD4+ cells; nonspecific symptoms, including weight loss, fatigue, night sweats, fevers related to altered function of CD4+ cells, immunodeficiency, and infection of other CD4+ antigen-bearing cells; neurologic symptoms resulting from HIV encephalopathy and infection of neuroglial cells; and opportunistic infection or cancer related to immunodeficiency.

Opportunistic infections in AIDS

This chart shows the complicating infections that may occur in acquired immunodeficiency syndrome (AIDS).

MICROBIOLOGICAL AGENT	ORGANISM	CONDITION
Protozoa	*Pneumocystis carinii* *Cryptosporidium* *Toxoplasma gondii* *Histoplasma*	*Pneumocystis carinii* pneumonia Cryptosporidiosis Toxoplasmosis Histoplasmosis
Fungi	*Candida albicans* *Cryptococcus neoformans*	Candidiasis Cryptococcosis
Viruses	Herpes Cytomegalovirus	Herpes simplex 1 and 2 Cytomegalovirus retinitis
Bacteria	*Mycobacterium tuberculosis* *M. avium-intracellulare*	Tuberculosis Mycobacteriosis

Other opportunistic conditions include:
+ Kaposi's sarcoma
+ wasting disease
+ AIDS dementia complex.

CLINICAL ALERT In children, HIV infection has a mean incubation time of 17 months. Signs and symptoms resemble those in adults, except for findings related to sexually transmitted diseases. Children have a high incidence of opportunistic bacterial infections: otitis media, sepsis, chronic salivary gland enlargement, lymphoid interstitial pneumonia, *Mycobacterium avium-intracellulare* complex function, and pneumonias, including *Pneumocystis carinii*.

COMPLICATIONS

Complications of AIDS are repeated opportunistic infections. (See *Opportunistic infections in AIDS*.)

DIAGNOSIS

The CDC has developed an HIV/AIDS classification matrix defining AIDS as an illness characterized by one or more indicator diseases, coexisting with laboratory evidence of HIV infection and other possible causes of immunosuppression. Diagnosis of AIDS includes confirmed presence of HIV infection, CD4$^+$ T-cell count of less than 200 cells/µl, or the presence of one or more conditions specified by the CDC as Categories A, B, or C. (See *Conditions associated with AIDS*, page 470.)

TREATMENT

No cure has yet been found for AIDS. Primary therapy includes the use of various combinations of three different types of antiretroviral agents to try to gain the maximum benefit of inhibiting HIV viral replication with the fewest adverse reactions. Current recommendations include the use of two nucleosides plus one pro-

Microbiological agents in AIDS
+ Protozoa
+ Fungi
+ Viruses
+ Bacteria

Alert!
+ In children, HIV infection has a mean incubation time of 17 months.
+ Signs and symptoms resemble those in adults, except for findings related to sexually transmitted diseases.

Complications
+ Repeated opportunistic infections

Diagnosis
+ Confirmed presence of HIV infection
+ CD4$^+$ T-cell count of less than 200 cells/µl
+ Presence of one or more conditions specified by CDC as Categories A, B, or C

AIDS-associated conditions

Category A
+ Asymptomatic HIV infection
+ Persistent generalized lymph node enlargement
+ Acute primary HIV infection

Category B
+ Bacillary angiomatosis
+ Moderate or severe cervical abnormalities or cervical cancer
+ Oropharyngeal or persistent vulvovaginal candidiasis that lasts longer than 1 month

Category C
+ Candidiasis of the bronchi, trachea, lungs, or esophagus
+ Invasive cervical cancer
+ Disseminated or extrapulmonary coccidioidomycosis

Treatment
+ No cure
+ Various combinations of three different types of antiretroviral agents
+ Combination of nucleosides, protease inhibitors
+ Immunomodulatory agents
+ Human granulocyte colony-stimulating growth factor
+ Anti-infective and antineoplastic agents
+ Nutritional support, fluid, electrolyte replacement therapy
+ Pain relief
+ Psychological support

Conditions associated with AIDS

The Centers for Disease Control and Prevention (CDC) lists acquired immunodeficiency syndrome (AIDS)–associated diseases under three categories. Periodically, the CDC adds to these lists.

CATEGORY A
+ Asymptomatic human immunodeficiency virus (HIV) infection
+ Persistent generalized lymph node enlargement
+ Acute primary HIV infection with accompanying illness
+ History of acute HIV infection

CATEGORY B
+ Bacillary angiomatosis
+ Oropharyngeal or persistent vulvovaginal candidiasis lasting longer than 1 month
+ Moderate or severe cervical abnormalities or cervical cancer
+ Symptoms such as fever or diarrhea lasting longer than 1 month
+ Herpes zoster involving at least 2 distinct episodes or more than one dermatome
+ Listeriosis
+ Oral hairy leukoplakia
+ Idiopathic thrombocytopenic purpura
+ Pelvic inflammatory disease, especially with a tubo-ovarian abscess
+ Peripheral neuropathy

CATEGORY C
+ Candidiasis of the bronchi, trachea, lungs, or esophagus
+ Invasive cervical cancer
+ Disseminated or extrapulmonary coccidioidomycosis
+ Extrapulmonary cryptococcosis
+ Chronic interstitial cryptosporidiosis
+ Cytomegalovirus (CMV) disease affecting organs other than the liver, spleen, or lymph nodes
+ CMV retinitis with vision loss
+ Encephalopathy related to HIV
+ Herpes simplex infection with chronic ulcers or herpetic bronchitis, pneumonitis, or esophagitis
+ Disseminated or extrapulmonary histoplasmosis
+ Chronic intestinal isosporiasis
+ Kaposi's sarcoma
+ Burkitt's lymphoma or its equivalent
+ Immunoblastic lymphoma or its equivalent
+ Primary brain lymphoma
+ Disseminated or extrapulmonary *Mycobacterium avium* complex or *M. kansasii*
+ Pulmonary or extrapulmonary *M. tuberculosis*
+ Disseminated or extrapulmonary infection with any other species of *Mycobacterium*
+ *Pneumocystis carinii* pneumonia
+ Recurrent pneumonia
+ Progressive multifocal leukoencephalopathy
+ Recurrent *Salmonella* septicemia
+ Toxoplasmosis of the brain
+ Wasting disease caused by HIV

tease inhibitor, or two nucleosides and one nonnucleoside to help inhibit the production of resistant, mutant strains. The drugs include protease inhibitors to block replication of virus particles formed through the action of viral protease (reducing the number of new virus particles produced), nucleoside reverse-transcriptase inhibitors to interfere with the copying of viral RNA into DNA by the enzyme reverse transcriptase, and nonnucleoside reverse-transcriptase inhibitors to interfere with the action of reverse transcriptase.

Additional treatment may include immunomodulatory agents to boost the immune system weakened by AIDS and retroviral therapy, human granulocyte colony-stimulating growth factor to stimulate neutrophil production (retroviral therapy causes anemia, so patients may receive epoetin alfa), and anti-infective and antineoplastic agents to combat opportunistic infections and associated cancers (some prophylactically to help resist opportunistic infections). Supportive therapy, including nutritional support, fluid and electrolyte replacement therapy, pain relief, and psychological support is essential.

Nursing considerations

✦ Advise health care workers and the public to use precautions in all situations that risk exposure to blood, body fluids, and secretions. Diligent practice of standard precautions can prevent the inadvertent transmission of AIDS and other infectious diseases transmitted by similar routes.

✦ Recognize that a diagnosis of AIDS is profoundly distressing because of the disease's social impact and discouraging prognosis. The patient may lose his job and financial security as well as the support of family and friends. Do your best to help the patient cope with an altered body image, the emotional burden of serious illness, and the threat of death. Encourage and assist the patient in learning about AIDS societies and support programs.

▼ *LIFE-THREATENING DISORDER*

ANAPHYLAXIS

Anaphylaxis is an acute, potentially life-threatening type I (immediate) hypersensitivity reaction marked by the sudden onset of rapidly progressive urticaria (vascular swelling in skin accompanied by itching) and respiratory distress. With prompt recognition and treatment, the prognosis is good. However, a severe reaction may precipitate vascular collapse, leading to systemic shock and, sometimes, death. The reaction typically occurs within minutes but can occur up to 1 hour after reexposure to the antigen.

Causes

The cause of anaphylaxis is usually the ingestion of or other systemic exposure to sensitizing drugs or other substances. Such substances may include serums (usually horse serum); vaccines; allergen extracts; enzymes such as L-asparaginase; hormones; penicillin or other antibiotics; sulfonamides; local anesthetics; salicylates; polysaccharides; diagnostic chemicals such as sulfobromophthalein sodium; sodium dehydrocholate; and radiographic contrast media; food proteins, such as those in legumes, nuts, berries, seafood, and egg albumin; food additives containing sulfite; and insect venom.

The most common anaphylaxis-causing antigen is penicillin. The drug induces a reaction in 1 to 4 of every 10,000 patients treated with it. Penicillin is most likely to induce anaphylaxis after parenteral administration or prolonged therapy and in patients with an inherited tendency to food or drug allergy, or atopy.

Pathophysiology

Anaphylaxis requires previous sensitization or exposure to the specific antigen, resulting in immunoglobulin (Ig) E production by plasma cells in the lymph nodes and enhancement by helper T cells. IgE antibodies then bind to membrane receptors on mast cells in connective tissue and to basophils.

On reexposure, the antigen binds to adjacent IgE antibodies or cross-linked IgE receptors, activating a series of cellular reactions that trigger mast cell degranulation. With degranulation, powerful chemical mediators, such as histamine, eosinophil chemotactic factor of anaphylaxis, and platelet-activating factor, are released from the mast cells. IgG or IgM enters into the reaction and activates the complement cascade, leading to the release of the complement fractions.

Key nursing actions

✦ Advise health care workers and the public to use precautions in all situations that risk exposure.

✦ Recognize that a diagnosis of AIDS is profoundly distressing.

Characteristics of anaphylaxis

✦ Life-threatening disorder

✦ Acute type I hypersensitivity reaction

✦ Sudden onset of rapidly progressive urticaria, respiratory distress

✦ Prognosis is good with treatment

✦ Severe reaction may precipitate vascular collapse

Causes

✦ Ingestion or systemic exposure to sensitizing drugs, other substances

How it happens

✦ Requires previous sensitization or exposure to specific antigen

✦ IgE production by plasma cells in the lymph nodes and enhancement by helper T cells

✦ IgE antibodies bind to membrane receptors on mast cells in connective tissue

✦ On reexposure, cellular reactions trigger mast cell degranulation

✦ Histamine, eosinophil chemotactic factor of anaphylaxis, and platelet-activating factor released

✦ Bradykinin, leukotrienes induce vascular collapse

✦ Reduction of blood volume causes hypotension, hypovolemic shock, cardiac dysfunction

At the same time, two other chemical mediators, bradykinin and leukotrienes, induce vascular collapse by stimulating contraction of certain groups of smooth muscles and increasing vascular permeability. These substances, together with the other chemical mediators, cause vasodilation, smooth-muscle contraction, enhanced vascular permeability, and increased mucus production. Continued release, along with the spread of these mediators through the body by way of the basophils in the circulation, triggers the systemic responses. Also, increased vascular permeability leads to decreased peripheral resistance and plasma leakage from the circulation to the extravascular tissues. Consequent reduction of blood volume causes hypotension, hypovolemic shock, and cardiac dysfunction.

SIGNS AND SYMPTOMS

An anaphylactic reaction produces sudden physical distress within seconds or minutes after exposure to an allergen. A delayed or persistent reaction may occur up to 24 hours later. The severity of the reaction is inversely related to the interval between exposure to the allergen and the onset of symptoms.

Immediately after exposure, the patient may complain of a feeling of impending doom or fright due to activation of IgE and subsequent release of chemical mediators. He may experience sweating due to release of histamine and vasodilation and sneezing, shortness of breath, nasal pruritus, urticaria, and angioedema (swelling of nerves and blood vessels) secondary to histamine release and increased capillary permeability.

Cardiovascular symptoms include hypotension, shock, and sometimes cardiac arrhythmias due to increased vascular permeability and subsequent decrease in peripheral resistance and leakage of plasma fluids.

Respiratory symptoms commonly include nasal mucosal edema; profuse watery rhinorrhea; itching; nasal congestion; and sudden sneezing attacks due to histamine release, vasodilation, and increased capillary permeability. Edema of the upper respiratory tract results in hypopharyngeal and laryngeal obstruction, due to increased capillary permeability and mast cell degranulation. The respiratory obstruction causes hoarseness, stridor, wheezing, and accessory muscle use secondary to bronchiole smooth muscle contraction and increased mucus production.

GI and genitourinary symptoms include severe stomach cramps, nausea, diarrhea, and urinary urgency and incontinence resulting from smooth-muscle contraction of the intestines and bladder.

COMPLICATIONS

Untreated anaphylaxis can cause respiratory obstruction, systemic vascular collapse, and death minutes to hours after the first symptoms (although a delayed or persistent reaction may occur for up to 24 hours).

DIAGNOSIS

No single diagnostic test can identify anaphylaxis. Anaphylaxis can be diagnosed by the rapid onset of severe respiratory or cardiovascular symptoms after ingestion or injection of a drug, vaccine, diagnostic agent, food, or food additive, or after an insect sting. If these symptoms occur without a known allergic stimulus, other possible causes of shock (such as acute myocardial infarction, status asthmaticus, or heart failure) must be ruled out.

Skin tests showing hypersensitivity to a specific allergen or elevated serum IgE levels may show clues to the patient's risk of anaphylaxis.

Key signs and symptoms

+ Sudden physical distress within minutes after allergen exposure
+ Delayed reaction may occur up to 24 hours later
+ Feeling of impending doom or fright
+ Sweating
+ Sneezing
+ Shortness of breath
+ Nasal pruritus
+ Urticaria
+ Angioedema

Complications

+ Respiratory obstruction
+ Systemic vascular collapse
+ Death minutes to hours after first symptoms

Diagnosis

+ Rapid onset of severe respiratory or cardiovascular symptoms after exposure
+ Rule out other causes of shock
+ Skin tests may show clues to risk of anaphylaxis

TREATMENT

Always an emergency, anaphylaxis requires an immediate administration of epinephrine 1:1,000 aqueous solution to reverse bronchoconstriction and cause vasoconstriction. It may be given I.M. or subcutaneously if the patient hasn't lost consciousness and is normotensive, or I.V. if the reaction is severe (repeating dosage every 5 to 20 minutes as needed).

Tracheostomy or endotracheal intubation and mechanical ventilation may be necessary to maintain a patent airway and oxygen therapy may be needed to increase tissue perfusion. After the initial emergency, administer longer-acting epinephrine, corticosteroids, and diphenhydramine (Benadryl) to reduce the allergic response (long-term management).

An albuterol mini-nebulizer treatment is administered or cimetidine or other histamine-2 blocker. As ordered, aminophylline is administered to reverse bronchospasm. Administer volume expanders to maintain and restore circulating plasma volume. As prescribed, administer I.V. vasopressors such as norepinephrine (Levophed) and dopamine (Intropin) to stabilize blood pressure. If cardiac arrest occurs, begin cardiopulmonary resuscitation.

NURSING CONSIDERATIONS

✦ To prevent anaphylaxis, teach the patient to avoid exposure to known allergens. A person allergic to certain foods or drugs must learn to avoid the offending food or drug in all its forms. A person allergic to insect stings should avoid open fields and wooded areas during the insect season. An anaphylaxis kit (epinephrine, antihistamine, and tourniquet) should also be carried whenever the patient with known severe allergic reactions goes outdoors. In addition, every patient prone to anaphylaxis should wear a medical identification bracelet identifying his allergies.
✦ If a patient must receive a drug to which he's allergic, prevent a severe reaction by making sure he receives careful desensitization with gradually increasing doses of the antigen or advance administration of steroids. Of course, a person with a known allergic history should receive a drug with a high anaphylactic potential only after cautious pretesting for sensitivity. Closely monitor the patient during testing, and make sure you have resuscitative equipment and epinephrine ready. When any patient needs a drug with a high anaphylactic potential (particularly parenteral drugs), make sure he receives each dose under close medical observation.
✦ Closely monitor a patient undergoing diagnostic tests that use radiographic contrast media, such as excretory urography, cardiac catheterization, and angiography.

LATEX ALLERGY

Latex allergy is a hypersensitivity reaction to products that contain natural latex, a substance found in an increasing number of products at home and at work, that's derived from the sap of a rubber tree, not synthetic latex. The hypersensitivity reactions can range from local dermatitis to life-threatening anaphylactic reaction.

CAUSES

Exposure to latex proteins found in natural rubber products produces a true latex allergy. Those in frequent contact with latex-containing products are at risk for developing a latex allergy. More frequent exposure leads to a higher risk.

Treatment
✦ Always an emergency
✦ Immediate administration of epinephrine 1:1,000 aqueous solution
✦ Tracheostomy or endotracheal intubation and mechanical ventilation
✦ Administer longer-acting epinephrine, corticosteroids, diphenhydramine

Key nursing actions
✦ Teach the patient to avoid exposure to known allergens.
✦ An anaphylaxis kit should be carried whenever the patient with known severe allergic reactions goes outdoors.
✦ Patient should wear a medical identification bracelet identifying his allergies.
✦ When any patient needs a drug with a high anaphylactic potential, make sure he receives each dose under close medical observation.
✦ Closely monitor a patient undergoing diagnostic tests that use radiographic contrast media.

Characteristics of latex allergy
✦ Hypersensitivity reaction to products containing natural latex
✦ Reactions range from local dermatitis to anaphylactic reaction

Causes
✦ Exposure to latex proteins produces latex allergy
✦ Frequent exposure leads to higher risk

How it happens

+ IgE-mediated immediate hyper-sensitivity reaction
+ Mast cells release histamine, other secretory products
+ Vascular permeability increases, vasodilation, bronchoconstriction occur

Key signs and symptoms

+ Signs and symptoms of anaphylaxis

Complications

+ Respiratory obstruction
+ Systemic vascular collapse
+ Death

Diagnosis

+ Based on history and physical assessment
+ Radioallergosorbent test shows specific IgE antibodies to latex
+ Patch test results in hives, itching, redness

Treatment

+ Prevention of exposure
+ Corticosteroids, antihistamines, histamine-2-receptor blockers before and after possible exposure

Acute emergency

+ Epinephrine 1:1,000 aqueous solution
+ Tracheostomy or endotracheal intubation

The populations at highest risk are medical and dental professionals, workers in latex companies, and patients with spina bifida or other conditions that require multiple surgeries involving latex material.

Other individuals at risk include patients with a history of asthma or other allergies, especially to bananas, avocados, tropical fruits, or chestnuts; multiple intra-abdominal or genitourinary surgeries; and frequent intermittent urinary catheterization.

PATHOPHYSIOLOGY

A true latex allergy is an immunoglobulin (Ig) E-mediated immediate hypersensitivity reaction. Mast cells release histamine and other secretory products. Vascular permeability increases and vasodilation and bronchoconstriction occur.

Chemical sensitivity dermatitis is a type IV delayed hypersensitivity reaction to the chemicals used in processing rather than the latex itself. In a cell-mediated allergic reaction, sensitized T-lymphocytes are triggered, stimulating the proliferation of other lymphocytes and mononuclear cells. This results in tissue inflammation and contact dermatitis.

SIGNS AND SYMPTOMS

With a true latex allergy, the patient shows signs and symptoms of anaphylaxis, including hypotension due to vasodilation and increased vascular permeability, tachycardia secondary to hypotension, and oxygen desaturation.

Other clinical findings include urticaria and pruritus due to histamine release, difficulty breathing, bronchospasm, wheezing, and stridor secondary to bronchoconstriction, and angioedema from increased vascular permeability and loss of water to tissues.

COMPLICATIONS

Like anaphylaxis, a true latex allergy may lead to respiratory obstruction, systemic vascular collapse, or death.

DIAGNOSIS

Diagnosis of latex allergy is based mainly on history and physical assessment. A radioallergosorbent test showing specific IgE antibodies to latex is safest for use in patients with history of type I hypersensitivity. The patch test results in hives with itching or redness as a positive response.

TREATMENT

The best treatment is prevention of exposure, including use of latex-free products to decrease possible exacerbation of hypersensitivity. When a latex allergy is suspected, the patient receives drug therapy, such as corticosteroids, antihistamines, and histamine-2-receptor blockers before and after possible exposure to latex to depress immune response and block histamine release.

If the patient is experiencing an acute emergency, treatment includes immediate administration of epinephrine 1:1,000 aqueous solution to reverse bronchoconstriction and cause vasoconstriction. The drug is given I.M. or subcutaneously if the patient hasn't lost consciousness and is normotensive, or I.V. if the reaction is severe (repeating dosage every 5 to 20 minutes as needed).

Tracheostomy or endotracheal intubation and mechanical ventilation may be necessary to maintain a patent airway and oxygen therapy may be needed to increase tissue perfusion. As ordered, administer volume expanders to maintain and restore circulating plasma volume. As prescribed, administer I.V. vasopressors such as norepinephrine (Levophed) and dopamine (Intropin) to stabilize blood pressure. If cardiac arrest occurs, begin cardiopulmonary resuscitation.

After the initial emergency, administer longer-acting epinephrine, corticosteroids, and diphenhydramine (Benadryl) to reduce the allergic response (long-term management). As ordered, administer drugs to reverse bronchospasm, including aminophylline and albuterol.

NURSING CONSIDERATIONS

✦ Make sure items that aren't available latex-free, such as stethoscopes and blood pressure cuffs, are wrapped in cloth before they come in contact with a hypersensitive patient's skin.
✦ Place the patient in a private room or with another patient who requires a latex-free environment.
✦ When adding medication to an I.V. bag, inject the drug through the spike port, not the rubber latex port.
✦ Urge the patient to wear medical identification jewelry mentioning his latex allergy.
✦ Teach the patient and his family how to use an epinephrine autoinjector.
✦ Teach the patient to be aware of all latex-containing products and to use vinyl or silicone products instead. Advise him that Mylar balloons don't contain latex.

LUPUS ERYTHEMATOSUS

Lupus erythematosus is a chronic inflammatory disorder of the connective tissues that appears in two forms: discoid lupus erythematosus, which affects only the skin, and systemic lupus erythematosus (SLE), which affects multiple organ systems as well as the skin and can be fatal. SLE is characterized by recurring remissions and exacerbations, which are especially common during the spring and summer.

The prognosis improves with early detection and treatment but remains poor for patients who develop cardiovascular, renal, or neurologic complications, or severe bacterial infections.

CAUSES

The exact cause of SLE remains unknown, but available evidence points to interrelated immunologic, environmental, hormonal, and genetic factors.

Certain predisposing factors may make a person susceptible to SLE. Physical or mental stress, streptococcal or viral infections, exposure to sunlight or ultraviolet light, immunization, pregnancy, and abnormal estrogen metabolism may all affect the development of this disease. SLE may also be triggered or aggravated by treatment with certain drugs, such as procainamide (Pronestyl), hydralazine (Apresoline), anticonvulsants and, less commonly, penicillins, sulfa drugs, and hormonal contraceptives.

Key nursing actions

✦ Make sure items that aren't available latex-free are wrapped in cloth before they come in contact with a hypersensitive patient's skin.
✦ Place the patient in a private room or with another patient who requires a latex-free environment.
✦ When adding medication to an I.V. bag, inject the drug through the spike port, not the rubber latex port.
✦ Urge the patient to wear medical identification jewelry mentioning his latex allergy.

Characteristics of lupus erythematosus

✦ Chronic inflammatory disorder of the connective tissues
✦ Two forms: discoid lupus erythematosus, systemic lupus erythematosus
✦ SLE characterized by recurring remissions and exacerbations
✦ Prognosis improves with early detection and treatment
✦ Prognosis poor for patients with cardiovascular, renal, neurologic complications, severe bacterial infections

Causes

✦ Unknown
✦ Evidence points to immunologic, environmental, hormonal, genetic factors
✦ Possible predisposing factors
✦ May be triggered or aggravated by treatment with certain drugs

Signs of SLE

+ Malar or discoid rash
+ Photosensitivity
+ Oral or nasopharyngeal ulcerations
+ Nonerosive arthritis
+ Pleuritis or pericarditis
+ Profuse proteinuria
+ Seizures, psychoses
+ Hemolytic anemia, leukopenia, lymphopenia, thrombocytopenia

How it happens

+ Autoimmunity believed to be prime mechanism
+ Body produces antibodies against components of own cells
+ Immune complex disease follows
+ Patients may produce antibodies against many tissue components

Key signs and symptoms

+ Onset acute or insidious, produces no characteristic clinical pattern
+ Signs and symptoms relate to tissue injury, inflammation, necrosis
+ Fever, weight loss, malaise, fatigue, rashes, polyarthralgia
+ Joint involvement
+ Skin lesions
+ Classic butterfly rash over nose and cheeks in < 50% of patients

---

Signs of systemic lupus erythematosus

Diagnosing systemic lupus erythematosus (SLE) is difficult because it commonly mimics other diseases; symptoms may be vague and vary greatly among patients.

For these reasons, the American Rheumatism Association issued a list of criteria for classifying SLE to be used primarily for consistency in epidemiologic surveys. Commonly, four or more of these signs are present at some time during the course of the disease:

+ malar or discoid rash
+ photosensitivity
+ oral or nasopharyngeal ulcerations
+ nonerosive arthritis (of two or more peripheral joints)
+ pleuritis or pericarditis
+ profuse proteinuria (more than 0.5 g/day) or excessive cellular casts in the urine
+ seizures or psychoses
+ hemolytic anemia, leukopenia, lymphopenia, or thrombocytopenia
+ anti–double-stranded deoxyribonucleic acid or positive findings of antiphospholipid antibodies (elevated immunoglobulin [Ig] G or IgM anticardiolipin antibodies, positive test result for lupus anticoagulant, or false-positive serologic test results for syphilis)
+ abnormal antinuclear antibody titer.

PATHOPHYSIOLOGY

Autoimmunity is believed to be the prime mechanism involved with SLE. The body produces antibodies against components of its own cells, such as the antinuclear antibody (ANA), and immune complex disease follows.

Patients with SLE may produce antibodies against many different tissue components, such as RBCs, neutrophils, platelets, lymphocytes, or almost any organ or tissue in the body.

SIGNS AND SYMPTOMS

The onset of SLE may be acute or insidious and produces no characteristic clinical pattern. (See *Signs of systemic lupus erythematosus.*)

Although SLE may involve any organ system, signs and symptoms all relate to tissue injury and subsequent inflammation and necrosis resulting from the invasion by immune complexes. They commonly include fever, weight loss, malaise, fatigue, rashes, and polyarthralgia. In 90% of patients, joint involvement is similar to rheumatoid arthritis, although the arthritis of lupus is usually nonerosive.

Skin lesions are most commonly erythematous rash in areas exposed to light. The classic butterfly rash over the nose and cheeks occurs in less than 50% of the patients. A scaly, papular rash mimics psoriasis, especially in sun-exposed areas. Vasculitis (especially in the digits), possibly leads to infarctive lesions, necrotic leg ulcers, or digital gangrene.

Other signs and symptoms include Raynaud's phenomenon, which appears in about 20% of patients, and patchy alopecia and painless ulcers of the mucous membranes, which are common. Pulmonary abnormalities, such as pleurisy, pleural effusions, pneumonitis, pulmonary hypertension and, rarely, pulmonary hemorrhage may occur.

In addition, cardiac involvement, such as pericarditis, myocarditis, endocarditis, and early coronary atherosclerosis may also occur. Renal effects may include microscopic hematuria, pyuria, and urine sediment with cellular casts due to glomerulonephritis, possibly progressing to kidney failure (particularly when untreated).

Urinary tract infections may result from a heightened susceptibility to infection. Seizure disorders and mental dysfunction may indicate neurologic damage. Central nervous system (CNS) involvement may produce emotional instability, psychosis, and organic brain syndrome. Headaches, irritability, and depression are common.

Constitutional symptoms of SLE include aching, malaise, fatigue, low-grade or spiking fever and chills, anorexia and weight loss, lymph node enlargement (diffuse or local, and nontender), and abdominal pain. Nausea, vomiting, diarrhea, and constipation may also occur. Women may experience irregular menstrual periods or amenorrhea during the active phase of SLE.

COMPLICATIONS

Possible complications of SLE include concomitant infections, urinary tract infections, renal failure, and osteonecrosis of the hip from long-term steroid use.

DIAGNOSIS

Test results that may indicate SLE include complete blood count with differential possibly showing anemia and a decreased white blood cell (WBC) count, platelet count, which may be decreased, erythrocyte sedimentation rate, which is usually elevated, and serum electrophoresis, which may show hypergammaglobulinemia.

Other diagnostic tests include ANA and lupus erythematosus cell tests showing positive results in active SLE. The anti–double-stranded deoxyribonucleic acid antibody (anti-dsDNA) is the most specific test for SLE. It correlates with disease activity, especially renal involvement, and helps monitor response to therapy. It may be low or absent in remission.

Urine studies may show RBCs and WBCs, urine casts and sediment, and significant protein loss (more than 0.5 g/24 hours). Serum complement blood studies show decreased serum complement (C3 and C4) levels indicating active disease.

In addition, a chest X-ray may disclose pleurisy or lupus pneumonitis. Electrocardiography may show a conduction defect with cardiac involvement or pericarditis. Kidney biopsy can determine the disease stage and extent of renal involvement. Lupus anticoagulant and anticardiolipin tests may be positive in some patients (usually in patients prone to antiphospholipid syndrome of thrombosis, abortion, and thrombocytopenia).

TREATMENT

The mainstay of SLE treatment is drug therapy. Aspirin or nonsteroidal anti-inflammatory compounds usually control arthritis symptoms. Skin lesions need topical corticosteroid creams such as hydrocortisone buteprate (Acticort) or triamcinolone (Aristocort). Intralesional corticosteroids or antimalarials such as hydroxychloroquine sulfate (Plaquenil) are used to treat refractory skin lesions.

Systemic corticosteroids are administered to reduce systemic symptoms of SLE, for acute generalized exacerbations, or for serious disease related to vital organ systems, such as pleuritis, pericarditis, lupus nephritis, vasculitis, and CNS involvement. High-dose steroids and cytotoxic therapy (such as cyclophosphamide [Cytoxan]) are administered to treat diffuse proliferative glomerulonephritis.

Dialysis or kidney transplant may be necessary for renal failure. When treatment is ineffective, antihypertensive drugs and dietary changes can also be effective to minimize effects of renal involvement.

NURSING CONSIDERATIONS

Careful assessment, supportive measures, emotional support, and patient education are all important parts of the care plan for patients with SLE.

Complications
+ Concomitant infections
+ UTI
+ Renal failure
+ Osteonecrosis of hip

Diagnosis
+ Complete blood count with differential showing anemia, decreased WBC and platelet count
+ ANA and lupus erythematosus cell tests show positive results
+ Anti-dsDNA test correlates with disease activity
+ Urine studies show RBCs and WBCs, urine casts, sediment, significant protein loss
+ Decreased serum C3 and C4 levels
+ Pleurisy, lupus pneumonitis
+ Cardiac involvement, pericarditis
+ Positive lupus anticoagulant and anticardiolipin tests

Treatment
+ Aspirin or nonsteroidal anti-inflammatory compounds
+ Corticosteroids
+ High-dose steroids and cytotoxic therapy
+ Dialysis or kidney transplant
+ Antihypertensive drugs and dietary changes

Key nursing actions

- Watch for constitutional symptoms.
- Observe for dyspnea, chest pain, and edema of the extremities.
- Note the size, type, and location of skin lesions.
- Check urine for hematuria, scalp for hair loss, and skin and mucous membranes for petechiae, bleeding, ulceration, pallor, and bruising.
- Advise the patient receiving cyclophosphamide to maintain adequate hydration.
- Offer cosmetic tips and refer the patient to a hairdresser who specializes in scalp disorders.

Characteristics of RA

- Chronic, systemic, inflammatory, potentially crippling disease
- Attacks peripheral joints, surrounding muscles, tendons, ligaments, blood vessels
- Partial remissions and unpredictable exacerbations
- Three times more common in women than in men
- Follows an intermittent course
- 10% of affected people have total disability
- Prognosis worsens with development of nodules, vasculitis, high titers of RF

Alert!

- RA can occur at any age.
- The peak onset is between ages 35 and 50.

- Watch for constitutional symptoms: joint pain or stiffness, weakness, fever, fatigue, and chills. Observe for dyspnea, chest pain, and edema of the extremities. Note the size, type, and location of skin lesions. Check urine for hematuria, scalp for hair loss, and skin and mucous membranes for petechiae, bleeding, ulceration, pallor, and bruising.
- Provide a balanced diet. Renal involvement may mandate a low-sodium, low-protein diet.
- Urge the patient to get plenty of rest. Schedule diagnostic tests and procedures to allow adequate rest. Explain all tests and procedures. Tell the patient that several blood samples are needed initially, then periodically, to monitor progress.
- Apply heat packs to relieve joint pain and stiffness. Encourage regular exercise to maintain full range of motion (ROM) and prevent contractures. Teach ROM exercises as well as body alignment and postural techniques. Arrange for physical therapy and occupational counseling as appropriate.
- Explain the expected benefit of prescribed medications. Watch for adverse effects, especially when the patient is taking high doses of corticosteroids.
- Advise the patient receiving cyclophosphamide to maintain adequate hydration. If prescribed, give mesna to prevent hemorrhagic cystitis and ondansetron to prevent nausea and vomiting.
- Monitor vital signs, intake and output, weight, and laboratory reports. Check pulse rates and observe for orthopnea. Check stools and GI secretions for blood.
- Observe for hypertension, weight gain, and other signs of renal involvement.
- Assess for signs of neurologic damage: personality change, paranoid or psychotic behavior, ptosis, or diplopia. Take seizure precautions. If Raynaud's phenomenon is present, warm and protect the patient's hands and feet.
- Offer cosmetic tips, such as suggesting the use of hypoallergenic makeup, and refer the patient to a hairdresser who specializes in scalp disorders.
- Advise the patient to purchase medications in quantity, if possible. Warn against "miracle" drugs for relief of arthritis symptoms.
- Refer the patient to the Lupus Foundation of America and the Arthritis Foundation as necessary.

RHEUMATOID ARTHRITIS

Rheumatoid arthritis (RA) is a chronic, systemic inflammatory disease that primarily attacks peripheral joints and the surrounding muscles, tendons, ligaments, and blood vessels. Partial remissions and unpredictable exacerbations mark the course of this potentially crippling disease. RA is three times more common in women than in men.

RA occurs worldwide, affecting more than 6.5 million people in the United States alone.

CLINICAL ALERT RA can occur at any age. The peak onset is between ages 35 and 50.

This disease usually requires lifelong treatment and sometimes surgery. (See *Drug therapy for rheumatoid arthritis,* pages 480 and 481.)

In most patients, it follows an intermittent course and allows normal activity between flares, although 10% of affected people have total disability from severe joint deformity, associated extra-articular symptoms, such as vasculitis, or both. The prognosis worsens with the development of nodules, vasculitis, and high titers of rheumatoid factor (RF).

CAUSES

The cause of the chronic inflammation characteristic of RA isn't known. Possible theories include an abnormal immune activation occurring in a genetically susceptible individual leading to inflammation, complement activation, and cell proliferation within joints and tendon sheaths.

Possible infection (viral or bacterial), hormone action, or lifestyle factors may influence disease onset. Some patients develop an immunoglobulin (Ig) M antibody against the body's own IgG (also called *rheumatoid factor*). RF aggregates into complexes, generates inflammation, causing eventual cartilage damage and triggering other immune responses.

PATHOPHYSIOLOGY

If not arrested, the inflammatory process in the joints occurs in four stages. First, synovitis develops from congestion and edema of the synovial membrane and joint capsule. Infiltration by lymphocytes, macrophages, and neutrophils continues the local inflammatory response. These cells, as well as fibroblast-like synovial cells, produce enzymes that help to degrade bone and cartilage. Formation of pannus—thickened layers of granulation tissue—marks the onset of the second stage. Pannus covers and invades cartilage and eventually destroys the joint capsule and bone.

Progression to the third stage is characterized by fibrous ankylosis—fibrous invasion of the pannus and scar formation that occludes the joint space. Bone atrophy and misalignment cause visible deformities and disrupt the articulation of opposing bones, which cause muscle atrophy and imbalance and, possibly, partial dislocations (subluxations).

In the fourth stage, fibrous tissue calcifies, resulting in bony ankylosis and total immobility.

SIGNS AND SYMPTOMS

RA usually develops insidiously and initially causes nonspecific signs and symptoms, most likely related to the initial inflammatory reactions before the inflammation of the synovium, including fatigue, malaise, anorexia and weight loss, persistent low-grade fever, lymphadenopathy, and vague articular symptoms.

As the disease progresses, signs and symptoms include specific localized, bilateral, and symmetric articular symptoms. These commonly occur in the fingers at the proximal interphalangeal, metacarpophalangeal, and metatarsophalangeal joints, possibly extending to the wrists, knees, elbows, and ankles from inflammation of the synovium. The affected joints stiffen after inactivity, especially on arising in the morning, due to progressive synovial inflammation and destruction.

Spindle-shaped fingers develop from marked edema and congestion in the joints. Joint pain and tenderness occur at first only with movement but eventually even at rest, due to prostaglandin release, edema, and synovial inflammation and destruction. The patient experiences a feeling of warmth at the joint from inflammation. Ultimately, diminished joint function and deformities occur as synovial destruction continues.

Deformities are common if active disease continues. Flexion deformities or hyperextension of metacarpophalangeal joints, subluxation of the wrist, and stretching of tendons pulling the fingers to the ulnar side (ulnar drift), or characteristic swan-neck or boutonnière deformity from joint swelling and loss of joint space may occur. Carpal tunnel syndrome may develop from synovial pressure on the median nerve causing paresthesia in the fingers.

(Text continues on page 482.)

Causes
+ Cause of chronic inflammation characteristic unknown

Theories
+ Abnormal immune activation
+ Infection
+ Hormone action
+ Lifestyle factors

How it happens
+ Inflammatory process occurs in four stages

First stage
+ Synovitis from congestion, edema of synovial membrane and joint capsule
+ Lymphocytes, macrophages, neutrophils continue inflammatory response
+ Enzymes produced that help degrade bone, cartilage

Second stage
+ Pannus covers, invades cartilage, destroys joint capsule and bone

Third stage
+ Fibrous ankylosis
+ Bone atrophy, misalignment cause visible deformities, disrupt articulation of opposing bones

Fourth stage
+ Bony ankylosis, total immobility

Key signs and symptoms
+ Develops insidiously, initially causes nonspecific signs
+ Fatigue, malaise, anorexia, persistent low-grade fever, lymphadenopathy, articular symptoms
+ Joints stiffen after inactivity
+ Spindle-shaped fingers
+ Carpal tunnel syndrome

Drug therapy for rheumatoid arthritis

This flowchart identifies the major pathophysiologic events in rheumatoid arthritis and shows where in this chain of events the major drug therapies act to control the disease.

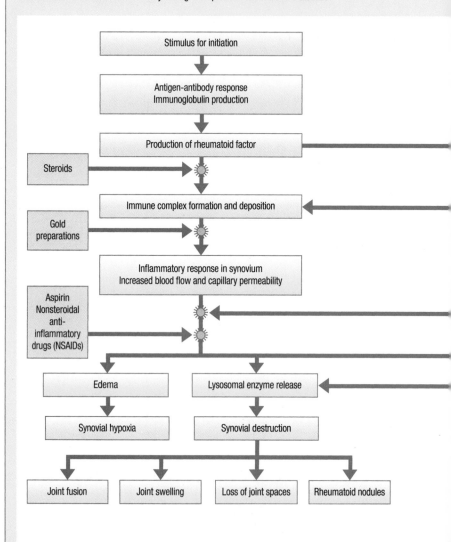

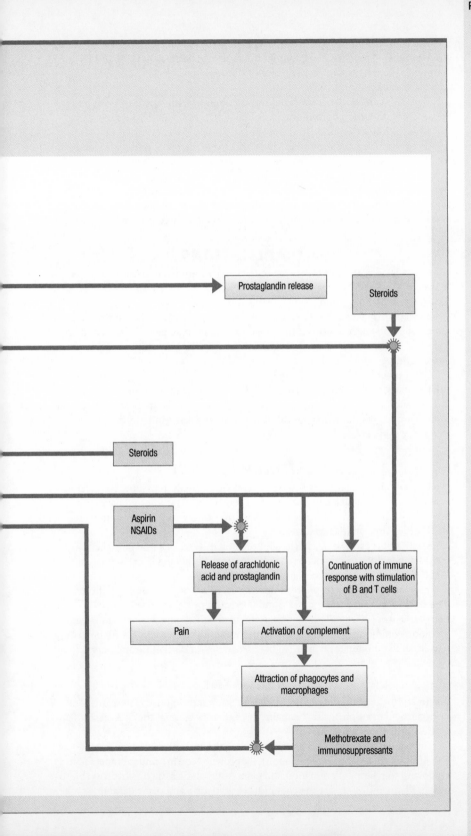

The most common extra-articular finding is the gradual appearance of rheumatoid nodules — subcutaneous, round or oval, nontender masses (20% of RF-positive patients), usually on the patient's elbows, hands, or Achilles tendon, from destruction of the synovium.

Vasculitis can lead to skin lesions, leg ulcers, and multiple systemic complications from infiltration of immune complexes and subsequent tissue damage and necrosis in the vasculature.

Other common extra-articular effects include pericarditis, pulmonary nodules or fibrosis, pleuritis, or inflammation of the sclera and overlying tissues of the eye from immune complex invasion and subsequent tissue damage and necrosis. Peripheral neuropathy may produce numbness or tingling in the feet or weakness and loss of sensation in the fingers from infiltration of the nerve fibers. Stiff, weak, or painful muscles secondary to limited mobility and decreased use are common.

COMPLICATIONS

Pain associated with movement may restrict active joint use and cause fibrous or bony ankylosis, soft-tissue contractures, and joint deformities. Vasculitis can lead to skin lesions, leg ulcers, and multisystem complications.

Between 15% and 20% of patients develop Sjögren's syndrome with keratoconjunctivitis sicca. RA can also destroy the odontoid process, part of the second cervical vertebra. Rarely, spinal cord compression can occur, particularly in patients with long-standing deforming RA.

Other complications include subluxations, popliteal (Baker's) cysts, osteoporosis, vasculitis, amyloidosis, recurrent infections, anemia, necrosis of the hip joint, cardiac and pulmonary disorders, renal insufficiency, GI disturbances, pleural effusions, lymphadenopathy, peripheral neuritis, and myositis (inflammation of the voluntary muscles).

DIAGNOSIS

No test definitively diagnoses RA, but several are useful. X-rays show bone demineralization and soft-tissue swelling in early stages. Cartilage loss and narrowed joint spaces, and, lastly, cartilage and bone destruction and erosion, subluxations, and deformities are seen in later stages.

An RF test is positive in 75% to 80% of patients (titer of 1:160 or higher). Synovial fluid analysis shows increased volume and turbidity but decreased viscosity and elevated WBC counts (usually greater than 10,000/µl).

A serum protein electrophoresis test may show elevated serum globulin levels. The erythrocyte sedimentation rate and C-reactive protein levels show elevations in 85% to 90% of patients. This may be useful to monitor response to therapy because elevation commonly parallels disease activity. Additionally, a complete blood count usually shows moderate anemia, slight leukocytosis, and slight thrombocytosis.

TREATMENT

Treatment for RA involves pharmacologic therapy and supportive measures. Salicylates, particularly aspirin, are the mainstay of therapy because they decrease inflammation and relieve joint pain.

The patient may also receive other nonsteroidal anti-inflammatory drugs (NSAIDs), such as fenoprofen (Nalfon), ibuprofen (Motrin), and indomethacin (Indocin), to relieve inflammation and pain. Antimalarials, such as hydroxychloroquine (Plaquenil), sulfasalazine (Azulfidine), gold salts, and penicillamine

Complications
+ Fibrous or bony ankylosis, soft-tissue contractures, joint deformities
+ Skin lesions, leg ulcers, multisystem complications
+ Sjögren's syndrome with keratoconjunctivitis sicca
+ Spinal cord compression
+ Recurrent infections
+ Anemia
+ Necrosis of the hip joint

Diagnosis
+ X-rays show bone demineralization, soft-tissue swelling
+ Positive RF test
+ Increased synovial fluid volume, turbidity; decreased viscosity, elevated WBC counts
+ Elevated serum globulin
+ Elevated erythrocyte sedimentation rate and C-reactive protein levels
+ Moderate anemia, slight leukocytosis, slight thrombocytosis

Treatment
+ Salicylates
+ NSAIDs
+ Antimalarials
+ Immunosuppressants
+ Synovectomy
+ Osteotomy
+ Tendon transfers
+ Joint reconstruction, arthroplasty

(Cuprimine), are administered to reduce acute and chronic inflammation. Corticosteroids such as prednisone are administered in low doses for anti-inflammatory effects, in higher doses for immunosuppressive effect on T cells.

Other therapeutic drugs include azathioprine (Imuran), cyclosporine (Neoral), and methotrexate (Folex) in early disease for immunosuppression by suppressing T- and B-lymphocyte proliferation causing destruction of the synovium.

Synovectomy (removal of destructive, proliferating synovium, usually in the wrists, knees, and fingers) can halt or delay the course of the disease. Osteotomy (cutting of bone or excision of a wedge of bone) can realign joint surfaces and redistribute stress. Tendon transfers can prevent deformities or relieve contractures.

The patient may need joint reconstruction or total joint arthroplasty, including metatarsal head and distal ulnar resectional arthroplasty, insertion of a Silastic prosthesis between metacarpophalangeal and proximal interphalangeal joints in severe disease. In some cases, arthrodesis (joint fusion) is performed, which may help with stability and relief from pain, but may sacrifice joint mobility.

NURSING CONSIDERATIONS

✦ Assess all joints carefully. Look for deformities, contractures, immobility, and inability to perform everyday activities.
✦ Monitor vital signs, and note weight changes, sensory disturbances, and level of pain. Administer analgesics, as ordered, and watch for adverse effects.
✦ Provide meticulous skin care. Check for rheumatoid nodules as well as pressure ulcers and breakdowns due to immobility, vascular impairment, corticosteroid treatment, or improper splinting. Use lotion or cleansing oil, not soap, for dry skin.
✦ Explain all diagnostic tests and procedures. Tell the patient to expect multiple blood samples to allow firm diagnosis and accurate monitoring of therapy.
✦ Monitor the duration, not the intensity, of morning stiffness because duration more accurately reflects the severity of the disease. Encourage the patient to take hot showers or baths at bedtime or in the morning to reduce the need for pain medication.
✦ Apply splints carefully and correctly. Observe for pressure ulcers if the patient is in traction or wearing splints.
✦ Explain the nature of the disease. Make sure the patient and his family understand that RA is a chronic disease that requires major changes in lifestyle. Emphasize that there are no miracle cures, despite claims to the contrary.
✦ Encourage a balanced diet, but make sure the patient understands that special diets won't cure RA. Stress the need for weight control because obesity adds further stress to joints.
✦ Urge the patient to perform activities of daily living, such as dressing and feeding himself (supply easy-to-open cartons, lightweight cups, and unpackaged silverware). Allow the patient enough time to calmly perform these tasks.
✦ Provide emotional support. Remember that the patient with chronic illness easily becomes depressed, discouraged, and irritable. Encourage the patient to discuss his fears concerning dependency, sexuality, body image, and self-esteem. Refer him to an appropriate social service agency as needed.
✦ Discuss sexual aids: alternative positions, pain medication, and moist heat to increase mobility.
✦ Before discharge, make sure the patient knows how and when to take prescribed medication and how to recognize possible adverse effects.
✦ Teach the patient how to stand, walk, and sit correctly. Tell him to sit in chairs with high seats and armrests; he'll find it easier to get up from a chair if his knees are lower than his hips. If he doesn't own a chair with a high seat, recommend

Key nursing actions

✦ Assess all joints carefully.
✦ Monitor vital signs, and note weight changes, sensory disturbances, and level of pain.
✦ Provide meticulous skin care.
✦ Tell the patient to expect multiple blood samples to allow firm diagnosis and accurate monitoring of therapy.
✦ Monitor the duration of morning stiffness.
✦ Encourage the patient to take hot showers or baths at bedtime or in the morning.
✦ Apply splints carefully and correctly.
✦ Urge the patient to perform activities of daily living.
✦ Discuss sexual aids.
✦ Teach the patient how to stand, walk, and sit correctly.

Key nursing actions
(continued)

✦ Instruct the patient to pace daily activities.

✦ Teach him to avoid putting undue stress on joints.

✦ Suggest dressing aids and helpful household items.

✦ Refer the patient to the Arthritis Foundation for more information on coping with the disease.

putting blocks of wood under the legs of a favorite chair. Suggest an elevated toilet seat.

✦ Instruct the patient to pace daily activities, resting for 5 to 10 minutes out of each hour and alternating sitting and standing tasks. Adequate sleep and correct sleeping posture are important. He should sleep on his back on a firm mattress and should avoid placing a pillow under his knees, which encourages flexion deformity.

✦ Teach him to avoid putting undue stress on joints by using the largest joint available for a given task, avoiding positions of flexion and promoting positions of extension, holding objects parallel to the knuckles as briefly as possible, always using his hands toward the center of his body, sliding—not lifting—objects whenever possible, and supporting weak or painful joints as much as possible. Enlist the aid of the occupational therapist to teach the patient how to simplify activities and protect arthritic joints. Stress the importance of shoes with proper support.

✦ Suggest dressing aids—long-handled shoehorn, reacher, elastic shoelaces, zipper-pull, and buttonhook—and helpful household items, such as easy-to-open drawers, handheld shower nozzle, handrails, and grab bars. The patient who has difficulty maneuvering fingers into gloves should wear mittens. Tell him to dress while in a sitting position as often as possible.

✦ Refer the patient to the Arthritis Foundation for more information on coping with the disease.

13

Endocrine system

The endocrine system consists of glands, specialized cell clusters, hormones, and target tissues. The glands and cell clusters secrete hormones and chemical transmitters in response to stimulation from the nervous system and other sites. Together with the nervous system, the endocrine system regulates and integrates the body's metabolic activities and maintains internal homeostasis. Each target tissue has receptors for specific hormones. Hormones connect with the receptors, and the resulting hormone-receptor complex triggers the target cell's response.

HORMONAL REGULATION

The hypothalamus, the main integrative center for the endocrine and autonomic nervous systems, helps control some endocrine glands by neural and hormonal pathways. Neural pathways connect the hypothalamus to the posterior pituitary gland, or neurohypophysis. Neural stimulation of the posterior pituitary causes the secretion of two effector hormones: antidiuretic hormone (ADH, also known as *vasopressin*) and oxytocin.

The hypothalamus also exerts hormonal control at the anterior pituitary gland, or adenohypophysis, by releasing and inhibiting hormones and factors, which arrive by a portal system. Hypothalamic hormones stimulate the pituitary gland to synthesize and release trophic hormones, such as corticotropin (ACTH, also called *adrenocorticotropic hormone*), thyroid-stimulating hormone (TSH), and gonadotropins, such as luteinizing hormone (LH) and follicle-stimulating hormone (FSH). Secretion of trophic hormones stimulates the adrenal cortex, thyroid gland, and gonads. Hypothalamic hormones also stimulate the pituitary gland to release or inhibit the release of effector hormones, such as growth hormone (GH) and prolactin.

In a patient with a possible endocrine disorder, this complex hormonal sequence requires careful assessment to identify the dysfunction, which may result from defects in the gland; defects of releasing, trophic, or effector hormones; or de-

Key facts about the endocrine system

+ Consists of glands, specialized cell clusters, hormones, tissues
+ Glands and cell clusters secrete hormones, chemical transmitters in response to stimulation
+ With nervous system, regulates metabolic activities, maintains internal homeostasis
+ Hormones connect with receptors in target tissues
+ Resulting hormone-receptor complex triggers target cell's response

Hormonal regulation

+ Hypothalamus helps control some endocrine glands
+ Neural stimulation of posterior pituitary causes secretion of ADH, oxytocin
+ Hypothalamic hormones stimulate pituitary gland to synthesize and release trophic hormones

Hormonal regulation
(continued)

✦ Trophic hormones stimulate adrenal cortex, thyroid gland, gonads
✦ Hypothalamic hormones stimulate pituitary to release or inhibit release of effector hormones
✦ Negative feedback system regulates endocrine system
✦ Simple feedback occurs when level of one substance regulates secretion of a hormone

Rhythms

✦ Circadian rhythm increases and decreases hormone levels by time of day
✦ Infradian rhythm: biorhythm that repeats in patterns > 24 hours

Hormonal effects

✦ Oxytocin: stimulates contraction of uterus, milk-letdown reflex
✦ ADH: controls concentration of body fluids
✦ Prolactin: controls milk secretion, GH
✦ GH: triggers growth
✦ Iodinated hormones: affect growth, development
✦ PTH: regulates calcium, phosphate metabolism

fects of the target tissue. Hyperthyroidism, for example, may result from excessive thyrotropin-releasing hormone, TSH, or thyroid hormones, or excessive response of the thyroid gland.

Besides hormonal and neural controls, a negative feedback system regulates the endocrine system. (See *Feedback mechanism of the endocrine system.*)

The feedback mechanism may be simple or complex. Simple feedback occurs when the level of one substance regulates secretion of a hormone. For example, a low serum calcium level stimulates the parathyroid glands to secrete parathyroid hormone (PTH), and a high serum calcium level inhibits PTH secretion.

One example of complex feedback occurs through the hypothalamic-pituitary target organ axis. Secretion of the hypothalamic corticotropin-releasing hormone releases pituitary corticotropin, which in turn stimulates adrenal cortisol secretion. Subsequently, an increase in serum cortisol levels inhibits corticotropin by decreasing corticotropin-releasing hormone secretion or corticotropin directly. Corticosteroid therapy disrupts the hypothalamic-pituitary-adrenal axis by suppressing the hypothalamic-pituitary secretion mechanism. Because abrupt withdrawal of steroids doesn't allow time for recovery of the hypothalamic-pituitary-adrenal axis to stimulate cortisol secretion, it can induce life-threatening adrenal crisis.

RHYTHMS

The endocrine system is also controlled by rhythms, many of which last 24 hours (circadian). Circadian rhythm control of corticotropin and cortisol increases levels of these hormones in the early morning hours and decreases them in the late afternoon. Stress, caused by pyrogens, surgery, hypoglycemia, exercise, severe emotional trauma, and other conditions, enhances corticotropin release and abolishes corticotropin circadian rhythmicity. High-dose glucocorticoid administration suppresses stress-related corticotropin release.

An infradian rhythm is a biorhythm that repeats in patterns greater than 24-hour periods. The menstrual cycle is an example of an infradian rhythm — in this case, 28 days.

Hormonal effects

The posterior pituitary gland secretes oxytocin and ADH. Oxytocin stimulates contraction of the uterus and causes the milk-letdown reflex in lactating women. ADH controls the concentration of body fluids by altering the permeability of the distal and collecting tubules of the kidneys to conserve water. ADH secretion depends on plasma osmolality, the characteristic of a solution determined by the ionic concentration of the dissolved substance and the solution, which is monitored by hypothalamic neurons. Hypovolemia and hypotension are the most powerful stimulators of ADH release. Other stimulators include trauma, nausea, morphine, tranquilizers, certain anesthetics, positive-pressure breathing, pain, and stress.

In addition to the trophic hormones, the anterior pituitary secretes prolactin, which stimulates milk secretion, and GH. GH affects most body tissues. It triggers growth by stimulating protein synthesis and fat mobilization, and by decreasing carbohydrate use by muscle and fat tissue. The thyroid gland synthesizes and secretes the iodinated hormones, thyroxine (T_4) and triiodothyronine (T_3). Thyroid hormones are necessary for normal growth and development, and act on many tissues to increase metabolic activity and protein synthesis.

The parathyroid glands secrete PTH, which regulates calcium and phosphate metabolism. PTH elevates serum calcium levels by stimulating resorption of calcium and excretion of phosphate from bone and — by stimulating the conversion of

Feedback mechanism of the endocrine system

The hypothalamus receives regulatory information (feedback) from its own circulating hormones (simple loop) and also from target glands (complex loop).

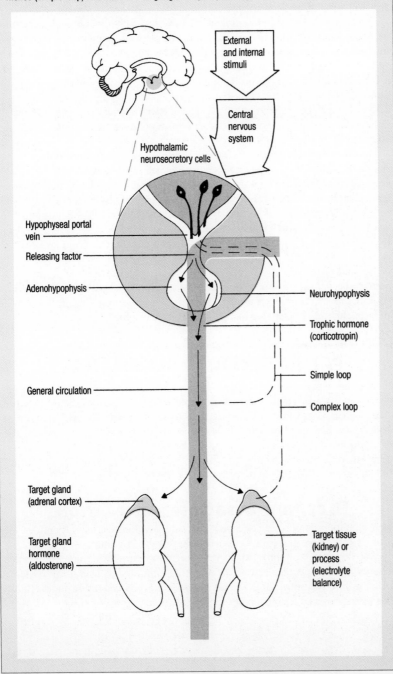

vitamin D to its most active form—enhances absorption of calcium from the GI tract. Calcitonin, another hormone secreted by the thyroid gland, affects calcium metabolism, although its precise role in humans is unknown.

The pancreas produces glucagon from the alpha cells and insulin from the beta cells. Glucagon, the hormone of the fasting state, releases stored glucose from the liver to increase blood glucose levels. Insulin, the hormone of the postprandial state, facilitates glucose transport into the cells, promotes glucose storage, stimulates protein synthesis, and enhances free fatty acid uptake and storage.

The adrenal cortex secretes mineralocorticoids, glucocorticoids, and sex steroid hormones (androgens). Aldosterone, a mineralocorticoid, regulates the reabsorption of sodium and the excretion of potassium by the kidneys. Although affected by corticotropin, aldosterone is mainly regulated by the renin-angiotensin system. Together, aldosterone, angiotensin II, and renin may be implicated in the pathogenesis of hypertension.

Cortisol, a glucocorticoid, stimulates gluconeogenesis, increases protein breakdown and free fatty acid mobilization, suppresses the immune response, and facilitates an appropriate response to stress.

The adrenal medulla is an aggregate of nervous tissue that produces the catecholamines epinephrine and norepinephrine, which cause vasoconstriction. In addition, epinephrine stimulates the fight-or-flight response—dilation of bronchioles and increased blood pressure, blood glucose level, and heart rate. The adrenal cortex as well as the gonads secretes androgens, which are steroid sex hormones. In males and premenopausal females, the contribution of adrenal androgens is very small, but in postmenopausal females, the adrenals are the major source of sex hormones.

The testes synthesize and secrete testosterone in response to gonadotropic hormones, especially LH, from the anterior pituitary gland; spermatogenesis occurs in response to FSH. The ovaries produce sex steroid hormones (primarily estrogen and progesterone) in response to anterior pituitary trophic hormones.

PATHOPHYSIOLOGIC CHANGES

Alterations in hormone levels, either significantly high or low, may result from various causes. Feedback systems may fail to function properly or may respond to the wrong signals. Dysfunction of an endocrine gland may manifest as either failure to produce adequate amounts of active hormone or excessive synthesis or release. After the hormones are released, they may be degraded at an altered rate or inactivated by antibodies before reaching the target cell. Abnormal target cell responses include receptor-associated alterations and intracellular alterations.

RECEPTOR-ASSOCIATED ALTERATIONS

These alterations have been associated with water-soluble hormones (peptides) and involve fewer receptors, resulting in diminished or defective hormone-receptor binding; impaired receptor function, resulting in insensitivity to the hormone; presence of antibodies against specific receptors, either reducing available binding sites or mimicking hormone action and suppressing or exaggerating target cell response; and unusual expression of receptor function.

Hormonal effects *(continued)*
- Glucagons: release stored glucose from liver
- Insulin: facilitates glucose transport, promotes glucose storage, stimulates protein synthesis, enhances free fatty acid uptake and storage
- Aldosterone: regulates reabsorption of sodium, excretion of potassium
- Cortisol: stimulates gluconeogenesis, increases protein breakdown, free fatty acid mobilization
- Epinephrine and norepinephrine: cause vasoconstriction

Pathophysiologic changes
- Result from various causes
- Feedback systems fail, respond to wrong signals
- Dysfunction may manifest as inadequate production of hormone or excessive synthesis or release
- Hormones may be degraded at altered rate, inactivated by antibodies

Receptor-associated alterations
- Associated with peptides, involve fewer receptors
- Result in diminished or defective hormone-receptor binding
- Impaired receptor function, insensitivity to hormone
- Presence of antibodies against specific receptors

INTRACELLULAR ALTERATIONS

These involve the inadequate synthesis of the second messenger needed to convert the hormonal signal into intracellular events. The two different mechanisms that may be involved include faulty response of target cells for water-soluble hormones to hormone-receptor binding and failure to generate the required second messenger, and abnormal response of the target cell to the second messenger and failure to express the usual hormonal effect.

Pathophysiologic aberrations affecting target cells for lipid-soluble (steroid) hormones occur less commonly or may be recognized less commonly.

ADDISON'S DISEASE

Addison's disease originates within the adrenal gland and is characterized by the decreased secretion of mineralocorticoids, glucocorticoids, and androgens. Secondary adrenal hypofunction is due to a disorder outside the gland such as impaired pituitary secretion of corticotropin. It's characterized by decreased glucocorticoid secretion. The secretion of aldosterone, the major mineralocorticoid, is commonly unaffected.

Addison's disease is relatively uncommon and can occur at any age and in both genders. Secondary adrenal hypofunction occurs when a patient abruptly stops long-term exogenous steroid therapy or when the pituitary is injured by a tumor or by infiltrative or autoimmune processes — these occur when circulating antibodies react specifically against adrenal tissue, causing inflammation and infiltration of the cells by lymphocytes. With early diagnosis and adequate replacement therapy, the prognosis for both primary and secondary adrenal hypofunction is good.

Adrenal crisis (addisonian crisis), a critical deficiency of mineralocorticoids and glucocorticoids, generally follows acute stress, sepsis, trauma, surgery, or the omission of steroid therapy in patients who have chronic adrenal insufficiency. Adrenal crisis is a medical emergency that needs immediate, vigorous treatment.

Autoimmune Addison's disease is most common in white females, and a genetic predisposition is likely. It's more common in patients with a familial predisposition to autoimmune endocrine diseases. Most people with Addison's disease are diagnosed between ages 30 and 60.

CAUSES

Addison's disease is the destruction of more than 90% of both adrenal glands, usually due to an autoimmune process in which circulating antibodies react specifically against the adrenal tissue.

Other causes include tuberculosis (once the chief cause, now responsible for less than 20% of adult cases), bilateral adrenalectomy, hemorrhage into the adrenal gland, neoplasms, and infections (histoplasmosis, cytomegalovirus [CMV]). Rarely, a family history of autoimmune disease may predispose the patient to Addison's disease and other endocrinopathies.

Causes of secondary hypofunction (glucocorticoid deficiency) include hypopituitarism, which can cause decreased corticotropin secretion. It can also stem from abrupt withdrawal of long-term corticosteroid therapy, as when long-term exogenous corticosteroid stimulation suppresses pituitary corticotropin secretion and causes adrenal gland atrophy. In addition, it can result from removal of a corticotropin-secreting tumor.

Intracellular alterations

+ Involve inadequate synthesis of second messenger
+ Faulty response of target cells
+ Abnormal response of target cell to second messenger
+ Failure to express usual hormonal effect
+ Aberrations affecting target cells for steroid hormones occur or are recognized less commonly

Characteristics of Addison's disease

+ Originates within adrenal glands
+ Destruction of more than 90% of both adrenal glands
+ Decreased secretion of mineralocorticoids, glucocorticoids, androgens
+ Secondary adrenal hypofunction due to disorder outside gland
+ Relatively uncommon
+ Can occur at any age in both genders
+ Prognosis for primary and secondary adrenal hypofunction good with early diagnosis and treatment
+ Most common in white females

Causes

+ Autoimmune process: antibodies react against adrenal tissue
+ Tuberculosis
+ Bilateral adrenalectomy
+ Hemorrhage into adrenal gland
+ Neoplasms
+ Infections

How it happens

+ Manifests as clinical syndrome
+ High corticotropin, corticotropin-releasing hormone levels, low glucocorticoid levels
+ Deficiencies of adrenocortical secretions, glucocorticoids, androgens, mineralocorticoids
+ Manifestations apparent when 90% of functional cells in glands lost
+ Dangerously low blood glucose in patients who take insulin routinely
+ Increased renal sodium loss, enhances potassium reabsorption
+ Normal blood pressure when supine, marked hypotension, tachycardia after standing
+ Increased production of angiotensin II
+ May decrease hair growth in axillary, pubic areas

Key signs and symptoms

Primary
+ Muscle weakness, fatigue, weight loss, GI disturbances
+ Conspicuous bronze skin color
+ Darkening of scars
+ Vitiligo
+ Orthostatic hypotension, decreased cardiac size and output
+ Weak, irregular pulse

Adrenal crisis is usually caused when body stores of glucocorticoids are exhausted in a person with adrenal hypofunction after trauma, surgery, or other physiologic stress.

PATHOPHYSIOLOGY

Addison's disease is a chronic condition that results from the partial or complete destruction of the adrenal cortex. It manifests as a clinical syndrome in which the symptoms are associated with deficient production of the adrenocortical hormones, cortisol, aldosterone, and androgens. High levels of corticotropin and corticotropin-releasing hormone accompany the low glucocorticoid levels.

Corticotropin acts primarily to regulate the adrenal release of glucocorticoids (primarily cortisol); mineralocorticoids, including aldosterone; and sex steroids that supplement those produced by the gonads. Corticotropin secretion is controlled by corticotropin-releasing hormone from the hypothalamus and by negative feedback control by the glucocorticoids.

Addison's disease involves all zones of the cortex, causing deficiencies of the adrenocortical secretions, glucocorticoids, androgens, and mineralocorticoids.

Manifestations of adrenocortical hormone deficiency become apparent when 90% of the functional cells in both glands are lost. Usually, cellular atrophy is limited to the cortex, although medullary involvement may occur, resulting in catecholamine deficiency. Cortisol deficiency causes decreased liver gluconeogenesis (the formation of glucose from molecules that aren't carbohydrates). The resulting low blood glucose levels can become dangerously low in patients who take insulin routinely.

Aldosterone deficiency causes increased renal sodium loss and enhances potassium reabsorption. Sodium excretion causes a reduction in water volume that leads to hypotension. Patients with Addison's disease may have normal blood pressure when supine, but show marked hypotension and tachycardia after standing for several minutes. Low plasma volume and arteriolar pressure stimulate renin release and a resulting increased production of angiotensin II.

Androgen deficiency may decrease hair growth in axillary and pubic areas as well as on the extremities of women. The metabolic effects of testicular androgens make decreased hair growth less noticeable in men.

Addison's disease is a decrease in the biosynthesis, storage, or release of adrenocortical hormones. In about 80% of the patients, an autoimmune process causes partial or complete destruction of both adrenal glands. Autoimmune antibodies can block the corticotropin receptor or bind with corticotropin, preventing it from stimulating adrenal cells. Infection is the second most common cause of Addison's disease, specifically tuberculosis, which causes about 20% of the cases.

Other diseases that can cause Addison's disease include acquired immunodeficiency syndrome, systemic fungal infections, CMV, adrenal tumor, and metastatic cancers. Infection can impair cellular function and affect corticotropin at any stage of regulation.

SIGNS AND SYMPTOMS

Clinical features vary with the type of adrenal hypofunction. Signs and symptoms of primary hypofunction include muscle weakness, fatigue, weight loss, and various GI disturbances, such as nausea, vomiting, and anorexia.

The patient with Addison's disease typically has a conspicuous bronze color of the skin, especially in the creases of the hands and over the metacarpophalangeal joints (hand and finger), elbows, and knees. The patient may also exhibit the darkening of scars, areas of vitiligo (absence of pigmentation), and increased pigmentation of the mucous membranes, especially the buccal mucosa. This is due to decreased secretion of cortisol, causing simultaneous secretion of excessive amounts of corticotropin and melanocyte-stimulating hormone by the pituitary gland.

In Addison's disease, associated cardiovascular abnormalities include orthostatic hypotension, decreased cardiac size and output, and a weak, irregular pulse. Other clinical effects include decreased tolerance for even minor stress, fasting hypoglycemia due to decreased gluconeogenesis, and a craving for salty foods due to decreased mineralocorticoid secretion, which normally causes salt retention.

Secondary hypofunction produces clinical effects similar to primary hypofunction, but without hyperpigmentation due to low corticotropin and melanocyte-stimulating hormone levels. This condition doesn't necessarily cause hypotension and electrolyte abnormalities due to fairly normal aldosterone secretion. Normal androgen secretion will continue.

Addisonian crisis produces profound weakness and fatigue; nausea, vomiting, and dehydration; hypotension; and, occasionally, high fever followed by hypothermia.

COMPLICATIONS

Possible complications of adrenal hypofunction include hyperpyrexia, psychotic reactions, deficient or excessive steroid treatment, shock, and profound hypoglycemia, as well as ultimate vascular collapse, renal shutdown, coma, and death (if untreated).

DIAGNOSIS

Diagnosis of adrenal hypofunction is based on plasma cortisol levels confirming adrenal insufficiency. The corticotropin stimulation test differentiates between primary and secondary adrenal hypofunction. The metyrapone test is indicated for suspicion of secondary adrenal hypofunction. This test requires oral or I.V. metyrapone, which blocks cortisol production and should stimulate the release of corticotropin from the hypothalamic-pituitary system. In Addison's disease, the hypothalamic-pituitary system responds normally and plasma corticotropin levels are high. Because the adrenal glands are destroyed, plasma concentrations of the cortisol precursor 11-deoxycortisol increase, as do urinary 17-hydroxycorticosteroids.

To differentiate between primary and secondary hypofunction, rapid corticotropin stimulation test is performed by I.V. or I.M. administration of cosyntropin, a synthetic form of corticotropin after baseline sampling for cortisol and corticotropin. Samples are drawn for cortisol 30 and 60 minutes after injection. A low corticotropin level indicates a secondary disorder. An elevated level is indicative of a primary disorder.

In a patient with typical addisonian symptoms, a decreased plasma cortisol level (less than 10 mcg/dl in the morning; less in the evening); decreased serum sodium and fasting blood glucose levels; increased serum potassium, calcium, and blood urea nitrogen levels; an elevated hematocrit; and increased lymphocyte and eosinophil counts strongly suggest acute adrenal insufficiency. In addition, X-rays may show adrenal calcification if the cause is infectious.

TREATMENT

The main treatment for primary and secondary adrenal hypofunction is lifelong corticosteroid replacement, usually with cortisone or hydrocortisone. Both have a

Key signs and symptoms

Secondary
✦ Clinical effects similar to primary without hyperpigmentation

Complications
✦ Hyperpyrexia
✦ Psychotic reactions
✦ Deficient or excessive steroid treatment
✦ Shock
✦ Profound hypoglycemia
✦ Renal shutdown
✦ Coma
✦ Death

Diagnosis
✦ Based on plasma cortisol levels confirming adrenal insufficiency
✦ Decreased serum sodium and fasting blood glucose levels
✦ Increased serum potassium, calcium, blood urea nitrogen levels
✦ Elevated hematocrit
✦ Increased lymphocyte and eosinophil counts
✦ X-rays may show adrenal calcification

Treatment

+ Lifelong corticosteroid replacement

Adrenal crisis

+ Prompt I.V. bolus of hydrocortisone, 100 mg every 6 hours for 24 hours
+ Then, 50 to 100 mg I.M. or diluted hydrocortisone with dextrose in saline solution I.V. until stable

Key nursing actions

+ If the patient has diabetes, check blood glucose levels periodically.
+ Record weight and intake and output carefully.
+ Until onset of mineralocorticoid effect, encourage fluids to replace excessive fluid loss.

To manage the patient receiving maintenance steroid therapy

+ Arrange for a diet that maintains sodium and potassium balances.
+ If the patient is anorexic, suggest six small meals per day to increase caloric intake.
+ Observe the patient receiving steroids for cushingoid signs.
+ Warn that infection, injury, or profuse sweating in hot weather may precipitate adrenal crisis.
+ Instruct the patient to always carry a medical identification card with the name of the steroid he takes and the dosage.
+ Tell the patient to keep an emergency kit available containing hydrocortisone in a prepared syringe for use in times of stress.

mineralocorticoid effect. Patients with Addison's disease may need oral fludrocortisone (Florinef), a synthetic mineralocorticoid, to prevent dangerous dehydration, hypotension, hyponatremia, and hyperkalemia.

Treatment for a patient with adrenal crisis is prompt I.V. bolus of hydrocortisone, 100 mg every 6 hours for 24 hours; then, 50 to 100 mg I.M. or diluted with dextrose in saline solution and given I.V. until the patient's condition stabilizes. Up to 300 mg/day of hydrocortisone and 3 to 5 L of I.V. saline and glucose solutions may be needed during the acute stage.

With proper treatment, adrenal crisis usually subsides quickly; blood pressure stabilizes, and water and sodium levels return to normal. After the crisis, maintenance doses of hydrocortisone preserve physiologic stability.

NURSING CONSIDERATIONS

In adrenal crisis, monitor vital signs carefully, especially for hypotension, volume depletion, and other signs of shock (decreased level of consciousness and urine output). Watch for hyperkalemia before treatment and for hypokalemia after treatment (from excessive mineralocorticoid effect). Watch for cardiac arrhythmias (may be caused by a serum potassium disturbance).

+ If the patient also has diabetes, check blood glucose levels periodically because steroid replacement may require adjustment of insulin dosage.
+ Record weight and intake and output carefully because the patient may have volume depletion. Until onset of mineralocorticoid effect, encourage fluids to replace excessive fluid loss.

To manage the patient receiving maintenance steroid therapy

+ Arrange for a diet that maintains sodium and potassium balances.
+ If the patient is anorexic, suggest six small meals per day to increase caloric intake. Ask the dietitian to provide a diet high in protein and carbohydrates. Keep a late-morning snack available in case the patient becomes hypoglycemic.
+ Observe the patient receiving steroids for cushingoid signs, such as fluid retention around the eyes and face. Watch for fluid and electrolyte imbalance, especially if the patient is receiving mineralocorticoids. Monitor weight and check blood pressure to assess body fluid status. Remember, steroids administered in the late afternoon or evening may cause stimulation of the central nervous system and insomnia in some patients. Check for petechiae because these patients bruise easily.
+ If the patient receives glucocorticoids alone, observe for orthostatic hypotension or electrolyte abnormalities, which may indicate a need for mineralocorticoid therapy.
+ Explain that lifelong steroid therapy is necessary.
+ Teach the patient the symptoms of steroid overdose (swelling, weight gain) and steroid underdose (lethargy, weakness).
+ Tell the patient that dosage may need to be increased during times of stress (when he has a cold, for example).
+ Warn that infection, injury, or profuse sweating in hot weather may precipitate adrenal crisis.
+ Instruct the patient to always carry a medical identification card stating that he takes a steroid and giving the name of the drug and the dosage.
+ Teach the patient and his family how to give a hydrocortisone injection.
+ Tell the patient to keep an emergency kit available containing hydrocortisone in a prepared syringe for use in times of stress.
+ Explain to the patient the importance of taking antacids while on steroids. Antacids will help decrease the gastric irritation caused by steroids.

✦ Warn the patient that stress may necessitate additional cortisone to prevent adrenal crisis. Review stress management techniques. Encourage adequate rest and nutrition.

CUSHING'S SYNDROME

Cushing's syndrome is a cluster of clinical abnormalities caused by excessive adrenocortical hormones (particularly cortisol) or related corticosteroids and, to a lesser extent, androgens and aldosterone. Cushing's disease (pituitary corticotropin excess) accounts for about 80% of endogenous cases of Cushing's syndrome. Cushing's disease occurs most commonly between ages 20 and 40 and is three to eight times more common in females.

 CLINICAL ALERT Cushing's syndrome caused by ectopic corticotropin secretion is more common in adult men, with the peak incidence between ages 40 and 60. In 20% of patients, Cushing's syndrome results from a cortisol-secreting tumor. Adrenal tumors, rather than pituitary tumors, are more common in children, especially girls.

The annual incidence of endogenous cortisol excess in the United States is two to four cases per 1 million people per year. The incidence of Cushing's syndrome resulting from exogenous administration of cortisol is uncertain, but it's known to be much greater than that of endogenous types.

The prognosis for endogenous Cushing's syndrome is guardedly favorable with surgery, but morbidity and mortality are high without treatment. About 50% of individuals with untreated Cushing's syndrome die within 5 years of onset as a result of overwhelming infection, suicide, complications from generalized arteriosclerosis (coronary artery disease), and severe hypertensive disease.

CAUSES

In about 70% of patients, Cushing's syndrome results from excess production of corticotropin and consequent hyperplasia of the adrenal cortex. Corticotropin overproduction may stem from pituitary hypersecretion (Cushing's disease), a corticotropin-producing tumor in another organ (usually malignant, commonly oat cell carcinoma of the lung), or administration of synthetic glucocorticoids or corticotropin.

In the remaining 30% of patients, Cushing's syndrome results from a cortisol-secreting adrenal tumor, which is usually benign. In infants, the usual cause of Cushing's syndrome is adrenal carcinoma.

PATHOPHYSIOLOGY

Cushing's syndrome is caused by prolonged exposure to excess glucocorticoids. Cushing's syndrome can be exogenous, resulting from chronic glucocorticoid or corticotropin administration, or endogenous, resulting from increased cortisol or corticotropin secretion. Cortisol excess results in anti-inflammatory effects and excessive catabolism of protein and peripheral fat to support hepatic glucose production. The mechanism may be corticotropin dependent (elevated plasma corticotropin levels stimulate the adrenal cortex to produce excess cortisol), or corticotropin independent (excess cortisol is produced by the adrenal cortex or exogenously administered). Excess cortisol suppresses the hypothalamic-pituitary-adrenal axis, also present in ectopic corticotropin-secreting tumors.

Characteristics of Cushing's syndrome
✦ Cluster of clinical abnormalities
✦ Caused by excessive adrenocortical hormones, related corticosteroids, androgens, aldosterone
✦ Cushing's disease accounts for 80% of endogenous cases of Cushing's syndrome
✦ Occurs most commonly between ages 20 and 40
✦ Prognosis favorable with surgery
✦ Morbidity and mortality high without treatment

Alert!
✦ Cushing's syndrome caused by ectopic corticotropin secretion is more common in adult men, with the peak incidence between ages 40 and 60.

Causes
✦ Excess production of corticotropin, consequent hyperplasia of adrenal cortex
✦ Overproduction caused by pituitary hypersecretion, tumor, synthetic glucocorticoids or corticotropin

How it happens
✦ Caused by prolonged exposure to excess glucocorticoids
✦ Exogenous: chronic glucocorticoid or corticotropin administration
✦ Endogenous: increased cortisol or corticotropin secretion
✦ Cortisol excess results in anti-inflammatory effects, excessive catabolism of protein and peripheral fat
✦ Mechanism may be corticotropin dependent or independent

SIGNS AND SYMPTOMS

Like other endocrine disorders, Cushing's syndrome induces changes in many body systems. Signs and symptoms depend on the degree and duration of hypercortisolism, the presence or absence of androgen excess, and additional tumor-related effects (adrenal carcinoma or ectopic corticotropin syndrome). Specific clinical effects vary with the system affected.

The endocrine and metabolic systems exhibit diabetes mellitus, with decreased glucose tolerance, fasting hyperglycemia, and glucosuria due to cortisol-induced insulin resistance and increased gluconeogenesis in the liver.

The musculoskeletal system exhibits muscle weakness due to hypokalemia or loss of muscle mass from increased catabolism, pathologic fractures due to decreased bone mineral ionization, osteopenia, osteoporosis, and skeletal growth retardation in children.

Inspection of the skin reveals purple striae; facial plethora (edema and blood vessel distention); acne; fat pads above the clavicles, over the upper back (buffalo hump), on the face (moon facies), and throughout the trunk (truncal obesity) with slender arms and legs; little or no scar formation; poor wound healing due to decreased collagen and weakened tissues; spontaneous ecchymosis; hyperpigmentation; and fungal skin infections.

GI system effects include a peptic ulcer due to increased gastric secretions and pepsin production and decreased gastric mucus, abdominal pain, increased appetite, and weight gain.

Central nervous system effects include irritability and emotional lability, ranging from euphoric behavior to depression or psychosis; insomnia due to the cortisol's role in neurotransmission; and headache.

Cardiovascular system effects include hypertension due to sodium and secondary fluid retention; heart failure; left ventricular hypertrophy; capillary weakness from protein loss, which leads to bleeding and ecchymosis; dyslipidemia; and ankle edema.

Immunologic system effects include increased susceptibility to infection due to decreased lymphocyte production and suppressed antibody formation; decreased resistance to stress; and a suppressed inflammatory response masking even severe infection.

Effects of the renal and urologic systems include fluid retention, increased potassium excretion, and ureteral calculi from increased bone demineralization with hypercalciuria.

Increased androgen production with clitoral hypertrophy, mild virilism, hirsutism, and amenorrhea or oligomenorrhea in women; sexual dysfunction; decreased libido; and impotence are effects of the reproductive system.

COMPLICATIONS

The stimulating and catabolic effects of cortisol produce the complications of Cushing's syndrome. Increased calcium resorption from bone may lead to osteoporosis and pathologic fractures. Frequent infections or slow wound healing due to decreased lymphocyte production and suppressed antibody formation may occur. Suppressed inflammatory response may mask even a severe infection.

Other complications include hirsutism, ureteral calculi, and metastasis of malignant tumors.

DIAGNOSIS

Initial screening may consist of a 24-hour urine test to determine free cortisol excretion rate and a low-dose dexamethasone test. Failure to suppress plasma and urine cortisol levels (urinary free cortisol levels more than 150 μg/24 hours) confirms the diagnosis of Cushing's syndrome. A low-dose dexamethasone suppression test can be used to confirm the diagnosis and determine the cause, possibly an adrenal tumor or a nonendocrine, corticotropin-secreting tumor.

Blood chemistry may show hyperglycemia, hypernatremia, hypokalemia, hypocalcemia, metabolic alkalosis, and elevated lymphocyte counts. Blood levels of corticotropin-releasing hormone, corticotropin, and different glucocorticoids can also help diagnose and localize the cause to the pituitary or adrenal gland.

TREATMENT

Differentiation among pituitary, adrenal, and ectopic causes of hypercortisolism is essential for effective treatment, which is specific for the cause of cortisol excess and includes medication, radiation, and surgery.

Surgery may be required for tumors of the adrenal and pituitary glands or other tissue such as the lung. Tumors may require radiation therapy for treatment.

The patient may require drug therapy, which may include ketoconazole, metyrapone, and aminoglutethimide to inhibit cortisol synthesis; mitotane to destroy the adrenocortical cells that secrete cortisol; and bromocriptine and cyproheptadine to inhibit corticotropin secretion.

NURSING CONSIDERATIONS

Patients with Cushing's syndrome require painstaking assessment and vigorous supportive care:
✦ Frequently monitor vital signs, especially blood pressure. Carefully observe the hypertensive patient who also has cardiac disease.
✦ Check laboratory reports for hypernatremia, hypokalemia, hyperglycemia, and glycosuria.
✦ Because the cushingoid patient is likely to retain sodium and water, check for edema and monitor daily weight and intake and output carefully. To minimize weight gain, edema, and hypertension, ask the dietary department to provide a diet that's high in protein and potassium but low in calories, carbohydrates, and sodium.
✦ Watch for infection, which is a particular problem in Cushing's syndrome.
✦ If the patient has osteoporosis and is bedridden, perform passive range-of-motion exercises carefully because of the severe risk of pathologic fractures.
✦ Remember, Cushing's syndrome produces emotional lability. Record situations that upset the patient and try to prevent them from occurring if possible. Help him get the physical and mental rest he needs—by sedation, if necessary. Offer support to the emotionally labile patient throughout the difficult testing period.

After bilateral adrenalectomy and pituitary surgery
✦ Report wound drainage or temperature elevation to the patient's physician immediately. Use strict sterile technique in changing the patient's dressings.
✦ Administer analgesics and replacement steroids as ordered.
✦ Monitor urine output and check vital signs carefully, watching for signs of shock (decreased blood pressure, increased pulse rate, pallor, and cold, clammy skin). To counteract shock, give vasopressors and increase the rate of I.V. fluids, as ordered.

Diagnosis
✦ Failure to suppress plasma and urine cortisol levels confirms diagnosis
✦ Low-dose dexamethasone suppression test confirms diagnosis, determines cause
✦ Hyperglycemia, hypernatremia, hypokalemia, hypocalcemia, metabolic alkalosis, elevated lymphocyte counts
✦ Blood levels can help diagnose and localize cause to pituitary or adrenal gland

Treatment
✦ Differentiation among causes essential for effective treatment
✦ Medication
✦ Radiation
✦ Surgery
✦ Drug therapy

Key nursing actions
✦ Frequently monitor vital signs.
✦ Check laboratory reports for hypernatremia, hypokalemia, hyperglycemia, and glycosuria.
✦ Check for edema and monitor daily weight and intake and output carefully.
✦ Watch for infection.

After bilateral adrenalectomy and pituitary surgery
✦ Report wound drainage or temperature elevation immediately.
✦ Use strict sterile technique in changing the patient's dressings.
✦ Monitor urine output and vital signs for signs of shock.

Key nursing actions
(continued)

✦ Check laboratory reports for hypoglycemia.
✦ Check for abdominal distention and return of bowel sounds after adrenalectomy.
✦ Check regularly for signs of adrenal hypofunction.
✦ In the patient undergoing pituitary surgery, check for and immediately report signs of increased intracranial pressure.

Characteristics of diabetes insipidus

✦ Disorder of water metabolism
✦ Pituitary diabetes insipidus caused by deficiency of vasopressin
✦ Nephrogenic diabetes insipidus caused by resistance of renal tubules to vasopressin
✦ Diabetes insipidus characterized by excessive fluid intake, hypotonic polyuria
✦ Decrease in ADH levels leads to renal excretion of large amount of urine
✦ Disorder may start at any age
✦ Incidence greater today than in past
✦ Prognosis good with adequate water replacement

Causes

✦ May be acquired, familial, idiopathic, neurogenic, nephrogenic
✦ Associated with stroke, hypothalamic or pituitary tumors, cranial trauma or surgery
✦ X-linked recessive trait or end-stage renal failure
✦ Certain drugs or alcohol

Because mitotane, aminoglutethimide, and metyrapone decrease mental alertness and produce physical weakness, assess neurologic and behavioral status, and warn the patient of adverse CNS effects. Also watch for severe nausea, vomiting, and diarrhea.

✦ Check laboratory reports for hypoglycemia due to removal of the source of cortisol, a hormone that maintains blood glucose levels.

✦ Check for abdominal distention and return of bowel sounds after adrenalectomy.

✦ Check regularly for signs of adrenal hypofunction (orthostatic hypotension, apathy, weakness, fatigue), which indicate that steroid replacement is inadequate.

✦ In the patient undergoing pituitary surgery, check for and immediately report signs of increased intracranial pressure (confusion, agitation, changes in level of consciousness, nausea, and vomiting). Watch for hypopituitarism.

✦ Provide comprehensive teaching to help the patient cope with lifelong treatment.

✦ Advise the patient to take replacement steroids with antacids or meals to minimize gastric irritation. (Usually, it's helpful to take two-thirds of the dosage in the morning and the remaining one-third in the early afternoon to mimic diurnal adrenal secretion.)

✦ Tell the patient to carry medical identification and to immediately report physiologically stressful situations such as infections, which necessitate increased dosage.

✦ Instruct the patient to watch closely for signs of inadequate steroid dosage (fatigue, weakness, dizziness) and of overdosage (severe edema, weight gain). Emphatically warn against abrupt discontinuation of steroid dosage because this may produce a fatal adrenal crisis.

DIABETES INSIPIDUS

A disorder of water metabolism, diabetes insipidus results from a deficiency of circulating vasopressin (also called *antidiuretic hormone,* or ADH) or from renal resistance to this hormone. Pituitary diabetes insipidus is caused by a deficiency of vasopressin, and nephrogenic diabetes insipidus is caused by the resistance of renal tubules to vasopressin. Diabetes insipidus is characterized by excessive fluid intake and hypotonic polyuria. A decrease in ADH levels leads to altered intracellular and extracellular fluid control, causing renal excretion of a large amount of urine.

The disorder may start at any age and is slightly more common in men than in women. The incidence is slightly greater today than in the past.

In uncomplicated diabetes insipidus, the prognosis is good with adequate water replacement, and patients usually lead normal lives.

CAUSES

The cause of diabetes insipidus may be acquired, familial, idiopathic, neurogenic, or nephrogenic; associated with stroke, hypothalamic or pituitary tumors, and cranial trauma or surgery (neurogenic diabetes insipidus); X-linked recessive trait or end-stage renal failure (nephrogenic diabetes insipidus, less common); and certain drugs, such as lithium (Duralith), phenytoin (Dilantin), or alcohol (transient diabetes insipidus).

PATHOPHYSIOLOGY

Diabetes insipidus is related to an insufficiency of ADH, leading to polyuria and polydipsia. The three forms of diabetes insipidus are neurogenic, nephrogenic, and psychogenic.

Neurogenic, or central, diabetes insipidus is an inadequate response of ADH to plasma osmolarity, which occurs when an organic lesion of the hypothalamus, infundibular stem, or posterior pituitary partially or completely blocks ADH synthesis, transport, or release. The many organic lesions that can cause diabetes insipidus include brain tumors, hypophysectomy, aneurysms, thrombosis, skull fractures, infections, and immunologic disorders. Neurogenic diabetes insipidus has an acute onset. A three-phase syndrome can occur, which involves progressive loss of nerve tissue and increased diuresis, normal diuresis, and polyuria and polydipsia, the manifestation of permanent loss of the ability to secrete adequate ADH.

Nephrogenic diabetes insipidus is caused by an inadequate renal response to ADH. The collecting duct permeability to water doesn't increase in response to ADH. Nephrogenic diabetes insipidus is generally related to disorders and drugs that damage the renal tubules or inhibit the generation of cyclic adenosine monophosphate in the tubules, preventing activation of the second messenger. Causative disorders include pyelonephritis, amyloidosis, destructive uropathies, polycystic disease, and intrinsic renal disease. Drugs include lithium (Eskalith), general anesthetics such as methoxyflurane, and demeclocycline (Declomycin). In addition, hypokalemia or hypercalcemia impairs the renal response to ADH. A rare genetic form of nephrogenic diabetes insipidus is an X-linked recessive trait.

Psychogenic diabetes insipidus is caused by an extremely large fluid intake, which may be idiopathic or related to psychosis or sarcoidosis. The polydipsia and resultant polyuria wash out ADH more quickly than it can be replaced. Chronic polyuria may overwhelm the renal medullary concentration gradient, rendering patients partially or totally unable to concentrate urine.

Regardless of the cause, insufficient ADH causes the immediate excretion of large volumes of dilute urine and consequent plasma hyperosmolality. In conscious individuals, the thirst mechanism is stimulated, usually for cold liquids. With severe ADH deficiency, urine output may be greater than 12 L/day, with a low specific gravity. Dehydration develops rapidly if fluids aren't replaced.

SIGNS AND SYMPTOMS

The patient's history shows an abrupt onset of polydipsia (cardinal symptom) — fluid intake of 5 to 20 L/day and polyuria (cardinal symptom) — urine output of 2 to 20 L/24-hour period of dilute urine. This disorder may result in nocturia, leading to sleep disturbance and fatigue. Urinalysis reveals almost colorless urine with a low urine specific gravity of less than 1.006.

Other symptoms include fever, changes in level of consciousness, hypotension, tachycardia, and headache and visual disturbance due to electrolyte disturbance and dehydration. The patient may report abdominal fullness, anorexia, and weight loss due to almost continuous fluid consumption.

COMPLICATIONS

Untreated diabetes insipidus can produce hypovolemia, hyperosmolality, circulatory collapse, loss of consciousness, central nervous system (CNS) damage, shock, and renal failure. These complications are most likely if the patient has an impaired or absent thirst mechanism.

How it happens
+ Related to insufficiency of ADH, leading to polyuria and polydipsia
+ Regardless of cause, causes immediate excretion of large volumes of dilute urine
+ Neurogenic diabetes insipidus due to block of ADH function
+ Nephrogenic diabetes insipidus due to inadequate renal response to ADH
+ Psychogenic diabetes insipidus due to extremely large fluid intake

Key signs and symptoms
+ Patient's history shows abrupt onset of polydipsia
+ Polyuria
+ Urine output of 2 to 20 L/24-hour period of dilute urine
+ Nocturia
+ Colorless urine with low specific gravity
+ Fever
+ Changes in level of consciousness
+ Hypotension
+ Tachycardia
+ Headache and vision disturbances
+ Abdominal fullness

Complications
+ Hypovolemia
+ Hyperosmolality
+ Circulatory collapse
+ Loss of consciousness
+ CNS damage
+ Shock
+ Renal failure

A prolonged urinary flow increase may produce chronic complications, such as bladder distention, enlarged caliceal, hydroureter, and hydronephrosis. Complications may result from underlying conditions, such as metastatic brain lesions, head trauma, and infections.

Diagnosis

◆ Urinalysis reveals almost colorless urine of low osmolality, low specific gravity
◆ Water deprivation test differentiates vasopressin deficiency from other forms of polyuria

DIAGNOSIS

To distinguish diabetes insipidus from other types of polyuria, urinalysis and a dehydration test may be ordered. Urinalysis reveals almost colorless urine of low osmolality (50 to 200 mOsm/kg, less than that of plasma) and of low specific gravity (less than 1.005).

The water deprivation test differentiates vasopressin deficiency from other forms of polyuria, resulting in renal inability to concentrate urine.

Treatment

◆ Administration of vasopressin
◆ Hydrochlorothiazide with potassium supplement
◆ S.C. vasopressin aqueous preparation administration
◆ DDAVP orally, by nasal spray, S.C. or I.V. injection
◆ Chlorpropamide

TREATMENT

Until the cause of diabetes insipidus can be identified and eliminated, the administration of vasopressin (Pitressin) can control fluid balance and prevent dehydration. Hydrochlorothiazide with potassium supplement can be used both for central and nephrogenic diabetes insipidus.

Vasopressin aqueous preparation is administered subcutaneously (S.C.) several times daily. It's effective for only 2 to 6 hours and is used as a diagnostic agent and, rarely, in acute disease. Desmopressin acetate (DDAVP) may be given orally, by nasal spray absorbed through the mucous membranes, or by S.C. or I.V. injection. It's effective for 8 to 20 hours depending on the dosage. Chlorpropamide (Diabinese) is sometimes used to decrease thirst sensation in patients with continued hypernatremia.

Key nursing actions

◆ Record fluid intake and output carefully.
◆ Watch for signs of hypovolemic shock, and monitor blood pressure and heart and respiratory rates regularly.
◆ Keep the rails up on his bed and assist the patient with walking.
◆ Monitor urine specific gravity between doses.
◆ Monitor serum electrolytes closely.
◆ If constipation develops, add high-fiber foods and fruit juices to his diet.

NURSING CONSIDERATIONS

Patient care includes monitoring symptoms to ensure that fluid balance is restored and maintained.

◆ Record fluid intake and output carefully. Maintain adequate fluid intake to prevent severe dehydration. Watch for signs of hypovolemic shock, and monitor blood pressure and heart and respiratory rates regularly, especially during the water deprivation test. Check the patient's weight daily.

◆ If the patient is dizzy or has muscle weakness, keep the side rails up on his bed and assist him with walking.

◆ Monitor urine specific gravity between doses. Watch for a decrease in specific gravity accompanied by increased urine output, indicating the recurrence of polyuria and necessitating administration of the next dose of medication or a dosage increase.

◆ Monitor serum electrolytes closely. Report abnormal values and treat them as ordered.

◆ If constipation develops, add more high-fiber foods and fruit juices to the patient's diet. If necessary, obtain an order for a mild laxative such as milk of magnesia.

◆ Provide meticulous skin and mouth care; apply petroleum jelly as needed to cracked or sore lips.

◆ Urge the patient to verbalize his feelings. Offer encouragement and a realistic assessment of his situation.

◆ Help the patient identify strengths that he can use in developing coping strategies.

✦ Refer the patient to a mental health professional for additional counseling if necessary.

✦ Before discharge, teach the patient how to monitor intake and output.

✦ Instruct the patient to administer desmopressin by nasal spray only after the onset of polyuria — not before — to prevent excess fluid retention and water intoxication.

✦ Tell the patient to report weight gain, which may indicate that his medication dose is too high. Recurrence of polyuria, as reflected on the intake and output sheet, indicates that the dosage is too low.

✦ Teach the parents of a child with diabetes insipidus about normal growth and development. Discuss how their child may differ from others at his developmental stage.

✦ Encourage the parents to help identify the child's strengths and to use them in developing coping strategies.

✦ Refer the family for counseling if necessary.

✦ Advise the patient with diabetes insipidus to wear a medical identification bracelet and to carry his medication with him at all times.

DIABETES MELLITUS

Diabetes mellitus is a metabolic disorder characterized by hyperglycemia (elevated serum glucose level) resulting from lack of insulin, lack of insulin effect, or both. Three general classifications are recognized. Type I is characterized by an absolute insulin insufficiency. Insulin resistance with varying degrees of insulin secretory defects characterizes type 2. Gestational diabetes emerges during pregnancy.

Onset of type 1 (insulin-dependent) usually occurs before age 30 (although it may occur at any age); the patient is usually thin and requires exogenous insulin and dietary management to achieve control. Conversely, type 2 (non–insulin-dependent) usually occurs in obese adults after age 40 and is treated with diet and exercise in combination with various oral antidiabetic drugs, although treatment may include insulin therapy.

Medical advances permit increased longevity and improved quality of life if the patient carefully monitors blood glucose levels, uses the data to make pharmacologic and lifestyle changes, and uses new insulin delivery systems, such as subcutaneous (S.C.) insulin pumps. In addition, medications now available enhance the body's own glucose metabolism and insulin sensitivity to optimize glycemic control and prevent progression to long-term complications.

CAUSES

The etiology of type 1 and type 2 diabetes remains unknown. Genetic factors may play a part in the development of all types. Autoimmune disease and viral infections may be risk factors in type 1.

Other risk factors include obesity, which contributes to the resistance to endogenous insulin, and physiologic or emotional stress, which can cause prolonged elevation of stress hormone levels (cortisol, epinephrine, glucagon, and growth hormone). This elevation increases blood glucose levels, which, in turn, places increased demands on the pancreas. Pregnancy causes weight gain and increases levels of estrogen and placental hormones, which antagonize insulin. Some medications antagonize the effects of insulin, including thiazide diuretics, adrenal corticosteroids, and hormonal contraceptives.

Key nursing actions
(continued)

✦ Refer the patient to a mental health professional for additional counseling.

✦ Teach the parents of a child with diabetes insipidus about normal growth and development.

✦ Refer the family for counseling if necessary.

✦ Advise the patient with diabetes insipidus to wear a medical identification bracelet and to carry medication at all times.

Characteristics of diabetes mellitus

✦ Metabolic disorder characterized by hyperglycemia resulting from lack of insulin or insulin effect

✦ Three general classifications: type I, type 2, gestational diabetes

✦ Type 1 occurs before age 30

✦ Type 2 occurs in obese adults after age 40

Causes

✦ Etiology of type 1 and type 2 unknown

✦ Genetic factors may play role

✦ Autoimmune disease, viral infections may be risk factors in type 1

✦ Obesity

✦ Physiologic or emotional stress

✦ Pregnancy causes weight gain, increases levels of hormones, which antagonize insulin

✦ Medications that antagonize effects of insulin

How it happens

Type 1

✦ Triggering event in susceptible person causes production of autoantibodies against pancreas beta cells

✦ Leads to decline in and lack of insulin secretion

✦ Leads to hyperglycemia, enhanced lipolysis, protein catabolism

✦ Characteristics occur when more than 90% of beta cells destroyed

Type 2

✦ Impaired insulin secretion, inappropriate hepatic glucose production, peripheral insulin receptor insensitivity

✦ Genetic factors significant

✦ Onset accelerated by obesity, sedentary lifestyle

Gestational

✦ Woman without diabetes shows glucose intolerance during pregnancy

✦ May occur if placental hormones counteract insulin

✦ Significant risk factor for future occurrence of type 2

Alert!

✦ Type 1 diabetes usually presents rapidly.

✦ Type 2 diabetes is typically slow and insidious in onset.

Key signs and symptoms

✦ Polyuria and polydipsia

✦ Anorexia or polyphagia

✦ Headaches, fatigue, lethargy, reduced energy levels

✦ Muscle cramps, irritability, emotional lability

✦ Vision changes

✦ Numbness and tingling

PATHOPHYSIOLOGY

In persons genetically susceptible to type 1 diabetes, a triggering event, possibly a viral infection, causes production of autoantibodies against the beta cells of the pancreas. The resultant destruction of the beta cells leads to a decline in and ultimate lack of insulin secretion. Insulin deficiency leads to hyperglycemia, enhanced lipolysis (decomposition of fat), and protein catabolism. These characteristics occur when more than 90% of the beta cells have been destroyed.

Type 2 diabetes mellitus is a chronic disease caused by one or more of the following factors: impaired insulin secretion, inappropriate hepatic glucose production, or peripheral insulin receptor insensitivity. Genetic factors are significant, and onset is accelerated by obesity and a sedentary lifestyle. Added stress can be a pivotal factor.

Gestational diabetes mellitus occurs when a woman not previously diagnosed with diabetes shows glucose intolerance during pregnancy. This may occur if placental hormones counteract insulin, causing insulin resistance. Gestational diabetes mellitus is a significant risk factor for the future occurrence of type 2 diabetes mellitus.

SIGNS AND SYMPTOMS

 CLINICAL ALERT Type 1 diabetes usually presents rapidly, typically with polydipsia, polyuria, polyphagia, weakness, weight loss, dry skin, and ketoacidosis. Type 2 diabetes is typically slow and insidious in onset and usually unaccompanied by symptoms.

Signs and symptoms of diabetes mellitus include polyuria and polydipsia due to high serum osmolality caused by high serum glucose levels. The patient may report anorexia (common) or polyphagia (occasional). Weight loss (usually 10% to 30%; persons with type 1 diabetes typically have almost no body fat at time of diagnosis) is due to prevention of normal metabolism of carbohydrates, fats, and proteins caused by impaired or absent insulin function.

CNS symptoms include headaches, fatigue, lethargy, reduced energy levels, and impaired school and work performance due to low intracellular glucose levels. The patient may report muscle cramps, irritability, and emotional lability due to electrolyte imbalance; vision changes, such as blurring, due to glucose-induced swelling; and numbness and tingling due to neural tissue damage.

GI symptoms include abdominal discomfort and pain due to autonomic neuropathy (causing gastroparesis, constipation), and nausea, diarrhea, or constipation due to dehydration and electrolyte imbalances or autonomic neuropathy.

Inspection may reveal slowly healing skin infections or wounds and itchy skin. The patient may need treatment for recurrent monilial infections of the vagina or anus.

COMPLICATIONS

Two acute metabolic complications of diabetes are ketoacidosis and hyperosmolar coma (hyperosmolar nonketotic diabetic coma). These life-threatening conditions require immediate medical intervention.

Patients with diabetes mellitus also have a higher risk of various chronic illnesses affecting virtually all body systems. The most common chronic complications include cardiovascular disease, peripheral vascular disease, retinopathy, nephropathy, diabetic dermopathy, and peripheral and autonomic neuropathy. Nearly two-thirds of persons with diabetes die because of cardiovascular disease. It's also the leading cause of renal failure and blindness.

Peripheral neuropathy usually affects the hands and feet and may cause numbness or pain. Autonomic neuropathy manifests itself in several ways, including gastroparesis (leading to delayed gastric emptying and a feeling of nausea and fullness after meals), nocturnal diarrhea, impotence, and postural hypotension.

Hyperglycemia impairs the patient's resistance to infection because the glucose content of the epidermis and urine encourages bacterial growth. The patient is susceptible to skin and urinary tract infections and vaginitis. The patient with diabetes mellitus also has an increased incidence of cognitive depression.

DIAGNOSIS

In adult men and nonpregnant women, diabetes mellitus is diagnosed by two of these criteria obtained more than 24 hours apart, using the same test twice or any combination: laboratory tests revealing fasting plasma glucose level of 126 mg/dl or more on at least two occasions; documentation showing typical symptoms of uncontrolled diabetes and random blood glucose level of 200 mg/dl or more; findings reveal blood glucose level of 200 mg/dl or more 2 hours after ingesting 75 g of oral dextrose during the oral glucose tolerance test.

Diagnosis may also be based on diabetic retinopathy found on ophthalmologic examination. Other diagnostic and monitoring tests include urinalysis for acetone and glycosylated hemoglobin (reflects glycemic control over the past 2 to 3 months).

TREATMENT

Effective treatment of all types of diabetes optimizes blood glucose control and decreases complications. Treatment for type 1 diabetes includes insulin replacement, meal planning, and exercise. Current forms of insulin replacement include mixed-dose, split mixed-dose, and multiple daily injection regimens and continuous S.C. insulin infusions.

Pancreas transplantation is available and currently requires chronic immunosuppression. (See *Treatment of type 1 diabetes mellitus,* pages 502 and 503.)

Treatment of type 2 diabetes mellitus includes oral antidiabetic drugs to stimulate endogenous insulin production, increase insulin sensitivity at the cellular level, suppress hepatic gluconeogenesis, and delay GI absorption of carbohydrates (drug combinations may be used). Treatment of both types of diabetes mellitus includes careful monitoring of blood glucose levels.

Patients need individualized meal plans designed to meet nutritional needs, control blood glucose and lipid levels, and reach and maintain appropriate body weight. The plan must be followed consistently with meals eaten at regular times. Weight reduction is the goal in obese patients with type 2 diabetes mellitus. The calorie allotment may be high, depending on growth stage and activity level in type 1 diabetes mellitus.

Treatment of gestational diabetes involves medical nutrition therapy and injectable insulin if controlled glucose isn't achieved with diet alone. Oral antidiabetic agents are teratogenic and, therefore, are contraindicated during pregnancy. Postpartum counseling addresses the high risk of gestational diabetes in subsequent pregnancies and type 2 diabetes later in life. Regular exercise and prevention of weight gain may help prevent type 2 diabetes.

Complications
+ Ketoacidosis and hyperosmolar coma
+ Cardiovascular disease
+ Peripheral vascular disease
+ Retinopathy
+ Nephropathy

Diagnosis

In adult men and nonpregnant women
+ Fasting plasma glucose level of 126 mg/dl or more on at least two occasions
+ Documentation showing typical symptoms of uncontrolled diabetes
+ Random blood glucose level of 200 mg/dl or more
+ Blood glucose level of 200 mg/dl or more 2 hours after ingesting 75 g of oral dextrose
+ Urinalysis for acetone and glycosylated hemoglobin

Treatment

Type 1
+ Insulin replacement
+ Meal planning
+ Exercise

Type 2
+ Oral antidiabetic drugs
+ Meal planning
+ Maintain appropriate body weight

Gestational
+ Medical nutrition therapy
+ Injectable insulin if needed
+ Postpartum counseling, regular exercise, prevention of weight gain

(Text continues on page 504.)

Treatment of type 1 diabetes mellitus

This algorithm shows the pathophysiologic process of diabetes and points for treatment intervention.

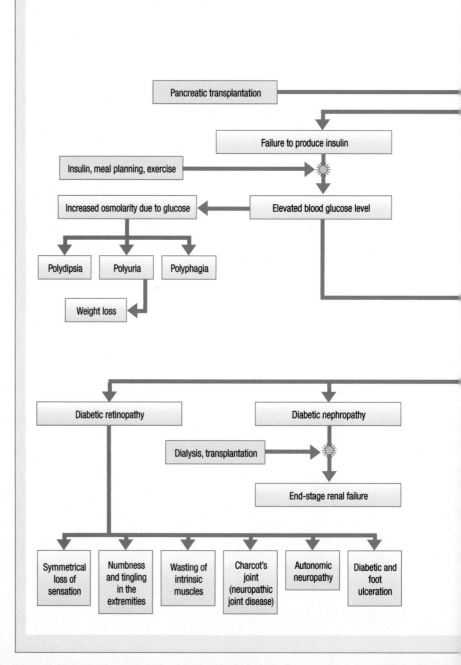

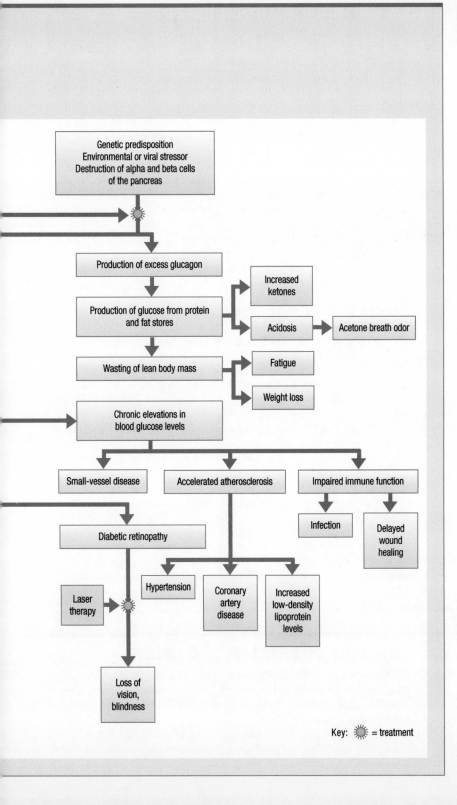

Key: ☀ = treatment

NURSING CONSIDERATIONS

Stress the importance of complying with the prescribed treatment program. Tailor your teaching to the patient's needs, abilities, and developmental stage. Include diet; purpose, administration, and possible adverse effects of medications; exercise; monitoring; hygiene; and the prevention, recognition, and treatment of hypoglycemia and hyperglycemia. Stress the effect of blood glucose control on long-term health.

♦ Watch for acute complications of diabetic therapy, especially hypoglycemia (vagueness, slow cerebration, dizziness, weakness, pallor, tachycardia, diaphoresis, seizures, and coma); immediately give carbohydrates, ideally in the form of fruit juice, hard candy, honey or, if the patient is unconscious, glucagon or dextrose I.V. Also be alert for signs of ketoacidosis (acetone breath, dehydration, weak and rapid pulse, Kussmaul's respirations) and hyperosmolar coma (polyuria, thirst, neurologic abnormalities, stupor). These hyperglycemic crises require I.V. fluids and regular insulin.

♦ Monitor diabetes control by obtaining blood glucose, glycosylated hemoglobin, lipid levels, and blood pressure measurements regularly.

♦ Watch for diabetic effects on the cardiovascular system, such as cerebrovascular, coronary artery, and peripheral vascular impairment, and the peripheral and autonomic nervous systems. Treat all injuries, cuts, and blisters (particularly on the legs or feet) meticulously. Monitor for signs and symptoms of cellulitis. Be alert for signs of urinary tract infection and renal disease.

♦ Urge regular ophthalmologic examinations to detect diabetic retinopathy.

♦ Assess for signs of diabetic neuropathy (numbness or pain in hands and feet, footdrop, neurogenic bladder). Stress the need for personal safety precautions because decreased sensation can mask injuries. Minimize complications by maintaining strict blood glucose control.

♦ Teach the patient to care for his feet by washing them daily, drying carefully between toes, and inspecting for corns, calluses, redness, swelling, bruises, and breaks in the skin. Urge him to report any changes to the physician. Advise him to wear nonconstricting shoes and to avoid walking barefoot. Instruct him to use over-the-counter athlete's foot remedies and seek professional care should athlete's foot not improve. Encourage periodic visits to a podiatrist.

♦ Teach the patient how to manage his diabetes when he has a minor illness, such as a cold, flu, or upset stomach.

♦ To delay the clinical onset of diabetes, teach people at high risk to avoid risk factors. Advise genetic counseling for young adults with diabetes who are planning families.

♦ Further information may be obtained from the Juvenile Diabetes Foundation, the American Diabetes Association, and the American Association of Diabetes Educators.

Key nursing actions

♦ Stress the importance of complying with the prescribed treatment program.
♦ Be alert for signs of ketoacidosis and hyperosmolar coma.
♦ Watch for complications of diabetic therapy, especially hypoglycemia.
♦ Obtain blood glucose, glycosylated hemoglobin, lipid levels, and blood pressure measurements regularly.
♦ Watch for diabetic effects on the cardiovascular system.
♦ Treat all injuries, cuts, and blisters meticulously.
♦ Urge regular ophthalmologic examinations to detect diabetic retinopathy.
♦ Assess for signs of diabetic neuropathy.
♦ Advise genetic counseling for young adults with diabetes who are planning families.

Characteristics of hyperparathyroidism

♦ Results from excessive secretion of PTH
♦ Leads to hypercalcemia and hypophosphatemia
♦ Renal, GI absorption of calcium increase
♦ Commonly diagnosed based on elevated calcium levels
♦ More common in women

HYPERPARATHYROIDISM

Hyperparathyroidism results from excessive secretion of parathyroid hormone (PTH) from one or more of the four parathyroid glands. PTH promotes bone resorption, and hypersecretion leads to hypercalcemia and hypophosphatemia. Renal and GI absorption of calcium increase.

Primary hyperparathyroidism is commonly diagnosed based on elevated calcium levels found on laboratory test results in asymptomatic patients. It's two to three times more common in women than in men.

CAUSES

Hyperparathyroidism may be primary or secondary. In primary hyperparathyroidism, one or more parathyroid glands enlarge and increase PTH secretion and serum calcium levels. It's most commonly caused by a single adenoma, but this may be a component of multiple endocrine neoplasia (all four glands usually involved).

In secondary hyperparathyroidism, a hypocalcemia-producing abnormality outside the parathyroids causes excessive compensatory production of PTH. Causes include rickets, vitamin D deficiency, chronic renal failure, and osteomalacia due to phenytoin (Dilantin).

PATHOPHYSIOLOGY

Overproduction of PTH by a tumor or hyperplastic tissue increases intestinal calcium absorption, reduces renal calcium clearance, and increases bone calcium release. Response to this excess varies for each patient for an unknown reason.

Hypophosphatemia results when excessive PTH inhibits renal tubular phosphate reabsorption. The hypophosphatemia aggravates hypercalcemia by increasing the sensitivity of the bone to PTH.

SIGNS AND SYMPTOMS

Signs and symptoms of primary hyperparathyroidism result from hypercalcemia and are typically present in several body systems. Renal system manifestations include polyuria, nephrocalcinosis, nocturia, polydipsia, dehydration, uremia symptoms, renal colic pain, nephrolithiasis, and renal insufficiency. The patient may report vague aches and pains, arthralgia, and localized swellings.

Skeletal and articular system effects include chronic low back pain and easy fracturing due to bone degeneration; bone tenderness; chondrocalcinosis (decreased bone mass); osteopenia and osteoporosis, especially on the vertebrae; erosions of the juxta-articular (adjoining joint) surface; subchondral fractures; traumatic synovitis; and pseudogout. The patient may also report muscle weakness and atrophy, particularly in the legs.

GI system effects include pancreatitis causing constant, severe epigastric pain that radiates to the back and peptic ulcers, causing abdominal pain, anorexia, nausea, and vomiting.

In addition, central nervous system effects include psychomotor and personality disturbances, emotional lability, depression, slow mentation, poor memory, drowsiness, ataxia, overt psychosis, stupor and, possibly, coma.

The patient may complain of pruritus caused by ectopic calcifications in the skin and skin necrosis, cataracts, calcium microthrombi to lungs and pancreas, anemia, and subcutaneous calcification.

Secondary hyperparathyroidism may produce the same features of calcium imbalance with skeletal deformities of the long bones (such as rickets) as well as symptoms of the underlying disease.

COMPLICATIONS

Untreated hyperparathyroidism damages the skeleton and kidneys from hypercalcemia. Bone and articular problems include pathologic fractures. Renal complications include renal damage and urinary tract infections (UTIs).

Other possible complications include hypertension, cardiac arrhythmias, insulin hypersecretion, decreased insulin sensitivity, and pseudogout.

Causes

Primary
+ Parathyroid glands enlarge, increase PTH secretion, serum calcium levels
+ Single adenoma

Secondary
+ Hypocalcemia-producing abnormality outside parathyroids causes excessive production of PTH
+ Rickets, vitamin D deficiency, and chronic renal failure

How it happens
+ Overproduction of PTH increases intestinal calcium absorption
+ Reduces renal calcium clearance, increases bone calcium release
+ Response varies for each patient
+ PTH inhibits renal tubular phosphate reabsorption; hypophosphatemia results
+ Aggravates hypercalcemia by increasing sensitivity of bone to PTH

Key signs and symptoms

Renal system
+ Polyuria
+ Nephrocalcinosis

Skeletal and articular systems
+ Chronic low back pain
+ Easy fracturing

GI system
+ Pancreatitis
+ Peptic ulcers

CNS
+ Psychomotor disturbances
+ Emotional lability

Complications
+ Untreated, damages skeleton
+ Renal damage, UTIs

Diagnosis

Primary

+ Hypercalcemia and high concentrations of serum PTH on radioimmunoassay
+ Diffuse demineralization of bones, bone cysts
+ Increased bone turnover
+ Elevated urine and serum calcium, chloride, alkaline phosphatase levels

Secondary

+ Normal or slightly decreased serum calcium level
+ Variable serum phosphorus level
+ Familial kidney disease, seizure disorders, drug ingestion

Treatment

Primary

+ Surgery to remove adenoma or all but one-half of one gland
+ Encouraging consumption of fluids
+ Limiting dietary intake of calcium
+ Promoting sodium and calcium excretion
+ Furosemide
+ Ethacrynic acid

Secondary

+ Correct underlying cause of parathyroid hypertrophy
+ Vitamin D for parathyroid hyperplasia
+ Aluminum hydroxide preparation for hyperphosphatemia
+ Dialysis
+ Administration of calcitonin
+ Initiation of pamidronate

DIAGNOSIS

Findings differ in primary and secondary disease. In primary disease, diagnosis is confirmed by hypercalcemia and high concentrations of serum PTH on radioimmunoassay. X-rays may show diffuse demineralization of bones, bone cysts, outer cortical bone absorption, and subperiosteal erosion of the phalanges and distal clavicles. A microscopic bone examination by X-ray spectrophotometry typically demonstrates increased bone turnover.

Laboratory tests reveal elevated urine and serum calcium, chloride, and alkaline phosphatase levels, and decreased serum phosphorus levels. Hyperparathyroidism may cause elevated uric acid and creatinine levels, which may also increase basal gastric acid secretion and serum immunoreactive gastrin. Increased serum amylase levels may indicate acute pancreatitis.

Diagnosis of secondary disease is based on normal or slightly decreased serum calcium level and variable serum phosphorus level, especially when the cause is rickets, osteomalacia, or kidney disease. Patient history may reveal familial kidney disease, seizure disorders, or drug ingestion.

TREATMENT

Effective treatment varies, depending on the cause of the disease. In primary hyperparathyroidism, surgery is the only definitive therapy. The only effective long-term medical therapy is maintaining hydration in mild hyperparathyroidism.

Treatment of primary disease may include surgery to remove the adenoma or, depending on the extent of hyperplasia, all but one-half of one gland. The remaining part of the gland is necessary to maintain normal PTH levels. Surgery may relieve bone pain within 3 days, but renal damage may be irreversible.

Other treatments can decrease calcium levels preoperatively if surgery isn't feasible or necessary. These treatments include encouraging the consumption of fluids, limiting dietary intake of calcium, and promoting sodium and calcium excretion through forced diuresis (using as much as 6 qt [6 L] of urine output in life-threatening circumstances), and use of furosemide (Lasix) or ethacrynic acid (Edecrin).

Treatments also include oral sodium or potassium phosphate, subcutaneous calcitonin (Calcimar), and I.V. plicamycin. I.V. magnesium and phosphate or sodium phosphate solution by mouth or retention enema may be administered for potential postoperative magnesium and phosphate deficiencies. Supplemental calcium, vitamin D, or calcitriol (Calcijex) may be administered because serum calcium level decreases to low-normal range during the first 4 to 5 days after surgery.

Treatment of secondary disease must correct the underlying cause of parathyroid hypertrophy. Vitamin D is administered to correct the underlying cause of parathyroid hyperplasia. Aluminum hydroxide preparation is used to correct hyperphosphatemia in the patient with kidney disease.

Dialysis may be necessary in the patient with renal failure to decrease phosphorus levels and may be lifelong. The enlarged glands may not revert to normal size and function even after calcium levels have been controlled in the patient with chronic secondary hyperparathyroidism.

For severe hypercalcemia (serum calcium greater than 14 mg/dl) or for the patient with severe symptoms, administration of calcitonin, a rapid-acting agent, along with hydration is necessary. Possible initiation of pamidronate, a slower-acting agent, may provide a longer-lasting effect.

Nursing considerations

Care emphasizes prevention of complications from the underlying disease and its treatment.

✦ Obtain pretreatment baseline serum potassium, calcium, phosphate, and magnesium levels because these values may change abruptly during treatment.

✦ During hydration to reduce serum calcium level, record intake and output accurately. Strain urine to check for calculi. Provide at least 3 qt (3 L) of fluid per day, including cranberry or prune juice to increase urine acidity and help prevent calculus formation. As ordered, obtain blood samples and urine specimens to measure sodium, potassium, and magnesium levels, especially for the patient taking furosemide.

✦ Auscultate for breath sounds often. Listen for signs of pulmonary edema in the patient receiving large amounts of saline solution I.V., especially if he has pulmonary or cardiac disease. Monitor the patient on cardiac glycosides carefully because elevated calcium levels can rapidly produce toxic effects.

✦ Because the patient is predisposed to pathologic fractures, take safety precautions to minimize the risk of injury. Assist him with walking, keep the bed at its lowest position, and raise the side rails. Lift the immobilized patient carefully to minimize bone stress. Schedule care to allow the patient with muscle weakness as much rest as possible.

✦ Watch for signs of peptic ulcer and administer antacids as appropriate.

After parathyroidectomy

✦ Check frequently for respiratory distress, and keep a tracheotomy tray at the bedside. Watch for postoperative complications, such as laryngeal nerve damage or, rarely, hemorrhage. Monitor intake and output carefully.

✦ Check for swelling at the operative site. Place the patient in semi-Fowler's position, and support his head and neck with sandbags to decrease edema, which may cause pressure on the trachea.

✦ Watch for signs of mild tetany such as complaints of tingling in the hands and around the mouth. These symptoms should subside quickly but may be prodromal signs of tetany, so keep calcium gluconate or calcium chloride I.V. available for emergency administration. Watch for increased neuromuscular irritability and other signs of severe tetany, and report them immediately.

✦ Ambulate the patient as soon as possible postoperatively, even though he may find this uncomfortable, because pressure on bones speeds up bone recalcification.

✦ Check laboratory results for low serum calcium and magnesium levels.

✦ Monitor mental status and watch for listlessness. In the patient with persistent hypercalcemia, check for muscle weakness and psychiatric symptoms.

✦ Before discharge, advise the patient of the possible adverse effects of drug therapy. Emphasize the need for periodic follow-up through laboratory blood tests. If hyperparathyroidism wasn't corrected surgically, warn the patient to avoid calcium-containing antacids and thiazide diuretics.

HYPOPARATHYROIDISM

Hypoparathyroidism is caused by disease, injury, or congenital malfunction of the parathyroid glands. Because the parathyroid glands primarily regulate calcium balance, hypoparathyroidism causes hypocalcemia and consequent neuromuscular symptoms ranging from paresthesia to tetany.

Key nursing actions

✦ Obtain pretreatment baseline serum potassium, calcium, phosphate, and magnesium levels.

✦ During hydration to reduce serum calcium level, record intake and output accurately.

✦ Strain urine to check for calculi.

✦ Schedule care to allow the patient with muscle weakness as much rest as possible.

After parathyroidectomy

✦ Check frequently for respiratory distress, and keep a tracheotomy tray at the bedside.

✦ Check for swelling at the operative site.

✦ Place the patient in semi-Fowler's position.

✦ Watch for signs of tetany.

✦ Ambulate the patient as soon as possible postoperatively.

✦ Check laboratory results for low serum calcium and magnesium levels.

✦ Monitor mental status and watch for listlessness.

✦ If hyperparathyroidism wasn't corrected surgically, warn the patient to avoid calcium-containing antacids and thiazide diuretics.

Characteristics of hypoparathyroidism

✦ Caused by disease, injury, congenital malfunction of parathyroid glands

✦ Causes hypocalcemia, neuromuscular symptoms

✦ Clinical effects usually correctable with replacement therapy

✦ Some complications irreversible

Causes

Idiopathic or acquired
✦ Acute pancreatitis or malabsorption
✦ Renal failure
✦ Osteomalacia

Idiopathic
✦ Autoimmune genetic disorder
✦ Congenital absence of parathyroid gland

Acquired
✦ Accidental removal of or injury to parathyroid glands during surgery, thyroid irradiation
✦ Ischemic infarction of parathyroid glands

Alert!
✦ The incidence of the idiopathic and reversible forms of hypoparathyroidism is greatest in children.

How it happens
✦ Underproduction of PTH causes hypocalcemia, hyperphosphatemia
✦ Surgical manipulation of neck may damage parathyroid glands
✦ Degree can vary from decreased reserve to frank tetany
✦ Hypomagnesemia can prevent PTH secretion in some patients

Key signs and symptoms
✦ Usually causes hypocalcemia and high serum phosphate levels
✦ Neuromuscular irritability
✦ Increased deep tendon reflexes
✦ Chvostek's sign
✦ Dysphagia

The clinical effects of hypoparathyroidism are usually correctable with replacement therapy. Some complications of long-term hypocalcemia, such as cataracts and basal ganglion calcifications, are irreversible.

CAUSES

Hypoparathyroidism may be acute or chronic and is classified as idiopathic or acquired. Possible causes include acute pancreatitis or malabsorption, renal failure, and osteomalacia. Idiopathic hypoparathyroidism may result from an autoimmune genetic disorder or congenital absence of the parathyroid glands.

Acquired hypoparathyroidism commonly results from accidental removal of or injury to the parathyroid glands during thyroidectomy or other neck surgery or, rarely, from massive thyroid irradiation.

It may also result from ischemic infarction of the parathyroid glands during surgery or from amyloidosis, neoplasms, or trauma.

An acquired, reversible hypoparathyroidism may result from impairment of hormone synthesis and release due to hypomagnesemia, suppression of normal gland function due to hypercalcemia, and delayed maturation of parathyroid function.

Parathyroid hormone (PTH) is regulated directly by serum calcium levels, not by the pituitary or hypothalamus. It normally maintains normocalcemia by regulating bone resorption and GI absorption of calcium. It also maintains an inverse relationship between serum calcium and phosphate levels by inhibiting phosphate reabsorption in the renal tubules.

 CLINICAL ALERT The incidence of the idiopathic and reversible forms of hypoparathyroidism is greatest in children; the incidence of the irreversible acquired form is greatest in adults who have undergone surgery for hyperthyroidism or other head and neck conditions.

PATHOPHYSIOLOGY

Underproduction of PTH causes hypocalcemia and hyperphosphatemia. Surgical manipulation of the neck may damage the parathyroid glands, possibly by causing ischemia. The degree of hypoparathyroidism can vary from decreased reserve to frank tetany. Hypomagnesemia can prevent PTH secretion in patients with chronic GI magnesium losses, nutritional deficiencies, and renal magnesium wasting.

SIGNS AND SYMPTOMS

Mild hypoparathyroidism may not produce symptoms but usually causes hypocalcemia and high serum phosphate levels affecting the central nervous system (CNS) and other systems.

Signs and symptoms of chronic hypoparathyroidism typically include neuromuscular irritability, increased deep tendon reflexes, Chvostek's sign (spasm of the hyperirritable facial nerve when it's tapped), dysphagia, organic brain syndrome, psychosis, mental deficiency in children, and tetany. Chronic tetany may cause difficulty walking and a tendency to fall.

Signs and symptoms of acute hypoparathyroidism include tingling in the fingertips, around the mouth, and occasionally in the feet (first symptom). The tingling begins to spread and becomes more severe, producing muscle tension and spasms and consequent adduction of the thumbs, wrists, and elbows. Pain varies with the degree of muscle tension but seldom affects the face, legs, and feet. Both forms of tetany can lead to laryngospasm, stridor, cyanosis, and seizures. These

CNS abnormalities tend to be exaggerated during hyperventilation, pregnancy, infection, withdrawal of thyroid hormone, or administration of diuretics and before menstruation.

Other clinical effects include abdominal pain; intestinal malabsorption with steatorrhea; dry, lusterless hair; spontaneous hair loss; brittle fingernails developing ridges or falling out; dry, scaly skin; exfoliative dermatitis; candidal infections; cataracts; and weakened tooth enamel, causing teeth to stain, crack, and decay easily.

COMPLICATIONS

In hypoparathyroidism, complications are related to hypocalcemia. Decreased calcium levels can cause neuromuscular excitability and delayed cardiac repolarization, which may lead to heart failure. Lens calcification leads to cataract formation that may persist despite calcium replacement therapy. Papillary edema and increased intracranial pressure, irreversible calcification of basal ganglia, and bone deformities also occur. Parkinson's symptoms, hypothyroidism, laryngospasm, respiratory stridor, anoxia, paralysis of the vocal cords, seizures, and death may occur in severe forms of tetany. Hypoparathyroidism that develops during childhood results in malformed teeth.

DIAGNOSIS

Radioimmunoassay for PTH shows decreased serum PTH level. Blood and urine tests reveal decreased serum and urine calcium levels, increased serum phosphorus level (more than 5.4 mg/dl), and reduced creatinine levels.

Electrocardiography (ECG) changes disclose prolonged QT and ST intervals due to hypocalcemia. Inflating a blood pressure cuff on the upper arm to between diastolic and systolic blood pressure and maintaining this inflation for 3 minutes elicits Trousseau's sign (carpal spasm) to show clinical evidence of hypoparathyroidism.

TREATMENT

Acute, life-threatening tetany calls for immediate I.V. calcium salts, such as 10% calcium gluconate, to increase ionized serum calcium levels. Breathing into a paper bag and inhaling one's own carbon dioxide causes a mild respiratory acidosis that increases serum calcium levels. The patient must be awake and able to cooperate.

Sedatives and anticonvulsants may control spasms until calcium levels increase. Patients require an increased dietary intake of calcium and maintenance therapy with oral calcium and vitamin D supplements.

Treatment includes vitamin D and calcium supplements because of calcium absorption from the small intestine requiring the presence of vitamin D. Except for the reversible form of the disease, treatment is usually lifelong. Calcitriol (Calcijex) may be used if hepatic or renal problems cause the patient to not tolerate vitamin D.

NURSING CONSIDERATIONS

While awaiting diagnosis of hypoparathyroidism in a patient with a history of tetany, maintain a patent I.V. line and keep I.V. calcium available. Because the patient is vulnerable to seizures, maintain seizure precautions. Also, keep a tracheotomy tray and endotracheal tube at the bedside because laryngospasm may result from hypocalcemia.
◆ Instruct the patient to follow a high-calcium, low-phosphorus diet.

Complications
◆ Neuromuscular excitability
◆ Delayed cardiac repolarization
◆ Cataract formation that may persist
◆ Papillary edema
◆ Increased intracranial pressure
◆ Irreversible calcification of basal ganglia
◆ Bone deformities
◆ Parkinson's symptoms
◆ Hypothyroidism

Diagnosis
◆ Decreased serum PTH level
◆ Decreased serum and urine calcium levels
◆ Increased serum phosphorus level
◆ Reduced creatinine levels

Treatment
◆ Immediate I.V. calcium salts
◆ Breathing into a paper bag if awake and cooperative
◆ Sedatives and anticonvulsants
◆ Increased dietary intake of calcium
◆ Maintenance therapy with oral calcium and vitamin D supplements
◆ Vitamin D and calcium supplements

Key nursing actions
◆ Maintain a patent I.V. line and keep I.V. calcium available while awaiting diagnosis.
◆ Maintain seizure precautions.
◆ Keep a tracheotomy tray and endotracheal tube at the bedside.
◆ Instruct the patient to follow a high-calcium, low-phosphorus diet.

Key nursing actions
(continued)

✦ Stay alert for minor muscle twitching and for signs of laryngospasm.
✦ For the patient on drug therapy, emphasize the importance of checking serum calcium levels at least three times per year.
✦ Instruct the patient with scaly skin to use creams to soften his skin.
✦ For the patient with tetany, administer 10% calcium gluconate by slow I.V. infusion and maintain a patent airway.

Characteristics of hyperthyroidism

✦ Metabolic imbalance from overproduction of thyroid hormone
✦ Most common form is Graves' disease
✦ With treatment, most patients lead normal lives
✦ Thyroid storm is a life-threatening medical emergency

Alert!

✦ The incidence of Graves' disease is greatest in women between ages 30 and 60, especially those with a family history of thyroid abnormalities.
✦ Only 5% of the patients are younger than age 15.

Causes

✦ Thyrotoxicosis from genetic, immunologic factors
✦ Probably autosomal recessive gene
✦ Occasionally exists with other endocrine abnormalities
✦ Medications, toxic nodules, tumors

✦ When caring for the patient with chronic disease, particularly a child, stay alert for minor muscle twitching and for signs of laryngospasm because these effects may signal the onset of tetany.
✦ For the patient on drug therapy, emphasize the importance of checking serum calcium levels at least three times per year. Instruct the patient to watch for signs of hypercalcemia and to keep medications away from light and heat.
✦ Dental changes, cataracts, and brain calcifications are permanent. These can be prevented with early detection and periodic calcium determinations.
✦ Because the patient with chronic disease has prolonged QT intervals on ECG, watch for heart block and signs of decreasing cardiac output. Because calcium potentiates the effect of cardiac glycosides, closely monitor the patient receiving both a cardiac glycoside and calcium. Stay alert for signs of digoxin toxicity (arrhythmias, nausea, fatigue, visual changes).
✦ Instruct the patient with scaly skin to use creams to soften his skin. Also tell him to keep his nails trimmed to prevent them from splitting.
✦ Hyperventilation or recent blood transfusions may worsen tetany. (Anticoagulant in stored blood binds calcium.)
✦ For the patient with tetany, administer 10% calcium gluconate by slow I.V. infusion (1 ml/minute), and maintain a patent airway. The patient may also require intubation and sedation with I.V. diazepam. Monitor vital signs often after administration of diazepam to make certain that blood pressure and heart rate return to normal.

HYPERTHYROIDISM

Hyperthyroidism, or thyrotoxicosis, is a metabolic imbalance that results from the overproduction of thyroid hormone. The most common form is Graves' disease, which increases thyroxine (T_4) production, enlarges the thyroid gland (goiter), and causes multiple system changes. (See *Other forms of hyperthyroidism.*)

 CLINICAL ALERT The incidence of Graves' disease is greatest in women between ages 30 and 60, especially those with a family history of thyroid abnormalities; only 5% of the patients are younger than age 15.

With treatment, most patients can lead normal lives. However, thyroid storm—an acute, severe exacerbation of thyrotoxicosis—is a medical emergency that may have life-threatening cardiac, hepatic, or renal consequences.

CAUSES

Thyrotoxicosis may result from both genetic and immunologic factors. An increased incidence in monozygotic twins points to an inherited factor, probably autosomal recessive gene. This disease occasionally exists with other endocrine abnormalities, such as type 1 diabetes mellitus, thyroiditis, and hyperparathyroidism.

Due to a defect in suppressor T-lymphocyte function, the production of autoantibodies (thyroid-stimulating immunoglobulin and thyroid-stimulating hormone [TSH]-binding inhibitory immunoglobulin) is permitted.

Clinical thyrotoxicosis can be precipitated by excessive dietary intake of iodine or possibly stress in patients with latent disease. In people with inadequately treated hyperthyroidism, stress, such as surgery, infection, toxemia of pregnancy, or diabetic ketoacidosis, can precipitate thyroid storm. Other causes include medications, such as lithium and amiodarone and toxic nodules or tumors.

Other forms of hyperthyroidism

♦ *Toxic adenoma,* a small, benign nodule in the thyroid gland that secretes thyroid hormone, is the second most common cause of hyperthyroidism. The cause of toxic adenoma is unknown; incidence is highest in the elderly. Clinical effects are essentially similar to those of Graves' disease, except that toxic adenoma doesn't induce ophthalmopathy, pretibial myxedema, or acropachy. Presence of adenoma is confirmed by radioactive iodine (^{131}I) uptake and thyroid scan, which shows a single hyperfunctioning nodule suppressing the rest of the gland. Treatment includes ^{131}I therapy or surgery to remove adenoma after antithyroid drugs achieve a euthyroid state.

♦ *Thyrotoxicosis factitia* results from chronic ingestion of thyroid hormone for thyrotropin suppression in patients with thyroid carcinoma, or from thyroid hormone abuse by people who are trying to lose weight.

♦ *Functioning metastatic thyroid carcinoma* is a rare disease that causes excess production of thyroid hormone.

♦ *Thyroid-stimulating hormone-secreting pituitary tumor* causes overproduction of thyroid hormone.

♦ *Subacute thyroiditis* is a virus-induced granulomatous inflammation of the thyroid, producing transient hyperthyroidism associated with fever, pain, pharyngitis, and tenderness in the thyroid gland.

♦ *Silent thyroiditis* is a self-limiting, transient form of hyperthyroidism, with histologic thyroiditis but no inflammatory symptoms.

PATHOPHYSIOLOGY

The thyroid gland secretes the thyroid precursor, T_4, thyroid hormone or triiodothyronine (T_3), and calcitonin. T_4 and T_3 stimulate protein, lipid, and carbohydrate metabolism primarily through catabolic pathways. Calcitonin removes calcium from the blood and incorporates it into bone.

Biosynthesis, storage, and release of thyroid hormones are controlled by the hypothalamic-pituitary axis through a negative-feedback loop. Thyrotropin-releasing hormone (TRH) from the hypothalamus stimulates the release of TSH by the pituitary. Circulating T_3 levels provide negative feedback through the hypothalamus to decrease TRH levels, and through the pituitary to decrease TSH levels.

Although the exact mechanism isn't understood, hyperthyroidism has a hereditary component, and it's usually associated with other autoimmune endocrinopathies.

Graves' disease is an autoimmune disorder characterized by the production of autoantibodies that attach to and then stimulate TSH receptors on the thyroid gland. A goiter is an enlarged thyroid gland, either the result of increased stimulation or a response to increased metabolic demand. The latter occurs in iodine-deficient areas of the world, where the incidence of goiter increases during puberty (a time of increased metabolic demand). These goiters commonly regress to normal size after puberty in males, but not in females. Sporadic goiter in non–iodine-deficient areas is of unknown origin. Endemic and sporadic goiters are nontoxic and may be diffuse or nodular. Toxic goiters may be uninodular or multinodular and may secrete excess thyroid hormone.

Pituitary tumors with TSH-producing cells are rare, as is hypothalamic disease causing TRH excess.

SIGNS AND SYMPTOMS

The classic features of hyperthyroidism are enlarged thyroid (goiter), nervousness, heat intolerance and sweating, weight loss despite increased appetite, frequent bow-

Other forms of hyperthyroidism

♦ Toxic adenoma
♦ Thyrotoxicosis
♦ Functioning metastatic thyroid carcinoma
♦ Thyroid-stimulating hormone-secreting pituitary tumor
♦ Subacute thyroiditis
♦ Silent thyroiditis

How it happens

♦ Hereditary component, usually associated with other autoimmune endocrinopathies
♦ Graves' disease: autoantibodies attach to and stimulate TSH receptors on thyroid gland
♦ Goiter result of increased stimulation or response to increased metabolic demand
♦ Latter occurs in iodine-deficient areas
♦ Sporadic goiter in non–iodine-deficient areas of unknown origin
♦ Endemic or sporadic goiters nontoxic, may be diffuse or nodular
♦ Toxic goiters may be uninodular or multinodular; may secrete excess thyroid hormone
♦ Pituitary tumors with TSH-producing cells rare

Key signs and symptoms

+ Goiter
+ Nervousness
+ Heat intolerance and sweating
+ Weight loss despite increased appetite
+ Frequent bowel movements
+ Tremor and palpitations
+ Exophthalmos considered most characteristic, absent in many patients with thyrotoxicosis
+ CNS effects
+ Effects on the skin, hair, nails
+ Cardiovascular system effects
+ GI system effects
+ Musculoskeletal system effects
+ Reproductive system effects
+ Effects on the eyes

el movements, and tremor and palpitations. Exophthalmos is considered most characteristic but absent in many patients with thyrotoxicosis.

Other signs and symptoms are common because thyrotoxicosis profoundly affects virtually every body system. Central nervous system effects include difficulty concentrating due to accelerated cerebral function; excitability or nervousness caused by increased basal metabolic rate from T_4; fine tremor, shaky handwriting, and clumsiness from increased activity in the spinal cord area that controls muscle tone; emotional instability and mood swings ranging from occasional outbursts to overt psychosis.

Effects on the skin, hair, and nails include moist, smooth, warm, flushed skin (patient sleeps with minimal covers and little clothing); fine, soft hair; premature patchy graying and increased hair loss in both sexes; friable nails and onycholysis (distal nail separated from the bed); pretibial myxedema (nonpitting edema of the anterior surface of the legs, dermopathy), producing thickened skin; accentuated hair follicles; sometimes itchy or painful raised red patches of skin with occasional nodule formation; microscopic examination showing increased mucin deposits.

Systolic hypertension, tachycardia, full bounding pulse, wide pulse pressure, cardiomegaly, increased cardiac output and blood volume, visible point of maximal impulse, paroxysmal supraventricular tachycardia and atrial fibrillation (especially in elderly people), and occasional systolic murmur at the left sternal border characterize the cardiovascular system effects.

In addition, an increased respiratory rate and dyspnea on exertion and at rest, possibly due to cardiac decompensation and increased cellular oxygen use, occur in the respiratory system.

Effects on other body systems

GI system effects include excessive oral intake with weight loss; nausea and vomiting due to increased GI motility and peristalsis; increased defecation; soft stools or, in severe disease, diarrhea; liver enlargement.

Musculoskeletal system effects include weakness, fatigue, and muscle atrophy; rare coexistence with myasthenia gravis; possibly generalized or localized paralysis associated with hypokalemia; and, rarely, acropachy (soft-tissue swelling accompanied by underlying bone changes where new bone formation occurs).

Effects on the reproductive system include oligomenorrhea or amenorrhea, decreased fertility, increased incidence of spontaneous abortion (females), gynecomastia due to increased estrogen levels (males), and diminished libido (both sexes).

Effects on the eyes include exophthalmos due to combined effects of accumulated mucopolysaccharides and fluids in the retro-orbital tissues, forcing the eyeball outward and lid retraction, thereby producing a characteristic staring gaze; occasional inflammation of conjunctivae, corneas, or eye muscles; diplopia; and increased tearing.

When thyrotoxicosis escalates to thyroid storm, symptoms that may occur include extreme irritability, hypertension, tachycardia, vomiting, temperature of up to 106° F (41.1° C), delirium, and coma. Thyrotoxicosis can escalate to thyroid storm, a life-threatening medical emergency. Signs and symptoms may include high fever (up to 106° F), tachycardia, pulmonary edema, hypertension, shock, tremors, emotional lability, extreme irritability, confusion, delirium, psychosis, apathy, stupor, coma, diarrhea, abdominal pain, nausea and vomiting, jaundice, and hyperglycemia.

 CLINICAL ALERT Consider apathetic thyrotoxicosis, a morbid condition resulting from overactive thyroid, in elderly patients with atrial fibrillation or depression.

Alert!

+ Consider apathetic thyrotoxicosis, a morbid condition resulting from overactive thyroid, in elderly patients with atrial fibrillation or depression.

COMPLICATIONS

Thyroid hormones have widespread effects on almost all body tissues, so the complications of hypersecretion may be far-reaching and varied. Cardiovascular complications are most common in elderly persons and include arrhythmias, especially atrial fibrillation; cardiac insufficiency; cardiac decompensation; and resistance to the usual therapeutic dose of a cardiac glycoside. Additional complications include muscle weakness and atrophy, paralysis, visual loss or diplopia, hypoparathyroidism after surgical removal of the thyroid, and hypothyroidism after radioiodine treatment.

DIAGNOSIS

The diagnosis of thyrotoxicosis is usually straightforward. It depends on a careful clinical history and physical examination, a high index of suspicion, and routine hormone determinations. Radioimmunoassay shows increased serum T_4 and T_3 levels. TSH levels are decreased. Thyroid scan reveals increased uptake of radioactive iodine (^{131}I) in Graves' disease and, usually, in toxic multinodular goiter and toxic adenoma. The test reveals low radioactive uptake in thyroiditis and thyrotoxic factitia; however, the test is contraindicated in pregnancy. Ultrasonography confirms subclinical ophthalmopathy.

TREATMENT

The primary forms of therapy include antithyroid drugs, single oral dose of ^{131}I, and surgery. Appropriate treatment depends on severity of thyrotoxicosis, causes, patient age and parity, and how long surgery will be delayed (if patient is appropriate candidate for surgery).

Antithyroid therapy includes antithyroid drugs for children, young adults, pregnant women, and patients who refuse surgery or ^{131}I treatment. Antithyroid drugs are preferred in patients with new-onset Graves' disease because of spontaneous remission in many of these patients; they're also used to correct the thyrotoxic state in preparation for ^{131}I treatment or surgery.

Thyroid hormone antagonists, including propylthiouracil (PTU) and methimazole (Tapazole), block thyroid hormone synthesis. Although hypermetabolic symptoms subside within 4 to 8 weeks after therapy begins, remission of Graves' disease requires continued therapy for 6 months to 2 years.

Propranolol (Inderal) may be given concurrently until antithyroid drugs reach their full effect to manage tachycardia and other peripheral effects of excessive hypersympathetic activity resulting from blocking the conversion of T_4 to the active T_3 hormone.

During pregnancy, antithyroid medications should be kept at a minimum dosage to keep maternal thyroid function within the high-normal range until delivery and to minimize the risk of fetal hypothyroidism. PTU is the preferred agent during pregnancy. Neonatal thyrotoxicosis may necessitate treatment with antithyroid medications and propranolol for 2 to 3 months because most infants of hyperthyroid mothers are born with mild and transient thyrotoxicosis caused by placental transfer of thyroid-stimulating immunoglobulins.

Continuous control of maternal thyroid function is essential because thyrotoxicosis is sometimes exacerbated in the puerperal period. Antithyroid drugs can be gradually tapered and thyroid function reassessed after 3 to 6 months postpartum. Periodic checks of infant's thyroid function are necessary with a breast-feeding mother on low-dose antithyroid treatment due to possible presence of small

Complications
- May be far-reaching and varied
- Cardiovascular complications most common in elderly
- Muscle weakness and atrophy
- Paralysis
- Visual loss or diplopia
- Hypoparathyroidism after surgical removal of thyroid
- Hypothyroidism after radioiodine treatment

Diagnosis
- Depends on a careful clinical history, physical examination, high index of suspicion, routine hormone determinations
- Increased serum T_4 and T_3 levels
- TSH levels decreased
- Increased uptake of ^{131}I
- Subclinical ophthalmopathy

Treatment
- Antithyroid drugs
- Thyroid hormone antagonists
- Single oral dose of ^{131}I
- Surgery
- Local application of topical medications
- Calcium channel blockers
- External-beam radiation therapy

amounts of the drug in breast milk, which can rapidly lead to thyrotoxicity in the infant.

A single oral dose of ^{131}I is the treatment of choice for patients not planning to have children. Patients of reproductive age must give informed consent for this treatment, because ^{131}I concentrates in the gonads. During treatment with ^{131}I, the thyroid gland picks up the radioactive element as it would regular iodine. The radioactivity destroys some of the cells that normally concentrate iodine and produce T_4, thus decreasing thyroid hormone production and normalizing thyroid size and function.

In most patients, hypermetabolic symptoms diminish 6 to 8 weeks after such treatment. However, some patients may require a second dose. Almost all patients treated with ^{131}I eventually become hypothyroid. Subtotal thyroidectomy, which decreases the thyroid gland's capacity for hormone production, is indicated for patients who refuse or aren't candidates for ^{131}I treatment.

The patient may receive iodides (Lugol's solution or saturated solution of potassium iodide), antithyroid drugs, and propranolol to relieve hyperthyroidism preoperatively. If the patient doesn't become euthyroid, surgery should be delayed, and antithyroid drugs and propranolol should be given to decrease the systemic effects (cardiac arrhythmias) of thyrotoxicosis. Lifelong regular medical supervision is required because most patients become hypothyroid, sometimes as long as several years after surgery.

Treatment of ophthalmopathy includes local application of topical medications, such as prednisone acetate suspension, but may require high doses of corticosteroids. Calcium channel blockers, such as diltiazem and verapamil, may be administered to block the peripheral effects of thyroid hormones. External-beam radiation therapy or surgical decompression may be required for severe exophthalmos that causes pressure on optic nerve and orbital contents.

Emergency treatment of thyroid storm includes administering an antithyroid drug to stop conversion of T_4 to T_3 and to block sympathetic effect; corticosteroids to inhibit the conversion of T_4 to T_3; and iodide to block the release of thyroid hormone. Supportive measures include the administration of nutrients, vitamins, fluids, oxygen, hypothermia blankets, and sedatives.

NURSING CONSIDERATIONS

Patients with hyperthyroidism require vigilant care to prevent acute exacerbations and complications.

✦ Record vital signs and weight.
✦ Monitor serum electrolyte levels, and check periodically for hyperglycemia and glycosuria.
✦ Carefully monitor cardiac function if the patient is elderly or has coronary artery disease. If the heart rate is more than 100 beats/minute, check blood pressure and pulse rate often. Monitor the patient's ECG for arrhythmias and changes in the ST segment.
✦ Check level of consciousness and urine output.
✦ If the patient is pregnant, tell her to watch closely during the first trimester for signs of spontaneous abortion and to report such signs immediately.
✦ Encourage bed rest, and keep the patient's room cool, quiet, and dark. The patient with dyspnea will be most comfortable sitting upright or in high Fowler's position.
✦ Remember, extreme nervousness may produce bizarre behavior. Reassure the patient and his family that such behavior will probably subside with treatment. Provide sedatives as necessary.

Key nursing actions
✦ Record vital signs and weight.
✦ Monitor serum electrolyte levels, and check periodically for hyperglycemia and glycosuria.
✦ Carefully monitor cardiac function if the patient is elderly or has coronary artery disease.
✦ Check level of consciousness and urine output.
✦ If the patient is pregnant, tell her to watch closely during the first trimester for signs of spontaneous abortion and to report such signs immediately.
✦ Encourage bed rest, and keep the patient's room cool, quiet, and dark.
✦ Provide sedatives as necessary.

✦ To promote weight gain, provide a balanced diet with six meals per day. If the patient has edema, suggest a low-sodium diet.

✦ If iodide is part of the treatment, mix it with milk, juice, or water to prevent GI distress, and administer it through a straw to prevent tooth discoloration.

✦ Watch for signs of thyroid storm (tachycardia, hyperkinesis, fever, vomiting, hypertension).

✦ Check intake and output to ensure adequate hydration and fluid balance.

✦ Closely monitor blood pressure, heart rate and rhythm, and temperature. If the patient has a high fever, reduce it with appropriate hypothermic measures. Maintain an I.V. line and give drugs as ordered.

✦ If the patient has exophthalmos or other ophthalmopathy, suggest sunglasses or eye patches to protect his eyes from light. Moisten the conjunctivae often with isotonic eye drops. Warn the patient with severe lid retraction to avoid sudden physical movements that might cause the lid to slip behind the eyeball.

✦ Avoid excessive palpation of the thyroid to avoid precipitating thyroid storm.

Thyroidectomy postoperative care

✦ Check often for respiratory distress, and keep a tracheotomy tray at the bedside.

✦ Watch for evidence of hemorrhage into the neck, such as a tight dressing with no blood on it. Change dressings and perform wound care as ordered; check the back of the dressing for drainage. Keep the patient in semi-Fowler's position, and support his head and neck with sandbags to ease tension on the incision.

✦ Check for dysphagia or hoarseness from possible laryngeal nerve injury.

✦ Watch for signs of hypocalcemia (tetany, numbness), a complication that results from accidental removal of the parathyroid glands during surgery.

✦ Stress the importance of regular medical follow-up after discharge because hypothyroidism may develop 2 to 4 weeks postoperatively.

Drug therapy and ^{131}I therapy

✦ After ^{131}I therapy, tell the patient not to expectorate or cough freely because his saliva will be radioactive for 24 hours. Stress the need for repeated measurement of serum T_4 levels. The patient shouldn't resume antithyroid therapy.

✦ If the patient is taking PTU and methimazole, monitor complete blood count periodically to detect leukopenia, thrombocytopenia, and agranulocytosis. Instruct him to take these medications with meals to minimize GI distress and to avoid over-the-counter cough preparations because many contain iodine.

✦ Tell him to report fever, enlarged cervical lymph nodes, sore throat, mouth sores, and other signs of blood dyscrasias and any rash or skin eruptions — signs of hypersensitivity.

✦ Watch the patient taking propranolol for signs of hypotension (dizziness, decreased urine output). Tell him to rise slowly after sitting or lying down to prevent orthostatic syncope.

✦ Instruct the patient receiving antithyroid drugs or ^{131}I therapy to report any symptoms of hypothyroidism.

HYPOTHYROIDISM IN ADULTS

Hypothyroidism results from hypothalamic, pituitary, or thyroid insufficiency or resistance to thyroid hormone. The disorder can progress to life-threatening

Key nursing actions
(continued)

✦ If iodide is part of the treatment, mix it with milk, juice, or water.

✦ Watch for signs of thyroid storm.

✦ Maintain an I.V. line and give drugs as ordered.

✦ Suggest sunglasses or eye patches to protect the patient's eyes from light.

✦ Avoid excessive palpation of the thyroid to avoid precipitating thyroid storm.

Thyroidectomy

✦ Check often for respiratory distress, and keep a tracheotomy tray at the bedside.

✦ Watch for evidence of hemorrhage into the neck.

✦ Change dressings and perform wound care as ordered; check the back of the dressing for drainage.

✦ Check for dysphagia or hoarseness from possible laryngeal nerve injury.

✦ Watch for signs of hypocalcemia (tetany, numbness)

Characteristics of hypothyroidism in adults

✦ Results from hypothalamic, pituitary, thyroid insufficiency, resistance to thyroid hormone

✦ Can progress to life-threatening myxedema coma

✦ More prevalent in women than in men

Alert!

+ Hypothyroidism occurs primarily after age 40.
+ After age 65, the prevalence increases to as much as 10% in females and 3% in males.

Causes

+ Inadequate production of thyroid hormone
+ Thyroidectomy
+ Radiation therapy
+ Inflammation
+ Chronic autoimmune thyroiditis
+ Amyloidosis
+ Sarcoidosis
+ Pituitary failure to produce TSH

How it happens

+ Autoantibodies destroy thyroid gland tissue
+ Heredity has a role
+ Antibodies reduce effect of thyroid hormone
+ Antibodies block TSH receptor, prevent production of TSH
+ Cytotoxic antithyroid antibodies may attack thyroid cells

Key signs and symptoms

+ Weakness
+ Fatigue
+ Forgetfulness
+ Sensitivity to cold
+ Unexplained weight gain
+ Constipation

---

myxedema coma. Hypothyroidism is more prevalent in women than in men; in the United States, the incidence is increasing significantly in people ages 40 to 50.

 CLINICAL ALERT Hypothyroidism occurs primarily after age 40. After age 65, the prevalence increases to as much as 10% in females and 3% in males.

CAUSES

Causes of hypothyroidism in adults include inadequate production of thyroid hormone, usually after thyroidectomy or radiation therapy (particularly with iodine 131 [^{131}I]), or due to inflammation, chronic autoimmune thyroiditis (Hashimoto's disease), or such conditions as amyloidosis and sarcoidosis (rare).

It may also result from pituitary failure to produce TSH, hypothalamic failure to produce thyrotropin-releasing hormone (TRH), inborn errors of thyroid hormone synthesis, iodine deficiency (usually dietary), or use of such antithyroid medications as propylthiouracil.

PATHOPHYSIOLOGY

Hypothyroidism may reflect a malfunction of the hypothalamus, pituitary, or thyroid gland, all of which are part of the same negative-feedback mechanism. However, disorders of the hypothalamus and pituitary rarely cause hypothyroidism. Primary hypothyroidism, a disorder of the gland itself, is most common.

Chronic autoimmune thyroiditis, also called chronic lymphocytic thyroiditis, occurs when autoantibodies destroy thyroid gland tissue. Chronic autoimmune thyroiditis associated with goiter is called Hashimoto's thyroiditis. The cause of this autoimmune process is unknown, although heredity has a role, and specific human leukocyte antigen subtypes are associated with greater risk.

Outside the thyroid, antibodies can reduce the effect of thyroid hormone in two ways. First, antibodies can block the thyroid-stimulating hormone (TSH) receptor and prevent the production of TSH. Second, cytotoxic antithyroid antibodies may attack thyroid cells.

Subacute thyroiditis, painless thyroiditis, and postpartum thyroiditis are self-limited conditions that usually follow an episode of hyperthyroidism. Untreated subclinical hypothyroidism in adults is likely to become overt at a rate of 5% to 20% per year.

SIGNS AND SYMPTOMS

Typically, the early clinical features of hypothyroidism are vague and include weakness, fatigue, forgetfulness, sensitivity to cold, unexplained weight gain, and constipation (see *Clinical findings in acquired hypothyroidism*).

As the disorder progresses, characteristic myxedematous signs and symptoms appear including decreasing mental stability; coarse, dry, flaky, inelastic skin; puffy face, hands, and feet; hoarseness; periorbital edema; upper eyelid droop; dry, sparse hair; and thick, brittle nails.

Cardiovascular involvement leads to decreased cardiac output, slow pulse rate, signs of poor peripheral circulation, and, occasionally, an enlarged heart.

Other common effects include anorexia, abdominal distention, menorrhagia, decreased libido, infertility, ataxia, and nystagmus. Reflexes show delayed relaxation time (especially in the Achilles tendon).

Progression to myxedema coma is usually gradual but may develop abruptly, with stress aggravating severe or prolonged hypothyroidism. Clinical effects include

---

Clinical findings in acquired hypothyroidism

Typical findings in acquired hypothyroidism are listed here:

HISTORY
+ Arthritis
+ Cold intolerance
+ Constipation
+ Decreased sociability
+ Drowsiness
+ Dry skin
+ Fatigue
+ Lethargy
+ Memory impairment
+ Menstrual disorders
+ Muscle cramps
+ Psychosis
+ Somnolence
+ Weakness

PHYSICAL EXAMINATION
+ Anemia
+ Bradycardia
+ Brittle hair
+ Cool skin
+ Delayed relaxation of reflexes
+ Dementia
+ Dry skin
+ Gravelly voice
+ Hypothermia
+ Large tongue
+ Loss of lateral third of eyebrow
+ Puffy face and hands
+ Slow speech
+ Weight changes

Adapted with permission from Martinez, M., et al. "Making Sense of Hypothyroidism: An Approach to Testing and Treatment," *Postgraduate Medicine* 93(6):143, May 1993.

---

progressive stupor, hypoventilation, hypoglycemia, hyponatremia, hypotension, and hypothermia.

COMPLICATIONS

Thyroid hormones affect almost every organ system in the body, so complications of hypothyroidism vary according to organs involved and the duration and severity of the condition.

Cardiovascular complications may include hypercholesterolemia with associated arteriosclerosis and ischemic heart disease. Poor peripheral circulation, heart enlargement, heart failure, and pleural and pericardial effusions may also occur.

GI complications include achlorhydria, pernicious anemia, and adynamic colon, resulting in megacolon and intestinal obstruction.

Anemia due to the generalized suppression of erythropoietin may result in bleeding tendencies and iron deficiency anemia. Other complications include conductive or sensorineural deafness, psychiatric disturbances, carpal tunnel syndrome, benign intracranial hypertension, and infertility.

DIAGNOSIS

Diagnosis of hypothyroidism is confirmed when radioimmunoassay shows low triiodothyronine (T_3) and thyroxine (T_4) levels. An increased TSH level is due to a thyroid disorder. A decreased TSH level is due to a hypothalamic or pituitary disorder.

A thyroid panel differentiates primary hypothyroidism (thyroid gland hypofunction), secondary hypothyroidism (pituitary hyposecretion of TSH), tertiary hypothyroidism (hypothalamic hyposecretion of TRH), and euthyroid sick syndrome (impaired peripheral conversion of thyroid hormone due to a suprathyroidal illness such as severe infection) (see *Thyroid test results in hypothyroidism,* page 518).

Key clinical findings in acquired hypothyroidism

History
+ Arthritis
+ Cold intolerance
+ Constipation
+ Drowsiness
+ Memory impairment
+ Weakness

Physical examination
+ Anemia
+ Bradycardia
+ Cool skin
+ Dementia
+ Loss of lateral third of eyebrow
+ Slow speech
+ Weight changes

Complications
+ Hypercholesterolemia
+ Cardiac complications
+ GI complications
+ Anemia
+ Conductive or sensorineural deafness
+ Psychiatric disturbances
+ Carpal tunnel syndrome
+ Benign intracranial hypertension
+ Infertility

Diagnosis
+ Low T_3 and T_4 levels
+ Thyroid panel differentiates primary, secondary, and tertiary hypothyroidism, euthyroid sick syndrome
+ Serum cholesterol, alkaline phosphatase, triglyceride levels elevated

Thyroid test results in hypothyroidism

DYSFUNCTION INVOLVES	THYROTROPIN-RELEASING HORMONE	THYROID-STIMULATING HORMONE	TH (T_3 AND T_4)
Hypothalamus	Low	Low	Low
Pituitary gland	High	Low	Low
Thyroid gland	High	High	Low
Peripheral conversion of thyroid hormone (TH)	High	Low or normal	T_3 and T_4 low, but reverse T_3 elevated

In addition, serum cholesterol, alkaline phosphatase, and triglyceride levels are elevated. Normocytic, normochromic anemia is present. In myxedema coma, laboratory tests also show low serum sodium levels, decreased pH, and increased partial pressure of carbon dioxide, indicating respiratory acidosis.

TREATMENT

In hypothyroidism, recommended treatment consists of gradual thyroid hormone replacement with synthetic T_4 and, occasionally, T_3. Surgical excision, chemotherapy, or radiation may be necessary for tumors.

 CLINICAL ALERT Elderly patients should be started on a very low dose of T_4 to avoid cardiac problems; TSH levels guide gradual increases in dosage.

NURSING CONSIDERATIONS

To manage the patient with hypothyroidism
✦ Provide a high-bulk, low-calorie diet and encourage activity to combat constipation and promote weight loss. Administer cathartics and stool softeners as needed.
✦ After thyroid replacement begins, watch for symptoms of hyperthyroidism, such as restlessness, sweating, and excessive weight loss.
✦ Tell the patient to report any signs of aggravated cardiovascular disease, such as chest pain and tachycardia.
✦ To prevent myxedema coma, tell the patient to continue his course of thyroid medication even if his symptoms subside.
✦ Warn the patient to report infection immediately and to make sure any physician who prescribes drugs for him knows about the underlying hypothyroidism.

Treatment of myxedema coma
✦ Check frequently for signs of decreasing cardiac output (such as decreased urine output).

Treatment
✦ Gradual thyroid hormone replacement with synthetic T_4, occasionally T_3
✦ Surgical excision
✦ Chemotherapy
✦ Radiation

Alert!
✦ Elderly patients should be started on a very low dose of T_4 to avoid cardiac problems.

Key nursing actions

Hypothyroidism
✦ Combat constipation and promote weight loss.
✦ After thyroid replacement begins, watch for symptoms of hyperthyroidism.
✦ Tell the patient to report any signs of aggravated cardiovascular disease.
✦ Tell the patient to continue his course of thyroid medication even if his symptoms subside.

◆ Monitor temperature until stable. Provide extra blankets and clothing and a warm room to compensate for hypothermia. Rapid rewarming may cause vasodilation and vascular collapse.

◆ Record intake and output and daily weight. As treatment begins, urine output should increase and body weight decrease; if not, report this immediately.

◆ Turn the edematous bedridden patient every 2 hours, and provide skin care, particularly around bony prominences, at least once per shift.

◆ Avoid sedation when possible or reduce dosage because hypothyroidism delays metabolism of many drugs.

◆ Maintain a patent I.V. line. Monitor serum electrolyte levels carefully when administering I.V. fluids.

◆ Monitor vital signs carefully when administering levothyroxine because rapid correction of hypothyroidism can cause adverse cardiac effects. Report chest pain or tachycardia immediately. Watch for hypertension and heart failure in the elderly patient.

◆ Check arterial blood gas values for hypercapnia, metabolic acidosis, and hypoxia to determine whether the patient who's severely myxedematous requires ventilatory assistance.

◆ Administer corticosteroids as ordered.

◆ Because myxedema coma may have been precipitated by an infection, check possible sources of the infection, such as blood and urine, and obtain sputum cultures.

HYPOTHYROIDISM IN CHILDREN

A deficiency of thyroid hormone secretion during fetal development and early infancy results in infantile cretinism (congenital hypothyroidism). Hypothyroidism in infants is seen as respiratory difficulties, cyanosis, persistent jaundice, lethargy, somnolence, large tongue, abdominal distention, poor feeding, and hoarse crying. Prompt treatment of hypothyroidism in infants prevents physical and mental retardation.

Older children who become hypothyroid have similar symptoms to those of adults, plus poor skeletal growth and late epiphyseal maturation and dental development. Sexual maturation may be accelerated in younger children and delayed in older children.

Cretinism is three times more common in girls than in boys. Early diagnosis and treatment allow the best prognosis; infants treated before age 3 months usually grow and develop normally. Athyroid children who remain untreated beyond age 3 months, and children with acquired hypothyroidism who remain untreated beyond age 2 years, have irreversible mental retardation; their skeletal abnormalities are reversible with treatment.

CAUSES

Hypothyroidism usually results from defective embryonic development that causes congenital absence or underdevelopment of the thyroid gland (cretinism in infants). The next most common cause is an inherited autosomal recessive defect in the synthesis of thyroxine. Less commonly, an iodine deficiency or antithyroid drugs taken during pregnancy produce cretinism in infants.

In children older than age 2, hypothyroidism usually results from chronic autoimmune thyroiditis.

Key nursing actions

Myxedema coma

◆ Check frequently for signs of decreasing cardiac output.
◆ Maintain patent I.V. line
◆ Monitor temperature until stable.
◆ Provide extra blankets and clothing and a warm room to compensate for hypothermia.
◆ Record intake and output.
◆ Avoid sedation or reduce dosage.

Characteristics of hypothyroidism in children

◆ Thyroid hormone secretion deficiency during fetal development or early infancy results in infantile cretinism
◆ Prompt treatment prevents physical and mental retardation
◆ Older children have similar symptoms to adults plus poor skeletal growth, late epiphyseal maturation and dental development
◆ Sexual maturation accelerated in young children, delayed in older
◆ Cretinism more common in girls

Causes

◆ Usually results from defective embryonic development
◆ Congenital absence or underdevelopment of thyroid gland
◆ Commonly inherited autosomal recessive defect in synthesis of thyroxine
◆ Less commonly: iodine deficiency or antithyroid drugs during pregnancy
◆ Usually results from chronic autoimmune thyroiditis in children older than age 2

How it happens

+ Related to decreased thyroid hormone production or secretion
+ Autoimmune process can cause loss of functional thyroid tissue
+ Defective thyroid synthesis may be related to congenital defects
+ Iodine deficiency or antithyroid drugs used during pregnancy can contribute
+ May also be related to decreased secretion or resistance to TSH

Key signs and symptoms

+ Infant with infantile cretinism will have normal weight and length at birth
+ Characteristic signs develop within 3 to 6 months
+ Onset of most symptoms may be delayed due to thyroid hormone in breast milk
+ Sleeps excessively, seldom cries, inactive

Complications

+ Skeletal malformations
+ Irreversible mental retardation for hypothyroid infants not treated by age 3 months; early treatment helps prevent retardation
+ Accelerated or delayed sexual maturation

Diagnosis

+ High TSH level associated with low T_3 and T_4 levels
+ Thyroid scan and ^{131}I uptake tests show decreased uptake
+ Gonadotropin levels increased, compatible with sexual precocity
+ Delayed skeletal development

PATHOPHYSIOLOGY

Hypothyroidism in infants and children is related to decreased thyroid hormone production or secretion. An autoimmune process can cause loss of functional thyroid tissue. Defective thyroid synthesis may be related to congenital defects, with thyroid dysgenesis (defective development) the most common. Iodine deficiency or antithyroid drugs used by the mother during pregnancy can also contribute. Hypothyroidism may also be related to decreased thyroid-stimulating hormone (TSH) secretion or resistance to TSH.

SIGNS AND SYMPTOMS

An infant with infantile cretinism will have normal weight and length at birth, with characteristic signs developing within 3 to 6 months. The onset of most symptoms may be delayed until weaning from breast-feeding due to small amounts of thyroid hormone in breast milk.

Typically, an infant with cretinism sleeps excessively, seldom cries (except for occasional hoarse crying), and is inactive. Because of this, parents may describe the infant as a "good baby—no trouble at all." Such behavior actually results from reduced metabolism and progressive mental impairment. The infant with cretinism also exhibits abnormal deep tendon reflexes, hypotonic abdominal muscles, protruding abdomen, and slow, awkward movements.

He has feeding difficulties, constipation, and jaundice because the immature liver can't conjugate bilirubin. His large, protruding tongue obstructs respiration, making loud and noisy breathing and forcing him to open his mouth. He may have dyspnea on exertion; anemia; abnormal facial features, such as a short forehead, puffy wide-set eyes (periorbital edema), wrinkled eyelids, a broad short and upturned nose; and a dull expression reflecting mental retardation.

In addition, the infant with cretinism has cold, mottled skin due to poor circulation; and dry, brittle, and dull hair. His teeth erupt late and decay early, and he has a body temperature that's below normal and a slow pulse rate.

Growth retardation becomes apparent in short stature due to delayed epiphyseal maturation, particularly in the legs; obesity; and a head appearing abnormally large due to stunted arms and legs. An older child may show delayed or accelerated sexual development. Mental retardation can be prevented by appropriate treatment if the child acquires hypothyroidism after age 2 years.

COMPLICATIONS

Complications include skeletal malformations and irreversible mental retardation for hypothyroid infants not treated by age 3 months. Early treatment helps prevent retardation. Older children may exhibit learning disabilities and accelerated or delayed sexual maturation.

DIAGNOSIS

TSH level is high and associated with low T_3 and T_4 levels pointing to cretinism. Because early detection and treatment can minimize the effects of cretinism, many states require measurement of infant thyroid hormone levels at birth.

Thyroid scan and ^{131}I uptake tests show decreased uptake and confirm the absence of thyroid tissue in athyroid children. Gonadotropin levels are increased and compatible with sexual precocity in older children.

An electrocardiogram shows bradycardia and flat or inverted T waves in untreated infants. In addition, hip, knee, and thigh X-rays reveal the absence of the femoral or tibial epiphyseal line and markedly delayed skeletal development relative to chronological age.

Low T_4 and normal TSH levels suggest hypothyroidism secondary to hypothalamic or pituitary disease (rare).

TREATMENT

Early detection is mandatory to prevent irreversible mental retardation and permit normal physical development. Treatment includes oral levothyroxine (Synthroid), beginning with moderate doses. Dosages gradually increase to levels sufficient for lifelong maintenance. A rapid increase in dosage may precipitate thyrotoxicity. Children require proportionately higher doses than adults because children metabolize thyroid hormone more quickly.

NURSING CONSIDERATIONS

Prevention, early detection, comprehensive parent teaching, and psychological support are essential. Know the early signs. Be especially wary if parents emphasize how good and how quiet their new baby is.

✦ During early management of infantile cretinism, monitor blood pressure and pulse rate; report hypertension and tachycardia immediately; however, remember that normal infant heart rate is approximately 120 beats/minute. If the infant's tongue is unusually large, position him on his side and observe him frequently to prevent airway obstruction. Check rectal temperature every 2 to 4 hours. Keep the infant warm and his skin moist.

✦ Inform parents that the child will require lifelong treatment with thyroid supplements. Teach them to recognize signs of overdose: rapid pulse rate, irritability, insomnia, fever, sweating, and weight loss. Stress the need to comply with the treatment regimen to prevent further mental impairment.

✦ Provide support to help parents deal with a child who may be mentally retarded. Help them adopt a positive but realistic attitude and focus on their child's strengths rather than his weaknesses. Encourage them to provide stimulating activities to help the child reach his maximal potential. Refer them to appropriate community resources for support.

✦ To prevent infantile cretinism, emphasize the importance of adequate nutrition during pregnancy, including iodine-rich foods and the use of iodized salt or, in case of sodium restriction, an iodine supplement.

Treatment
✦ Oral levothyroxine

Key nursing actions
✦ Note if parents emphasize how good and quiet their new baby is.
✦ Monitor blood pressure and pulse rate; report hypertension and tachycardia immediately.
✦ If the infant's tongue is unusually large, position him on his side and observe him frequently to prevent airway obstruction.
✦ Check rectal temperature every 2 to 4 hours.
✦ Keep the infant warm and his skin moist.
✦ Inform parents that the child will require lifelong treatment with thyroid supplements.
✦ Teach parents to recognize signs of overdose.

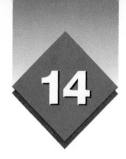

Renal system

Key facts about the renal system

- Kidneys produce and excrete urine to maintain homeostasis
- Ureters transport urine to bladder from kidneys
- Bladder: reservoir for urine until it leaves body through urethra

The components of the renal system are the kidneys, ureters, bladder, and urethra. The kidneys, located retroperitoneally in the lumbar area, produce and excrete urine to maintain homeostasis. They regulate the volume, electrolyte concentration, and acid-base balance of body fluids; detoxify the blood and eliminate wastes; regulate blood pressure; and support red blood cell (RBC) production (erythropoiesis). The ureters are tubes that extend from the kidneys to the bladder; their only function is to transport urine to the bladder. The bladder is a muscular bag that serves as a reservoir for urine until it leaves the body through the urethra.

PATHOPHYSIOLOGIC CHANGES

Pathophysiologic changes

- Filtration and reabsorption changes affect total filtration effort
- Capillary pressure and interstitial fluid colloid osmotic pressure affect filtration
- Interstitial fluid pressure and plasma colloid osmotic pressure affect filtration
- Altered renal perfusion; disease affecting vessels, glomeruli, tubules; obstruction to urine slow the GFR

Wastes are eliminated from the body by urine formation—glomerular filtration, tubular reabsorption, and tubular secretion—and excretion. Glomerular filtration is the process of filtering the blood as it flows through the kidneys. The glomerulus of the renal tubule filters plasma and then reabsorbs the filtrate. Glomerular function depends on the permeability of the capillary walls, vascular pressure, and filtration pressure. The normal glomerular filtration rate (GFR) is about 120 ml/minute. To prevent too much fluid from leaving the vascular system, tubular reabsorption opposes capillary filtration. Reabsorption takes place as capillary filtration progresses. When fluid filters through the capillaries, albumin, which doesn't pass through capillary walls, remains behind. As the albumin concentration inside the capillaries increases, the capillaries begin to draw water back in by osmosis. This osmotic force controls the quantities of water and diffusible solutes that enter and leave the capillaries.

Anything that affects filtration or reabsorption affects total filtration effort. Capillary pressure and interstitial fluid colloid osmotic pressure affect filtration. Interstitial fluid pressure and plasma colloid osmotic pressure affect reabsorption.

Altered renal perfusion; renal disease affecting the vessels, glomeruli, or tubules; or obstruction to urine flow can slow the GFR. The results are retention of nitrogenous wastes (azotemia), such as blood urea nitrogen and creatinine, which can lead to acute renal failure.

CAPILLARY PRESSURE

The renal arteries branch into five segmental arteries, which supply different areas of the kidneys. The segmental arteries then branch into several divisions from which the afferent arterioles and vasa recta arise. Renal veins follow a similar branching pattern — characterized by stellate vessels and segmental branches — and empty into the inferior vena cava. The tubular system receives its blood supply from a peritubular capillary network. The ureteral veins follow the arteries and drain into the renal vein. The bladder receives blood through vesical arteries. Vesical veins unite to form the pudendal plexus, which empties into the iliac veins. A rich lymphatic system drains the renal cortex, kidneys, ureters, and bladder.

Capillary pressure reflects mean arterial pressure (MAP). Increased MAP increases capillary pressure, which in turn increases the GFR. When MAP decreases, so do capillary pressure and GFR. Autoregulation of afferent and efferent arterioles minimizes and controls changes in capillary pressure, unless MAP exceeds 180 mm Hg or is less than 80 mm Hg.

Sympathetic branches from the celiac plexus, upper lumbar splanchnic and thoracic nerves; the intermesenteric and superior hypogastric plexuses surround and innervate the kidneys. Similar numbers of sympathetic and parasympathetic nerves from the renal plexus, superior hypogastric plexus, and intermesenteric plexus innervate the ureters. Nerves that arise from the inferior hypogastric plexus innervate the bladder. The parasympathetic nerve supply to the bladder controls urination.

The effects of changes

Increased sympathetic activity and angiotensin II constrict afferent and efferent arterioles, decreasing the capillary pressure. Because these changes affect both the afferent and efferent arterioles, they have no net effect on GFR.

Inadequate renal perfusion accounts for 40% to 80% of acute renal failure. Volume loss (as with GI hemorrhage, burns, diarrhea, and diuretic use), volume sequestration (as in pancreatitis, peritonitis, and rhabdomyolysis), or decreased effective circulating volume (as in cardiogenic shock and sepsis) may reduce circulating blood volume. Decreased cardiac output due to peripheral vasodilatation (by sepsis or drugs) or profound renal vasoconstriction (as in severe heart failure, hepatorenal syndrome, or with such drugs as nonsteroidal anti-inflammatories [NSAIDs]) also diminishes renal perfusion.

Hypovolemia causes a decrease in MAP that triggers a series of neural and humoral responses: activation of the sympathetic nervous system and renin-angiotensin-aldosterone system, and release of arginine vasopressin. Prostaglandin-mediated relaxation of afferent arterioles and angiotensin II–mediated constriction of efferent arterioles maintain GFR. GFR decreases steeply if MAP decreases to less than 80 mm Hg. Drugs that block prostaglandin production (such as NSAIDs) can cause severe vasoconstriction and acute renal failure during hypotension.

Prolonged renal hypoperfusion causes acute tubular necrosis. Processes involving large renal vessels, microvasculature, glomeruli, or tubular interstitium cause intrinsic renal disease. Emboli or thrombi, aortic dissection, or vasculitis can occlude renal arteries. Cholesterol-rich atheroemboli can occur spontaneously or follow aortic instrumentation. If they lodge in medium and small renal arteries, they trigger an eosinophil-rich inflammatory reaction.

After age 40, a person's renal function begins to diminish. If he lives to age 90, it may have decreased by as much as 50%. This change is reflected in a decreased GFR

Capillary pressure
+ Reflects MAP
+ Increased MAP increases capillary pressure and GFR
+ Decreased MAP decreases capillary pressure and GFR
+ Increased sympathetic activity and angiotensin II decrease capillary pressure but not GFR
+ Inadequate renal perfusion accounts for 40% to 80% of acute renal failure
+ Hypovolemia causes a decrease in MAP
+ Prolonged renal hypoperfusion causes acute tubular necrosis

and is caused by age-related changes in the renal vasculature that disturb glomerular hemodynamics as well as by reduced cardiac output and atherosclerotic changes that reduce renal blood flow by more than 50%.

INTERSTITIAL FLUID COLLOID OSMOTIC PRESSURE

Few plasma proteins and RBCs are filtered out of the glomeruli, so interstitial fluid colloid osmotic pressure (the force of albumin in the interstitial fluid) remains low. Large quantities of plasma protein flow through glomerular capillaries. Size and surface charge keep albumin, globulin, and other large proteins from crossing the glomerular wall. Smaller proteins leave the glomerulus but are absorbed by the proximal tubule.

Injury to the glomeruli or peritubular capillaries can increase interstitial fluid colloid osmotic pressure, drawing fluid out of the glomerulus and the peritubular capillaries. Swelling and edema occur in Bowman's space and the interstitial space surrounding the tubule. Increased interstitial fluid pressure opposes glomerular filtration, causes collapse of the surrounding nephrons and peritubular capillaries, and leads to hypoxia and renal cell injury or death. When cells die, intracellular enzymes are released that stimulate immune and inflammatory reactions. This further contributes to swelling and edema.

The resulting increase in interstitial fluid pressure can interfere with glomerular filtration and tubular reabsorption. Loss of glomerular filtration renders the kidney incapable of regulating blood volume and electrolyte composition. Diseases that damage the tubules alter their permeability, causing tubular proteinuria because small proteins can move from capillaries into tubules.

Normal glomerular cells, which are endothelial in nature, form a barrier that prevents cells and other particles from crossing the membrane. The basement membrane typically traps larger proteins. The channels of the basement membrane are coated with glycoproteins that are rich in glutamate, aspartate, and sialic acid. This produces a negative charge barrier that impedes the passage of such anionic molecules as albumin. (See *The glomerulus.*)

Glomerular disease disrupts the basement membrane, allowing large proteins to leak out. Damage to epithelial cells permits albumin leakage. Hypoalbuminemia, as in nephrotic syndrome, is the result of excessive loss of albumin in the urine, increased renal catabolism, and inadequate hepatic synthesis of albumin. Plasma oncotic pressure decreases and edema results as fluid moves from capillaries into the interstitium. Consequent activation of the renin-angiotensin system, arginine-vasopressin, and sympathetic nervous system increases renal salt and water reabsorption, which further contributes to edema. The severity of edema is directly related to the degree of hypoalbuminemia and is exacerbated by heart disease or peripheral vascular disease.

PLASMA COLLOID PRESSURE

Protein concentration of the plasma determines the plasma colloid pressure (the pulling force of albumin in the intravascular fluid), the major force influencing reabsorption of fluid into the capillaries. Plasma protein levels can decrease as a result of liver disease, protein loss in the urine, and protein malnutrition.

As oncotic pressure decreases, less fluid moves back into the capillaries and fluid begins to accumulate in the tubular and peritubular areas. Swelling around the tubule causes collapse of the tubule and peritubular capillaries, hypoxia, and death of the nephrons.

Interstitial fluid colloid osmotic pressure

+ Normally remains low
+ Injury to the glomeruli or peritubular capillaries can increase it
+ Swelling, edema occur in Bowman's space, interstitial space surrounding tubule
+ Opposes glomerular filtration, causes collapse of surrounding nephrons, peritubular capillaries
+ Leads to hypoxia, renal cell injury or death
+ Intracellular enzymes released to stimulate immune and inflammatory reactions
+ Further contributes to swelling, edema
+ Loss of glomerular filtration hinders kidney function

Plasma colloid pressure

+ Protein concentration of plasma determines plasma colloid
+ Major force influencing fluid reabsorption into capillaries
+ Plasma protein levels decrease as result of liver disease, protein loss in urine, protein malnutrition

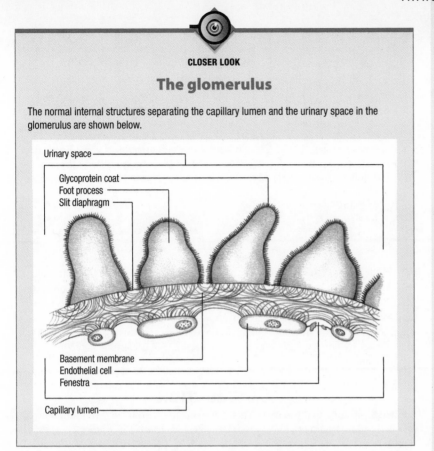

The glomerulus

The normal internal structures separating the capillary lumen and the urinary space in the glomerulus are shown below.

Urinary space

Glycoprotein coat
Foot process
Slit diaphragm

Basement membrane
Endothelial cell
Fenestra

Capillary lumen

Diminished plasma oncotic pressure and urine protein loss stimulate hepatic lipoprotein synthesis, and the resulting hyperlipidemia manifests as lipid bodies (fatty casts, oval fat bodies) in the urine. As other proteins are lost in the urine, including thyroxine-binding globulin, cholecalciferol-binding protein, transferrin, and metal-binding proteins, metabolic disturbances result. Urine losses of antithrombin III, decreased serum levels of proteins S and C, hyperfibrinogenemia, and enhanced platelet aggregation lead to a hypercoagulable state, as in nephrotic syndrome. Some patients also develop severe immunoglobulin G deficiency, which increases susceptibility to infection.

STRUCTURAL VARIATIONS

Variations in normal anatomic structure of the urinary tract occur in 10% to 15% of the total population and range from minor and easily correctable to lethal. Ectopic kidneys, which result if the embryonic kidneys don't ascend from the pelvis to the abdomen, function normally. If the embryonic kidneys fuse as they ascend, a single U-shaped kidney results, causing no symptoms in about one-third of affected people. The most common problems associated with horseshoe kidneys include hydronephrosis, infection, and calculus formation.

 CLINICAL ALERT Structural abnormalities of the renal system account for about 45% of renal failure in children.

Structural variations

✦ Variations in normal anatomic structure of urinary tract occur in 10% to 15% of total population
✦ Range from minor to lethal
✦ Ectopic kidneys function normally
✦ Embryonic kidneys fuse into U-shaped kidney as they ascend
✦ Urinary tract malformations commonly associated with nonrenal anomalies

Alert!

✦ Structural abnormalities of the renal system account for about 45% of renal failure in children.

Congenital conditions affecting kidney function

- ✦ Renal hypoplasia
- ✦ Renal dysplasia
- ✦ Renal malrotation
- ✦ Ectopic kidney
- ✦ Horseshoe kidney
- ✦ Obstructive uropathy
- ✦ Ureterocele

Congenital nephropathies and uropathies

The following congenital conditions can affect kidney function:
- ✦ Renal hypoplasia — the kidney is small because of a reduction in the number of normally developed nephrons, and it may be unilateral or bilateral.
- ✦ Renal dysplasia — the kidney is abnormally shaped, and the involved areas are nonfunctional.
- ✦ Renal malrotation — the kidney is positioned abnormally.
- ✦ Ectopic kidney — the kidney is located in the pelvic or thoracic area, causing reflux from the bladder into the ureters.
- ✦ Horseshoe kidney — the lower poles of the kidneys are fused by an isthmus.
- ✦ Obstructive uropathy — a pathologic condition (abnormal vasculature, adhesions, kinks, or masses) that blocks the flow of urine, usually causing hydronephrosis.
- ✦ Ureterocele — a prolapse of the end portion of the ureter into the bladder, leading to an obstruction in urine flow.

Urinary tract malformations are commonly associated with certain nonrenal anomalies. These characteristics include low-set and malformed ears, chromosomal disorders (especially trisomies 13 and 18), absent abdominal muscles, spinal cord and lower extremity anomalies, imperforate anus or genital deviation, Wilms' tumor, congenital ascites, cystic disease of the liver, and positive family history of renal disease (hereditary nephritis or cystic disease). (See *Congenital nephropathies and uropathies*.)

OBSTRUCTION

Obstruction along the urinary tract causes urine to accumulate behind the source of obstruction, leading to infection or damage. (See *Sources of urinary tract obstruction*.)

Obstructions may be congenital or acquired. Causes include tumors, calculi (stones), trauma, strictures (secondary to surgical intervention and scarring), edema, pregnancy, benign prostatic hyperplasia or carcinoma, inflammation of the GI tract, and loss of ureteral peristaltic activity or bladder muscle function.

Consequences of obstruction depend on the location and whether it's unilateral or bilateral, partial or complete, and acute or chronic, as well as the cause. For example, obstruction of a ureter causes hydroureter, or an accumulation of urine within the ureter, which increases retrograde pressure to the renal pelvis and calyces. As urine accumulates in the renal collection system, hydronephrosis results. If the obstruction is complete and acute, increasing pressure transmitted to the proximal tubule inhibits glomerular filtration. If GFR declines to zero, the result is renal failure.

Chronic partial obstruction compresses structures as urine accumulates, resulting in papillary and medullary infarct. The kidneys initially increase in size, but progressive atrophy follows, with eventual loss of renal mass. The underlying tubular damage decreases the kidney's ability to conserve sodium and water and excrete hydrogen ions and potassium; sodium and bicarbonate are wasted. Urine volume is excessive, even though GFR has declined. The result is an increased risk of dehydration and metabolic acidosis.

Tubular obstruction caused by renal calculi or scarring from repeated infection can increase interstitial fluid pressure. As fluid accumulates in the nephron, it backs up into Bowman's capsule and space. If the obstruction is unrelieved, nephrons and

Obstruction

- ✦ Obstruction along urinary tract causes urine to accumulate behind obstruction
- ✦ May be congenital or acquired
- ✦ Can result in infection or renal failure

CLOSER LOOK

Sources of urinary tract obstruction

Shown below are the major sites of urinary tract obstruction.

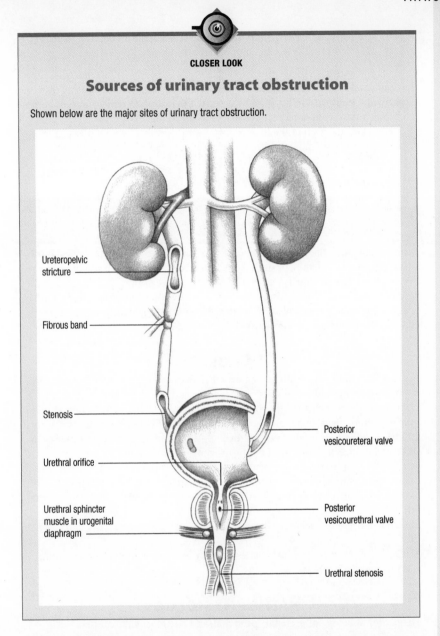

Ureteropelvic stricture

Fibrous band

Stenosis

Urethral orifice

Urethral sphincter muscle in urogenital diaphragm

Posterior vesicoureteral valve

Posterior vesicourethral valve

Urethral stenosis

capillaries collapse, and renal damage is irreversible. The papillae, which are the final site of urine concentration, are particularly affected.

Relief of the obstruction is usually followed by copious diuresis of sodium and water retained during the period of obstruction, and a return to normal GFR. Excessive loss of sodium and water (more than 10 L/day) is uncommon. If GFR doesn't recover quickly, diuresis may not be significant after relief of the obstruction.

Unresolved obstruction can result in infection or even renal failure. Obstructions below the bladder cause urine to accumulate, forming a medium for bacterial growth.

Alert!

+ Urinary tract infections are most common in girls ages 7 to 11.
+ This is a result of bacteria ascending the urethra.

Characteristics of acute renal failure

+ Life-threatening disorder
+ Sudden interruption of renal function
+ Caused by obstruction, poor circulation, underlying kidney disease
+ Usually passes through three distinct phases: oliguric, diuretic, recovery
+ 5% of hospitalized patients develop acute renal failure
+ Usually reversible with treatment
+ May progress to end-stage renal disease, prerenal azotemia, death
+ Prerenal, intrarenal, postrenal

Causes

+ Cardiac problems
+ Burns
+ Dehydration
+ Hemorrhage
+ Trauma
+ Antihypertensive drugs
+ Sepsis
+ Arterial embolism, thrombosis
+ Tumor

How it happens

Prerenal failure

+ Condition diminishing blood flow to kidneys leads to hypoperfusion

CLINICAL ALERT Urinary tract infections are most common in girls ages 7 to 11. This is a result of bacteria ascending the urethra.

Cystitis is an infection of the bladder that results in mucosal inflammation and congestion. The detrusor muscle becomes hyperactive, decreasing bladder capacity and leading to reflux into the ureters. This transient reflux can cause acute or chronic pyelonephritis if bacteria ascend to the kidney.

Bilateral obstruction of the ureters not relieved within 1 week of onset causes acute or chronic renal failure. Chronic renal failure progresses over weeks to months without symptoms until 90% of renal function is lost.

▼ **LIFE-THREATENING DISORDER**

ACUTE RENAL FAILURE

Acute renal failure, the sudden interruption of renal function, can be caused by obstruction, poor circulation, or underlying kidney disease. Whether prerenal, intrarenal, or postrenal, it usually passes through three distinct phases: oliguric, diuretic, and recovery. About 5% of hospitalized patients develop acute renal failure. The condition is usually reversible with treatment, but if not treated, it may progress to end-stage renal disease, prerenal azotemia, and death.

CAUSES

Acute renal failure may be prerenal, intrarenal, or postrenal. Causes of prerenal failure include arrhythmias that cause reduced cardiac output, cardiac tamponade, cardiogenic shock, heart failure, myocardial infarction, burns, dehydration, diuretic overuse, hemorrhage, hypovolemic shock, trauma, antihypertensive drugs, sepsis, arterial embolism, arterial or venous thrombosis, tumor, disseminated intravascular coagulation, eclampsia, malignant hypertension, and vasculitis.

Causes of intrarenal failure include poorly treated prerenal failure, nephrotoxins, obstetric complications, crush injuries, myopathy, transfusion reaction, acute glomerulonephritis, acute interstitial nephritis, acute pyelonephritis, bilateral renal vein thrombosis, malignant nephrosclerosis, papillary necrosis, polyarteritis nodosa, renal myeloma, sickle cell disease, systemic lupus erythematosus, and vasculitis.

Causes of postrenal failure include bladder obstruction, ureteral obstruction, and urethral obstruction.

PATHOPHYSIOLOGY

The pathophysiology of prerenal, intrarenal, and postrenal failure differs.

Prerenal failure

Prerenal failure ensues when a condition that diminishes blood flow to the kidneys leads to hypoperfusion. Examples include hypovolemia, hypotension, vasoconstriction, or inadequate cardiac output. Azotemia (excess nitrogenous waste products in the blood) develops in 40% to 80% of acute renal failure cases.

When renal blood flow is interrupted, so is oxygen delivery. The ensuing hypoxemia and ischemia can rapidly and irreversibly damage the kidney. The tubules are most susceptible to hypoxemia's effects.

Azotemia is a consequence of renal hypoperfusion. The impaired blood flow results in decreased glomerular filtration rate (GFR) and increased tubular reabsorption of sodium and water. A decrease in GFR causes electrolyte imbalance and metabolic acidosis. Usually, restoring renal blood flow and glomerular filtration reverses azotemia.

Intrarenal failure

Intrarenal failure, also called intrinsic or parenchymal renal failure, results from damage to the filtering structures of the kidneys. Causes of intrarenal failure are classified as nephrotoxic, inflammatory, or ischemic. When the damage is caused by nephrotoxicity or inflammation, the delicate layer under the epithelium (the basement membrane) becomes irreparably damaged, typically leading to chronic renal failure. Severe or prolonged lack of blood flow caused by ischemia may lead to renal damage (ischemic parenchymal injury) and excess nitrogen in the blood (intrinsic renal azotemia).

Acute tubular necrosis, the precursor to intrarenal failure, can result from ischemic damage to renal parenchyma during unrecognized or poorly treated prerenal failure, or from obstetric complications, such as eclampsia, postpartum renal failure, septic abortion, or uterine hemorrhage.

The fluid loss causes hypotension, which leads to ischemia. The ischemic tissue generates toxic oxygen-free radicals, which cause swelling, injury, and necrosis.

Another cause of acute failure is the use of nephrotoxins, including analgesics, anesthetics, heavy metals, radiographic contrast media, organic solvents, and antimicrobials, particularly aminoglycoside antibiotics. These drugs accumulate in the renal cortex, causing renal failure that manifests well after treatment or other toxin exposure. The necrosis caused by nephrotoxins tends to be uniform and limited to the proximal tubules, whereas ischemia necrosis tends to be patchy and distributed along various parts of the nephron.

Postrenal failure

Bilateral obstruction of urine outflow leads to postrenal failure. The cause may be in the bladder, ureters, or urethra. Bladder obstruction can result from anticholinergic drugs, autonomic nerve dysfunction, infection, and tumors. Ureteral obstructions, which restrict urine flow from kidneys to bladder, can result from blood clots, calculi, edema or inflammation, necrotic renal papillae, retroperitoneal fibrosis or hemorrhage, surgery (accidental ligation and strictures), and tumor or uric acid crystals. Urethral obstruction can be the result of prostatic hyperplasia, tumor, or strictures.

The three types of acute renal failure (prerenal, intrarenal, or postrenal) usually pass through three distinct phases: oliguric, diuretic, and recovery.

Oliguric phase

Oliguria may be the result of one or several factors. Necrosis of the tubules can cause sloughing of cells, cast formations, and ischemic edema. The resulting tubular obstruction causes a retrograde increase in pressure and a decrease in GFR. Renal failure can occur within 24 hours from this effect. Glomerular filtration may remain normal in some cases of renal failure, but tubular reabsorption of filtrate may be accelerated. In this instance, ischemia may increase tubular permeability and cause backleak. Another concept is that intrarenal release of angiotensin II or redistribution of blood flow from the cortex to the medulla may constrict the afferent arterioles, increasing glomerular permeability and decreasing GFR.

Urine output may remain at less than 30 ml/hour or 400 ml/day for a few days to weeks. Before damage occurs, the kidneys respond to decreased blood flow by conserving sodium and water.

How it happens

Intrarenal failure
+ Damage to filtering structures of kidneys
+ Nephrotoxic, inflammatory, ischemic

Postrenal failure
+ Bilateral obstruction of urine outflow leads to postrenal failure

Oliguric phase
+ May be the result of one or several factors
+ Necrosis of tubules causes sloughing of cells, cast formations, ischemic edema
+ Resulting tubular obstruction causes retrograde increase in pressure, decrease in GFR
+ Renal failure can occur within 24 hours
+ Damage impairs kidneys ability to conserve sodium
+ Fluid volume excess, azotemia, and electrolyte imbalance occur

How it happens

Diuretic phase

+ Marked by increased urine secretion of more than 400 ml/24 hours
+ GFR may be normal or increased, tubular support mechanisms abnormal
+ High BUN levels produce osmotic diuresis, deficits of potassium and sodium
+ May last days or weeks

Recovery phase

+ Gradual return to normal or near-normal renal function over 3 to 12 months

Alert!

+ Even with treatment, the elderly patient is particularly susceptible to volume overload, precipitating acute pulmonary edema, hypertensive crisis, hyperkalemia, and infection.

Key signs and symptoms

+ Oliguria
+ Azotemia
+ Anuria (rare)
+ Electrolyte imbalance
+ Metabolic acidosis
+ Anorexia, nausea, vomiting, diarrhea or constipation
+ Stomatitis
+ Bleeding
+ Hematemesis

Damage impairs the kidney's ability to conserve sodium. Fluid (water) volume excess, azotemia (elevated serum levels of urea, creatinine, and uric acid), and electrolyte imbalance occur. Ischemic or toxic injury leads to the release of mediators and intrarenal vasoconstriction. Medullary hypoxia results in the swelling of tubular and endothelial cells, adherence of neutrophils to capillaries and venules, and inappropriate platelet activation. Increasing ischemia and vasoconstriction further limit perfusion.

Injured cells lose polarity, and the ensuing disruption of tight junctions between the cells promotes backleak of filtrate. Ischemia impairs the function of energy-dependent membrane pumps, and calcium accumulates in the cells. This excess calcium further stimulates vasoconstriction and activates proteases and other enzymes. Untreated prerenal oliguria may lead to acute tubular necrosis.

Diuretic phase

As the kidneys become unable to conserve sodium and water, the diuretic phase, marked by increased urine secretion of more than 400 ml/24 hours, ensues. GFR may be normal or increased, but tubular support mechanisms are abnormal. Excretion of dilute urine causes dehydration and electrolyte imbalances. High blood urea nitrogen (BUN) levels produce osmotic diuresis and consequent deficits of potassium, sodium, and water. The diuretic phase may last days or weeks.

Recovery phase

If the cause of the diuresis is corrected, azotemia gradually disappears and recovery occurs. The recovery phase is a gradual return to normal or near-normal renal function over 3 to 12 months.

 CLINICAL ALERT **Even with treatment, the elderly patient is particularly susceptible to volume overload, precipitating acute pulmonary edema, hypertensive crisis, hyperkalemia, and infection.**

SIGNS AND SYMPTOMS

Acute renal failure is a critical illness, and its early signs are oliguria, azotemia and, rarely, anuria. Electrolyte imbalance, metabolic acidosis, and other severe effects follow, as the patient becomes increasingly uremic and renal dysfunction disrupts other body systems.

Signs and symptoms of acute renal failure involving the GI system include anorexia, nausea, vomiting, diarrhea or constipation, stomatitis, bleeding, hematemesis, dry mucous membranes, and uremic breath. Those related to the central nervous system include headache, drowsiness, irritability, confusion, peripheral neuropathy, seizures, and coma. Cutaneous signs and symptoms are dryness, pruritus, pallor, purpura and, rarely, uremic frost.

Early in the disease, hypotension may occur. Later, other cardiovascular problems surface; the signs and symptoms include hypertension, arrhythmias, fluid overload, heart failure, systemic edema, anemia, and altered clotting mechanisms. In the late stages, the patient may also experience pulmonary edema and Kussmaul's respirations.

COMPLICATIONS

Renal failure affects many body processes. One common complication is fever and chills, which may indicate infection; another is metabolic acidosis, which is due to decreased excretion of hydrogen ions.

Numerous other complications are caused by changes in the blood: Anemia is due to decreased erythropoietin levels, glomerular filtration of erythrocytes, or bleeding associated with platelet dysfunction, and the resulting tissue hypoxia can increase ventilation and the work of breathing. Decreased white blood cell–mediated immunity may lead to sepsis. Abnormalities in quantities or function of anticoagulant proteins, coagulation factor, platelet, or endothelial mediators may cause a hypercoagulable state that may end in bleeding or clotting difficulties. Eventually, heart failure may result from fluid overload and anemia, which cause additional workload to the heart.

An altered mental status and altered peripheral sensation are due to effects on the highly sensitive cells of nerves secondary to retained toxins, hypoxia, electrolyte imbalance, and acidosis.

DIAGNOSIS

In acute renal failure, blood studies show elevated BUN, serum creatinine, and potassium levels; decreased bicarbonate level, hematocrit, and hemoglobin levels; and low blood pH.

Urine studies show casts, cellular debris, and decreased specific gravity. In glomerular diseases, urine studies reveal proteinuria and urine osmolality close to serum osmolality. If oliguria results from decreased perfusion, the urine sodium level is less than 20 mEq/L; it's greater than 40 mEq/L if the cause is intrarenal. A creatinine clearance test measures GFR and reflects the number of remaining functioning nephrons.

Electrocardiogram (ECG) shows tall, peaked T waves; widened QRS complex; and disappearing P waves if hyperkalemia is present.

The diagnosis of acute renal failure is also supported by ultrasonography, plain films of the abdomen, kidney-ureter-bladder radiography, excretory urography, renal scan, retrograde pyelography, computed tomographic scans, and nephrotomography.

TREATMENT

A high-calorie diet that's low in protein, sodium, and potassium helps meet the metabolic needs of a patient in renal failure.

Other treatments include I.V. therapy to maintain and correct fluid. The patient's electrolyte balance and electrolytes are carefully monitored, and fluid restriction is used to minimize edema. Diuretic therapy helps treat the oliguric phase of acute renal failure, and sodium polystyrene sulfonate (Kayexalate) by mouth or enema is administered to reverse hyperkalemia with mild hyperkalemic symptoms (malaise, loss of appetite, muscle weakness), while hypertonic glucose, insulin, and sodium bicarbonate I.V. are administered for more severe hyperkalemic symptoms (numbness and tingling and ECG changes).

Hemodialysis or peritoneal dialysis is performed to correct electrolyte and fluid imbalances.

NURSING CONSIDERATIONS

Patient care includes careful monitoring and dietary education.
+ Measure and record intake and output, including body fluids, such as wound drainage, nasogastric output, and diarrhea. Weigh the patient daily.
+ Assess hemoglobin levels and hematocrit and replace blood components, as ordered. Don't use whole blood if the patient is prone to heart failure and can't toler-

Complications
+ Fever and chills
+ Metabolic acidosis
+ Anemia
+ Sepsis
+ Bleeding or clotting difficulties
+ Heart failure
+ Altered mental status
+ Altered peripheral sensation

Diagnosis
+ Elevated BUN, serum creatinine, potassium levels
+ Decreased bicarbonate, hematocrit, and hemoglobin levels
+ Low blood pH
+ Casts, cellular debris, decreased specific gravity in urine
+ Proteinuria and urine osmolality close to serum osmolality
+ Urine sodium level < 20 mEq/L; > 40 mEq/L if cause is intrarenal

Treatment
+ High-calorie diet low in protein, sodium, potassium
+ I.V. therapy
+ Fluid restriction
+ Diuretic
+ Kayexalate by mouth or enema
+ Hypertonic glucose, insulin, sodium bicarbonate I.V.
+ Hemodialysis or peritoneal dialysis

ate extra fluid volume. Packed red cells deliver the necessary blood components without added volume.

✦ Monitor vital signs. Watch for and report signs of pericarditis (pleuritic chest pain, tachycardia, pericardial friction rub), inadequate renal perfusion (hypotension), and acidosis.

✦ Maintain proper electrolyte balance. Strictly monitor potassium levels. Watch for symptoms of hyperkalemia (malaise, anorexia, paresthesia, muscle weakness) and ECG changes (tall, peaked T waves; widening QRS segment; disappearing P waves); report them immediately. Avoid administering medications containing potassium.

✦ Assess the patient frequently, especially during emergency treatment to lower potassium levels. If the patient receives hypertonic glucose and insulin infusions, monitor potassium and glucose levels. If you give sodium polystyrene sulfonate rectally, make sure the patient doesn't retain it and become constipated, to prevent bowel perforation.

✦ Maintain nutritional status. Provide a high-calorie, low-protein, low-sodium, and low-potassium diet, with vitamin supplements. Give the anorexic patient small, frequent meals.

✦ Use sterile technique because the patient with acute renal failure is highly susceptible to infection. Don't allow personnel with upper respiratory tract infections to care for the patient.

✦ Prevent complications of immobility by encouraging coughing and deep breathing and by performing passive range-of-motion exercises. Help the patient walk as soon as possible. Add lubricating lotion to bath water to combat skin dryness.

Patient care and precautions

✦ Provide good mouth care frequently because mucous membranes are dry. If stomatitis occurs, an antibiotic solution may be ordered. Have the patient swish the solution around in his mouth before swallowing.

✦ Monitor for GI bleeding by guaiac-testing stools for blood. Administer medications carefully, especially antacids and stool softeners. Use aluminum hydroxide–based antacids; magnesium-based antacids can cause serum magnesium levels to rise to critical levels.

✦ Use appropriate safety measures, such as side rails and restraints, because the patient with central nervous system involvement may be dizzy or confused.

✦ Provide emotional support to the patient and his family. Clearly explain procedures.

✦ During peritoneal dialysis, position the patient carefully. Elevate the head of the bed to reduce pressure on the diaphragm and aid respiration. Be alert for signs of infection (cloudy drainage, elevated temperature) and, rarely, bleeding. If pain occurs, reduce the amount of dialysate. Monitor the diabetic patient's blood glucose periodically and administer insulin, as ordered. Watch for complications, such as peritonitis, atelectasis, hypokalemia, pneumonia, and shock.

✦ If the patient requires hemodialysis, check the blood access site (arteriovenous fistula, subclavian or femoral catheter) every 2 hours for patency and signs of clotting. Don't use the arm with the shunt or fistula for taking blood pressures or drawing blood. Weigh the patient before beginning dialysis. During dialysis, monitor vital signs, clotting times, blood flow, the function of the vascular access site, and arterial and venous pressures. Watch for complications, such as septicemia, embolism, hepatitis, and rapid fluid and electrolyte loss. After dialysis, monitor vital signs and the vascular access site, weigh the patient, and watch for signs of fluid and electrolyte imbalances.

✦ Use standard precautions when handling blood and body fluids.

Key nursing actions

✦ Measure and record intake and output, including body fluids.

✦ Weigh the patient daily.

✦ Maintain proper electrolyte balance.

✦ Use sterile technique because the patient with acute renal failure is highly susceptible to infection.

✦ Provide good mouth care frequently because mucous membranes are dry.

✦ Monitor for GI bleeding by guaiac-testing stools for blood.

✦ If the patient requires hemodialysis, check the blood access site every 2 hours for patency and signs of clotting.

✦ After dialysis, monitor vital signs and the vascular access site, weigh the patient, and watch for signs of fluid and electrolyte imbalances.

✦ Use standard precautions when handling blood and body fluids.

CHRONIC RENAL FAILURE

Chronic renal failure is usually the end result of gradual tissue destruction and loss of renal function. It can also result from a rapidly progressing disease of sudden onset that destroys the nephrons and causes irreversible kidney damage.

Few symptoms develop until less than 25% of glomerular filtration remains. The normal parenchyma then deteriorates rapidly, and symptoms worsen as renal function decreases. This syndrome is fatal without treatment, but maintenance on dialysis or a kidney transplant can sustain life.

CAUSES

Causes of chronic renal failure include chronic glomerular disease (glomerulonephritis), chronic infection (such as chronic pyelonephritis and tuberculosis), congenital anomalies (polycystic kidney disease), vascular disease (hypertension, nephrosclerosis), obstruction (renal calculi), collagen disease (lupus erythematosus), nephrotoxic agents (long-term aminoglycoside therapy), and endocrine disease (diabetic neuropathy).

PATHOPHYSIOLOGY

Chronic renal failure often progresses through four stages. Reduced renal reserve shows a glomerular filtration rate (GFR) of 35% to 50% of normal; renal insufficiency, a GFR of 20% to 35% of normal; renal failure, a GFR of 20% to 25% of normal; and end-stage renal disease, a GFR less than 20% of normal.

Nephron damage is progressive; damaged nephrons can't function and don't recover. The kidneys can maintain relatively normal function until about 75% of the nephrons are nonfunctional. Surviving nephrons hypertrophy and increase their rate of filtration, reabsorption, and secretion. Compensatory excretion continues as GFR diminishes.

Urine may contain abnormal amounts of protein, red blood cells (RBCs), and white blood cells or casts. The major end products of excretion remain essentially normal, and nephron loss becomes significant. As GFR decreases, plasma creatinine levels increase proportionately without regulatory adjustment. As sodium delivery to the nephron increases, less is reabsorbed, and sodium deficits and volume depletion follow. The kidney becomes incapable of concentrating and diluting urine.

If tubular interstitial disease is the cause of chronic renal failure, primary damage to the tubules — the medullary portion of the nephron — precedes failure, as do such problems as renal tubular acidosis, salt wasting, and difficulty diluting and concentrating urine. If vascular or glomerular damage is the primary cause, proteinuria, hematuria, and nephrotic syndrome are more prominent.

Changes in acid-base balance affect phosphorus and calcium balance. Renal phosphate excretion and $1,25(OH)_2$ vitamin D_3 synthesis are diminished. Hypocalcemia results in secondary hypoparathyroidism, diminished GFR, and progressive hyperphosphatemia, hypocalcemia, and dissolution of bone. In early renal insufficiency, acid excretion and phosphate reabsorption increase to maintain normal pH. When GFR decreases by 30% to 40%, progressive metabolic acidosis ensues and tubular secretion of potassium increases. Total-body potassium levels may increase to life-threatening levels requiring dialysis.

In glomerulosclerosis, distortion of filtration slits and erosion of the glomerular epithelial cells lead to increased fluid transport across the glomerular wall. Large proteins traverse the slits but become trapped in glomerular basement membranes,

Characteristics of chronic renal failure
- Usually end result of gradual tissue destruction, loss of renal function
- Can also result from rapidly progressing disease of sudden onset
- Few symptoms develop until less than 25% of glomerular filtration remains
- Normal parenchyma deteriorates rapidly
- Symptoms worsen as renal function decreases
- Syndrome is fatal without treatment
- Maintenance on dialysis or kidney transplant can sustain life

Causes
- Glomerular disease
- Chronic infection
- Congenital anomalies
- Vascular disease
- Obstruction

How it happens
- Often progresses through four stages: reduced renal reserve, renal insufficiency, renal failure, end-stage renal disease
- Nephron damage is progressive
- Kidneys maintain relatively normal function until about 75% of nephrons are nonfunctional
- Compensatory excretion continues as GFR diminishes
- Urine may contain abnormal amounts of protein, RBCs, white blood cells or casts
- Plasma creatinine levels increase without regulatory adjustment

How it happens
(continued)

+ Tubulointerstitial injury occurs from toxic or ischemic tubular damage, as with acute tubular necrosis.
+ The structural changes trigger an inflammatory response.
+ Eventually, the healthy glomeruli are so overburdened that they become sclerotic, stiff, and necrotic.

Extrarenal consequences

+ Hypertension occurs
+ Irregular distant heart sounds
+ Bibasilar crackles in lungs
+ Peripheral edema
+ Reduced macrophage activity
+ Decreased breath sounds
+ Kussmaul's respirations
+ GI mucosa becomes inflamed, ulcerated
+ Stomatitis
+ Uremic fetor
+ Pancreatitis in end-stage renal failure
+ Malnutrition

obstructing the glomerular capillaries. Epithelial and endothelial injury causes proteinuria. Mesangial-cell proliferation, increased production of extracellular matrix, and intraglomerular coagulation cause the sclerosis.

Tubulointerstitial injury occurs from toxic or ischemic tubular damage, as with acute tubular necrosis. Debris and calcium deposits obstruct the tubules. The resulting defective tubular transport is associated with interstitial edema, leukocyte infiltration, and tubular necrosis. Vascular injury causes diffuse or focal ischemia of renal parenchyma, associated with thickening, fibrosis, or focal lesions of renal blood vessels. Decreased blood flow then leads to tubular atrophy, interstitial fibrosis, and functional disruption of glomerular filtration, medullary gradients, and concentration.

The structural changes trigger an inflammatory response. Fibrin deposits begin to form around the interstitium. Microaneurysms result from vascular wall damage and increased pressure secondary to obstruction or hypertension. Eventual loss of the nephron triggers compensatory hyperfunction of uninjured nephrons, which initiates a positive-feedback loop of increasing vulnerability.

Eventually, the healthy glomeruli are so overburdened that they become sclerotic, stiff, and necrotic. Toxins accumulate and potentially fatal changes ensue in all major organ systems.

Extrarenal consequences

Physiologic changes affect more than one system, and the presence and severity of manifestations depend on the duration of renal failure and its response to treatment. In some fluid and electrolyte imbalances, the kidneys can't retain salt, and hyponatremia results. Dry mouth, fatigue, nausea, hypotension, loss of skin turgor, and listlessness can progress to somnolence and confusion. Later, as the number of functioning nephrons decreases, so does the capacity to excrete sodium and potassium. Sodium retention leads to fluid overload and edema; the potassium overload leads to muscle irritability and weakness as well as life-threatening cardiac arrhythmias.

As the cardiovascular system becomes involved, hypertension occurs, and irregular distant heart sounds may be auscultated if pericardial effusion occurs. Bibasilar crackles in the lungs and peripheral edema reflect heart failure.

Pulmonary changes include reduced macrophage activity and increasing susceptibility to infection. Decreased breath sounds in areas of consolidation reflect the presence of pneumonia. As the pleurae become more involved, the patient may experience pleuritic pain and friction rubs.

Kussmaul's respirations may be noted as a result of metabolic acidosis. The GI mucosa becomes inflamed and ulcerated, and gums may also be ulcerated and bleeding. Stomatitis, uremic fetor (an ammonia smell to the breath), hiccups, peptic ulcer, and pancreatitis in end-stage renal failure are believed to be due to retention of metabolic acids and other metabolic waste products. Malnutrition may be secondary to anorexia, malaise, and reduced dietary intake of protein. The reduced protein intake also affects capillary fragility and results in decreased immune functioning and poor wound healing.

Normochromic normocytic anemia and platelet disorders with prolonged bleeding time ensue as diminished erythropoietin secretion leads to reduced RBC production in the bone marrow. Uremic toxins associated with chronic renal failure shorten RBC survival time. The patient experiences lethargy and dizziness.

Demineralization of the bone (renal osteodystrophy) manifested by bone pain and pathologic fractures is due to decreased renal activation of vitamin D (which decreases absorption of dietary calcium), retention of phosphate (which increases urinary loss of calcium), and increased circulation of parathyroid hormone (which is caused by decreased urinary excretion).

The skin acquires a grayish yellow tint as urine pigments (urochromes) accumulate. Inflammatory mediators released by retained toxins in the skin cause pruritus. Uric acid and other substances in the sweat crystallize and accumulate on the skin as uremic frost. High plasma calcium levels are also associated with pruritus.

Restless leg syndrome (abnormal sensation and spontaneous movement of the feet and lower legs), muscle weakness, and decreased deep tendon reflexes are believed to result from the effect of toxins on the nervous system.

 CLINICAL ALERT Restless leg syndrome is one of the first signs of peripheral neuropathy. This condition will eventually progress to paresthesia and motor nerve dysfunction (bilateral footdrop) unless dialysis is initiated.

Chronic renal failure increases the risk of death from infection. This is related to suppression of cell-mediated immunity and a reduction in the number and function of lymphocytes and phagocytes.

All hormone levels are impaired in excretion and activation. Females may be anovulatory, amenorrheic, or unable to carry pregnancy to full term. Males tend to have decreased sperm counts and impotence.

SIGNS AND SYMPTOMS

Chronic renal failure affects numerous areas of the body, and signs and symptoms are numerous. Hypervolemia, for example, is due to sodium retention, and hypocalcemia and hyperkalemia are caused by electrolyte imbalance. Azotemia results from retention of nitrogenous wastes, and metabolic acidosis (which causes Kussmaul's respirations) is due to loss of bicarbonate.

Other signs and symptoms include bone and muscle pain and fractures. These are caused by a calcium-phosphorus imbalance and consequent parathyroid hormone imbalances.

In addition, accumulated toxins may cause peripheral neuropathy and an altered mental state. Hyponatremia may also contribute to an altered mental state as well as cause such signs and symptoms as dry mouth, fatigue, nausea, and hypotension.

Other signs and symptoms may appear in the heart, circulatory system, and blood. For example, an irregular heart rate and muscle cramps and twitching, including cardiac irritability, may result from hypokalemia. Hypertension may be caused by fluid overload. Such additional problems as gum sores and bleeding are due to coagulopathies. Thrombocytopenia and platelet defects cause GI bleeding, hemorrhage, and bruising.

Additional signs and symptoms may be present in the skin: yellow-bronze skin is due to altered metabolic processes, and dry, scaly skin and severe itching may be caused by uremic frost.

 CLINICAL ALERT Growth retardation in children occurs from endocrine abnormalities induced by renal failure. Impaired bone growth and bowlegs in children are also due to rickets.

Alert!

+ Restless leg syndrome is one of the first signs of peripheral neuropathy.
+ This condition will eventually progress to paresthesia and motor nerve dysfunction unless dialysis is initiated.

Key signs and symptoms

+ Hypervolemia
+ Azotemia
+ Bone and muscle pain, fractures
+ Peripheral neuropathy, altered mental state
+ Dry mouth, fatigue, nausea, hypotension
+ Muscle cramps
+ Cardiac irritability
+ Thrombocytopenia
+ Yellow-bronze skin
+ Infertility
+ Decreased libido
+ Amenorrhea

Alert!

+ Growth retardation in children occurs from endocrine abnormalities induced by renal failure.
+ Impaired bone growth and bowlegs in children are also due to rickets.

Complications

+ Anemia
+ Peripheral neuropathy
+ Cardiopulmonary complications
+ GI complications
+ Sexual dysfunction
+ Skeletal defects
+ Paresthesias
+ Pathologic fractures
+ Motor nerve dysfunction

Diagnosis

+ Decreased arterial pH and bicarbonate
+ Low hemoglobin levels and hematocrit
+ Decreased RBC survival time
+ Mild thrombocytopenia
+ Platelet defects
+ Elevated blood urea nitrogen, serum creatinine, sodium, potassium levels
+ Renal biopsy reveals underlying disease

Treatment

+ Dietary therapy
+ Drug therapy
+ Iron and folate supplements
+ RBC transfusion
+ Conjugated estrogens
+ Dialysis
+ Emergency pericardiocentesis
+ Surgery for cardiac tamponade
+ Peritoneal or hemodialysis
+ Renal transplantation

Still other signs and symptoms, such as infertility, decreased libido, amenorrhea, and impotence, can result from endocrine disturbances. Pain, burning, and itching in the legs and feet are associated with the effects of peripheral neuropathy. Decreased macrophage activity results in infection.

COMPLICATIONS

Possible complications of chronic renal failure include anemia, peripheral neuropathy, cardiopulmonary complications, GI complications, sexual dysfunction, skeletal defects, paresthesias, pathologic fractures, and motor nerve dysfunction, such as footdrop and flaccid paralysis.

DIAGNOSIS

Blood study results that help diagnose chronic renal failure include a decreased arterial pH and bicarbonate; low hemoglobin levels and hematocrit; decreased RBC survival time; mild thrombocytopenia; platelet defects; elevated blood urea nitrogen, serum creatinine, sodium, and potassium levels; hyperglycemia (a sign of impaired carbohydrate metabolism); hypertriglyceridemia; and low levels of high-density lipoprotein. Increased renin production results in increased aldosterone secretion.

Several urinalysis results also aid in diagnosing. These include specific gravity fixed at 1.010, proteinuria, glycosuria, RBCs, leukocytes, casts, or crystals, depending on the cause.

Kidney-ureter-bladder radiography, excretory urography, nephrotomography, renal scan, or renal arteriography reveals reduced kidney size. Renal biopsy is commonly used to identify underlying disease, and EEG is performed to identify metabolic encephalopathy.

TREATMENT

Treatment of chronic renal failure may include dietary therapy such as a low-protein diet to limit the accumulation of end products of protein metabolism that the kidneys can't excrete. For patients on continuous peritoneal dialysis, however, a high-protein diet is recommended. A high-calorie diet may be used to help prevent ketoacidosis and tissue atrophy. For some patients, dietary restrictions are also implemented. Sodium and potassium restrictions, for example, prevent elevated levels of these minerals, and fluid restrictions help maintain fluid balance.

Drug therapy is commonly implemented as well. To mobilize fluids that cause edema, loop diuretics such as furosemide (Lasix) and cardiac glycosides such as digoxin are used. Calcium carbonate (Caltrate) or calcium acetate (PhosLo) is prescribed to treat renal osteodystrophy by binding phosphate and supplementing calcium. Blood pressure and edema are controlled with antihypertensives. Antiemetics relieve nausea and vomiting, famotidine (Pepcid) or ranitidine (Zantac) decrease gastric irritation, and methylcellulose or docusate prevents constipation.

To combat the hematologic effects of chronic renal failure, iron and folate supplements or RBC transfusion are prescribed to treat anemia, and synthetic erythropoietin is used to stimulate the bone marrow to produce RBCs. Supplemental iron, conjugated estrogens, and desmopressin are commonly administered as well.

For the itching that accompanies chronic renal failure, antipruritics, such as trimeprazine (Temaril) or diphenhydramine (Benadryl), are prescribed. Other supplemental therapies include aluminum hydroxide gel to reduce serum phosphate levels; supplementary vitamins, particularly B and D; and essential amino acids.

To treat hyperkalemia and fluid imbalances, dialysis may be performed. Cation exchange resins, such as sodium polystyrene sulfonate (Kayexalate), may be administered orally or rectally, and I.V. administration of calcium gluconate, sodium bicarbonate, 50% dextrose, and regular insulin are also used to reverse hyperkalemia.

Other therapies include emergency pericardiocentesis or surgery for cardiac tamponade, and intensive dialysis and thoracentesis for relieving pulmonary edema and pleural effusion. Peritoneal or hemodialysis may be performed to help control end-stage renal disease. Renal transplantation is usually the treatment of choice for chronic renal failure if a donor is available.

NURSING CONSIDERATIONS

Because chronic renal failure has such widespread clinical effects, it requires meticulous and carefully coordinated supportive care.

✦ Good skin care is important. Bathe the patient daily using superfatted soaps, oatmeal baths, and skin lotion without alcohol to ease pruritus. Don't use glycerin-containing soaps because they'll cause skin drying. Give good perineal care using mild soap and water. Pad the side rails to guard against ecchymoses. Turn the patient often, and use a convoluted foam mattress to prevent skin breakdown.

✦ Provide good oral hygiene. Brush the patient's teeth often with a soft brush or sponge tip to reduce breath odor. Sugarless hard candy and mouthwash minimize metallic taste in the mouth and alleviate thirst.

✦ Offer small, palatable meals that are also nutritious; try to provide favorite foods within dietary restrictions. Encourage intake of high-calorie foods. Instruct the outpatient to avoid high-sodium foods and high-potassium foods. Encourage adherence to fluid and protein restrictions. To prevent constipation, stress the need for exercise and sufficient dietary bulk.

✦ Watch for hyperkalemia. Observe for cramping of the legs and abdomen, and diarrhea. As potassium levels rise, watch for muscle irritability and a weak pulse rate. Monitor the electrocardiogram for tall, peaked T waves; widening QRS segment; prolonged PR interval; and disappearance of P waves, indicating hyperkalemia.

✦ Assess hydration status carefully. Check for jugular vein distention, and auscultate the lungs for crackles. Measure daily intake and output carefully, including drainage, emesis, diarrhea, and blood loss. Record daily weight, presence or absence of thirst, axillary sweat, dryness of tongue, hypertension, and peripheral edema.

✦ Monitor for bone or joint complications. Prevent pathologic fractures by turning the patient carefully and ensuring his safety. Provide passive range-of-motion exercises for the bedridden patient.

✦ Encourage deep breathing and coughing to prevent pulmonary congestion. Listen often for crackles, rhonchi, and decreased breath sounds. Be alert for clinical effects of pulmonary edema (dyspnea, restlessness, crackles). Administer diuretics and other medications as ordered.

✦ Maintain strict sterile technique. Use a micropore filter during I.V. therapy. Watch for signs of infection (listlessness, high fever, leukocytosis). Urge the outpatient to avoid contact with infected people during the cold and flu season.

✦ Carefully observe and document seizure activity. Infuse sodium bicarbonate for acidosis, and sedatives or anticonvulsants for seizures, as ordered. Pad the side rails, and keep an oral airway and suction setup at the bedside. Assess neurologic status periodically, and check for Chvostek's and Trousseau's signs, indicators of low serum calcium levels.

✦ Observe for signs of bleeding. Watch for prolonged bleeding at puncture sites and at the vascular access site used for hemodialysis. Monitor hemoglobin levels and hematocrit, and check stool, urine, and vomitus for blood.

Key nursing actions
✦ Good skin care is important.
✦ Provide good oral hygiene.
✦ Offer small, palatable meals that are also nutritious.
✦ Watch for hyperkalemia.
✦ Assess hydration status carefully.
✦ Monitor for bone or joint complications.
✦ Encourage deep breathing and coughing to prevent pulmonary congestion.
✦ Maintain strict sterile technique.
✦ Assess neurologic status periodically, and check for Chvostek's and Trousseau's signs, indicators of low serum calcium levels.
✦ Observe for signs of bleeding.
✦ Report signs of pericarditis, such as a pericardial friction rub and chest pain.

Alert!

✦ Watch for the disappearance of friction rub, with a drop of 15 to 20 mm Hg in blood pressure during inspiration—an early sign of pericardial tamponade.

Key nursing actions
(continued)

✦ Schedule medications carefully.
✦ If the patient requires a rectal infusion of sodium polystyrene sulfonate for dangerously high potassium levels, apply an emollient to soothe the perianal area.

If the patient requires dialysis

✦ Prepare the patient by fully explaining the procedure.
✦ Withhold the morning dose of antihypertensive on the morning of dialysis, and instruct the outpatient to do the same.
✦ After dialysis, check for disequilibrium syndrome, a result of sudden correction of blood chemistry abnormalities.

Characteristics of glomerulonephritis

✦ Bilateral inflammation of glomeruli after streptococcal infection

Acute glomerulonephritis

✦ Most common in boys ages 3 to 7, but can occur at any age
✦ Prognosis good except in elderly

RPGN

✦ Commonly occurs between ages 50 and 60
✦ May be idiopathic or associated with proliferative glomerular

Chronic glomerulonephritis

✦ Slowly progressive disease
✦ Characterized by inflammation, sclerosis, scarring, renal failure

---

✦ Report signs of pericarditis, such as a pericardial friction rub and chest pain.

 CLINICAL ALERT **Watch for the disappearance of friction rub, with a drop of 15 to 20 mm Hg in blood pressure during inspiration (paradoxical pulse)—an early sign of pericardial tamponade.**

✦ Schedule medications carefully. Give iron before meals, aluminum hydroxide gels after meals, and antiemetics, as necessary, half an hour before meals. Administer antihypertensives at appropriate intervals. If the patient requires a rectal infusion of sodium polystyrene sulfonate for dangerously high potassium levels, apply an emollient to soothe the perianal area. Make sure the sodium polystyrene sulfonate enema is expelled; otherwise, it will cause constipation and won't lower potassium levels. Recommend antacid cookies as an alternative to aluminum hydroxide gels needed to bind GI phosphate.

If the patient requires dialysis

✦ Prepare the patient by fully explaining the procedure. Make sure that he understands how to protect and care for the arteriovenous shunt, fistula, or other vascular access. Check the vascular access site every 2 hours for patency, and check the extremity for adequate blood supply and intact nervous function (temperature, pulse rate, capillary refill, and sensation). If a fistula is present, feel for a thrill and listen for a bruit. Use a gentle touch to avoid occluding the fistula. Report signs of possible clotting. Don't use the arm with the vascular access site to take blood pressure readings, draw blood, insert I.V. lines, or give injections because these procedures may rupture the fistula or occlude blood flow.
✦ Withhold the 6 a.m. (or morning) dose of antihypertensive on the morning of dialysis, and instruct the outpatient to do the same.
✦ Use standard precautions when handling body fluids and needles.
✦ Monitor hemoglobin levels and hematocrit. Assess the patient's tolerance of his levels. Some individuals are more sensitive to lower levels than others. Instruct the anemic patient to conserve energy and to rest frequently.
✦ After dialysis, check for disequilibrium syndrome, a result of sudden correction of blood chemistry abnormalities. Symptoms range from a headache to seizures. Also, check for excessive bleeding from the dialysis site. Apply a pressure dressing or an absorbable gelatin sponge as indicated. Monitor blood pressure carefully after dialysis.
✦ A patient undergoing dialysis is under a great deal of stress, as is his family. Refer him to appropriate counseling agencies for assistance in coping with chronic renal failure.

GLOMERULONEPHRITIS

Glomerulonephritis is a bilateral inflammation of the glomeruli, typically following a streptococcal infection. Acute glomerulonephritis is also called *acute poststreptococcal glomerulonephritis.*

Acute glomerulonephritis is most common in boys ages 3 to 7, but it can occur at any age. Up to 95% of children and 70% of adults recover fully; the rest, especially elderly patients, may progress to chronic renal failure within months.

Rapidly progressive glomerulonephritis (RPGN)—also called *subacute, crescentic,* or *extracapillary glomerulonephritis*—most commonly occurs between ages 50 and 60. It may be idiopathic or associated with a proliferative glomerular disease such as poststreptococcal glomerulonephritis.

Characteristics of glomerular lesions

The types of glomerular lesions and their characteristics include:
+ diffuse lesions — relatively uniform, involve most or all glomeruli (for example, glomerulonephritis)
+ focal lesions — involve only some glomeruli; others normal
+ segmental-local — involve only one part of the glomerulus
+ mesangial — deposits of immunoglobulins in mesangial matrix
+ membranous — thickening of glomerular capillary wall
+ proliferative lesions — increased number of glomerular cells
+ sclerotic lesions — glomerular scarring from previous glomerular injury
+ crescent lesions — accumulation of proliferating cells in Bowman's space.

 CLINICAL ALERT Goodpasture's syndrome, a type of rapidly progressive glomerulonephritis, is rare but occurs most commonly in men ages 20 to 30.

Chronic glomerulonephritis is a slowly progressive disease characterized by inflammation, sclerosis, scarring and, eventually, renal failure. It usually remains undetected until the progressive phase, which is usually irreversible.

CAUSES

Causes of acute glomerulonephritis and RPGN include a streptococcal infection of the respiratory tract, impetigo, immunoglobulin (Ig) A nephropathy (Berger's disease), and lipoid nephrosis.

Chronic glomerulonephritis is caused by membranoproliferative glomerulonephritis, membranous glomerulopathy, focal glomerulosclerosis, RPGN, poststreptococcal glomerulonephritis, systemic lupus erythematosus, Goodpasture's syndrome, and hemolytic uremic syndrome.

PATHOPHYSIOLOGY

In nearly all types of glomerulonephritis, the epithelial or podocyte layer of the glomerular membrane is disturbed. This results in a loss of negative charge. (See *Characteristics of glomerular lesions*.)

Acute poststreptococcal glomerulonephritis results from the entrapment and collection of antigen-antibody complexes in the glomerular capillary membranes after infection with a group A beta-hemolytic streptococcus. The antigens, which are endogenous or exogenous, stimulate the formation of antibodies. Circulating antigen-antibody complexes become lodged in the glomerular capillaries. (See *Glomerulonephritis,* page 540.)

Glomerular injury occurs when the complexes initiate complement activation and the release of immunologic substances that lyse cells and increase membrane permeability. Antibody damage to basement membranes causes crescent formation. The severity of glomerular damage and renal insufficiency is related to the size, number, location (focal or diffuse), duration of exposure, and type of antigen-antibody complexes.

Antibody or antigen-antibody complexes in the glomerular capillary wall activate biochemical mediators of inflammation — complement, leukocytes, and fibrin. Activated complement attracts neutrophils and monocytes, which release lysosomal enzymes that damage the glomerular cell walls and cause a proliferation of

Key types of glomerular lesions
+ Diffuse
+ Focal
+ Segmental-local

Alert!
+ Goodpasture's syndrome is rare but occurs most commonly in men ages 20 to 30.

Causes

Acute glomerulonephritis and RPGN
+ Streptococcal infection of respiratory tract
+ Impetigo

Chronic glomerulonephritis
+ Membranoproliferative glomerulonephritis
+ Membranous glomerulopathy

How it happens
+ Epithelial layer of glomerular membrane is disturbed
+ Loss of negative charge

Acute poststreptococcal glomerulonephritis
+ Entrapment and collection of antigen-antibody complexes in glomerular capillary membranes
+ Occurs after group A beta-hemolytic streptococcus infection
+ Antigens stimulate formation of antibodies
+ Circulating antigen-antibody complexes become lodged in glomerular capillaries
+ Complexes initiate complement activation, release of immunologic substances that lyse cells, increase membrane permeability
+ Severity is related to size, number, location, duration of exposure, type of antigen-antibody complexes

CLOSER LOOK

Glomerulonephritis

The immune complex depositions that occur in glomerulonephritis are shown here.

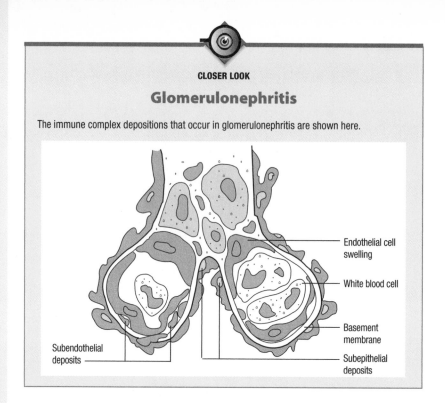

Endothelial cell swelling

White blood cell

Basement membrane

Subepithelial deposits

Subendothelial deposits

How it happens
(continued)

+ Membrane damage leads to platelet aggregation, and platelet degranulation releases substances that increase glomerular permeability
+ Proteinuria and hematuria result
+ Fibrin deposits in Bowman's space, leading to diminished renal blood flow and GFR
+ Fluid retention and decreased urine output, extracellular fluid volume expansion, and hypertension result

Goodpasture's syndrome
+ An RPGN in which antibodies are produced against the pulmonary capillaries and glomerular basement membrane

IgA nephropathy
+ Berger's disease is usually idiopathic; plasma IgA level is elevated, and IgA and inflammatory cells are deposited into Bowman's space
+ The result is sclerosis and fibrosis of the glomerulus and a reduced GFR

Lipid nephrosis
+ Lipid nephrosis causes disruption of the capillary filtration membrane and loss of its negative charge

the extracellular matrix, affecting glomerular blood flow. Those events increase membrane permeability, which causes a loss of negative charge across the glomerular membrane as well as enhanced protein filtration.

Membrane damage leads to platelet aggregation, and platelet degranulation releases substances that increase glomerular permeability. Protein molecules and red blood cells (RBCs) can now pass into the urine, resulting in proteinuria or hematuria. Activation of the coagulation system leads to fibrin deposits in Bowman's space. The result is crescent formation and diminished renal blood flow and glomerular filtration rate (GFR). Glomerular bleeding causes acidic urine, which transforms hemoglobin to methemoglobin and results in brown urine without clots.

The inflammatory response decreases GFR, which causes fluid retention and decreased urine output, extracellular fluid volume expansion, and hypertension. Gross proteinuria is associated with nephrotic syndrome. After 10 to 20 years, renal insufficiency develops, followed by nephrotic syndrome and end-stage renal failure.

Goodpasture's syndrome is an RPGN in which antibodies are produced against the pulmonary capillaries and glomerular basement membrane. Diffuse intracellular antibody proliferation in Bowman's space leads to a crescent-shaped structure that obliterates the space. The crescent is composed of fibrin and endothelial, mesangial, and phagocytic cells, which compress the glomerular capillaries, diminish blood flow, and cause extensive scarring of the glomeruli. GFR is reduced, and renal failure occurs within weeks or months.

IgA nephropathy, or Berger's disease, is usually idiopathic. Plasma IgA level is elevated, and IgA and inflammatory cells are deposited into Bowman's space. The result is sclerosis and fibrosis of the glomerulus and a reduced GFR.

Lipid nephrosis causes disruption of the capillary filtration membrane and loss of its negative charge. This increased permeability with resultant loss of protein leads to nephrotic syndrome.

Systemic diseases, such as hepatitis B virus, systemic lupus erythematosus, or solid malignant tumors, cause a membranous nephropathy. An inflammatory process causes thickening of the glomerular capillary wall. Increased permeability and proteinuria lead to nephrotic syndrome.

Sometimes the immune complement further damages the glomerular membrane. The damaged and inflamed glomeruli lose the ability to be selectively permeable, so that RBCs and proteins filter through as GFR decreases. Uremic poisoning may result. Renal function may deteriorate, especially in adults with sporadic acute poststreptococcal glomerulonephritis, commonly in the form of glomerulosclerosis accompanied by hypertension. The more severe the disorder, the more likely its complications will occur. Hypervolemia leads to hypertension, resulting from either sodium and water retention (caused by the decreased GFR) or inappropriate renin release. The patient develops pulmonary edema and heart failure. (See *Averting renal failure in glomerulonephritis,* page 542.)

SIGNS AND SYMPTOMS

Patients with glomerulonephritis experience various signs and symptoms. They have, for instance, decreased urination or oliguria caused by decreased GFR and have smoky or coffee-colored urine due to hematuria.

They may also have dyspnea and orthopnea, which result from pulmonary edema (which is secondary to hypervolemia). Hypervolemia also causes periorbital edema. In addition, patients with decreased GFR have mild to severe hypertension, sodium or water retention, and inappropriate release of renin. In these patients, heart failure causes bibasilar crackles.

 CLINICAL ALERT The presenting features of glomerulonephritis in children may be encephalopathy with seizures and local neurologic deficits. An elderly patient with glomerulonephritis may report vague, nonspecific symptoms, such as nausea, malaise, and arthralgia.

COMPLICATIONS

Possible complications of glomerulonephritis include pulmonary edema, heart failure, sepsis, renal failure, severe hypertension, and cardiac hypertrophy.

DIAGNOSIS

In patients with glomerulonephritis, blood study results reveal elevated electrolyte, blood urea nitrogen, and creatinine levels; decreased serum protein level; decreased hemoglobin levels in chronic glomerulonephritis; elevated antistreptolysin-O titers in 80% of patients; elevated streptozyme (a hemagglutination test that detects antibodies to several streptococcal antigens) and anti-DNase B (a test to determine a previous infection of group A beta-hemolytic streptococcus) titers, and low serum complement levels indicating recent streptococcal infection.

Urinalysis results in these patients show RBCs, white blood cells, mixed cell casts, and protein indicating renal failure and fibrin-degradation products and C3 protein.

CLINICAL ALERT Significant proteinuria isn't a common finding in an elderly patient.

Other studies that help confirm a diagnosis of glomerulonephritis include a throat culture that shows group A beta-hemolytic streptococcus, and a kidney-ureter-bladder X-ray that reveals bilateral kidney enlargement in acute

Key signs and symptoms
+ Decreased urination or oliguria
+ Smoky, coffee-colored urine
+ Dyspnea
+ Orthopnea
+ Hypertension

Alert!
+ The presenting features of glomerulonephritis in children may be encephalopathy with seizures and local neurologic deficits.
+ An elderly patient with glomerulonephritis may report vague, nonspecific symptoms, such as nausea, malaise, and arthralgia.

Complications
+ Pulmonary edema
+ Heart failure
+ Sepsis
+ Renal failure

Diagnosis
+ Elevated electrolyte, blood urea nitrogen, creatinine levels
+ Decreased serum protein level
+ Decreased hemoglobin levels in chronic glomerulonephritis
+ Elevated antistreptolysin-O titers
+ Elevated streptozyme

Alert!
+ Significant proteinuria isn't a common finding in an elderly patient.

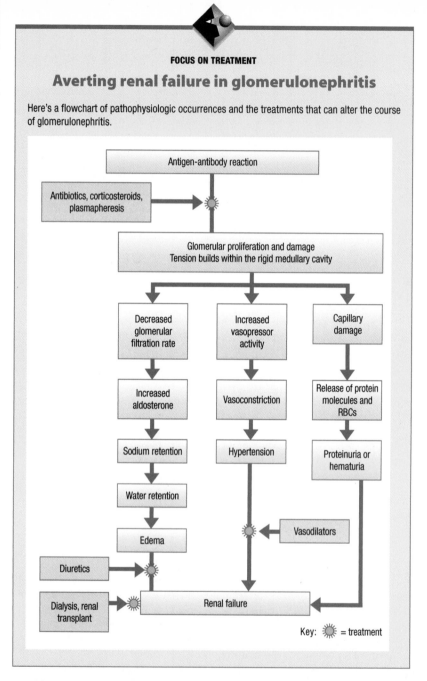

FOCUS ON TREATMENT

Averting renal failure in glomerulonephritis

Here's a flowchart of pathophysiologic occurrences and the treatments that can alter the course of glomerulonephritis.

Antigen-antibody reaction

Antibiotics, corticosteroids, plasmapheresis

Glomerular proliferation and damage
Tension builds within the rigid medullary cavity

Decreased glomerular filtration rate

Increased vasopressor activity

Capillary damage

Increased aldosterone

Vasoconstriction

Release of protein molecules and RBCs

Sodium retention

Hypertension

Proteinuria or hematuria

Water retention

Vasodilators

Edema

Diuretics

Dialysis, renal transplant

Renal failure

Key: ☀ = treatment

glomerulonephritis. Symmetric contraction with normal pelves and calyces (chronic glomerulonephritis) is also seen on X-ray. A renal biopsy confirms the diagnosis or assesses renal tissue status.

TREATMENT

Treatment of glomerulonephritis and the primary disease involves altering the immunologic cascade. Patients are given antibiotics for 7 to 10 days to treat infections contributing to ongoing antigen-antibody response. Anticoagulants are prescribed as well to control fibrin crescent formation in RPGN. Bed rest reduces metabolic demands, fluid restrictions decrease edema, and dietary sodium restriction prevents fluid retention.

Additional treatment includes loop diuretics, such as metolazone (Zaroxolyn) or furosemide (Lasix), to reduce extracellular fluid overload. Vasodilators, such as hydralazine (Apresoline) or nifedipine (Procardia), are used to decrease hypertension. Throughout the course of treatment, electrolytes are carefully monitored and corrected.

To treat chronic glomerulonephritis, dialysis or kidney transplantation is used. In both cases, corticosteroids are administered to decrease antibody synthesis and suppress inflammatory response, and plasmapheresis suppresses rebound antibody production in RPGN. Plasmapheresis can be combined with corticosteroids and cyclophosphamide (Cytoxan).

NURSING CONSIDERATIONS

For patients with acute or chronic glomerulonephritis, care is primarily supportive.
+ Check vital signs and electrolyte values. Monitor intake and output and daily weight. Assess renal function daily through serum creatinine, blood urea nitrogen, and urine creatinine clearance levels. Watch for and immediately report signs of acute renal failure (oliguria, azotemia, and acidosis). Monitor for ascites and edema.
+ Consult the dietitian to provide a diet high in calories and low in protein, sodium, potassium, and fluids.
+ Administer medications as ordered, and provide good skin care (because of pruritus and edema) and oral hygiene. Instruct the patient to continue taking prescribed antihypertensives as scheduled, even if he's feeling better, and to report any adverse effects. Advise him to take diuretics in the morning, so he won't have to disrupt his sleep to void. Teach him how to assess ankle edema.
+ Protect the debilitated patient against secondary infection by providing good nutrition, using good hygienic technique, and preventing contact with infected people.
+ Bed rest is necessary during the acute phase. Allow the patient to gradually resume normal activities as symptoms subside.
+ Advise the patient with a history of chronic upper respiratory tract infections to immediately report signs of infection (fever, sore throat).
+ Tell the patient that follow-up examinations are necessary to detect chronic renal failure. Stress the need for regular blood pressure, urinary protein, and renal function assessments during the convalescent months to detect recurrence. After acute glomerulonephritis, gross hematuria may recur during nonspecific viral infections; abnormal urinary findings may persist for years.
+ Encourage pregnant women with a history of glomerulonephritis to have frequent medical evaluations because pregnancy further stresses the kidneys and increases the risk of chronic renal failure.
+ Help the patient adjust to this illness by encouraging him to express his feelings. Explain all necessary procedures beforehand, and answer the patient's questions about them.

Treatment
+ Antibiotics
+ Anticoagulants
+ Bed rest
+ Loop diuretics
+ Vasodilators
+ Dialysis or kidney transplantation

Key nursing actions
+ Check vital signs and electrolyte values.
+ Consult the dietitian to provide a diet high in calories and low in protein, sodium, potassium, and fluids.
+ Administer medications as ordered.
+ Protect the debilitated patient against secondary infection by providing good nutrition, using good hygienic technique, and preventing contact with infected people.
+ Bed rest is necessary during the acute phase.
+ Advise the patient with a history of chronic upper respiratory tract infections to immediately report signs of infection.
+ Encourage pregnant women with a history of glomerulonephritis to have frequent medical evaluations.

Characteristics of nephrotic syndrome

- Marked proteinuria, hypoalbuminemia, hyperlipidemia, edema
- Results from a defect in permeability of glomerular vessels
- 75% of cases result from primary glomerulonephritis
- Prognosis highly variable
- More common in boys

Alert!

- Age has no part in the progression or prognosis of nephrotic syndrome.

Causes

- Lipid nephrosis
- Membranous glomerulonephritis
- Focal glomerulosclerosis
- Membranoproliferative glomerulonephritis

Alert!

- Lipid nephrosis is the main cause of nephrotic syndrome in children younger than age 8.
- Membranous glomerulonephritis is the most common lesion in adult idiopathic nephrotic syndrome.

How it happens

- Characterized by appearance of immune complexes
- Uniform thickening of basement membrane
- Progresses to renal failure
- Focal glomerulosclerosis: lesions cause slowly progressive deterioration in renal function
- Membranoproliferative glomerulonephritis: slowly progressive lesions in subendothelial region of basement membrane

NEPHROTIC SYNDROME

Marked proteinuria, hypoalbuminemia, hyperlipidemia, and edema characterize nephrotic syndrome. It results from a defect in the permeability of glomerular vessels. About 75% of the cases result from primary (idiopathic) glomerulonephritis. The prognosis is highly variable, depending on the underlying cause.

 CLINICAL ALERT Age has no part in the progression or prognosis of nephrotic syndrome. Primary nephrotic syndrome is found predominantly in the preschool child. Incidence peaks between ages 2 and 3 and is rare after age 8.

Primary nephrotic syndrome is more common in boys than in girls; incidence is 3 per 100,000 children per year. Some forms of nephrotic syndrome may eventually progress to end-stage renal failure.

CAUSES

Causes of nephrotic syndrome include lipid nephrosis (nil lesions), membranous glomerulonephritis, focal glomerulosclerosis, membranoproliferative glomerulonephritis, metabolic diseases such as diabetes mellitus, and collagen-vascular disorders, such as systemic lupus erythematosus and periarteritis nodosa.

 CLINICAL ALERT Lipid nephrosis is the main cause of nephrotic syndrome in children younger than age 8.

 CLINICAL ALERT Membranous glomerulonephritis is the most common lesion in adult idiopathic nephrotic syndrome.

Additional causes are circulatory diseases such as heart failure; sickle cell anemia; renal vein thrombosis; nephrotoxins, such as mercury, gold, and bismuth; infections, such as tuberculosis and enteritis; allergic reactions; pregnancy; hereditary nephritis; and neoplastic diseases such as multiple myeloma.

PATHOPHYSIOLOGY

In lipid nephrosis, the glomeruli appear normal by light microscopy, and some tubules may contain increased lipid deposits. Membranous glomerulonephritis is characterized by the appearance of immune complexes, seen as dense deposits in the glomerular basement membrane, and by the uniform thickening of the basement membrane. It eventually progresses to renal failure.

Focal glomerulosclerosis can develop spontaneously at any age, can occur after kidney transplantation, or may result from heroin injection. Ten percent of children and up to 20% of adults with nephrotic syndrome develop this condition. Lesions initially affect some of the deeper glomeruli, causing hyaline sclerosis. Involvement of the superficial glomeruli occurs later. These lesions usually cause slowly progressive deterioration in renal function, although remission may occur in children.

Membranoproliferative glomerulonephritis causes slowly progressive lesions in the subendothelial region of the basement membrane. This disorder may follow infection, particularly streptococcal infection, and occurs primarily in children and young adults.

Regardless of the cause, the injured glomerular filtration membrane allows the loss of plasma proteins, especially albumin and immunoglobulin. In addition, metabolic, biochemical, or physiochemical disturbances in the glomerular basement membrane result in the loss of negative charge as well as increased permeability to protein. Hypoalbuminemia results not only from urinary loss but also from decreased hepatic synthesis of replacement albumin. Increased plasma concentration and low molecular weight accentuate albumin loss. Hypoalbuminemia stimulates the liver to synthesize lipoprotein, with consequent hyperlipidemia. Decreased dietary intake, as with anorexia, malnutrition, or concomitant disease, further contributes to decreased plasma albumin levels. Loss of immunoglobulin also increases susceptibility to infections.

Extensive proteinuria (more than 3.5 g/day) and a low serum albumin level, secondary to renal loss, lead to low serum colloid osmotic pressure and edema. The low serum albumin level also leads to hypovolemia and compensatory salt and water retention. Consequent hypertension may precipitate heart failure in compromised patients.

SIGNS AND SYMPTOMS

Patients with nephrotic syndrome may present with a variety of signs and symptoms. From fluid overload (which generally occurs in the morning), they may have periorbital edema. Or they may show mild to severe dependent edema of the ankles or sacrum, and external genitalia from swelling in dependent areas. Orthostatic hypotension and ascites can occur as a result of fluid imbalance.

Other signs and symptoms include pleural effusions, which cause respiratory difficulty, and a susceptibility to infections may result in pneumonia. Anorexia and diarrhea are caused by edema of the intestinal mucosa. Cutaneous findings include pallor, shiny skin with prominent veins, and change in quality of hair from protein deficiency. Children may have frothy urine.

COMPLICATIONS

Possible complications include malnutrition, infection, coagulation disorders, thromboembolic vascular occlusion (especially in the lungs and legs), accelerated atherosclerosis, hypochromic anemia caused by excessive urinary excretion of transferrin, and acute renal failure.

DIAGNOSIS

Diagnosis of nephrotic syndrome is based on more than one test: a urinalysis that shows hyaline, granular and waxy fatty casts, and oval fat bodies, and 24-hour urine collections that show consistent heavy proteinuria (more than 3.5 mg/dl). Other studies include blood tests that reveal increased serum cholesterol, phospholipid (especially low-density and very low-density lipoproteins), and triglyceride levels, and decreased albumin levels, and a renal biopsy that allows for histologic identification of the lesion.

TREATMENT

Treatment for nephrotic syndrome begins with correction of the underlying cause, if possible. The patient should consume a nutritious diet, including 0.6 g of protein/kg of body weight per day. Restricted sodium intake and diuretics help the patient reduce edema, and antibiotics are prescribed to treat infection.

In addition, an 8-week course of a corticosteroid, such as prednisone (Deltasone), followed by maintenance therapy or a combination of prednisone and aza-

How it happens
(continued)

+ Hypoalbuminemia: stimulates liver to synthesize lipoprotein, with hyperlipidemia
+ Loss of immunoglobulin also increases susceptibility to infections
+ Extensive proteinuria, low serum albumin level, lead to low serum colloid osmotic pressure, edema

Key signs and symptoms

+ Fluid overload
+ Periorbital edema
+ Orthostatic hypotension
+ Pleural effusions
+ Pneumonia
+ Anorexia and diarrhea

Complications

+ Malnutrition
+ Infection
+ Coagulation disorders
+ Thromboembolic vascular occlusion
+ Accelerated atherosclerosis

Diagnosis

+ Urinalysis shows hyaline, granular and waxy fatty casts, oval fat bodies
+ 24-hour urine collections with consistent heavy proteinuria
+ Increased serum cholesterol, phospholipid, triglyceride levels
+ Decreased albumin levels
+ Histologic identification of lesion

Treatment
+ Nutritious diet
+ Restricted sodium intake
+ Diuretics
+ Antibiotics

Key nursing actions
+ Frequently check urine protein.
+ Measure blood pressure with the patient supine and standing; immediately report a drop in blood pressure exceeding 20 mm Hg.
+ Monitor intake and output and daily weight.
+ After kidney biopsy, watch for bleeding and shock.
+ Offer the patient and his family reassurance and support, especially during the acute phase.

Characteristics of polycystic kidney disease
+ Inherited disorder
+ Multiple, bilateral, grapelike clusters of fluid-filled cysts
+ Enlarged kidneys that compress and replace functioning renal tissue
+ Appears in two distinct forms: ADPKD and rare infantile form
+ Adult form has insidious onset, usually becomes obvious between ages 30 and 50
+ Can remain asymptomatic into 70s (rare)
+ Prognosis in adults extremely variable
+ Three genetic variants of autosomal dominant form

Alert!
+ Renal deterioration is more gradual in adults than in infants.

thioprine (Imuran) or cyclophosphamide (Cytoxan) may be prescribed to combat inflammation.

Other treatments include paracentesis to treat ascites and thoracentesis to treat pleural effusion. Although treating hyperlipidemia is generally unsuccessful, an attempt is usually made.

NURSING CONSIDERATIONS
Patient care includes identification and treatment of the underlying cause accompanied by supportive care during treatment.
+ Frequently check urine protein. (Urine containing protein appears frothy.)
+ Measure blood pressure while the patient is supine and while he's standing; immediately report a drop in blood pressure that exceeds 20 mm Hg.
+ Monitor and document the location and degree of edema.
+ After kidney biopsy, watch for bleeding and shock.
+ Monitor intake and output and check weight at the same time each morning— after the patient voids and before he eats—and while he's wearing the same kind of clothing. Ask the dietitian to plan a moderate-protein, low-sodium diet.
+ Provide good skin care because the patient with nephrotic syndrome usually has edema.
+ To avoid thrombophlebitis, encourage activity and exercise, and provide antiembolism stockings as ordered.
+ Watch for and teach the patient and family how to recognize adverse drug effects, such as bone marrow toxicity from cytotoxic immunosuppressants, and cushingoid symptoms (muscle weakness, mental changes, acne, moon face, hirsutism, girdle obesity, purple striae, amenorrhea) from long-term steroid therapy. Other steroid complications include masked infections, increased susceptibility to infections, ulcers, GI bleeding, and steroid-induced diabetes; a steroid crisis may occur if the drug is discontinued abruptly. To prevent GI complications, administer steroids with an antacid or with cimetidine or ranitidine. Explain that steroid adverse effects will subside when therapy stops.
+ Offer the patient and his family reassurance and support, especially during the acute phase, when edema is severe and the patient's body image changes.

POLYCYSTIC KIDNEY DISEASE
Polycystic kidney disease is an inherited disorder characterized by multiple, bilateral, grapelike clusters of fluid-filled cysts that enlarge the kidneys, compressing and eventually replacing functioning renal tissue. (See *Polycystic kidney*.)

The disease affects males and females equally and appears in two distinct forms. Autosomal dominant polycystic kidney disease (ADPKD) occurs in 1 in 1,000 to 1 in 3,000 people and accounts for about 10% of end-stage renal disease in the United States. The rare infantile form causes stillbirth or early neonatal death. The adult form has an insidious onset but usually becomes obvious between ages 30 and 50; rarely, it remains asymptomatic until the patient is in his 70s.

 CLINICAL ALERT Renal deterioration is more gradual in adults than in infants, but in both age-groups, the disease progresses relentlessly to fatal uremia.

The prognosis in adults is extremely variable. Progression may be slow, even after symptoms of renal insufficiency appear. After uremia symptoms develop, polycystic disease usually is fatal within 4 years, unless the patient receives dialysis.

CLOSER LOOK

Polycystic kidney

This cross-sectional drawing shows multiple areas of cystic damage. Each indentation depicts a cyst.

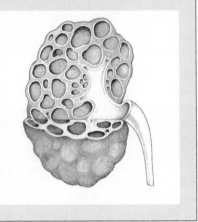

Three genetic variants of the autosomal dominant form have been identified (see below).

CAUSES

Polycystic kidney disease is inherited as an autosomal dominant trait (adult type), or an autosomal recessive trait (infantile type).

PATHOPHYSIOLOGY

ADPKD occurs as ADPKD-1, mapped to the short arm of chromosome 16 and encoded for a 4,300–amino acid protein; as ADPKD-2, mapped to the short arm of chromosome 4 with later onset of symptoms; and as a third variety not yet mapped. Autosomal recessive polycystic kidney disease occurs in 1 in 10,000 to 1 in 40,000 live births and has been localized to chromosome 6.

Grossly enlarged kidneys are caused by multiple spherical cysts, which are a few millimeters to centimeters in diameter and contain straw-colored or hemorrhagic fluid. The cysts are distributed evenly throughout the cortex and medulla. Hyperplastic polyps and renal adenomas are common. Renal parenchyma may have varying degrees of tubular atrophy, interstitial fibrosis, and nephrosclerosis. The cysts cause elongation of the pelvis, flattening of the calyces, and indentations in the kidney.

Characteristically, an affected infant shows signs of respiratory distress, heart failure and, eventually, uremia and renal failure. Accompanying hepatic fibrosis and intrahepatic bile duct abnormalities may cause portal hypertension and bleeding varices.

In most cases, progressive compression of kidney structures by the enlarging mass causes renal failure about 10 years after symptoms appear.

Cysts also form elsewhere — such as on the liver, spleen, pancreas, and ovaries. Intracranial aneurysms, colonic diverticula, and mitral valve prolapse also occur.

In the autosomal recessive form, death in the neonatal period is most commonly due to pulmonary hypoplasia.

Causes

+ Inherited as autosomal dominant trait (adult type) or autosomal recessive trait (infantile)

How it happens

+ Grossly enlarged kidneys caused by multiple spherical cysts
+ Cysts contain straw-colored or hemorrhagic fluid
+ Distributed evenly throughout cortex and medulla
+ Cysts cause elongation of pelvis, flattening of calyces, indentations in kidney
+ Progressive compression of kidney structures causes renal failure within 10 years

SIGNS AND SYMPTOMS

Neonates with polycystic kidney disease due to genetic abnormalities commonly have these signs and symptoms: pronounced epicanthic folds (vertical fold of skin on either side of the nose), a pointed nose, a small chin, and floppy, low-set ears (Potter facies). These neonates also have huge, bilateral, symmetrical masses on the flanks that are tense and can't be transilluminated. The masses are caused by kidney enlargement. Other signs and symptoms include respiratory distress, and uremia, caused by renal failure.

In adults, signs and symptoms include hypertension from activation of the renin-angiotensin system. These adults also have enlarged kidney mass that causes lumbar pain and widening abdominal girth. On palpation, the kidneys are grossly enlarged, and the abdomen is swollen and tender. The swelling and tenderness is caused by the enlarging kidney mass; both discomforts may worsen with exertion and be relieved by lying down.

COMPLICATIONS

 CLINICAL ALERT A few infants with this disease survive for 2 years and then die of hepatic complications or renal, heart, or respiratory failure.

Possible complications of polycystic kidney disease in adults include pyelonephritis, recurrent hematuria, life-threatening retroperitoneal bleeding from cyst rupture, proteinuria, colicky abdominal pain from ureteral passage of clots or calculi, and renal failure.

DIAGNOSIS

These tests aid diagnosis of polycystic kidney disease: excretory or retrograde urography (which shows enlarged kidneys, with elongation of the pelvis, flattening of the calyces, and indentations in the kidney caused by cysts); ultrasonography, tomography, and radioisotope scans (which show kidney enlargement and cysts); tomography, computed tomography, and magnetic resonance imaging (which show multiple areas of cystic damage); and urinalysis and creatinine clearance tests (which show nonspecific results indicating abnormalities). In the neonate, excretory urography shows poor excretion of contrast medium.

TREATMENT

Treatment for patients with polycystic kidney disease includes adequate hydration for maintaining fluid balance, antibiotics for infections, and surgical drainage of cystic abscesses or retroperitoneal bleeding, or surgery for intractable pain (uncommon symptom). Analgesics may also be prescribed for abdominal pain.

Progressive renal failure is treated with dialysis or kidney transplantation. Polycystic kidney disease occurs bilaterally, and the infection could recur in the remaining kidney. For this reason, nephrectomy is not a recommended treatment.

NURSING CONSIDERATIONS

Because polycystic kidney disease is usually relentlessly progressive, comprehensive patient teaching and emotional support are essential.
+ Refer the young adult patient or the parents of infants with polycystic kidney disease for genetic counseling. Parents will probably have many questions about the risk to other offspring.

✦ Provide supportive care to minimize any associated symptoms. Carefully assess the patient's lifestyle and his physical and mental status; determine how rapidly the disease is progressing. Use this information to plan individualized patient care.

✦ Acquaint yourself with all aspects of end-stage renal disease, including dialysis and transplantation, so you can provide appropriate care and patient teaching as the disease progresses.

✦ Explain all diagnostic procedures to the patient, or to his family if the patient is an infant. Before beginning excretory urography or other procedures that use an iodine-based contrast medium, determine whether the patient has ever had an allergic reaction to iodine or shellfish. Even if the patient has no history of allergy, watch him for an allergic reaction during and after undergoing the procedures.

✦ Administer antibiotics as ordered for urinary tract infection. Stress to the patient the need to take the medication exactly as prescribed, even if symptoms are minimal or absent.

RENAL CALCULI

Renal calculi, or stones (nephrolithiasis), can form anywhere in the urinary tract, although they most commonly develop on the renal pelves or calyces. They may vary in size and may be solitary or multiple. (See *Renal calculi,* page 550.)

Renal calculi are more common in men than in women and rarely occur in children. Calcium calculi generally occur in middle-age men with a familial history of calculus formation.

Renal calculi rarely occur in blacks. They're prevalent in certain geographic areas, such as the southeastern United States (called the *stone belt*), possibly because a hot climate promotes dehydration and concentrates calculus-forming substances, or because of regional dietary habits.

CAUSES

Although the exact cause of renal calculi is unknown, predisposing factors include dehydration, infection, and changes in urine pH (calcium carbonate calculi, high pH; uric acid calculi, lower pH). Other possible causes are obstruction to urine flow (which leads to stasis in the urinary tract), immobilization (which causes calcium to be released into the blood, and the blood is filtered by the kidneys), metabolic factors, dietary factors, renal disease, and gout (a disease of increased uric acid production or decreased excretion).

PATHOPHYSIOLOGY

The major types of renal calculi are calcium oxalate and calcium phosphate, accounting for 75% to 80% of calculi; struvite (magnesium, ammonium, and phosphate), 15%; and uric acid, 7%. Cystine calculi are relatively rare, making up 1% of all renal calculi.

Calculi form when substances that are normally dissolved in the urine, such as calcium oxalate and calcium phosphate, precipitate. Dehydration may lead to renal calculi as calculus-forming substances concentrate in urine.

Calculi form around a nucleus or nidus in the appropriate environment. A crystal evolves in the presence of calculus-forming substances (calcium oxalate, calcium carbonate, magnesium, ammonium, phosphate, or uric acid) and becomes trapped

Key nursing actions
✦ Provide patient teaching and emotional support.
✦ Refer the young adult patient or the parents of infants with polycystic kidney disease for genetic counseling.
✦ Explain all diagnostic procedures to the patient or to his family if the patient is an infant.
✦ Even if the patient has no history of allergy, watch him for an allergic reaction during and after undergoing the procedures.

Characteristics of renal calculi
✦ Stones or nephrolithiasis
✦ Commonly develop on renal pelves or calyces
✦ May be solitary or multiple
✦ More common in men; rarely occur in children or in blacks
✦ Prevalent in certain geographic areas

Causes
✦ Exact cause unknown
✦ Predisposing factors: dehydration, infection, changes in urine pH
✦ Possible causes: obstruction to urine flow, immobilization, metabolism, diet, renal disease, gout

How it happens
✦ Calculi form when substances that are normally dissolved in urine precipitate
✦ Dehydration may lead to calculi
✦ Calculi form around nucleus or nidus

CLOSER LOOK

Renal calculi

Renal calculi vary in size and type. Small calculi may remain in the renal pelvis or pass down the ureter. A staghorn calculus (a cast of the calyceal and pelvic collecting system) may develop from a calculus that stays in the kidney.

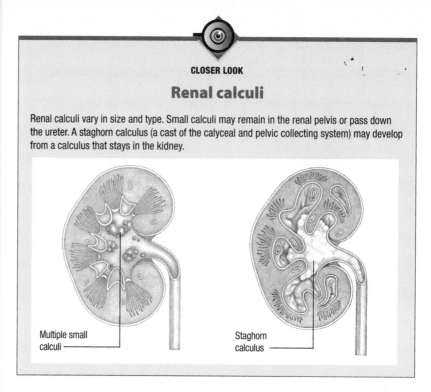

Multiple small calculi

Staghorn calculus

How it happens
(continued)

+ Crystal evolves in presence of forming substances; becomes trapped in urinary tract
+ Attracts other crystals to form calculus
+ Cacium calculi commonly occur with hyperuricuria
+ Struvite calculi are typically precipitated by an infection
+ Gout results in high uric acid production, hyperuricuria, and uric acid calculi

in the urinary tract, where it attracts other crystals to form a calculus. A high urine saturation of these substances encourages crystal formation and results in calculus growth.

Calculi may be composed of different substances, and the pH of the urine affects the solubility of many calculus-forming substances. Formation of calcium oxalate and cystine calculi is independent of urine pH.

Calculi may occur on the papillae, renal tubules, calyces, renal pelves, ureter, or bladder. Many calculi are less than 5 mm in diameter and are usually passed in the urine. Staghorn calculi can continue to grow in the pelvis, extending to the calyces, forming a branching calculus, and ultimately resulting in renal failure if not surgically removed.

Calcium calculi are the smallest. Most are calcium oxalate or a combination of oxalate and phosphate. Although 80% are idiopathic, they commonly occur with hyperuricuria (a high level of uric acid in the urine). Prolonged immobilization can lead to bone demineralization, hypercalciuria, and calculus formation. In addition, hyperparathyroidism, renal tubular acidosis, and excessive intake of vitamin D or dietary calcium may predispose to renal calculi.

Struvite calculi are typically precipitated by an infection, particularly with *Pseudomonas* or *Proteus* species. These urea-splitting organisms are more common in women. Struvite calculi can destroy renal parenchyma.

Gout results in a high uric acid production, hyperuricuria, and uric acid calculi. Diets high in purine (such as meat, fish, and poultry) elevate levels of uric acid in the body. Regional enteritis and ulcerative colitis can precipitate the formation of uric acid calculi. These diseases commonly result in fluid loss and loss of bicarbonate, leading to metabolic acidosis. Acidic urine enhances the formation of uric acid calculi.

Cystinuria is a rare hereditary disorder in which a metabolic error causes decreased tubular reabsorption of cystine. This causes an increased amount of cystine in the urine. Because cystine is a relatively insoluble substance, its presence contributes to calculus formation.

Infected, scarred tissue may be an ideal site for calculus development. In addition, infected calculi (usually magnesium ammonium phosphate or staghorn calculi) may develop if bacteria serve as the nucleus in calculus formation.

Urinary stasis allows calculus constituents to collect and adhere and encourages infection, which compounds the obstruction.

Calculi may either enter the ureter or remain in the renal pelvis, where they damage or destroy renal parenchyma and may cause pressure necrosis.

In ureters, calculi cause obstruction with resulting hydronephrosis, and they tend to recur. Intractable pain and serious bleeding also can result from calculi and the damage they cause. Large, rough calculi occlude the opening to the ureteropelvic junction and increase the frequency and force of peristaltic contractions, causing hematuria from trauma.

The patient usually reports pain traveling from the costovertebral angle to the flank and then to the suprapubic region and external genitalia (classic renal colic pain). Pain intensity fluctuates and may be excruciating at its peak. The patient with calculi in the renal pelvis and calyces may report a constant, dull pain. He may also report back pain if calculi are causing obstruction within a kidney and severe abdominal pain from calculi traveling down a ureter. Infection can develop in static urine or after trauma as the calculus abrades surfaces. If the calculus lodges and blocks urine, hydronephrosis can occur.

SIGNS AND SYMPTOMS

Possible signs and symptoms of renal calculi include nausea and vomiting and abdominal distention. Fever and chills occur because of infection. When the calculi abrade a ureter, the patient may experience hematuria. Obstruction causes severe pain, and bilateral obstruction of a patient's only kidney results in anuria.

COMPLICATIONS

Complications include damage or destruction of renal parenchyma, pressure necrosis, obstruction by the calculus, hydronephrosis, bleeding, pain, and infection.

DIAGNOSIS

These studies help diagnose renal calculi: kidney-ureter-bladder (KUB) radiography (which shows most renal calculi) and excretory urography (which helps confirm the diagnosis and determine the size and location of calculi). To detect obstructive changes, such as unilateral or bilateral hydronephrosis and radiolucent calculi not seen on KUB radiography, kidney ultrasonography is performed.

Other helpful studies are urine culture (which shows pyuria, a sign of urinary tract infection) and 24-hour urine collection (which is used to obtain calcium oxalate, phosphorus, and uric acid excretion levels). In addition, calculus analysis is performed to determine mineral content. Serial blood calcium and phosphorus levels diagnose hyperparathyroidism and increased calcium relative to normal serum protein. Blood protein levels determine the level of free calcium unbound to protein.

How it happens
(continued)

+ Infected, scarred tissue may be an ideal site for calculus development; infected calculi may develop if bacteria serve as the nucleus in calculus formation
+ Urinary stasis allows calculus constituents to collect and adhere and encourages infection, which compounds the obstruction
+ Calculi may either enter the ureter or remain in the renal pelvis, where they damage or destroy renal parenchyma and may cause pressure necrosis

Key signs and symptoms

+ Nausea, vomiting, abdominal distention
+ Fever
+ Hematuria

Complications

+ Damage or destruction of renal parenchyma
+ Pressure necrosis
+ Obstruction by calculus

Diagnosis

+ KUB radiography shows most renal calculi
+ Excretory urography confirms diagnosis, determines size and location
+ Kidney ultrasonography
+ Urine culture shows pyuria
+ Calculus analysis to determine mineral content
+ Serial blood calcium and phosphorus levels
+ Blood protein levels to determine free calcium unbound to protein

Treatment

+ Increase fluid intake
+ Antimicrobial agents
+ Analgesics
+ Diuretics
+ Maintain a low-calcium diet

Key nursing actions

+ To aid diagnosis, maintain a 24- to 48-hour record of urine pH, with Nitrazine paper.
+ Strain all urine through gauze or a tea strainer, and save all solid material recovered for analysis.
+ Encourage the patient to walk and promote sufficient intake of fluids.
+ Stress the importance of proper diet and compliance with drug therapy.
+ After surgery, expect bloody drainage from the catheter.
+ Never irrigate the catheter without a physician's order.

TREATMENT

Treatment for renal calculi includes several options: The patient's fluid intake is increased to more than 3 qt/day (3 L) to promote hydration, and antimicrobial agents, which vary with the cultured organism, are prescribed to treat infection. For pain, analgesics such as meperidine (Demerol) or morphine are administered. Diuretics are used to prevent urinary stasis and further calculus formation; thiazides are given to decrease calcium excretion into the urine. When infection is present, methenamine is used to suppress calculus formation.

To help prevent recurrence, treatment is typically as follows: The patient is advised to maintain a low-calcium diet. Oxalate-binding cholestyramine is given for absorptive hypercalciuria, and parathyroidectomy is performed to treat hyperparathyroidism. Uric acid calculi are treated with allopurinol (Zyloprim), and daily small doses of ascorbic acid are prescribed to acidify urine.

Renal calculi themselves may be removed in one of several ways. Calculi too large for natural passage are manipulated and removed in cystoscopy. Percutaneous ultrasonic lithotripsy, for example, and extracorporeal shock wave lithotripsy or laser therapy are used to shatter the calculus into fragments for removal by suction or natural passage. Obstruction is relieved through surgical removal of cystine calculi or large calculi or by placement of urinary diversion around the calculus.

NURSING CONSIDERATIONS

Patient care includes confirming the diagnosis, facilitating passage of the calculus, and helping to prevent future occurrences.

+ To aid diagnosis, maintain a 24- to 48-hour record of urine pH, with Nitrazine paper; strain all urine through gauze or a tea strainer, and save all solid material recovered for analysis.
+ To facilitate spontaneous passage of calculi, encourage the patient to walk, if possible. Also promote sufficient intake of fluids to maintain a urine output of 2 to 4 qt/day (2 to 4 L) (urine should be very dilute and colorless). To help acidify urine, offer fruit juices, particularly cranberry juice. If the patient can't drink the required amount of fluid, supplemental I.V. fluids may be given. Record intake and output and daily weight to assess fluid status and renal function.
+ Administer pain medication as needed and as ordered.
+ Stress the importance of proper diet and compliance with drug therapy. For example, if the patient's calculus is caused by a hyperuricemic condition, advise the patient or whoever prepares his meals which foods are high in purine.
+ If surgery is necessary, give reassurance by supplementing and reinforcing what the surgeon has told the patient about the procedure. The patient is apt to be fearful, especially if surgery includes removal of a kidney, so emphasize the fact that the body can adapt well to one kidney. If he is to have an abdominal or flank incision, teach deep-breathing and coughing exercises.
+ After surgery, the patient will probably have an indwelling catheter or a nephrostomy tube. Unless one of his kidneys was removed, expect bloody drainage from the catheter. Never irrigate the catheter without a physician's order. Check dressings regularly for bloody drainage, and know how much drainage to expect. Immediately report suspected hemorrhage (excessive drainage, rising pulse rate). Use sterile technique when changing dressings or providing catheter care.

✦ Watch for signs of infection (rising fever, chills), and give antibiotics as ordered. To prevent pneumonia, encourage frequent position changes, and ambulate the patient as soon as possible. Have him hold a small pillow over the operative site to splint the incision and thereby facilitate deep-breathing and coughing exercises.

✦ Before discharge, teach the patient and his family the importance of following the prescribed dietary and medication regimens to prevent recurrence of calculi. Encourage increased fluid intake. If appropriate, show the patient how to check his urine pH, and instruct him to keep a daily record. Tell him to immediately report symptoms of acute obstruction (pain, inability to void).

Key nursing actions
(continued)

✦ To prevent pneumonia, encourage frequent position changes, and ambulate the patient as soon as possible.

✦ Before discharge, teach the patient and his family the importance of following the prescribed dietary and medication regimens.

15

Integumentary system

Key facts about the integumentary system

◆ Largest and heaviest body system
◆ Includes skin, epidermal appendages, sebaceous, eccrine, apocrine glands
◆ Protects body against injury, microorganisms, substances
◆ Regulates body temperature
◆ Acts as reservoir for food, water

Skin

◆ Epidermis outermost layer; contains sensory receptors for pain, temperature, touch
◆ Dermis contains connective tissue, sebaceous glands
◆ Subcutaneous tissue beneath dermis; contains fat, sweat glands, hair follicles
◆ Skin color depends on four pigments: melanin, carotene, oxyhemoglobin, deoxyhemoglobin
◆ Each pigment unique in function, effect on skin

The integumentary system, the largest and heaviest body system, includes the skin—the integument, or external covering of the body—and the epidermal appendages, including the hair, nails, and sebaceous, eccrine, and apocrine glands. It protects the body against injury and invasion of microorganisms, harmful substances, and radiation; regulates body temperature; serves as a reservoir for food and water; and synthesizes vitamin D. Emotional well-being, including one's responses to the daily stresses of life, is reflected in the skin.

SKIN

The skin is composed of three layers: the epidermis, dermis, and subcutaneous tissues. The epidermis is the outermost layer. It's thin and contains sensory receptors for pain, temperature, touch, and vibration. The epidermal layer has no blood vessels and relies on the dermal layer for nutrition. The dermis contains connective tissue, the sebaceous glands, and some hair follicles. The subcutaneous tissue lies beneath the dermis; it contains fat and sweat glands and the rest of the hair follicles. The subcutaneous layer can store calories for future use in the body. (See *Close-up view of the skin.*)

Skin color depends on four pigments: melanin, carotene, oxyhemoglobin, and deoxyhemoglobin. Each pigment is unique in its function and effect on the skin. For example, melanin, the brownish pigment of the skin, is genetically determined, though it can be altered by sunlight exposure. Excessive dietary carotene causes a yellowing of the skin. Excessive oxyhemoglobin in the blood causes a reddening of the skin, and excessive deoxyhemoglobin causes a bluish discoloration.

Close-up view of the skin

The skin is composed of three major layers—the epidermis, the dermis, and the subcutaneous tissue. The epidermis consists of five strata, shown below. Subcutaneous tissue lying beneath the dermis consists of loose connective tissue that attaches the skin to underlying structures.

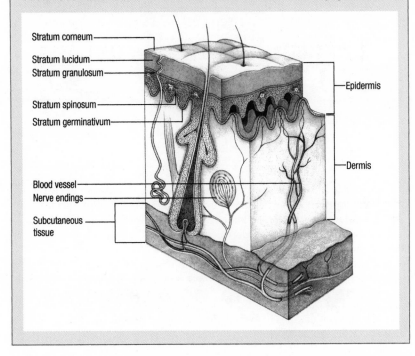

Stratum corneum
Stratum lucidum
Stratum granulosum
Stratum spinosum
Stratum germinativum
Blood vessel
Nerve endings
Subcutaneous tissue
Epidermis
Dermis

HAIR AND NAILS

The hair and nails are considered appendages of the skin. Both have protective functions in addition to their cosmetic appeal. For example, the cuticle of the nail functions as a seal, protecting the area between two portions of the nail from external hazards. (See *Nail structure*, page 556.)

GLANDS

The sebaceous glands, found on all areas of the skin except the palms and soles, produce sebum, a semifluid material composed of fat and epithelial cells. Sebum is secreted into the hair follicle and exits to the skin surface. It helps waterproof the hair and skin and promotes the absorption of fat-soluble substances into the dermis.

The eccrine glands produce sweat, an odorless, watery fluid. Glands in the palms and soles secrete sweat primarily in response to emotional stress. The other remaining eccrine glands respond mainly to thermal stress, effectively regulating temperature.

Hair and nails

+ Considered appendages of skin
+ Have protective functions, cosmetic appeal

Glands

Sebaceous glands

+ Found on all skin areas except palms and soles
+ Produce sebum
+ Secreted into hair follicle, exits to skin surface; helps waterproof hair and skin

Eccrine glands

+ Produce sweat
+ Some respond to emotional and thermal stress

Apocrine glands

+ Located mainly in axillary and anogenital areas
+ Have coiled secretory portion that lies deeper in the than eccrine glands
+ Begin to function at puberty, have no known biological function

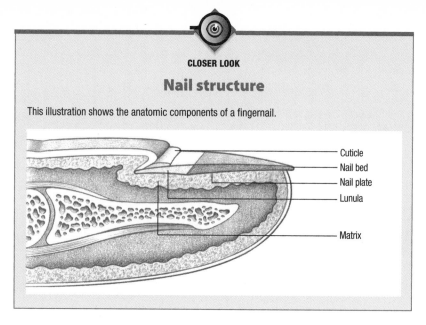

CLOSER LOOK

Nail structure

This illustration shows the anatomic components of a fingernail.

Cuticle
Nail bed
Nail plate
Lunula
Matrix

Located mainly in the axillary and anogenital areas, apocrine glands have a coiled secretory portion that lies deeper in the dermis than the eccrine glands. These glands begin to function at puberty and have no known biological function. Bacterial decomposition of the apocrine fluid produced by these glands causes body odor.

Pathophysiologic changes

◆ Inflammatory skin reaction
◆ Occurs with injury to skin
◆ Benficial, usually accompanied by some degree of discomfort
◆ Erythema, edema, warmth occur

Formation of lesions

◆ On previously healthy skin
◆ Response to disease or external irritation
◆ Classified by appearance
◆ Result from rupture, mechanical irritation, extension, invasion, or healing of primary lesions

PATHOPHYSIOLOGIC CHANGES

Clinical manifestations of skin dysfunction include the inflammatory reaction of the skin and the formation of lesions.

INFLAMMATORY REACTION OF THE SKIN

An inflammatory reaction occurs with injury to the skin. The reaction can only occur in living organisms. Although a beneficial response, it's usually accompanied by some degree of discomfort at the site. Irritation changes the epidermal structure and causes consequent increase of immunoglobulin E activity. Other classic signs of inflammatory skin responses are erythema, edema, and warmth, due to bioamines released from the granules of tissue mast cells and basophils.

FORMATION OF LESIONS

Primary skin lesions appear on previously healthy skin in response to disease or external irritation. They're classified by their appearance as macules, papules, plaques, patches, nodules, tumors, wheals, comedos, cysts, vesicles, pustules, or bullae. (See *Recognizing primary skin lesions.*)

Modified lesions are described as secondary skin lesions. These lesions occur as a result of rupture, mechanical irritation, extension, invasion, or normal or abnormal healing of primary lesions. These include atrophy, erosions, ulcers, scales, crusts, excoriation, fissures, lichenification, and scars. (See *Recognizing secondary skin lesions*, pages 559 and 560.)

Recognizing primary skin lesions

MACULE
Flat, pigmented, circumscribed area less than 1 cm in diameter (freckle, rubella)

PATCH
Flat, pigmented, circumscribed area more than 1 cm in diameter (herald patch [pityriasis rosea])

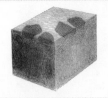

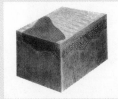

PAPULE
Firm, inflammatory, raised lesion up to 0.5 cm in diameter; may be the same color as skin or pigmented (acne papule, lichen planus)

NODULE
Firm, raised lesion; deeper than a papule, extending into dermal layer; 0.5 to 2 cm in diameter (intradermal nevus)

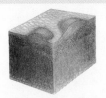

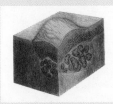

CYST
Semisolid or fluid-filled encapsulated mass extending deep into the dermis (sebaceous cyst, cystic acne)

TUMOR
Elevated solid lesion more than 2 cm in diameter, extending into dermal and subcutaneous layers (dermatofibroma)

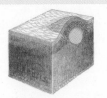

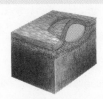

VESICLE
Raised, circumscribed, fluid-filled lesion less than 0.5 cm in diameter (chickenpox, herpes simplex)

COMEDO
Plugged pilosebaceous duct, exfoliative, formed from sebum and keratin (blackhead [open comedo], whitehead [closed comedo])

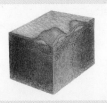

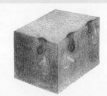

(continued)

Types of skin lesions
✦ Macule
✦ Patch
✦ Papule
✦ Nodule
✦ Cyst
✦ Tumor
✦ Vesicle
✦ Comedo
✦ Plaque
✦ Bulla
✦ Pustule
✦ Wheal

Recognizing primary skin lesions *(continued)*

PLAQUE
Circumscribed, solid, elevated lesion more than 1 cm in diameter; elevation above skin surface occupies larger surface area compared with height (psoriasis)

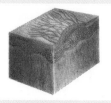

BULLA
Fluid-filled lesion more than 2 cm in diameter (also called a blister) (severe poison oak or ivy dermatitis, bullous pemphigoid, second-degree burn)

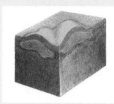

PUSTULE
Raised, circumscribed lesion usually less than 1 cm in diameter; contains purulent material, making it a yellow-white color (acne pustule, impetigo, furuncle)

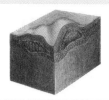

WHEAL
Raised, firm lesion with intense localized skin edema, varying in size and shape; color ranging from pale pink to red, disappears in hours (hive [urticaria], insect bite)

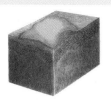

Characteristics of acne

+ Chronic inflammatory disease of sebaceous glands
+ Usually associated with high rate of sebum secretion
+ Occurs on areas of body with sebaceous glands
+ Two types of acne: inflammatory, noninflammatory
+ Severity and overall incidence usually greater in males
+ Tends to start earlier, last longer in females
+ Prognosis varies, depends on severity and underlying causes
+ Prognosis usually good with treatment

Alert!

+ Acne vulgaris develops in 80% to 90% of adolescents or young adults, primarily between ages 15 and 18.

ACNE

Acne is a chronic inflammatory disease of the sebaceous glands. It's usually associated with a high rate of sebum secretion and occurs on areas of the body that have sebaceous glands, such as the face, neck, chest, back, and shoulders. There are two types of acne: *inflammatory,* in which the hair follicle is blocked by sebum, causing bacteria to grow and eventually rupture the follicle; and *noninflammatory,* in which the follicle doesn't rupture but remains dilated.

 CLINICAL ALERT Acne occurs in both males and females. Acne vulgaris develops in 80% to 90% of adolescents or young adults, primarily between ages 15 and 18. Although the lesions can appear as early as age 8, acne primarily affects adolescents.

Although the severity and overall incidence of acne is usually greater in males, it tends to start at an earlier age and last longer in females.

The prognosis varies and depends on the severity and underlying causes; with treatment, the prognosis is usually good.

CLOSER LOOK

Recognizing secondary skin lesions

ATROPHY
Thinning of skin surface at site of disorder (striae, aging skin)

SCALE
Thin, dry flakes of shedding skin (psoriasis, dry skin, newborn desquamation)

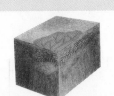

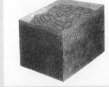

EROSION
Circumscribed lesion involving loss of superficial epidermis (rug burn, abrasion)

EXCORIATION
Linear, scratched or abraded areas, usually self-induced (abraded acne, eczema)

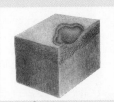

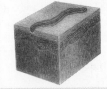

LICHENIFICATION
Thickened, prominent skin markings by constant rubbing (chronic atopic dermatitis)

FISSURE
Linear cracking of the skin extending into the dermal layer (hand dermatitis [chapped skin]

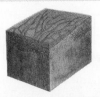

CRUST
Dried sebum, serous, sanguineous, or purulent exudate overlying an erosion or weeping vesicle, bulla, or pustule (impetigo)

ULCER
Epidermal and dermal destruction may extend into subcutaneous tissue; usually heals with scarring (pressure ulcer)

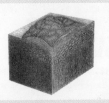

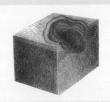

(continued)

Types of secondary skin lesions

✦ Atrophy
✦ Scale
✦ Erosion
✦ Excoriation
✦ Lichenification
✦ Fissure
✦ Crust
✦ Ulcer
✦ Scar

Causes

+ Multifactorial
+ Diet not believed to be precipitating factor
+ Increased activity of sebaceous glands
+ Blockage of pilosebaceous ducts
+ Heredity
+ Certain drugs
+ Emotional stress
+ Hormonal contraceptive use

How it happens

+ Androgens stimulate sebaceous gland growth
+ Sebum secreted into dilated hair follicles containing bacteria
+ Bacteria secrete lipase; interacts with sebum to produce free fatty acids, which provoke inflammation
+ Hair follicles produce keratin, joins with sebum to form plug in dilated follicle

Key signs and symptoms

+ Plug may appear as whitehead or blackhead
+ Rupture or leakage of enlarged plug into epidermis produces inflammation, pustules, papules
+ Cysts or abscesses in severe cases
+ Increased severity just before or during menstruation in women

Complications

+ Acne conglobata
+ Scarring
+ Impaired self-esteem
+ Abscesses or secondary bacterial infections

Recognizing secondary skin lesions *(continued)*

SCAR
Fibrous tissue caused by trauma, deep inflammation, or surgical incision; red and raised (recent), pink and flat (6 weeks), and depressed (old) (on a healed surgical incision)

CAUSES

The cause of acne is multifactorial. Diet isn't believed to be a precipitating factor. Possible causes of acne include increased activity of the sebaceous glands and blockage of the pilosebaceous ducts (hair follicles).

Factors that may predispose someone to acne include heredity, androgen stimulation, certain drugs (including corticosteroids, corticotropin [ACTH], androgens, iodides, bromides, trimethadione, phenytoin [Dilantin], isoniazid [Laniazid], lithium [Eskalith], and halothane), cobalt irradiation, hyperalimentation, trauma or rubbing from tight clothing, cosmetics, emotional stress, tropical climate, hormonal contraceptive use, and exposure to heavy oils, greases, or tars. (Many females experience acne flare-up during their first few menses after starting or discontinuing hormonal contraceptives.)

PATHOPHYSIOLOGY

Androgens stimulate sebaceous gland growth and the production of sebum, which is secreted into dilated hair follicles that contain bacteria. The bacteria, usually *Propionibacterium acnes* and *Staphylococcus epidermis,* are normal skin flora that secrete lipase. This enzyme interacts with sebum to produce free fatty acids, which provoke inflammation. Hair follicles also produce more keratin, which joins with the sebum to form a plug in the dilated follicle.

SIGNS AND SYMPTOMS

The acne plug may appear as a closed comedo, or whitehead (not protruding from the follicle and covered by the epidermis), or an open comedo, or blackhead (protruding from the follicle and not covered by the epidermis; melanin or pigment of the follicle causes the black color).

The rupture or leakage of an enlarged plug into the epidermis produces inflammation, characteristic acne pustules, and papules. In severe forms, acne cysts or abscesses (chronic, recurring lesions producing acne scars) occur.

In women, signs and symptoms may include increased severity just before or during menstruation, when estrogen levels are at their lowest.

COMPLICATIONS

Complications of acne may include acne conglobata, scarring (when acne is severe), impaired self-esteem, and abscesses or secondary bacterial infections.

DIAGNOSIS

Characteristic acne lesions, especially in adolescents, confirm diagnosis of acne vulgaris.

TREATMENT

Topical treatments of acne include the application of antibacterial agents, such as benzoyl peroxide (Benzac 5 or 10), clindamycin (Cleocin), or benzoyl peroxide plus erythromycin (Benzamycin) antibacterial agents. These may be applied alone or with tretinoin (Retin-A; retinoic acid), which is a keratolytic. Keratolytic agents, such as benzoyl peroxide and tretinoin, dry and peel the skin in order to help open blocked follicles, moving the sebum up to the skin level.

Systemic therapy may also be used. Antibiotics, usually tetracycline, are prescribed to decrease bacterial growth. Dosage is reduced for long-term maintenance when the patient is in remission. A culture is obtained to identify a possible secondary bacterial infection. (Look for exacerbation of pustules or abscesses while on tetracycline or erythromycin drug therapy.)

Oral isotretinoin (Accutane), another systemic therapy, inhibits sebaceous gland function and keratinization. (A 16- to 20-week course of isotretinoin is limited to patients with severe papulopustular or cystic acne not responding to conventional therapy; isotretinoin has severe adverse effects. Because this drug is known to cause birth defects, the manufacturer, with Food and Drug Administration approval, recommends these precautions: pregnancy testing before dispensing; dispensing only a 30-day supply; repeat pregnancy testing throughout treatment period; effective contraception during treatment; and informed consent. Because of its effects on the liver, a serum triglyceride level should be drawn before and periodically during treatment.)

For some females, birth control pills, such as norgestimate/ethinyl estradiol (Ortho Tri-Cyclen) or spironolactone may be prescribed. These are antiandrogens.

Other treatments may include the following: To dislodge superficial comedones, the patient should clean with an abrasive sponge. To remove comedones and to open and drain pustules, surgery may be performed (usually on an outpatient basis). For severe acne scarring, dermabrasion with a high-speed metal brush to smooth the skin is performed by a well-trained dermatologist or plastic surgeon. Bovine collagen injections into the dermis beneath the scarred area may be used to fill in affected areas and even out the skin surface. (This procedure isn't recommended by all dermatologists.)

NURSING CONSIDERATIONS

The main focus of care should be teaching about the disorder as well as its treatment and prevention.

✦ Check the patient's drug history because certain medications, such as hormonal contraceptives, may cause an acne flare-up.

✦ Try to identify predisposing factors that may be eliminated or modified.

✦ Try to identify eruption patterns (seasonal or monthly).

✦ Explain the causes of acne to the patient and his family. Make sure they understand that the prescribed treatment is more likely to improve acne than will a strict diet and fanatical scrubbing with soap and water. Provide written instructions regarding treatment.

✦ Describe the importance of not picking lesions and of practicing good personal hygiene in order to prevent secondary infections.

Diagnosis
✦ Characteristic acne lesions

Treatment
✦ Antibacterial agents
✦ Keratolytic agents
✦ Antibiotics
✦ Oral isotretinoin
✦ Birth control pills (for females)
✦ Good skin care
✦ Dermabrasion
✦ Bovine collagen injections

Key nursing actions
✦ Check the patient's drug history.
✦ Try to identify predisposing factors that may be eliminated or modified.
✦ Try to identify eruption patterns.
✦ Explain the causes of acne to the patient and his family.
✦ Describe the importance of not picking lesions and of practicing good personal hygiene in order to prevent secondary infections.

Key nursing actions
(continued)

✦ Instruct the patient receiving tretinoin to apply it at least 30 minutes after washing his face and at least 1 hour before bedtime.

✦ Instruct the patient to take tetracycline on an empty stomach and not to take it with antacids or milk.

✦ Tell the female patient about the severe risk of teratogenicity.

✦ Inform the patient that acne takes a long time to clear.

✦ Pay special attention to the patient's perception of his physical appearance, and offer emotional support.

Characteristics of burns

✦ Classified as first-degree, second-degree superficial partial thickness, second-degree deep partial thickness, third-degree full thickness, fourth degree.

✦ First-degree: limited to epidermis

✦ Second-degree: epidermis and part of dermis are damaged

✦ Third-degree: damages epidermis and dermis; vessels and tissue visible

✦ Fourth-degree: damage extends through deeply charred subcutaneous tissue to muscle, bone

✦ Major burns require painful treatment, a long rehabilitation

Causes

✦ Residential fires
✦ Automobile accidents
✦ Matches
✦ Improper handling of firecrackers or gasoline

✦ Instruct the patient receiving tretinoin to apply it at least 30 minutes after washing his face and at least 1 hour before bedtime. Warn against using it around the eyes or lips. After treatments, the skin should look pink and dry. If it appears red or starts to peel, the preparation may have to be weakened or applied less often. Advise the patient to avoid exposure to sunlight or to use a sunscreening agent. If the prescribed regimen includes tretinoin and benzoyl peroxide, avoid skin irritation by using one preparation in the morning and the other at night.

✦ Instruct the patient to take tetracycline on an empty stomach and not to take it with antacids or milk because it interacts with their metallic ions and is then poorly absorbed.

✦ Tell the patient who is taking isotretinoin to avoid vitamin A supplements, which can worsen any adverse effects. Also, teach the patient how to deal with the dry skin and mucous membranes that usually occur during treatment. Tell the female patient about the severe risk of teratogenicity. Monitor liver function and lipid levels.

✦ Inform the patient that acne takes a long time to clear — even years for complete resolution. Encourage continued local skin care even after acne clears. Explain the adverse effects of all drugs.

✦ Pay special attention to the patient's perception of his physical appearance, and offer emotional support.

BURNS

Burns are classified as first-degree, second-degree superficial partial thickness, second-degree deep partial thickness, third-degree full thickness, and fourth degree. A first-degree burn is limited to the epidermis. The most common example of a first-degree burn is sunburn, which results from exposure to the sun. In a second-degree burn, the epidermis and part of the dermis are damaged. A third-degree burn damages the epidermis and dermis, and vessels and tissue are visible. In fourth-degree burns, the damage extends through deeply charred subcutaneous tissue to muscle and bone. A major burn is a horrifying injury that requires painful treatment and a long period of rehabilitation.

Each year in the United States, about 2 million persons receive burn injuries. Of these, 300,000 are burned seriously, and more than 6,000 die, making burns this nation's third leading cause of accidental death. About 60,000 people are hospitalized each year for burns. Most significant burns occur in the home; home fires account for the highest burn fatality rate.

In victims younger than age 4 and older than age 60, a higher incidence of complications, and thus a higher mortality rate, exists. Immediate, aggressive burn treatment increases the patient's chance of survival. Later, supportive measures and strict sterile technique can minimize infection. Meticulous, comprehensive burn care can make the difference between life and death. Survival and recovery from a major burn are more likely once the burn wound is reduced to less than 20% of the total body surface area (BSA).

CAUSES

Thermal burns, the most common type, typically result from residential fires, automobile accidents, playing with matches, improper handling of firecrackers, improper handling of gasoline, scalding accidents and kitchen accidents (such as a child climbing on top of a stove or grabbing a hot iron), abuse (in children or elderly persons), and clothes that have caught on fire.

Chemical burns result from contact, ingestion, inhalation, or injection of acids, alkalis, or vesicants.

Electrical burns usually result from contact with faulty electrical wiring or high-voltage power lines. Sometimes young children chew electrical cords.

Friction or abrasion burns occur when the skin rubs harshly against a coarse surface.

Excessive exposure to sunlight causes sunburns.

PATHOPHYSIOLOGY

The injuring agent denatures cellular proteins. Some cells die because of traumatic or ischemic necrosis. Loss of collagen cross-linking also occurs with denaturation, creating abnormal osmotic and hydrostatic pressure gradients, which cause the movement of intravascular fluid into interstitial spaces. Cellular injury triggers the release of mediators of inflammation, contributing to local and, in the case of major burns, systemic increases in capillary permeability. Specific pathophysiologic events depend on the cause and classification of the burn. (See *Classifications of burns*.)

First-degree burns

A first-degree burn causes localized injury or destruction to the skin (epidermis only) by direct contact (such as a chemical spill) or indirect contact (such as sunlight). The barrier function of the skin remains intact, and these burns aren't life threatening.

Second-degree superficial partial-thickness burns

These burns involve destruction to the epidermis and some dermis. Thin-walled, fluid-filled blisters develop within a few minutes of the injury. As these blisters break, the nerve endings become exposed to the air. Because pain and tactile re-

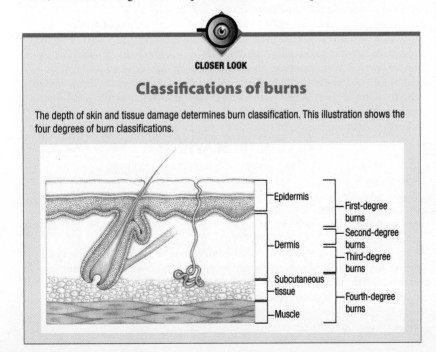

CLOSER LOOK

Classifications of burns

The depth of skin and tissue damage determines burn classification. This illustration shows the four degrees of burn classifications.

Epidermis — First-degree burns
Dermis — Second-degree burns
— Third-degree burns
Subcutaneous tissue
Muscle — Fourth-degree burns

Causes

Chemical burns
+ Contact
+ Ingestion
+ Inhalation

Electrical burns
+ Contact with faulty wiring, high-voltage lines

Friction or abrasion burns
+ Skin rubs harshly against coarse surface

Sunburns
+ Excessive sunlight exposure

How it happens

+ Injuring agent denatures cellular proteins
+ Some cells die of traumatic or ischemic necrosis
+ Abnormal osmotic or hydrostatic pressure gradients from denaturing
+ Intravascular fluid moves into interstitial spaces
+ Cellular injury leads to inflammation
+ Pathophysiologic events depend on burn cause and classification

First-degree burns
+ Causes localized injury or destruction to skin
+ Direct or indirect contact
+ Barrier function of skin remains intact

Second-degree superficial partial-thickness burns
+ Destruction to epidermis and some dermis
+ Fluid-filled blisters develop within minutes
+ Blisters break; nerve endings exposed to air
+ Pain and tactile responses intact, subsequent treatments painful
+ Barrier function of skin lost

How it happens

Second-degree deep partial-thickness burns
- Destruction of epidermis and dermis, blisters, mild to moderate edema, pain
- Hair follicles still intact
- Barrier function of skin lost

Third- and fourth-degree burns
- Affects every body system
- Extends through epidermis, dermis into subcutaneous tissue
- Fourth-degree burn involves muscle, bone, interstitial tissues
- Fluids shift to interstitial spaces within hours
- Immunologic response makes wound sepsis potential threat

Key signs and symptoms

First-degree
- Localized pain and erythema
- Chills, headache, localized edema, nausea and vomiting

Second-degree superficial partial-thickness
- Blisters
- Mild to moderate edema and pain

Second-degree deep partial-thickness
- White, waxy appearance

Third-degree
- White, brown, leathery tissue
- Visible thrombosed vessels
- Silver-colored, raised area is a sign of an electrical burn

Complications
- Total occlusion of circulation in extremity
- Restricted respiratory expansion
- Infection

sponses remain intact, subsequent treatments are very painful. The barrier function of the skin is lost.

Second-degree deep partial-thickness burns
These burns involve destruction of the epidermis and dermis, producing blisters and mild to moderate edema and pain. The hair follicles are still intact, so hair will grow again. Compared with second-degree superficial partial-thickness burns, less pain sensation exists with this burn because the sensory neurons have undergone extensive destruction. The areas around the burn injury remain very sensitive to pain. The barrier function of the skin is lost.

Third- and fourth-degree burns
A major burn affects every body system and organ. A third-degree burn extends through the epidermis and dermis and into the subcutaneous tissue layer. A fourth-degree burn involves muscle, bone, and interstitial tissues. Within only hours, fluids and protein shift from capillary to interstitial spaces, causing edema. An immediate immunologic response to a burn injury occurs, making burn wound sepsis a potential threat. Finally, an increase in calorie demand after a burn injury increases the metabolic rate.

SIGNS AND SYMPTOMS
Signs and symptoms depend on the type of burn.

In a first-degree burn, localized pain and erythema, usually without blisters, occurs in the first 24 hours. In many severe first-degree burns, the patient may experience chills, headache, localized edema, and nausea and vomiting.

In a second-degree superficial partial-thickness burn, thin-walled, fluid-filled blisters appear within minutes of the injury. The patient may have mild to moderate edema and pain. In second-degree deep partial-thickness burn, a white, waxy appearance is evident in the damaged area.

In a third-degree burn, white, brown, or black leathery tissue and visible thrombosed vessels occur as a result of destruction of skin elasticity (the dorsum of the hand is the most common site of thrombosed veins). There are no blisters in third-degree burns. A silver-colored, raised area, usually at the site of an electrical contact, is a sign of an electrical burn. In a fire, smoke inhalation and pulmonary damage cause singed nasal hairs, mucosal burns, voice changes, coughing, wheezing, soot in the mouth or nose, and darkened sputum.

COMPLICATIONS
Burns have many complications. For example, burns to face, hands, feet, and genitalia can cause loss of function. Edema from circumferential burns can result in total occlusion of circulation in an extremity, and neck burns can cause airway obstruction. Chest burns can cause restricted respiratory expansion, pulmonary injury from smoke inhalation or pulmonary embolism, and adult respiratory distress syndrome by left-sided heart failure or myocardial infarction.

In electrical and chemical burns, the damage may be greater than indicated by the surface burn, and there may be internal tissue damage along the conduction pathway in electrical burns. Electrical shock and fluid shifts cause cardiac arrhythmias and shock or hypovolemia. Burn wounds may become infected.

After burns, blood flow is slower and results in the formation of blood clots, which, in turn, causes stroke, heart attack, or pulmonary embolism. Burn shock is the result of fluid shifts out of the vascular compartments; it may lead to kidney damage and renal failure.

Decreased blood supply in the abdominal area causes peptic ulcer disease. In more severe burn sites, the patient may experience disseminated intravascular coagulation. Finally, with the psychological component of disfigurement, the patient experiences added pain, depression, and financial burden.

DIAGNOSIS

Diagnosis involves determining the size and classifying the wound.

Size is estimated in one of two ways: by using the Rule of Nines chart to arrive at the percentage of BSA covered by the burn or by using the Lund-Browder chart (more accurate because it allows BSA changes with age) to correlate the burn's depth and size to estimate its severity. (See *Using the Rule of Nines and the Lund-Browder chart,* pages 566 and 567.)

Major burns are classified as third-degree burns over more than 10% of BSA; second-degree burns over more than 25% of adult BSA (over 20% in children); burns of hands, face, feet, or genitalia; burns complicated by fractures or respiratory damage; electrical burns; and all burns in poor-risk patients.

Moderate burns are classified as third-degree burns over 2% to 10% of BSA, and second-degree burns over 15% to 25% of adult BSA (10% to 20% in children).

Minor burns are classified as third-degree burns over less than 2% of BSA, and second-degree burns over less than 15% of adult BSA (10% in children).

TREATMENT

Initial burn treatments are based on the type of burn.

Minor burns are treated by immersing the burned area in cool water (55° F [12.8° C]) or applying cool compresses. Pain medication or anti-inflammatory medications are administered as needed. After debridement, the area is covered with an antimicrobial agent and a nonstick bulky dressing. Prophylactic tetanus injections are provided as needed.

Hypoxia is prevented by maintaining an open airway and assessing airway, breathing, and circulation. The patient is checked for smoke inhalation immediately on receipt, and endotracheal intubation with 100% oxygen may be started as the first immediate treatment for moderate and major burns.

Smoldering clothing is removed by soaking it in a saline solution. In addition, any clothing stuck to the patient's skin, any rings, and any other constricting items are removed. Any active bleeding is adequately controlled.

Partial-thickness burns that are over 30% of BSA or full-thickness burns that are over 5% of BSA are covered with a clean, dry, sterile bed sheet. Large burns are covered with saline-soaked dressings because of the possibility of a drastic reduction in body temperature.

To prevent hypovolemic shock and maintain cardiac output, I.V. therapy is started immediately. Lactated Ringer's solution or a fluid replacement formula, and additional I.V. lines, may be used. In addition, all patients with major burns receive antimicrobial therapy.

To help determine additional treatments, various studies are done: A complete blood count and electrolytes, glucose, blood urea nitrogen, and serum creatinine level are obtained and monitored closely. Arterial blood gas analysis, typing and cross-matching, and urinalysis for myoglobinuria and hemoglobinuria are performed.

Diagnosis

+ Size: Rule of Nines chart, Lund-Browder chart to correlate depth and severity
+ Third-degree burns: > 10% of BSA
+ Second-degree burns: > 25% of adult BSA; hands, face, feet, genitalia; complicated by fractures or respiratory damage; electrical; poor-risk patients
+ Moderate (third-degree): > 2% to 10% of BSA; second-degree over 15% to 25% of adult BSA
+ Minor (third-degree): < 2% of BSA; second-degree < 15% of adult BSA

Treatment

+ Minor burns: immersion in cool water; use of cool compresses
+ Anti-inflammatory medications
+ Debridement
+ Antimicrobial agent
+ Prophylactic tetanus injections
+ Maintain airway, breathing, circulation
+ Endotracheal intubation with 100% oxygen for moderate and major burns
+ Bleeding control
+ Appropriate dressing for type of burn

Using the Rule of Nines and the Lund-Browder chart

You can quickly estimate the extent of an adult patient's burn by using the Rule of Nines. This method divides an adult's body surface area into percentages. To use this method, mentally transfer your patient's burns to the body chart shown below; then add up the corresponding percentages for each burned body section. The total, an estimate of the extent of your patient's burn, enters into the formula to determine his initial fluid replacement needs.

You can't use the Rule of Nines for infants and children because their body section percentages differ from those of adults. For example, an infant's head accounts for about 17% at the total body surface area compared with 7% for an adult. Instead, use the Lund-Browder chart.

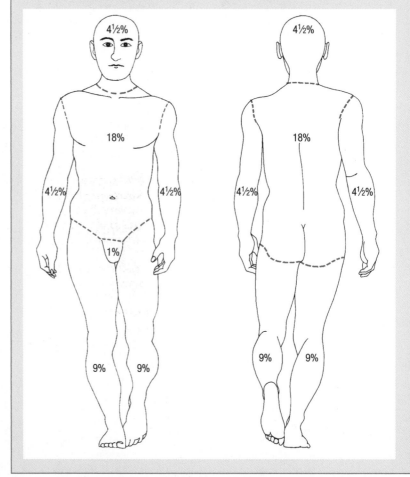

Intake and output are also closely monitored, and vital signs are checked frequently (every 15 minutes). If necessary to accurately track intake and output, an indwelling urinary catheter is used; to decompress the stomach and avoid aspiration of stomach contents, a nasogastric tube may be inserted. Copious amounts of normal saline solution are used to irrigate wounds from a chemical burn. Skin grafts and more thorough surgical cleaning may be performed on major burns.

LUND-BROWDER CHART

To determine the extent of an infant's or child's burns, use the Lund-Browder chart shown here.

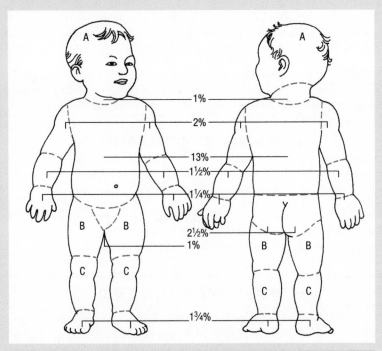

RELATIVE PERCENTAGES OF AREAS AFFECTED BY GROWTH

	At birth	0 to 1 yr	1 to 4 yrs	5 to 9 yrs	10 to 15 yrs	Adult
A: Half of head						
	9½%	8½%	6½%	5½%	4½%	3½%
B: Half of thigh						
	2¾%	3¼%	4%	4¼%	4½%	4¾%
C: Half of leg						
	2½%	2½%	2¾%	3%	3¼%	3½%

NURSING CONSIDERATIONS

✦ Don't treat the burn wound of a patient who will be transferred to a specialty facility within 4 hours. Wrap the patient in a sterile sheet and blanket for warmth, elevate the burned extremity, and prepare the patient for transport.

Key nursing actions

✦ Don't treat the burn wound of a patient who will be transferred to a specialty facility within 4 hours.

✦ Wrap the patient in a sterile sheet and blanket for warmth, elevate the burned extremity, and prepare the patient for transport.

Key nursing actions

Upon discharge or during prolonged care
+ Ensure increased caloric intake because of increased metabolic rate.
+ Stress the importance of keeping the dressing clean and dry and elevating the burned extremity for the first 24 hours.

Characteristics of dermatitis

+ Inflammation of skin
+ Atopic, seborrheic, nummular, contact, chronic, localized neurodermatitis, exfoliative, stasis

Key nursing actions

+ Warn the patient that drowsiness is possible with the use of antihistamines.
+ Suggest methods for inducing natural sleep to prevent overuse of sedatives.

Pressure ulcers

+ Also called *pressure sores*
+ Localized cellular necrosis
+ Occur most often in skin and subcutaneous tissue over bony prominences
+ Deep lesions commonly undetected until skin penetration
+ Usually develop over sacral area, greater trochanter, ischial tuberosity, heel, lateral malleolus
+ Partial-thickness ulcers involve dermis, epidermis
+ Wounds heal within weeks with treatment

Alert!

+ Age also has a role in the incidence of pressure ulcers.

Upon discharge or during prolonged care
+ To promote healing and recovery, ensure increased caloric intake because of increased metabolic rate.
+ Teach the patient and give complete discharge instructions for home care; stress the importance of keeping the dressing clean and dry, elevating the burned extremity for the first 24 hours, and having the wound rechecked in 1 to 2 days. Also stress the importance of taking pain medication as needed, especially before dressing changes.

DERMATITIS

Dermatitis is an inflammation of the skin that occurs in several forms: atopic, seborrheic, nummular, contact, chronic, localized neurodermatitis (lichen simplex chronicus), exfoliative, and stasis. (See *Types of dermatitis,* pages 570 to 573.)

NURSING CONSIDERATIONS

+ Warn the patient that drowsiness is possible with the use of antihistamines to relieve daytime itching. If nocturnal itching interferes with sleep, suggest methods for inducing natural sleep, such as drinking a glass of warm milk, to prevent overuse of sedatives.
+ Assist the patient in scheduling daily skin care. Keep his fingernails short to limit excoriation and secondary infections caused by scratching.
+ Apply cool, moist compresses to relieve itching and burning.

PRESSURE ULCERS

Pressure ulcers, commonly called *pressure sores* or *bedsores,* are localized areas of cellular necrosis that occur most often in the skin and subcutaneous tissue over bony prominences. These ulcers may be superficial, caused by local skin irritation with subsequent surface maceration, or deep, originating in underlying tissue. Deep lesions commonly go undetected until they penetrate the skin, but by then, they have usually caused subcutaneous damage. (See *Staging pressure ulcers,* pages 574 and 575.)

Most pressure ulcers develop over five body locations: sacral area, greater trochanter, ischial tuberosity, heel, and lateral malleolus. Collectively, these areas account for 95% of all pressure ulcer sites. Patients who have contractures are at increased risk for developing pressure ulcers because of the added pressure on the tissue and the alignment of the bones.

 CLINICAL ALERT Age also has a role in the incidence of pressure ulcers. Muscle is lost with aging, and skin elasticity decreases. Both of these factors increase the risk of developing pressure ulcers.

Partial-thickness ulcers usually involve the dermis and epidermis; with treatment, these wounds heal within a few weeks. Full-thickness ulcers also involve the dermis and epidermis, but in these wounds, the damage is more severe and complete. There may also be damage to the deeper tissue layers. Ulcers of the subcutaneous tissue and muscle may require several months to heal. If the damage has affected the bone in addition to the skin layers, osteomyelitis may occur, which will prolong healing time.

CAUSES

Possible causes of pressure ulcers include immobility and a decreased level of activity, friction or shearing forces causing damage to the epidermal and upper dermal skin layers, constant moisture on the skin causing tissue maceration, and impaired hygiene status, such as with urinary or fecal incontinence, leading to skin breakdown. Other causes are malnutrition (associated with pressure ulcer development), medical conditions such as diabetes, and orthopedic injuries (which may predispose the patient to pressure ulcer development). In some cases, psychological factors, such as depression and chronic emotional stresses, may have a role in pressure ulcer development.

PATHOPHYSIOLOGY

A pressure ulcer is caused by an injury to the skin and its underlying tissues. The pressure exerted on the area causes ischemia and hypoxemia to the affected tissues because of decreased blood flow to the site. As the capillaries collapse, thrombosis occurs, which subsequently leads to tissue edema and progression to tissue necrosis. Ischemia also adds to an accumulation of waste products at the site, which in turn leads to the production of toxins. The toxins further break down the tissue and eventually lead to the death of the cells.

SIGNS AND SYMPTOMS

The first clinical sign of a pressure ulcer is blanching erythema, varying from pink to bright red depending on the patient's skin color. In dark-skinned people, purple discoloration or a darkening of normal skin color is the first clinical sign. When the examiner presses a finger on the reddened area, the "pressed-on" area whitens, and color returns within 1 to 3 seconds if capillary refill is good. The patient complaints of pain at the site and in the surrounding area; localized edema may be evident because of the inflammatory response. Initially, the inflammatory response causes an increased body temperature; in more severe cases, the skin is cool because of more severe damage or necrosis.

In more severe cases, the patient may have nonblanching erythema ranging from dark red to purple or cyanotic. This indicates deep dermal involvement. Blisters, crusts, or scaling develop as the skin deteriorates and the ulcer progresses. A deep ulcer originating at the bony prominence below the skin surface usually has a dusky red appearance, doesn't bleed easily, is warm to the touch, and is possibly mottled. There may be a foul-smelling, purulent drainage from the ulcerated lesion and eschar tissue on and around the lesion because of the necrotic tissue that prevents healthy tissue growth.

COMPLICATIONS

Possible complications of pressure ulcers include progression of the pressure ulcer to a more severe state (greatest risk), secondary infections such as sepsis, and loss of limb from bone involvement (osteomyelitis).

(*Text continues on page 572.*)

Causes

+ Immobility or decreased level of activity
+ Friction or shearing forces
+ Constant moisture on skin
+ Impaired hygiene status
+ Malnutrition

How it happens

+ Pressure exerted on area causes ischemia and hypoxemia to affected tissues
+ Capillaries collapse, thrombosis occurs
+ Leads to tissue edema, progression to necrosis
+ Ischemia adds to accumulation of waste products at site
+ Toxins further break down tissue, lead to death of cells

Key signs and symptoms

+ Blanching erythema
+ Purple discoloration or darkening in darker skin
+ "Pressed-on" area whitens, color returns within 3 seconds if capillary refill good
+ Pain at site, surrounding area
+ Localized edema may be evident
+ Increased body temperature
+ Cool skin in more severe cases
+ Nonblanching erythema ranging from dark red to purple or cyanotic
+ Foul-smelling, purulent drainage from ulcerated lesion

Complications

+ Progression of the pressure ulcer to more severe state
+ Secondary infections
+ Loss of limb from bone involvement

Types of dermatitis
+ Seborrheic: subacute skin disease affecting the scalp and face
+ Nummular: chronic form characterized by inflammation
+ Contact: inflammation of the skin resulting from contact with a chemical or allergen
+ Hand or foot: inflammatory eruptions on the hands or feet

Types of dermatitis

TYPE	CAUSE
Seborrheic dermatitis	
A subacute skin disease affecting the scalp, face, and occasionally other areas that's characterized by lesions covered with yellow or brownish gray scales	✦ Unknown; stress, immunodeficiency, and neurologic conditions possibly predisposing factors; related to the yeast *Pityrosporum ovale* (normal flora)
Nummular dermatitis	
A chronic form of dermatitis characterized by inflammation in coin-shaped, scaling, or vesicular patches, usually pruriti	✦ Possibly precipitated by stress, dry skin, irritants, or scratching
Contact dermatitis	
Usually sharply demarcated inflammation of the skin resulting from contact with an irritating chemical or atopic allergen (a substance producing an allergic reaction in the skin) and irritation of the skin resulting from contact with concentrated substances to which the skin is sensitive, such as perfumes, soaps, or chemicals	✦ Mild irritants: chronic exposure to detergents or solvents ✦ Strong irritants: damage on contact with acids or alkalis ✦ Allergens: sensitization after repeated exposure
Hand or foot dermatitis	
A skin disease characterized by inflammatory eruptions of the hands or feet	✦ In many cases unknown but may result from irritant or allergic contact ✦ Excessively dry skin often a contributing factor ✦ 50% of patients are atopic

SIGNS AND SYMPTOMS	TREATMENT AND INTERVENTION
✦ Eruptions in areas with many sebaceous glands (usually scalp, face, chest, axillae, and groin) and in skin folds ✦ Itching, redness, and inflammation of affected areas; lesions possibly greasy looking; fissures possible ✦ Indistinct, occasionally yellowish scaly patches from excess stratum corneum (dandruff may be a mild seborrheic dermatitis)	✦ Removal of scales with frequent washing and shampooing with selenium sulfide suspension (most effective), zinc pyrithione, ketoconazole 2%, or tar and salicylic acid shampoo ✦ Application of topical corticosteroids and antifungals to involved area
✦ Round, nummular (coin-shaped), red lesions, usually on arms and legs, with distinct borders of crusts and scales ✦ Possible oozing and severe itching ✦ Summertime remissions common, with wintertime recurrence	✦ Elimination of known irritants ✦ Measures to relieve dry skin: increased humidification, limited frequency of baths, use of bland soap and bath oils, and application of emollients ✦ Application of wet dressings in acute phase ✦ Topical corticosteroids (occlusive dressings or intralesional injections) for persistent lesions ✦ Tar preparations and antihistamines to control itching ✦ Antibiotics for secondary infection
✦ Mild irritants and allergens: erythema and small vesicles that ooze, scale, and itch ✦ Strong irritants: blisters and ulcerations ✦ Classic allergic response: clearly defined lesions, with straight lines following points of contact ✦ Severe allergic reaction: marked erythema, blistering, and edema of affected areas	✦ Elimination of known allergens and decreased exposure to irritants, wearing protective clothing such as gloves, and washing immediately after contact with irritants or allergens ✦ Topical anti-inflammatory agents (including corticosteroids), systemic corticosteroids for edema and bullae, antihistamines, and local applications of Burow's solution (for blisters)
✦ Redness and scaling of the palms or soles ✦ May produce painful fissures ✦ In some cases, presenting with blisters (dyshidrotic eczema)	✦ Same as for nummular dermatitis ✦ In severe cases, systemic steroids possibly required

Key interventions for dermatitis
✦ Seborrheic: removal of scales with frequent washing and shampooing
✦ Nummular: elimination of known irritants
✦ Contact: elimination of known allergens and decreased exposure to irritants
✦ Hand or foot: elimination of known irritants; systemic steroids

(continued)

Types of dermatitis *(continued)*

TYPE	CAUSE
Localized neurodermatitis (lichen simplex chronicus, essential pruritus)	
Superficial inflammation of the skin characterized by itching and papular eruptions that appear on thickened, hyperpigmented skin	✦ Chronic scratching or rubbing of a primary lesion or insect bite or other skin irritation ✦ May be psychogenic
Exfoliative dermatitis	
Severe skin inflammation characterized by redness and widespread erythema and scaling, covering virtually the entire skin surface	✦ Preexisting skin lesions progressing to exfoliative stage, such as in contact dermatitis, drug reaction, lymphoma, leukemia, or atopic dermatitis ✦ May be idiopathic
Stasis dermatitis	
A condition usually caused by impaired circulation and characterized by eczema of the legs with edema, hyperpigmentation, and persistent inflammation	✦ Secondary to peripheral vascular diseases affecting the legs, such as recurrent thrombophlebitis and resultant chronic venous insufficiency

Types of dermatitis
(continued)

✦ Localized: superficial inflammation
✦ Exfoliative: severe skin inflammation
✦ Stasis: impaired circulation; eczema of the legs with edema

Diagnosis for pressure ulcers

✦ Physical examination shows presence of ulcer
✦ Wound culture reveals exudate or evidence of infection
✦ Elevated WBC count, erythrocyte sedimentation rate
✦ Temperature
✦ Total serum protein and serum albumin levels

DIAGNOSIS

To diagnose a pressure ulcer, a physical examination is performed and shows the presence of the ulcer. A wound culture then reveals exudate or evidence of infection, and elevated white blood cell (WBC) count and erythrocyte sedimentation rate and temperature indicate infection. Total serum protein and serum albumin levels show severe hypoproteinemia.

TREATMENT

Treatment for pressure ulcers includes repositioning the patient every 2 hours, or more often if indicated. Pillows are used to support immobile patients; patients

SIGNS AND SYMPTOMS	TREATMENT AND INTERVENTION
✦ Intense, sometimes continual scratching ✦ Thick, sharp-bordered, possibly dry, scaly lesions with raised papules and accentuated skin lines (lichenification) ✦ Usually affects easily reached areas, such as ankles, lower legs, anogenital area, back of neck, and ears ✦ One or several lesions present; asymmetric distribution	✦ Scratching stopped; then disappearance of lesions in about 2 weeks ✦ Fixed dressings or Unna's boot to cover affected areas ✦ Topical corticosteroids under occlusion or by intralesional injection ✦ Antihistamines and open wet dressings ✦ Emollients ✦ Patient informed about underlying cause
✦ Generalized dermatitis, with acute loss of stratum corneum, erythema, and scaling ✦ Sensation of tight skin ✦ Hair loss ✦ Possible fever, sensitivity to cold, shivering, gynecomastia, and lymphadenopathy	✦ Hospitalization, with protective isolation and hygienic measures to prevent secondary bacterial infection ✦ Open wet dressings, with colloidal baths ✦ Bland lotions over topical corticosteroids ✦ Maintenance of constant environmental temperature to prevent chilling or overheating ✦ Careful monitoring of renal and cardiac status ✦ Systemic antibiotics and steroids
✦ Varicosities and edema common, but obvious vascular insufficiency not always present ✦ Usually affects the lower leg just above internal malleolus or sites of trauma or irritation ✦ Early signs: dusky red deposits of hemosiderin in skin, with itching and dimpling of subcutaneous tissue ✦ Later signs: edema, redness, and scaling of large areas of legs ✦ Possible fissures, crusts, and ulcers	✦ Measures to prevent venous stasis: avoidance of prolonged sitting or standing, use of support stockings, weight reduction in obesity, and leg elevation ✦ Corrective surgery for underlying cause ✦ After ulcer develops, rest periods with legs elevated, open wet dressings, Unna's boot (zinc gelatin dressing provides continuous pressure to affected areas), and antibiotics for secondary infection after wound culture

Key interventions for dermatitis
✦ Localized: discontinue scratching; fixed dressings
✦ Exfoliative: hospitalization with protective isolation; open, wet dressings
✦ Stasis: measures to prevent venous stasis; corrective surgery for underlying cause

Treatment for pressure ulcers
✦ Reposition patient every 2 hours
✦ Pillows to support immobile patients
✦ Movement and ROM exercises encouraged
✦ Reduce pressure on ulcer site
✦ Maintain good skin care, hygiene practices
✦ Nutritional assessment, dietary consultation
✦ Increased fluids and fluid by I.V. if indicated
✦ Stage II or IV wound loosely filled with saline- or gel-moistened gauze
✦ Exudate management
✦ Surgical debridement

able to move are encouraged to do so. Both movement and range-of-motion (ROM) exercises are encouraged to promote circulation.

In addition to pillows for support, foam, gel, or air mattresses are used to reduce pressure on the ulcer site, to reduce the risk of more ulcers, and to aid in healing. These products may be used in chairs and wheelchairs as indicated.

The patient (and caregiver as necessary) receives instruction on maintaining good skin care and hygiene practices. For example, the incontinent patient requires meticulous hygiene and skin care to prevent breakdown of the affected tissue and skin.

Other treatments include a nutritional assessment and dietary consultation to determine the need for nutritional supplements, such as vitamin C and zinc. Monitoring serum albumin, protein markers, and body weight also helps determine if

Stages of pressure ulcers

Stage I
+ Observable pressure-related alteration of intact skin

Stage II
+ Partial-thickness skin loss
+ Ulcer is superficial and appears as an abrasion, blister, or crater

Stage III
+ Full-thickness skin loss
+ Damage or necrosis of subcutaneous tissue

Stage IV
+ Full-thickness skin loss with extensive destruction
+ Tunneling and sinus tracts may be associated

CLOSER LOOK

Staging pressure ulcers

The staging system described here is based on the recommendations of the National Pressure Ulcer Advisory Panel (NPUAP) (Consensus Conference, 1991) and the Agency for Health Care Policy and Research (*Clinical Practice Guidelines for Treatment of Pressure Ulcers,* 1992). The stage I definition was updated by the NPUAP in 1997.

STAGE I
A stage I pressure ulcer is an observable pressure-related alteration of intact skin. The indicators, compared with the adjacent or opposite area on the body, may include changes in one or more of the following factors: skin temperature (warmth or coolness), tissue consistency (firm or boggy feel), or sensation (pain or itching). The ulcer appears as a defined area of persistent redness in lightly pigmented skin; in darker skin, the ulcer may appear with persistent red, blue, or purple hues.

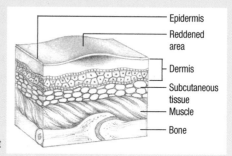

STAGE II
A stage II pressure ulcer is characterized by partial-thickness skin loss involving the epidermis or dermis. The ulcer is superficial and appears as an abrasion, blister, or shallow crater.

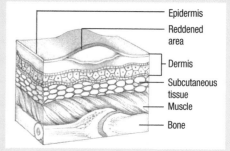

STAGE III
A stage III pressure ulcer is characterized by full-thickness skin loss involving damage or necrosis of subcutaneous tissue, which may extend down to, but not through, the underlying fascia. The ulcer appears as a deep crater with or without undermining of adjacent tissue.

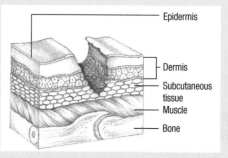

Staging pressure ulcers (continued)

STAGE IV

Full-thickness skin loss with extensive destruction, tissue necrosis, or damage to muscle, bone, or support structures (for example, tendon or joint capsule) characterizes a stage IV pressure ulcer. Tunneling and sinus tracts also may be associated with stage IV pressure ulcers.

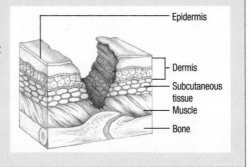

the patient is malnourished. A dehydrated patient is given increased fluids and fluid by I.V. if indicated.

Additional treatment is determined according to the stage of the pressure ulcer. Stage II pressure ulcers are covered with transparent film, polyurethane foam, or hydrocolloid dressing. A stage II or IV wound is loosely filled with saline- or gel-moistened gauze, and exudate is managed with absorbent dressing (moist gauze or foam) and covered with a secondary dressing. Certain types of ulcers, such as decubiti, are covered with clean, bulky dressings. For deeper wounds (stage III or IV), surgical debridement may be necessary.

NURSING CONSIDERATIONS

✦ During each shift, check the skin of bedridden or high-risk patients for possible changes in color, turgor, temperature, and sensation. Assess the patient for pain. Examine an existing ulcer for any change in size or degree of damage. When using pressure relief aids or topical agents, explain their function to the patient.

✦ Prevent pressure ulcers by repositioning the bedridden patient at least every 2 hours around the clock. To minimize the effects of a shearing force, use a footboard and raise the head of the bed to an angle not exceeding 60 degrees. Also, use a draw or pull sheet to turn the patient or to pull him up. Keep the patient's knees slightly flexed for short periods. Perform passive ROM exercises, or encourage the patient to do active exercises, if possible.

✦ To prevent pressure ulcers in immobilized patients, use support surface systems, such as compressive support mediums or fluid-filled and alternating pressure surfaces.

✦ Provide meticulous skin care. Keep the skin clean and dry without the use of harsh soaps. Gently massaging the skin around the affected area — not on it — promotes healing. Thoroughly rub moisturizing lotions into the skin to prevent maceration of the skin surface. Change bedding frequently for patients who are diaphoretic, incontinent, or have large amounts of drainage from wounds, suture lines, or drain sites. Use a fecal incontinence bag for incontinent patients.

✦ Clean open lesions with normal saline solution. Dressings, if needed, should be porous and lightly taped to healthy skin. Debridement of necrotic tissue may be necessary to allow healing. One method is to apply open wet dressings and allow them to dry on the ulcer. Removal of the dressings mechanically debrides exudate

Key nursing actions

✦ During each shift, check the skin of bedridden or high-risk patients.

✦ Assess the patient for pain.

✦ Examine an existing ulcer for any change in size or degree of damage.

✦ Prevent pressure ulcers by repositioning the bedridden patient at least every 2 hours around the clock.

✦ To prevent pressure ulcers in immobilized patients, use support surface systems.

✦ Provide meticulous skin care.

✦ Clean open lesions with normal saline solution.

✦ Dressings, if needed, should be porous and lightly taped to healthy skin.

Characteristics of psoriasis

✦ Chronic, recurrent epidermal proliferation
✦ Characterized by recurring partial remissions, exacerbations
✦ Flare-ups related to systemic or environmental factors, may be unpredictable
✦ Widespread involvement called *exfoliative*
✦ Usually affects young adults
✦ Genetic factors predetermine incidence
✦ Greater incidence of certain HLAs in families with history
✦ Appropriate treatment depends on type and extent of disease, patient response, effect on lifestyle
✦ No permanent cure

Causes

✦ Genetically determined
✦ Possible immune disorder
✦ Environmental factors
✦ Isomorphic effect
✦ Flare-up of guttate lesions

How it happens

✦ Life cycle of psoriatic skin cell only 4 days instead of normal 28
✦ Cell can't mature
✦ Stratum corneum becomes thick and flaky

Key signs and symptoms

✦ Itching and occasional pain from dry, cracked, encrusted lesions
✦ Lesions erythematous, usually well-defined plaques
✦ Scale removal can produce fine bleeding

and necrotic tissue. Other methods include surgical debridement with a fine scalpel blade and chemical debridement using proteolytic enzyme agents.
✦ Encourage adequate intake of nutritious food and fluids to maintain body weight and promote healing. Consult with the dietitian to provide a diet that promotes granulation of new tissue. Encourage the debilitated patient to eat frequent, small meals that provide protein- and calorie-rich supplements. Assist weakened patients with their meals.

PSORIASIS

Psoriasis is a chronic, recurrent disease marked by epidermal proliferation and characterized by recurring partial remissions and exacerbations. Flare-ups are commonly related to specific systemic and environmental factors but may be unpredictable. Widespread involvement is called *exfoliative* or *erythrodermic psoriasis*.

Psoriasis affects about 21% of the population in the United States. Although this disorder usually affects young adults, it may strike at any age, including infancy. Genetic factors predetermine the incidence of psoriasis; researchers have discovered a significantly greater incidence of certain human leukocyte antigens (HLAs) in families with psoriasis.

Flare-ups can usually be controlled with therapy. Appropriate treatment depends on the type of psoriasis, the extent of the disease, the patient's response, and the effect of the disease on the patient's lifestyle. No permanent cure exists, and all methods of treatment are palliative.

CAUSES

Causes of psoriasis include a genetically determined tendency to develop psoriasis, a possible immune disorder (as shown in the HLA type in families), and environmental factors. Other causes are isomorphic effect or Koebner's phenomenon (lesions develop at sites of injury because of trauma), flare-up of guttate (drop-shaped) lesions, and lesions resulting from infections, especially beta-hemolytic streptococci. Additional contributing factors include pregnancy, endocrine changes, climate (cold weather tends to exacerbate psoriasis), and emotional stress.

PATHOPHYSIOLOGY

A skin cell normally takes 14 days to move from the basal layer to the stratum corneum, where it's sloughed off after 14 days of normal wear and tear. Thus, the life cycle of a normal skin cell is 28 days compared with only 4 days for a psoriatic skin cell. This markedly shortened cycle doesn't allow time for the cell to mature. Consequently, the stratum corneum becomes thick and flaky, producing the cardinal manifestations of psoriasis.

SIGNS AND SYMPTOMS

The most common sign or symptom of psoriasis is itching and occasional pain from dry, cracked, encrusted lesions. Psoriatic lesions are erythematous and usually well-defined plaques, sometimes covering large areas of the body. The lesions most commonly occur on the scalp, chest, elbows, knees, back, and buttocks. Plaques have characteristic silver scales that either flake off easily or thicken, covering the lesion. Scale removal of the latter can produce fine bleeding. Occasional small guttate lesions (usually thin and erythematous, with few scales) appear either alone or with plaques.

COMPLICATIONS

This skin disorder has several complications. Psoriasis can spread to fingernails, producing small indentations or pits and yellow or brown discoloration (about 60% of patients). An accumulation of thick, crumbly debris under the nail can cause onycholysis (the nail separates from the nail bed). Itching and scratching may result in infection.

Rarely, psoriasis becomes pustular, taking one of two forms. In localized pustular psoriasis, pustules are found on the palms and soles. They remain sterile until opened. Generalized pustular (von Zumbusch's) psoriasis typically occurs with fever, leukocytosis, and malaise. Groups of pustules coalesce to form lakes of pus on red skin. They also remain sterile until opened and commonly involve the tongue and oral mucosa.

Erythrodermic psoriasis is the least common form. It's an inflammatory form of the disorder characterized by periodic fiery erythema and exfoliation of the skin with severe itching and pain. The patient may get arthritic symptoms that usually occur in one or more joints of the fingers or toes, the larger joints, or sometimes the sacroiliac joints. This may progress to spondylitis, and to morning stiffness in some patients.

DIAGNOSIS

A diagnosis of psoriasis is based on patient history, the appearance of the lesions and, if needed, the results of a skin biopsy. In psoriasis, the serum uric acid level is usually elevated in severe cases because of accelerated nucleic acid degradation, but an examination doesn't reveal indications of gout. HLA-Cw6, -B13, and -Bw57 may be present in early-onset familial psoriasis.

TREATMENT

Treatment of psoriasis may include ultraviolet B (UVB) or natural sunlight exposure to retard rapid cell production to the point of minimal erythema. Tar preparations may be applied as well to the affected areas about 15 minutes before exposure to UVB, or they may be left on overnight and wiped off the next morning. Exposure to UVB is gradually increased (outpatient treatment or day treatment avoids long hospitalizations and prolongs remission).

Other treatments include steroid creams and ointments applied twice daily, preferably after bathing to facilitate absorption. Overnight use of occlusive dressings also helps control symptoms of psoriasis. Caution is necessary when applying steroids to large areas of the body, especially the newer, more potent formulations. At higher dosages, the risk of percutaneous absorption increases, which could result in adrenal suppression.

Small, stubborn plaques are treated with an intralesional steroid injection; well-defined plaques are treated with anthralin ointment (Anthra-Derm) or a paste mixture (which is not applied to unaffected areas because of injury to and staining of normal skin). Before anthralin is used, petroleum jelly is applied around the affected skin. As an alternative, an anthralin (Anthra-Derm) and steroid combination may be used (anthralin is applied at night and the steroid during the day). Another drug treatment plan calls for calcipotriene ointment (Dovonex), a vitamin D analogue, which has its best results when alternated with a topical steroid.

Complications
+ Can spread to fingernails; debris under nail can cause onycholysis
+ Infection from scratching
+ May be pustular, cause infection when opened
+ Arthritic symptoms may occur in joints

Diagnosis
+ Based on patient history, appearance of lesions, results of skin biopsy
+ Serum uric acid level usually elevated in severe cases
+ Examination doesn't reveal indications of gout
+ HLA-Cw6, -B13, and -Bw57 may be present

Treatment
+ UVB or natural sunlight exposure
+ Tar preparations
+ Topical steroids
+ Intralesional steroid injection
+ Calcipotriene ointment

Treatment
(continued)

+ Goeckerman regimen
+ Psoralens with exposure to UVA
+ Cytotoxins
+ Immunosuppressants
+ NSAIDs
+ Biologics

In severe chronic psoriasis, the Goeckerman regimen (which combines tar baths and UVB treatments) helps achieve remission and clear the skin in 3 to 5 weeks. A variation of the Goeckerman regimen called the Ingram technique uses inhalation anthralin (Anthra-Derm) instead of tar.

Another treatment calling for exposure to light includes psoralens (plant extracts that accelerate exfoliation). It may be used in conjunction with exposure to high-intensity ultraviolet A (UVA) (psoralen plus UVA [PUVA] therapy).

A last-resort treatment for refractory psoriasis is using cytotoxin, usually methotrexate (Mexate); extensive psoriasis is treated with acitretin (Soriatane), a retinoid compound. In resistive cases, an immunosuppressant, cyclosporine (Neoral), is prescribed.

To relieve pruritus, low-dose antihistamines, oatmeal baths, emollients, and open wet dressings are prescribed. Aspirin and local heat help alleviate the pain of psoriatic arthritis, and nonsteroidal anti-inflammatory drugs (NSAIDs) may be used in severe cases. For psoriasis of the scalp, a tar shampoo followed by a steroid lotion is recommended. No effective topical treatment exists for psoriasis of the nails.

Recently, a new area of treatment called biologics has become available to treat psoriasis. The term *biologics* refers to substances derived from living sources. These substances must be injected or infused because they would be digested if taken by mouth. Alefacept (Amevive) and efalizumab (Raptiva) have been approved for use. Both of these agents interfere with immune system function. For example, alefacept blocks activation of T cells, which are believed to trigger accelerated skin cell development and maturation. Efalizumab, an antibody, isn't detected by the immune system because it's similar to other human antibodies in the body. It interferes with the actions of the immune system that promote the formation of psoriasis lesions.

NURSING CONSIDERATIONS

Design your patient's care plan to include patient teaching and careful monitoring for adverse effects of therapy.

+ Make sure the patient understands his prescribed therapy; provide written instructions to avoid confusion. Teach correct application of prescribed ointments, creams, and lotions. A steroid cream, for example, should be applied in a thin film and rubbed gently into the skin until the cream disappears. All topical medications, especially those containing anthralin and tar, should be applied with a downward motion to avoid rubbing them into the follicles. Gloves must be worn because anthralin stains and injures the skin. After application, the patient may dust himself with powder to prevent anthralin from rubbing off on his clothes. Warn the patient never to put an occlusive dressing over anthralin. Suggest use of mineral oil, then soap and water, to remove anthralin. Caution the patient to avoid scrubbing his skin vigorously to prevent Koebner's phenomenon. If a medication has been applied to the scales to soften them, suggest that the patient use a soft brush to remove them.

+ Watch for adverse effects, especially allergic reactions to anthralin; skin atrophy and acne from steroids; and burning, itching, nausea, and squamous cell epitheliomas from PUVA.

+ Initially evaluate the patient on methotrexate weekly, then monthly, for red blood cell, white blood cell, and platelet counts because cytotoxins may cause hepatic or bone marrow toxicity. Liver biopsy may be done to assess the effects of methotrexate. Patients taking methotrexate shouldn't drink alcohol because of the increased risk of hepatotoxicity.

Key nursing actions

+ Make sure the patient understands his prescribed therapy; provide written instructions to avoid confusion.
+ Teach correct application of prescribed ointments, creams, and lotions.
+ Initially evaluate the patient on methotrexate weekly, then monthly, for red blood cell, white blood cell, and platelet counts.

♦ Caution the patient receiving PUVA therapy to stay out of the sun on the day of treatment and to protect his eyes with sunglasses that block out UVA rays for 24 hours after treatment. Tell him to wear goggles during exposure to this light.

♦ Be aware that psoriasis can cause psychological problems. Assure the patient that psoriasis isn't contagious and that although exacerbations and remissions occur, they're controllable with treatment. However, make sure he understands that no cure exists. Also, because stressful situations tend to exacerbate psoriasis, help the patient learn effective stress management techniques and coping mechanisms. Explain the relationship between psoriasis and arthritis, but point out that psoriasis causes no other systemic disturbances. Refer all patients to the National Psoriasis Foundation, which provides information and directs patients to local chapters.

Key nursing actions
(continued)

♦ Caution the patient receiving PUVA therapy to stay out of the sun on the day of treatment.

♦ Assure the patient that psoriasis isn't contagious and that although exacerbations and remissions occur, they're controllable with treatment.

♦ Make sure he understands that no cure exists.

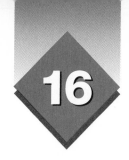

Reproductive system

Key facts about the reproductive system

+ Must function properly to ensure survival of species
+ Male reproductive system produces sperm, delivers them to female reproductive tract
+ Female reproductive system produces ova, nurtures and protects embryo and fetus; delivers it at birth
+ Functioning is determined by anatomic structure, hormonal, neurologic, vascular, psychogenic factors

Male reproductive system

+ Organs produce and maintain sperm, transfer sperm from testes, introduce sperm into female reproductive tract
+ Plays part in secretion of male sex hormones
+ Penis functions in urine elimination

The reproductive system must function properly to ensure survival of the species. The male reproductive system produces sperm and delivers them to the female reproductive tract. The female reproductive system produces the ovum. If a sperm fertilizes an ovum, this system also nurtures and protects the embryo and developing fetus and delivers it at birth. The functioning of the reproductive system is determined not only by anatomic structure but also by complex hormonal, neurologic, vascular, and psychogenic factors.

Anatomically, the main distinction between the male and the female is the presence of conspicuous external genitalia in the male, while the major reproductive organs of the female lie within the pelvic cavity.

MALE REPRODUCTIVE SYSTEM

The male reproductive system consists of the organs that produce and maintain sperm, transfer mature sperm from the testes, and introduce those sperm into the female reproductive tract, where fertilization occurs.

Besides supplying male sex cells (in a process called spermatogenesis), the male reproductive system plays a part in the secretion of male sex hormones. The penis also functions in urine elimination.

In males, the reproductive and urinary systems are structurally integrated; most disorders, therefore, affect both systems. Congenital abnormalities or prostate enlargement may impair both sexual and urinary function. Abnormal findings in the pelvic area may result from pathologic changes in other organ systems, such as the upper urinary and GI tracts, endocrine glands, and neuromusculoskeletal system.

REPRODUCTIVE ORGANS

The male reproductive organs include the penis, scrotum, testes, duct system, and accessory reproductive glands.

Penis

The penis consists of three cylinders of erectile tissue: two corpora cavernosa, and the corpus spongiosum, which contains the urethra. The glans, or tip, of the penis contains the urethral meatus, through which urine and semen pass to the exterior, and many nerve endings for sexual sensation.

Scrotum

The scrotum, which contains the testes, epididymis, and lower spermatic cords, maintains the proper testicular temperature for spermatogenesis through relaxation and contraction. This is important because excessive heat reduces the sperm count.

Testes

The testes (also called *gonads,* which is a term for any reproductive organ, or testicles) produce sperm in the seminiferous tubules. Complete spermatogenesis develops in most males by age 15 or 16.

The testes form in the abdominal cavity of the fetus and descend into the scrotum during the seventh month of gestation.

The testes produce and secrete hormones, especially testosterone, in their interstitial cells (Leydig's cells). Testosterone affects the development and maintenance of secondary sex characteristics and sex drive. It also regulates metabolism, stimulates protein anabolism (encouraging skeletal growth and muscular development), inhibits pituitary secretion of the gonadotropins (follicle-stimulating hormone and interstitial cell-stimulating hormone), promotes potassium excretion, and mildly influences renal sodium reabsorption.

Duct system

The vas deferens connects the epididymis, in which sperm mature and ripen for up to 6 weeks, and the ejaculatory ducts. The seminal vesicles — two convoluted membranous pouches — secrete a viscous liquid of fructose-rich semen, which provides energy for sperm, and prostaglandins that probably facilitate fertilization.

Accessory reproductive glands

The prostate gland secretes the thin alkaline substance that comprises most of the seminal fluid; this fluid also protects sperm from acidity in the male urethra and in the vagina, thus increasing sperm motility.

The bulbourethral (Cowper's) glands secrete an alkaline ejaculatory fluid, probably similar in function to that produced by the prostate gland. The spermatic cords are cylindrical fibrous coverings in the inguinal canal containing the vas deferens, blood vessels, and nerves.

FEMALE REPRODUCTIVE SYSTEM

Female reproductive structures include the mammary glands, external genitalia, and internal genitalia. Hormonal influences determine the development and function of these structures and affect fertility, childbearing, and the ability to experience sexual pleasure.

In no other part of the body do so many interrelated physiologic functions occur in such proximity as in the area of the female reproductive tract. Besides the internal genitalia, the female pelvis contains the organs of the urinary and GI systems (bladder, ureters, urethra, sigmoid colon, and rectum). The reproductive tract and

Reproductive organs

Penis
- Three cylinders of erectile tissue
- Two corpora cavernosa
- Glans contains urethral meatus through which urine and semen pass to exterior; contains nerve endings for sexual sensation

Scrotum
- Contains testes, epididymis, lower spermatic cords
- Maintains proper testicular temperature

Testes
- Produce sperm in seminiferous tubules
- Form in the abdominal cavity of fetus
- Descend into scrotum during seventh month of gestation
- Produce and secrete hormones

Duct system
- Vas deferens connects epididymis and ejaculatory ducts
- Seminal vesicles secrete semen

Accessory reproductive glands
- Prostate gland secretes alkaline substance comprising most of seminal fluid
- Bulbourethral glands secrete alkaline ejaculatory fluid
- Spermatic cords contain vas deferens, blood vessels, nerves

Female reproductive system
- External and internal genitalia
- Hormonal influences determine development and function of structures, affect fertility, childbearing, ability to experience sexual pleasure
- Female pelvis contains organs of urinary, GI systems
- Mammary glands in the breast secrete milk

its surrounding area are thus the site of urination, defecation, menstruation, ovulation, copulation, impregnation, and parturition.

MAMMARY GLANDS

Located in the breasts, the mammary glands are specialized accessory glands that secrete milk. Although present in both sexes, they normally function only in females.

EXTERNAL STRUCTURES

Female genitalia include these external structures, collectively known as the vulva: mons pubis (or mons veneris), labia majora, labia minora, clitoris, and vestibule. The perineum is the external region between the vulva and the anus. The size, shape, and color of these structures—as well as pubic hair distribution and skin texture and pigmentation—vary greatly among individuals. Furthermore, these external structures undergo distinct changes during the life cycle.

Mons pubis

The mons pubis is the pad of fat over the symphysis pubis (pubic bone), which is usually covered by the base of the inverted triangular patch of pubic hair that grows over the vulva after puberty.

Labia majora

The labia majora are the two thick, longitudinal folds of fatty tissue that extend from the mons pubis to the posterior aspect of the perineum. The labia majora protect the perineum and contain large sebaceous glands that help maintain lubrication. Virtually absent in the young child, their development is a characteristic sign of onset of puberty. The skin of the more prominent parts of the labia majora is pigmented and darkens after puberty.

Labia minora

The labia minora are the two thin, longitudinal folds of skin that border the vestibule. Firmer than the labia majora, they extend from the clitoris to the posterior fourchette.

Clitoris

The clitoris is the small, protuberant organ located just beneath the arch of the mons pubis. The clitoris contains erectile tissue, venous cavernous spaces, and specialized sensory corpuscles that are stimulated during coitus. It's homologous to the male penis.

Vestibule

The vestibule is the oval space bordered by the clitoris, labia minora, and fourchette. The urethral meatus is located in the anterior portion of the vestibule, and the vaginal meatus is in the posterior portion. The hymen is the elastic membrane that partially obstructs the vaginal meatus in virgins. Its absence doesn't necessarily imply a history of coitus, nor does its presence obstruct menstrual blood flow.

Several glands lubricate the vestibule. Skene's glands (also known as the paraurethral glands) open on both sides of the urethral meatus, and Bartholin's glands open on both sides of the vaginal meatus.

External structures

Mons pubis
+ Pad of fat over symphysis pubis
+ Usually covered by pubic hair

Labia majora
+ Two thick, longitudinal folds of fatty tissue
+ Extend from mons pubis to posterior aspect of perineum
+ Protect perineum, contain large sebaceous glands to maintain lubrication
+ Development characteristic of onset of puberty
+ Skin darkens after puberty

Labia minora
+ Two thin, longitudinal folds of skin that border vestibule
+ Firmer than labia majora
+ Extend from clitoris to posterior fourchette

Clitoris
+ Small, protuberant organ located beneath arch of mons pubis
+ Contains erectile tissue, venous cavernous spaces, specialized sensory corpuscles
+ Stimulated during coitus
+ Homologous to male penis

Vestibule
+ Oval space bordered by clitoris, labia minora, fourchette
+ Urethral meatus located in anterior portion
+ Vaginal meatus located in posterior portion
+ Hymen: elastic membrane partially obstructing vaginal meatus in virgins
+ Perineum: external surface of floor of pelvis; extends from fourchette to anus

The fourchette is the posterior junction of the labia majora and labia minora. The perineum, which includes the underlying muscles and fascia, is the external surface of the floor of the pelvis, extending from the fourchette to the anus.

INTERNAL STRUCTURES

The internal structures of the female genitalia include the vagina, cervix, uterus, fallopian tubes (or oviducts), and ovaries.

Vagina

The vagina occupies the space between the bladder and the rectum. A muscular, membranous tube approximately 2″ to 3″ (5 to 7.5 cm) in length, the vagina connects the uterus with the vestibule of the external genitalia. It serves as a passageway for sperm to the fallopian tubes, a conduit for the discharge of menstrual fluid, and the birth canal during parturition.

Cervix

The cervix, the narrow neck of the uterus, is the most inferior part of the vagina, protruding into the vaginal canal. The cervix provides a passageway between the vagina and the uterine cavity.

Uterus

The uterus is the hollow, pear-shaped organ in which the conceptus grows during pregnancy. The thick uterine wall consists of mucosal, muscular, and serous layers. The inner mucosal lining (the endometrium) undergoes cyclic changes (based on hormonal activity) to facilitate and maintain pregnancy.

The smooth muscular middle layer (the myometrium) interlaces the uterine and ovarian arteries and veins that circulate blood through the uterus. During pregnancy, this vascular system expands dramatically. After abortion or childbirth, the myometrium contracts to constrict the vasculature and control loss of blood.

The outer serous layer (the parietal peritoneum) covers all of the fundus and part of the corpus, but none of the cervix. This incompleteness allows surgical entry into the uterus without incision of the peritoneum, thus reducing the risk of peritonitis in the days before effective antibiotic therapy.

Fallopian tubes

The two fallopian tubes extend from the sides of the fundus and terminate near the ovaries. Each tube has a fimbriated (fringelike) end adjacent to the ovary that serves to capture an oocyte after ovulation. Through ciliary and muscular action, these small tubes carry ova from the ovaries to the uterus and facilitate the movement of sperm from the uterus toward the ovaries. The same ciliary and muscular action helps move a zygote (fertilized ovum) down to the uterus, where it may implant in the blood-rich inner uterine lining, the endometrium.

Ovaries

The ovaries are two almond-shaped organs, one on either side of the pelvis, situated behind and below the fallopian tubes. The ovaries produce ova and two primary hormones—estrogen and progesterone—in addition to small amounts of androgen. These hormones in turn produce and maintain secondary sex characteristics, prepare the uterus for pregnancy, and stimulate mammary gland development. The ovaries are connected to the uterus by the utero-ovarian ligament.

Internal structures

Vagina
+ Occupies space between bladder and rectum
+ Connects uterus with vestibule
+ Passageway for sperm to fallopian tubes
+ Conduit for discharge of menstrual fluid
+ Birth canal during parturition

Cervix
+ Narrow neck of uterus
+ Passageway between vagina and uterine cavity

Uterus
+ Hollow, pear-shaped organ where conceptus grows during pregnancy
+ Inner mucosal lining undergoes cyclic changes to facilitate and maintain pregnancy
+ Middle layer interlaces uterine and ovarian arteries and veins
+ Outer serous layer covers all of fundus, part of corpus, none of cervix

Fallopian tubes
+ Extend from sides of fundus, terminate near ovaries
+ Carry ova from ovaries to uterus, facilitate movement of sperm from uterus toward ovaries
+ Move zygote to uterus

Ovaries
+ Two almond-shaped organs on either side of pelvis, behind and below fallopian tubes
+ Produce ova, estrogen, progesterone, small amounts of androgen
+ Maintain secondary sex characteristics, prepare uterus for pregnancy, stimulate mammary gland development

The menstrual cycle

✦ Maturation of hypothalamus, increase in hormone levels initiate puberty
✦ Appearance of pubic, axillary hair and growth spurt follow breast development
✦ Reproductive system begins hormone-induced changes
✦ Result in menarche
✦ Menstrual cycle consists of menstrual, proliferative, secretory phases
✦ At end of secretory phase, uterine lining ready to receive and nourish a zygote

In the 30th week of gestation, the fetus has about 7 million follicles, which degenerate, leaving about 2 million present at birth. By puberty, only 400,000 remain, and these ova precursors become graafian follicles in response to the effects of pituitary gonadotropic hormones (follicle-stimulating hormone [FSH] and luteinizing hormone [LH]). Fewer than 500 of each woman's ova mature and become potentially fertile.

THE MENSTRUAL CYCLE

Maturation of the hypothalamus and the resultant increase in hormone levels initiate puberty. In the young girl, the appearance of pubic and axillary hair (pubarche) and the characteristic adolescent growth spurt follow breast development (thelarche)—the first sign of puberty. The reproductive system begins to undergo a series of hormone-induced changes that result in menarche, or the onset of menstruation (or menses).

The menstrual cycle consists of three different phases: menstrual, proliferative (estrogen dominated), and secretory (progesterone dominated). (See *Understanding the menstrual cycle*.)

At the end of the secretory phase, the uterine lining is ready to receive and nourish a zygote. If fertilization doesn't occur, increasing estrogen and progesterone lev-

3 phases of the menstrual cycle

Menstruation phase
✦ Starts on first day of menstruation
✦ Top layer of endometrium flows out of the body

Proliferative phase
✦ Endometrium thickens and level of estrogen in blood increases
✦ Estrogen production then decreases, and ovulation occurs

Secretory phase
✦ Endometrium thickens to nourish embryo, if fertilization occurs
✦ If it doesn't occur, top layer breaks down and cycle begins

CLOSER LOOK

Understanding the menstrual cycle

The menstrual cycle is divided into three distinct phases.

✦ During the menstrual phase, which starts on the first day of menstruation, the top layer of the endometrium breaks down and flows out of the body. This flow, the *menses*, consists of blood, mucus, and unneeded tissue.
✦ During the proliferative (follicular) phase, the endometrium begins to thicken and the level of estrogen in the blood increases,

surging at midcycle. Then estrogen production decreases, the follicle matures, and ovulation occurs.
✦ During the secretory (luteal) phase, the endometrium begins to thicken to nourish an embryo should fertilization occur. Without fertilization, the top layer of the endometrium breaks down and the menstrual phase of the cycle begins again.

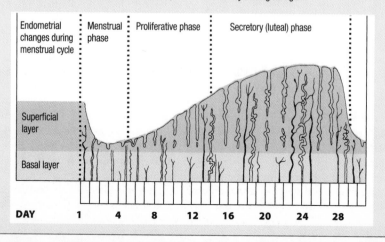

els decrease LH and FSH production. Because LH is needed to maintain the corpus luteum, a decrease in LH production causes the corpus luteum to atrophy and halt the secretion of estrogen and progesterone. The thickened uterine lining then begins to slough off, and menstruation begins.

In the nonpregnant female, LH controls the secretions of the corpus luteum, thereby increasing progesterone levels in the bloodstream. In the pregnant woman, human chorionic gonadotropin (hCG), produced by the nascent placenta, controls these secretions.

If fertilization and pregnancy occur, the endometrium grows even thicker and vascular ingrowth occurs. After implantation of the zygote (about 5 or 6 days after fertilization), the endometrium becomes the decidua. Trophoblastic cells produce hCG soon after implantation, stimulating the corpus luteum to continue secreting estrogen and progesterone, which prevents further ovulation and menstruation.

The hCG continues to stimulate the corpus luteum until the placenta (the vascular organ that develops to transport materials to and from the fetus) forms and starts producing its own estrogen and progesterone. After the placenta takes over hormonal production, secretions of the corpus luteum are no longer needed to maintain the pregnancy, and the corpus luteum gradually decreases its function and begins to degenerate. This is termed the luteoplacental shift and commonly occurs by the end of the first trimester.

PATHOPHYSIOLOGIC CHANGES

Alterations may occur in the structure, process, or function of both the male and the female reproductive systems.

SEXUAL MATURATION ALTERATION

Sexual maturation, or puberty, can be affected by various congenital and endocrine disorders. The timing of puberty may be too early (precocious puberty) or too late (delayed puberty). Precocious puberty is the onset of sexual maturation before age 9 in boys and before age 8 in girls. It occurs more often in girls than boys. In girls, the cause is most commonly idiopathic, whereas in boys it's more likely to be organic.

In delayed puberty, no evidence of the development of secondary sex characteristics exists in boys by age 14 or girls by age 13. There's usually no evidence of hormonal abnormalities. The hypothalamic-pituitary-ovarian axis, a system that stimulates and regulates the production of hormones necessary for normal sexual development and function, is intact, but maturation is slow. The cause is unknown.

HORMONAL ALTERATIONS

Complex hormonal interactions determine the normal function of the female reproductive tract and require an intact hypothalamic-pituitary-ovarian axis. A defect or malfunction of this system can cause infertility because of insufficient gonadotropin secretions (both LH and FSH). The ovary controls, and is controlled by, the hypothalamus through a system of negative and positive feedback mediated by estrogen production. Insufficient gonadotropin levels may result from infections, tumors, or neurologic disease of the hypothalamus or pituitary gland. A mild hormonal imbalance in gonadotropin production and regulation, possibly caused by polycystic disease of the ovary or abnormalities in the adrenal or thyroid gland that adversely affect hypothalamic-pituitary functioning, may sporadically inhibit ovu-

Hormonal alterations
(continued)

+ Male hypogonadism results from decreased androgen production in males
+ Secondary hypogonadism results from faulty interaction within the hypothalamic-pituitary axis
+ Symptoms vary depending on specific cause of hypogonadism

Menstrual alterations

+ Absence of menses
+ Abnormal bleeding patterns
+ Painful menstruation
+ Cessation of menstruation from declining ovarian function
+ Premature menopause occurs in about 5% of women in the United States
+ Ovarian failure may result from functional ovarian disorder from premature menopause

Alert!

+ The climacteric begins in most women between ages 40 and 50 and results in infrequent ovulation, decreased menstrual function and, eventually, cessation of menstruation.

lation. Because gonadotropins are released in a pulsatile fashion, a significant disturbance in this pulsatility will adversely affect ovulatory function.

Male hypogonadism, or an abnormal decrease in gonad size and function, results from decreased androgen production in males, which may impair spermatogenesis (causing infertility) and inhibit the development of normal secondary sex characteristics. The clinical effects of androgen deficiency depend on age at onset. Primary hypogonadism results directly from interstitial (Leydig's cell) cellular or seminiferous tubular damage of the testes due to faulty development or mechanical damage. Androgen deficiency causes increased secretion of gonadotropins by the pituitary in an attempt to increase the testicular functional state and is therefore termed hypergonadotropic hypogonadism. This form of hypogonadism includes Klinefelter's syndrome (47 XXY), Reifenstein's syndrome, male Turner's syndrome, Sertoli cell–only syndrome, anorchism, orchitis, and sequelae of irradiation.

Secondary hypogonadism is due to faulty interaction within the hypothalamic-pituitary axis, resulting in failure to secrete normal levels of gonadotropins, and is therefore termed hypogonadotropic hypogonadism. This form of hypogonadism includes hypopituitarism, isolated FSH deficiency, isolated LH deficiency, Kallmann's syndrome, and Prader-Willi syndrome. Depending on the patient's age at onset, hypogonadism may cause eunuchism (complete gonadal failure) or eunuchoidism (partial failure).

Symptoms vary depending on the specific cause of hypogonadism. Some characteristic findings may include delayed bone maturation; delayed puberty; infantile penis and small, soft testes; less than average muscle development and strength; fine, sparse facial hair; scant or absent axillary, pubic, and body hair; and a high-pitched, effeminate voice. In an adult, hypogonadism diminishes sex drive and potency and causes regression of secondary sex characteristics.

MENSTRUAL ALTERATIONS

Alterations in menstruation include the absence of menses, abnormal bleeding patterns, or painful menstruation. Menopause is the cessation of menstruation. It results from a complex continuum of physiologic changes—the climacteric—caused by declining ovarian function. The climacteric produces various changes in the body, the most dramatic being the cessation of menses.

 CLINICAL ALERT The climacteric, a normal gradual reduction in ovarian function caused by aging, begins in most women between ages 40 and 50 and results in infrequent ovulation, decreased menstrual function and, eventually, cessation of menstruation (usually between ages 45 and 55).

Premature menopause, the gradual or abrupt cessation of menstruation before age 35, occurs without apparent cause in about 5% of women in the United States. Certain diseases, especially autoimmune diseases such as premature ovarian failure, may cause pathologic menopause. Other factors that may precipitate premature menopause include malnutrition, debilitation, extreme emotional stress, pelvic irradiation, and surgical procedures that impair ovarian blood supply. Artificial menopause may follow radiation therapy or surgical procedures such as removal of both ovaries (bilateral oophorectomy). Hysterectomy decreases the interval before menopause even when the ovaries aren't removed. It's speculated that hysterectomy may decrease ovarian blood flow in some fashion.

Ovarian failure, in which no ova are produced, may result from a functional ovarian disorder from premature menopause. Amenorrhea is a natural consequence of ovarian failure.

Abnormal premenopausal bleeding

Causes of abnormal premenopausal bleeding vary with the type of bleeding:

◆ Oligomenorrhea (infrequent menses) and polymenorrhea (menses occurring too frequently) usually result from anovulation due to an endocrine or systemic disorder.

◆ Hypomenorrhea (decreased amount of menstrual fluid) results from local, endocrine, or systemic disorders or blockage caused by partial obstruction by the hymen or cervical obstruction.

◆ Hypermenorrhea (excessive bleeding occurring at regular intervals) usually results from local lesions, such as uterine leiomyomas, endometrial polyps, and endometrial hyperplasia. It may also result from endometritis, salpingitis, and anovulation.

◆ Cryptomenorrhea (no external bleeding, although menstrual symptoms are experienced) may result from an imperforate hymen or cervical stenosis.

◆ Metrorrhagia (bleeding occurring at irregular intervals) usually results from slight physiologic bleeding from the endometrium during ovulation but may also result from local disorders, such as uterine malignancy, cervical erosions, polyps (which tend to bleed after intercourse), or inappropriate estrogen therapy.

Complications of pregnancy can also cause premenopausal bleeding, which may be as mild as spotting or as severe as hypermenorrhea.

Types of abnormal premenopausal bleeding

◆ Oligomenorrhea: infrequent menses; polymenorrhea: menses occurring too frequently
◆ Hypomenorrhea: decreased amount of menstrual fluid
◆ Hypermenorrhea: excessive bleeding occurring at regular intervals
◆ Cryptomenorrhea: no external bleeding, although menstrual symptoms are experienced
◆ Metrorrhagia: bleeding occurring at irregular intervals

Pain is commonly associated with the menstrual cycle; in many common diseases of the female reproductive tract, such pain may follow a cyclic pattern. A patient with endometriosis, for example, may report increasing premenstrual pain that decreases at the end of menstruation. For a description of the types of abnormal menstrual bleeding, see *Abnormal premenopausal bleeding.*

SEXUAL DYSFUNCTION

Sexual dysfunction includes arousal problems, orgasmic problems, and sexual pain (dyspareunia, vaginismus). Dysfunction may be caused by a general medical condition, psychological condition, substance use or abuse, or a combination of these factors.

Arousal disorder is an inability to experience sexual pleasure. According to the *Diagnostic and Statistical Manual of Mental Disorders,* 4th ed. (*DSM-IV*), the essential feature is a persistent or recurrent inability to attain or to maintain an adequate lubrication-swelling response of sexual excitement until completion of the sexual act. Orgasmic disorder, according to the *DSM-IV*, is a persistent or recurrent delay in or absence of orgasm after a normal sexual excitement phase.

Both arousal and orgasmic disorders are considered primary if they exist in a female who has never experienced sexual arousal or orgasm; they are secondary when a physical, mental, or situational condition has inhibited or obliterated a previously normal sexual function. The prognosis is good for temporary or mild disorders resulting from misinformation or situational stress but is guarded for disorders that result from intense anxiety, chronically discordant relationships, psychological disturbances, or drug or alcohol abuse in either partner.

Many factors, alone or in combination, may cause an arousal or orgasmic disorder. For example, certain drugs, including central nervous system depressants, alcohol, street drugs and, rarely, hormonal contraceptives, contribute to such a disorder. General systemic illnesses, diseases of the endocrine or nervous system, or diseases that impair muscle tone or contractility also play a role. Arousal or orgasmic disorders can be caused by gynecologic factors, such as chronic vaginal or pelvic in-

Sexual dysfunction

◆ Arousal, orgasmic, and sexual problems
◆ Arousal disorder is inability to experience sexual pleasure
◆ May be primary or secondary
◆ Factors that may cause arousal or orgasmic disorder: alcohol, hormonal contraceptives, gynecologic factors

fection or pain, congenital anomalies, and genital cancers. Stress and fatigue and inadequate or ineffective stimulation are other factors. Psychological factors include performance anxiety, guilt, depression, or unconscious conflicts about sexuality. Relationship problems include poor communication, hostility, or ambivalence toward the partner, fear of abandonment or independence, or boredom with sex.

All of these factors may contribute to involuntary inhibition of the orgasmic reflex. Another crucial factor is the fear of losing control of feelings or behavior. Whether these factors produce sexual dysfunction and the type of dysfunction produced depend on how well the woman copes with the resulting pressures. Physical factors may also cause arousal or orgasmic disorder.

Female sexual dysfunction

Female sexual function and responses decline, along with estrogen levels, in the perimenopausal period. The decrease in estradiol levels during menopause affects nerve transmission and response in the peripheral vascular system. As a result, the timing and degree of vasoconstriction during the sexual response is affected, vasocongestion decreases, muscle tension decreases, lubrication decreases, and contractions are fewer and less intense during orgasm.

A female with arousal disorder has limited or absent sexual desire and experiences little or no pleasure from sexual stimulation. Physical signs of this disorder include lack of vaginal lubrication or absence of signs of genital vasocongestion.

Dyspareunia is genital pain associated with intercourse. Insufficient lubrication is the most common cause. Other physical causes of dyspareunia include endometriosis; genital, rectal, or pelvic scar tissue; acute or chronic infections of the genitourinary tract; and disorders of the surrounding viscera.

Other possible physical causes include deformities or lesions of the introitus or vagina, benign and malignant growths and tumors, intact hymen, radiation to the pelvis, and allergic reactions to diaphragms, condoms, or other contraceptives.

Psychological causes include fear of pain or injury during intercourse, previous painful experience including sexual abuse, guilty feelings about sex, fear of pregnancy or injury to the fetus during pregnancy, anxiety caused by a new sexual partner or technique, and mental or physical fatigue.

Vaginismus is an involuntary spastic constriction of the lower vaginal muscles, usually from fear of vaginal penetration. This disorder may coexist with dyspareunia and, if severe, may prevent intercourse (a common cause of unconsummated marriages). Vaginismus may be physical or psychological in origin. It may occur spontaneously as a protective reflex to pain or result from organic causes, such as hymenal abnormalities, genital herpes, obstetric trauma, and atrophic vaginitis.

Psychological causes may include childhood and adolescent exposure to rigid, punitive, and guilt-ridden attitudes toward sex; fear resulting from painful or traumatic sexual experiences, such as incest or rape; early traumatic experience with pelvic examinations; fear of pregnancy and sexually transmitted disease; or cancer.

Male sexual dysfunction

In males, the normal sexual response involves erection, emission, and ejaculation. Sexual dysfunction is the impairment of one or all of these processes.

Erectile disorder, or impotence, refers to an inability to attain or maintain penile erection sufficient to complete intercourse. Transient periods of impotence aren't considered dysfunction and probably occur in half of all adult males. Erectile disorder affects all age-groups but increases in frequency with age.

Psychogenic factors (guilt, fear, depression) are responsible for approximately 50% to 60% of the cases of erectile dysfunction; organic factors, for the rest. In

---

Sexual dysfunction

Female

✦ Arousal disorder: inability to experience sexual pleasure; persistent or recurrent inability to attain or maintain adequate lubrication

✦ Dyspareunia: genital pain associated with intercourse

✦ Vaginismus: involuntary spastic constriction of the lower vaginal muscles

✦ Causes of disorders may be psychological

Male

✦ Impairment of erection, emission, ejaculation

✦ Erectile disorder: inability to attain or maintain penile erection sufficient to complete intercourse

✦ Psychogenic factors in 50% to 60% of cases; organic for rest

some patients, psychogenic and organic factors (chronic disease, paralysis, consequence of a surgical procedure) coexist, making isolation of the primary cause difficult.

Most problems with emission and ejaculation usually have structural causes.

MALE STRUCTURAL ALTERATIONS

Structural defects of the male reproductive system may be congenital or acquired. Testicular disorders, such as cryptorchidism or torsion, may result in infertility.

In cryptorchidism, a congenital disorder, one or both testes fail to descend into the scrotum, remaining in the abdomen or inguinal canal or at the external ring. If bilateral cryptorchidism persists untreated into adolescence, it may result in sterility, make the testes more vulnerable to trauma, and significantly increase the risk of testicular cancer, particularly germ cell tumors. In about 80% of affected infants, the testes descend spontaneously during the 1st year; in the rest, the testes may descend later.

 CLINICAL ALERT The testes of an older male may be slightly smaller than those of a younger male, but they should be equal in size, smooth, freely moveable, and soft, without nodules. The left testis is commonly lower than the right.

Benign prostatic hyperplasia is a disorder of prostate enlargement caused by androgen-induced growth of prostate cells. It's more prevalent with aging and may result in urinary obstructive symptoms.

Hypospadias is the most common penile structural abnormality. The midline fusion of the urethral folds is incomplete, so the urethral meatus opens on the ventral (anterior, or "belly") surface of the penis. In epispadias, the urethral meatus is located on the dorsal (posterior, or "back") surface of the penis.

Priapism is prolonged, painful erection in the absence of sexual stimulation. It results from arteriovenous shunting within the corpus cavernosum that leads to obstructed venous outflow from the penis. In adults, it's usually idiopathic because of trauma. In children, it may be associated with sickle cell disease. Without prompt treatment, it can lead to ischemic fibrosis and infertility.

A urethral stricture is a narrowing of the urethra caused by scarring. It may result from trauma, surgery (adhesions), or infection. Common complications include prostatitis and secondary infection.

During the first 3 years of life, congenital adhesions between the foreskin and the glans penis separate naturally with penile erections. Phimosis is a condition in which the foreskin can't be retracted over the glans penis; poor hygiene and chronic infection can cause it. Paraphimosis is a condition in which the foreskin is retracted and can't be reduced to cover the glans; the penis becomes constricted, causing edema of the glans. Severe paraphimosis is a surgical emergency.

Another structural defect of the male results from the drug diethylstilbestrol (DES). To prevent threatened spontaneous abortion, millions of women took DES between 1946 and 1971. Men whose mothers took DES during their 8th to 16th weeks of pregnancy have experienced structural abnormalities, such as urethral meatal stenosis, hypospadias, epididymal cysts, varicoceles, cryptorchidism, and decreased fertility.

Male structural alterations

+ May be congenital or acquired
+ May result in infertility
+ Cryptorchidism: one or both testes fail to descend into the scotum
+ Benign prostatic hyperplasia: disorder of prostate enlargement
+ Priapism: prolonged, painful erection in absence of sexual stimulation
+ Urethral stricture: narrowing of urethra from scarring

Alert!

+ The testes of an older male may be slightly smaller than those of a younger male, but they should be equal in size, smooth, freely moveable, and soft, without nodules.
+ The left testis is commonly lower than the right.

Characteristics of amenorrhea

+ Abnormal absence or suppression of menstruation
+ Primary in adolescent; secondary if at least 3 months after normal onset of menarche
+ Prognosis variable, depending on specific cause
+ Surgical correction of outflow tract obstruction usually curative

Causes

+ Anovulation due to hormonal abnormalities
+ Absence of uterus
+ Endometrial damage
+ Ovarian, adrenal, pituitary tumors
+ Emotional disorders

How it happens

+ Mechanism varies depending on cause
+ Adequate estrogen but deficient progesterone; infertility results
+ Hypothalamic-pituitary-ovarian axis often dysfunctional in primary disease
+ Ovary doesn't receive hormonal signals from CNS
+ Secondary amenorrhea results from central factors, uterine factors, cervical stenosis, premature ovarian failure, others

Key signs and symptoms

+ Depend on specific cause
+ Absence of menstruation
+ Vasomotor flushes

Complications

+ Infertility
+ Endometrial adenocarcinoma

AMENORRHEA

Amenorrhea is the abnormal absence or suppression of menstruation. Absence of menstruation is normal before puberty, after menopause, or during pregnancy and lactation; it's abnormal, and therefore pathologic, at any other time. Primary amenorrhea is the absence of menarche in an adolescent (age 16 and older). Secondary amenorrhea is the failure of menstruation for at least 3 months after the normal onset of menarche. Primary amenorrhea occurs in 0.3% of women; secondary amenorrhea, in 1% to 3% of women. Prognosis is variable, depending on the specific cause. Surgical correction of outflow tract obstruction is usually curative.

CAUSES

Amenorrhea usually results from anovulation due to hormonal abnormalities, such as decreased secretion of estrogen, gonadotropins, luteinizing hormone, and follicle-stimulating hormone (FSH), lack of ovarian response to gonadotropins, and constant presence of progesterone or other endocrine abnormalities.

Amenorrhea may also result from absence of a uterus; endometrial damage; ovarian, adrenal, or pituitary tumors; emotional disorders (common in patients with severe disorders, such as depression and anorexia nervosa); mild emotional disturbances tending to distort the ovulatory cycle; severe psychic trauma abruptly changing the bleeding pattern or completely suppressing one or more full ovulatory cycles; and malnutrition and intense exercise, causing an inadequate hypothalamic response.

PATHOPHYSIOLOGY

The mechanism varies depending on the cause and whether the defect is structural, hormonal, or both. Women who have adequate estrogen levels but a progesterone deficiency don't ovulate and are thus infertile. In primary amenorrhea, the hypothalamic-pituitary-ovarian axis is dysfunctional. Because of anatomic defects of the central nervous system, the ovary doesn't receive the hormonal signals that normally initiate the development of secondary sex characteristics and the beginning of menstruation.

Secondary amenorrhea can result from several central factors (hypogonadotropic hypoestrogenic anovulation), uterine factors (as with Asherman's syndrome, in which the endometrium is sufficiently scarred such that no functional endometrium exists), cervical stenosis, premature ovarian failure, and others.

SIGNS AND SYMPTOMS

Amenorrhea may result from many disorders; signs and symptoms depend on the specific cause and include absence of menstruation, vasomotor flushes, vaginal atrophy, hirsutism (abnormal hairiness), and acne (secondary amenorrhea).

COMPLICATIONS

Complications of amenorrhea include infertility and endometrial adenocarcinoma (amenorrhea associated with anovulation that gives rise to unopposed estrogen stimulation of the endometrium).

DIAGNOSIS

A diagnosis of primary amenorrhea is confirmed by a history of failure to menstruate in females age 16 and older, if consistent with bone age. Secondary amenorrhea is diagnosed after absence of menstruation for 3 months in a previously established menstrual pattern.

Physical and pelvic examination and sensitive pregnancy test rule out pregnancy, as well as anatomic abnormalities (such as cervical stenosis) that may cause false amenorrhea (cryptomenorrhea), in which menstruation occurs without external bleeding.

The diagnosis is confirmed with the onset of menstruation (spotting) within 1 week after giving pure progestational agents such as medroxyprogesterone (Provera), indicating that enough estrogen exists to stimulate the lining of the uterus. If menstruation doesn't occur, special diagnostic studies, such as gonadotropin levels, are indicated.

In amenorrhea, blood and urine studies show hormonal imbalances, such as lack of ovarian response to gonadotropins (elevated pituitary gonadotropin levels), failure of gonadotropin secretion (low pituitary gonadotropin levels), and abnormal thyroid levels (without suspicion of premature ovarian failure or central hypogonadotropism, gonadotropin levels aren't clinically meaningful because they're released in a pulsatile fashion; at a given time of day, levels may be elevated, low, or average).

A complete medical workup, including appropriate X-rays, laparoscopy, and a biopsy to identify ovarian, adrenal, and pituitary tumors, is part of the diagnostic process. Tests to identify dominant or missing hormones include "ferning" of cervical mucus on microscopic examination (an estrogen effect); vaginal cytologic examination; endometrial biopsy; serum progesterone level; serum androgen levels; elevated urinary 17-ketosteroid levels with excessive androgen secretions; plasma FSH level more than 50 IU/L, depending on the laboratory (suggests primary ovarian failure); or normal or low FSH level (possible hypothalamic or pituitary abnormality, depending on the clinical situation).

TREATMENT

Amenorrhea is treated with appropriate hormone replacement to reestablish menstruation. If amenorrhea isn't related to a hormone deficiency, treatment focuses on the cause (for example, surgery for amenorrhea caused by a tumor or obstruction). Treatment may involve inducing ovulation; with an intact pituitary gland, clomiphene (Clomid) may induce ovulation in women with secondary amenorrhea due to gonadotropin deficiency, polycystic ovarian disease, or excessive weight loss or gain if it's reversed.

Women with pituitary disease may require FSH and human menopausal gonadotropins (Pergonal). Lifestyle changes to treat amenorrhea include improving nutritional status and modifying daily exercise routine.

NURSING CONSIDERATIONS

✦ Explain all diagnostic procedures.
✦ Provide reassurance and emotional support. Psychiatric counseling may be necessary if amenorrhea results from emotional disturbances.
✦ After treatment, teach the patient how to keep an accurate record of her menstrual cycles to aid early detection of recurrent amenorrhea.

Diagnosis

✦ Confirmed by history of failure to menstruate in females ages 16 and older
✦ Secondary disease diagnosed after absence of menses for 3 months in previously established pattern
✦ Rule out pregnancy and anatomic abnormalities
✦ Diagnosis confirmed with onset of menstruation within 1 week after giving pure progestational agents
✦ Blood and urine show hormonal imbalances

Treatment

✦ Appropriate hormone replacement
✦ Inducing ovulation
✦ FSH and human menopausal gonadotropins
✦ Improving nutritional status
✦ Modifying daily exercise routine

Key nursing actions

✦ Explain all diagnostic procedures.
✦ Provide reassurance and emotional support.
✦ Psychiatric counseling may be necessary if amenorrhea results from emotional disturbances.
✦ After treatment, teach the patient how to keep an accurate record of her menstrual cycles to aid early detection of recurrent amenorrhea.

BENIGN PROSTATIC HYPERPLASIA

Although most men age 50 and older have some prostatic enlargement, in benign prostatic hyperplasia (BPH) — also known as *benign prostatic hypertrophy* — the prostate gland enlarges enough to compress the urethra and cause overt urinary obstruction. Depending on the size of the enlarged prostate, the age and health of the patient, and the extent of obstruction, BPH is treated symptomatically or surgically. BPH is common, affecting up to 50% of men age 50 and older, and 75% of men age 80 and older.

CAUSES

The main cause of BPH may be age-associated changes in hormone activity. Androgenic hormone production decreases with age, causing imbalance in androgen and estrogen levels and high levels of dihydrotestosterone, the main prostatic intracellular androgen.

Other causes include arteriosclerosis, inflammation, and metabolic or nutritional disturbances.

PATHOPHYSIOLOGY

Regardless of the cause, BPH begins with nonmalignant changes in periurethral glandular tissue. The growth of the fibroadenomatous nodules (masses of fibrous glandular tissue) progresses to compress the remaining normal gland (nodular hyperplasia). The hyperplastic tissue is mostly glandular, with some fibrous stroma and smooth muscle. As the prostate enlarges, it may extend into the bladder and obstruct urinary outflow by compressing or distorting the prostatic urethra. There are periodic increases in sympathetic stimulation of the smooth muscle of the prostatic urethra and bladder neck. Progressive bladder distention may also cause a pouch to form in the bladder that retains urine when the rest of the bladder empties. This retained urine may lead to calculus formation or cystitis.

SIGNS AND SYMPTOMS

Clinical features of BPH depend on the extent of prostatic enlargement and the lobes affected. Characteristically, the condition starts with a group of symptoms known as prostatism, which includes reduced urinary stream caliber and force, urinary hesitancy, and difficulty starting micturition (resulting in straining, feeling of incomplete voiding, and an interrupted stream).

As the obstruction increases, it causes frequent urination with nocturia, sense of urgency, dribbling, urine retention, incontinence, and possible hematuria.

COMPLICATIONS

As BPH worsens, a common complication is complete urinary obstruction after infection or while using decongestants, tranquilizers, alcohol, antidepressants, or anticholinergics. Other complications include infection, hydronephrosis, renal insufficiency and, if untreated, renal failure, urinary calculi, hemorrhage, and shock.

DIAGNOSIS

Diagnosis includes a physical examination that reveals a visible midline mass above the symphysis pubis (the bulge is a sign of an incompletely emptied bladder) and a rectal palpation that reveals an enlarged prostate. Clinical features and a rectal examination are usually sufficient for diagnosis.

A diagnosis of BPH may be confirmed by a variety of tests. Excretory urography rules out urinary tract obstruction, hydronephrosis (distention of the renal pelvis and calices due to obstruction of the ureter and consequent retention of urine), calculi or tumors, and filling and emptying defects in the bladder. Alternatively, if the patient isn't cooperative, cystoscopy rules out other causes of urinary tract obstruction (neoplasm, calculi).

In addition, elevated blood urea nitrogen and serum creatinine levels suggest renal dysfunction. An elevated prostate-specific antigen (PSA) contributes to the diagnosis, but prostatic carcinoma must be ruled out.

Urinalysis and urine cultures show hematuria, pyuria and, with bacterial count more than 100,000/µl, urinary tract infection (UTI). Cystourethroscopy is performed for severe symptoms and can be used to make a definitive diagnosis — revealing prostate enlargement, bladder wall changes, and a raised bladder. (Typically, cystourethroscopy is only done immediately before surgery to help determine the best procedure.)

TREATMENT

Conservative therapy for BPH includes prostate massages, sitz baths, fluid restriction to prevent bladder distention, antimicrobials to treat infection, and regular ejaculation to help relieve prostatic congestion. Alpha-adrenergic blockers, such as terazosin (Hytrin) and prazosin (Minipress), improve urine flow rates to relieve bladder outlet obstruction by preventing contractions of the prostatic capsule and bladder neck.

In some patients, the size of the prostate is reduced using finasteride (Proscar). In high-risk patients, an indwelling urinary catheter is used to alleviate urine retention and to provide continuous drainage.

In many patients, surgery is the only effective therapy for relieving acute urine retention, hydronephrosis, severe hematuria, recurrent UTIs, and other intolerable symptoms. Open surgical removal of the prostate can be performed using a variety of techniques: If the prostate weighs less than 2 oz (56.7 g), a transurethral resection is performed and tissue is removed with a wire loop and electric current using a resectoscope. But for prostatic enlargement remaining within the bladder, a suprapubic (transvesical) resection is the most common and useful procedure. A retropubic (extravesical) resection, however, allows direct visualization and maintains potency and continence.

Other possible procedures include balloon dilation of the urethra and prostatic stents to maintain urethral patency. Laser excision can also relieve prostatic enlargement. Today, nerve-sparing surgical techniques reduce common complications such as erectile dysfunction.

NURSING CONSIDERATIONS

✦ Monitor and record the patient's vital signs, intake and output, and daily weight, watching closely for signs of postobstructive diuresis (such as increased urine output and hypotension) that may lead to serious dehydration, reduced blood volume, shock, electrolyte loss, and anuria.
✦ Insert an indwelling urinary catheter for urine retention (usually difficult in a patient with BPH). Using a coude catheter may make insertion easier.
✦ If the catheter can't be passed transurethrally, assist with suprapubic cystostomy under local anesthetic (watching for rapid bladder decompression).

Diagnosis
✦ Visible midline mass above symphysis pubis
✦ Rectal palpation reveals enlarged prostate
✦ Elevated blood urea nitrogen and serum creatinine levels
✦ Elevated PSA

Treatment
✦ Prostate massages
✦ Sitz baths
✦ Fluid restriction
✦ Antimicrobials
✦ Regular ejaculation
✦ Alpha-adrenergic blockers

Key nursing actions
✦ Monitor and record vital signs, intake and output, and daily weight.
✦ Watch closely for signs of postobstructive diuresis.
✦ Insert an indwelling urinary catheter for urine retention.
✦ If the catheter can't be passed transurethrally, assist with suprapubic cystostomy under local anesthetic.

Key nursing actions

After prostatic surgery

✦ Observe for immediate dangers of prostatic bleeding.

✦ Keep the catheter open at a rate sufficient to maintain clear, light pink returns.

✦ Irrigate a catheter with stopped drainage due to clots with 80 to 100 ml normal saline solution, as ordered, maintaining strict sterile technique.

✦ Administer belladonna and opium suppositories or other anticholinergics as ordered.

✦ Suppositories and rectal temperatures are sometimes contraindicated after open prostatic procedures; confirm orders with the physician.

✦ Administer stool softeners and laxatives as ordered to prevent straining.

✦ Reassure the patient that temporary frequency, dribbling, and occasional hematuria will likely occur after the catheter is removed.

✦ Encourage annual digital rectal exams and screening for PSA to identify a possible malignancy.

Characteristics of dysmenorrhea

✦ Painful menstruation associated with ovulation not related to pelvic disease

✦ Incidence peaks in early 20s and slowly decreases

✦ Can occur as a primary disorder or secondary to underlying disease

✦ Prognosis generally good

After prostatic surgery

✦ Maintain patient comfort; watch for and prevent postoperative complications; observe for immediate dangers of prostatic bleeding (shock, hemorrhage); check the catheter often (every 15 minutes for the first 2 to 3 hours) for patency and urine color; and check dressings for bleeding.

✦ Postoperatively, many urologists insert a three-way catheter and establish continuous bladder irrigation. Keep the catheter open at a rate sufficient to maintain clear, light pink returns; watch for fluid overload from absorption of the irrigating fluid into systemic circulation; observe an indwelling regular catheter closely (if used); and irrigate a catheter with stopped drainage due to clots with 80 to 100 ml normal saline solution, as ordered, maintaining strict sterile technique.

✦ Watch for septic shock (most serious complication of prostatic surgery); immediately report severe chills, sudden fever, tachycardia, hypotension, or other signs of shock; start rapid infusion of I.V. antibiotics as ordered; watch for signs and symptoms of a pulmonary embolus, heart failure, and renal failure; and monitor vital signs, central venous pressure, and arterial pressure continuously. (Supportive care in the intensive care unit may be needed.)

✦ Administer belladonna and opium suppositories or other anticholinergics as ordered to relieve painful bladder spasms that often occur after transurethral resection.

✦ After an open procedure, take patient comfort measures, such as providing suppositories (except after perineal prostatectomy), analgesic medication to control incisional pain, and frequent dressing changes. Suppositories and rectal temperatures are sometimes contraindicated after open prostatic procedures; confirm orders with the physician.

✦ Continue infusing I.V. fluids until the patient can drink sufficient fluids (2 to 3 qt/day [2 to 3 L]) to maintain adequate hydration.

✦ Administer stool softeners and laxatives as ordered to prevent straining. (Don't check for fecal impaction because a rectal examination may precipitate bleeding.)

✦ Reassure the patient that temporary frequency, dribbling, and occasional hematuria will likely occur after the catheter is removed.

✦ Reinforce prescribed limits on activity, such as lifting, strenuous exercise, and long automobile rides that increase bleeding tendency; caution the patient to restrict sexual activity for several weeks after discharge.

✦ Instruct the patient about the prescribed oral antibiotic drug regimen and indications for using gentle laxatives.

✦ Urge the patient to seek medical care immediately if he can't void, passes bloody urine, or develops a fever.

✦ Encourage annual digital rectal exams and screening for PSA to identify a possible malignancy.

DYSMENORRHEA

Dysmenorrhea is painful menstruation associated with ovulation that isn't related to pelvic disease. It's the most common gynecologic complaint and a leading cause of absenteeism from school (affecting 10% of high school girls each month) and work (estimated 140 million work hours lost annually). The incidence peaks in women in their early 20s and then slowly decreases.

Dysmenorrhea can occur as a primary disorder or secondary to an underlying disease. Because primary dysmenorrhea is self-limiting, the prognosis is generally good. The prognosis for secondary dysmenorrhea depends on the underlying disorder.

CAUSES

Although primary dysmenorrhea is unrelated to an identifiable cause, possible contributing factors include hormonal imbalance and psychogenic factors.

Dysmenorrhea may also be secondary to such gynecologic disorders as endometriosis, cervical stenosis, uterine leiomyomas (benign fibroid tumors), pelvic inflammatory disease, and pelvic tumors.

PATHOPHYSIOLOGY

The pain of dysmenorrhea probably results from increased prostaglandin secretion in menstrual blood, which intensifies normal uterine contractions. Prostaglandins intensify myometrial smooth muscle contraction and uterine blood vessel constriction, thereby worsening the uterine hypoxia normally associated with menstruation. This combination of intense muscle contractions and hypoxia causes the intense pain of dysmenorrhea. Prostaglandins and their metabolites can also cause GI disturbances, headache, and syncope.

Because dysmenorrhea almost always follows an ovulatory cycle, both the primary and secondary forms are rare during the anovulatory cycle of menses. After age 20, dysmenorrhea is generally secondary.

SIGNS AND SYMPTOMS

Possible signs and symptoms of dysmenorrhea include sharp, intermittent, cramping, lower abdominal pain that usually radiates to the back, thighs, groin, and vulva, and typically starts with or immediately before menstrual flow and peaks within 24 hours.

Dysmenorrhea may also be associated with signs and symptoms suggestive of premenstrual syndrome, including urinary frequency, nausea, vomiting, diarrhea, headache, backache, chills, abdominal bloating, painful breasts, depression, and irritability.

COMPLICATIONS

A possible but rare complication of dysmenorrhea is dehydration due to nausea, vomiting, and diarrhea.

DIAGNOSIS

To diagnose dysmenorrhea, a pelvic examination is performed and a detailed patient history is taken to help suggest the cause. A diagnosis of primary dysmenorrhea is made by ruling out secondary causes for menses that have been painful since menarche. Tests, such as laparoscopy, hysteroscopy, and pelvic ultrasound, are used to diagnose underlying disorders in secondary dysmenorrhea. Psychological evaluation and appropriate counseling help identify a psychogenic cause of persistently severe dysmenorrhea.

TREATMENT

The initial treatment of dysmenorrhea aims to relieve pain. Analgesics, such as nonsteroidal anti-inflammatory drugs, are suggested for mild to moderate pain; these are especially effective because they inhibit prostaglandin synthesis through inhibition of the enzyme cyclooxygenase and are most effective when taken 24 to 48 hours before the onset of menses. Opioids aren't frequently used but may be given for severe pain.

Causes
+ Primary form unrelated to identifiable cause
+ Hormonal imbalance and psychogenic factors are contributing factors
+ Secondary to endometriosis, cervical stenosis, uterine leiomyomas, pelvic inflammatory disease, pelvic tumors

How it happens
+ Pain probably results from increased prostaglandin secretion
+ Intensifies normal uterine contractions
+ Combination of intense muscle contractions and hypoxia causes intense pain
+ Can also cause GI disturbances, headache, syncope
+ Primary and secondary forms rare during anovulatory cycle of menses

Key signs and symptoms
+ Sharp, intermittent, cramping, lower abdominal pain
+ Urinary frequency
+ Nausea, vomiting, diarrhea
+ Headache

Complications
+ Dehydration (rare)

Diagnosis
+ Pelvic examination, detailed patient history
+ Rule out secondary causes
+ Tests to diagnose underlying disorders
+ Psychological evaluation

Treatment

+ Analgesics
+ Opioids
+ Prostaglandin inhibitors
+ Heat applied to lower abdomen
+ Sex steroids
+ Psychological counseling

Key nursing actions

+ Obtain a complete history focusing on the patient's gynecologic complaints.
+ Provide thorough patient teaching, including explanation of normal female anatomy and physiology as well as the nature of dysmenorrhea.
+ Encourage the patient to keep a detailed record of her menstrual cycle and symptoms and to seek medical care if symptoms persist.

Characteristics of endometriosis

+ Presence of endometrial tissue outside lining of uterine cavity
+ Ectopic tissue generally confined to pelvic area but can appear anywhere in body
+ May occur at any age
+ Abrupt or slow onset
+ Infertility occurs in 30% to 40% of cases
+ Usually manifests during menstrual years

Also suggested for relief of pain are prostaglandin inhibitors such as mefenamic acid and ibuprofen. These drugs work by decreasing the severity of uterine contractions. Heat applied to the lower abdomen may also relieve discomfort in mature women but should be used cautiously in young adolescents because appendicitis may mimic dysmenorrhea.

For primary dysmenorrhea, sex steroids, such as hormonal contraceptives, are effective alternatives to treatment with antiprostaglandins or analgesics. These steroids relieve pain by suppressing ovulation and inhibiting endometrial prostaglandin synthesis. Patients attempting pregnancy should rely on antiprostaglandin therapy.

If a psychogenic cause of persistently severe dysmenorrhea exists, appropriate psychological counseling is suggested. Treatment of secondary dysmenorrhea is designed to identify and correct the underlying cause and may include surgical treatment of underlying disorders, such as endometriosis or uterine leiomyomas (after conservative therapy fails).

NURSING CONSIDERATIONS

Effective management of the patient with dysmenorrhea focuses on relief of symptoms, emotional support, and appropriate patient teaching, especially for the adolescent.

+ Obtain a complete history focusing on the patient's gynecologic complaints, including detailed information on symptoms of pelvic disease, such as excessive bleeding, changes in bleeding pattern, vaginal discharge, and dyspareunia (painful intercourse).
+ Provide thorough patient teaching, including explanation of normal female anatomy and physiology as well as the nature of dysmenorrhea (depending on circumstances, providing the adolescent patient with information on pregnancy and contraception).
+ Encourage the patient to keep a detailed record of her menstrual cycle and symptoms and to seek medical care if symptoms persist.

ENDOMETRIOSIS

Endometriosis is the presence of endometrial tissue outside the lining of the uterine cavity. Ectopic tissue is generally confined to the pelvic area, usually around the ovaries, uterovesical peritoneum, uterosacral ligaments, and cul de sac, but it can appear anywhere in the body.

Active endometriosis may occur at any age, including adolescence. Up to 50% of infertile women may have endometriosis, although the true incidence in both fertile and infertile women remains unknown.

Severe symptoms of endometriosis may have an abrupt onset or may develop over many years. Infertility occurs in 30% to 40% of women with endometriosis. Endometriosis usually manifests during the menstrual years; after menopause, it tends to subside. Hormonal treatment of endometriosis (continuous use of hormonal contraceptives, danazol [Danocrine], and gonadotropin-releasing hormone [GnRH] antagonists) is potentially effective in relieving discomfort, although treatment for advanced stages of endometriosis usually isn't as successful because of impaired follicular development. However, nonsurgical treatment of endometriosis generally remains inadequate. Surgery appears to be the more effective way to enhance fertility, although definitive class I evidence doesn't currently exist. Pharmacologic and surgical treatment of endometriosis may help manage chronic pelvic pain.

CAUSES

The cause of endometriosis remains unknown, but several theories attempt to explain this disorder (one or more causes are perhaps true for certain populations of women).

One theory suggests that retrograde menstruation may implant ectopic sites (retrograde menstruation alone may not be sufficient for endometriosis to occur because it occurs in women with no clinical evidence of endometriosis). A second theory suggests that a genetic predisposition and depressed immune system may predispose a woman to endometriosis. A third theory blames coelomic metaplasia, repeated inflammation inducing metaplasia of mesothelial cells to the endometrial epithelium. A fourth theory says that lymphatic or hematogenous spread may cause the extraperitoneal disease.

PATHOPHYSIOLOGY

The ectopic endometrial tissue responds to normal stimulation in the same way as the endometrium, but more unpredictably. The endometrial cells respond to estrogen and progesterone with proliferation and secretion. During menstruation, the ectopic tissue bleeds, which causes inflammation of the surrounding tissues. This inflammation causes fibrosis, leading to adhesions that produce pain and infertility.

SIGNS AND SYMPTOMS

The classic symptoms of endometriosis include dysmenorrhea, abnormal uterine bleeding, and infertility. Pain typically begins 5 to 7 days before menses peaks and lasts for 2 to 3 days and varies among patients. Severity of pain doesn't indicate the extent of disease.

Other signs and symptoms depend on the location of the ectopic tissue. If located in the ovaries and oviducts, the patient experiences infertility and profuse menses. Deep-thrust dyspareunia occurs if the tissue is in the ovaries or cul de sac. Suprapubic pain, dysuria, and hematuria are a result of ectopic tissue in the bladder. Abdominal cramps, pain on defecation, constipation, and bloody stools due to bleeding of ectopic endometrium in the rectosigmoid musculature are caused by tissue in the large bowel and appendix. If the tissue is in the cervix, vagina, or perineum, bleeding from endometrial deposits in these areas during menses and pain on intercourse are the classic signs and symptoms.

COMPLICATIONS

Complications of endometriosis include infertility due to fibrosis, scarring and adhesions (major complication), chronic pelvic pain, and ovarian carcinoma (rare).

DIAGNOSIS

The only definitive way to diagnose endometriosis is through laparoscopy or laparotomy. Pelvic examination may suggest endometriosis or be unremarkable. Findings suggestive of endometriosis include multiple tender nodules on uterosacral ligaments or in the rectovaginal septum (in one-third of the patients), and ovarian enlargement in the presence of endometrial cysts on the ovaries.

Although laparoscopy is recommended to diagnose and determine the extent of disease, some clinicians recommend empiric trial of GnRH agonist therapy to confirm or refute the impression of endometriosis before resorting to laparoscopy (controversial, but may be cost-effective). A biopsy is done at the time of la-

Causes

Theories
- Retrograde menstruation implants ectopic sites
- Genetic predisposition, depressed immune system
- Coelomic metaplasia
- Lymphatic or hematogenous spread

How it happens
- Ectopic endometrial tissue responds to normal stimulation, but unpredictably
- Endometrial cells respond to estrogen and progesterone with proliferation and secretion
- Tissue bleeds during menstruation, causing inflammation of surrounding tissues
- Inflammation causes fibrosis, leading to adhesions

Key signs and symptoms
- Dysmenorrhea
- Abnormal uterine bleeding
- Infertility
- Suprapubic pain

Complications
- Infertility
- Chronic pelvic pain
- Ovarian carcinoma (rare)

Diagnosis
- Laparoscopy or laparotomy with biopsy
- Pelvic examination may suggest endometriosis
- Multiple tender nodules on uterosacral ligaments or in rectovaginal septum

paroscopy (helpful to confirm the diagnosis), although in some instances, diagnosis is confirmed by visual inspection.

TREATMENT

Treatment of endometriosis varies according to the stage of the disease and the patient's age and desire to have children. Conservative therapy for young women who want to have children includes androgens such as danazol (Danocrine); progestins and continuous combined hormonal contraceptives (pseudopregnancy regimen) to relieve symptoms by causing a regression of endometrial tissue; and GnRH agonists to induce pseudomenopause (medical oophorectomy), causing remission of the disease (commonly used).

No pharmacologic treatment has been shown to cure the disease or be effective in all women, and there are disadvantages of nonsurgical therapy. The woman may experience an adverse reaction to drug-induced menopause (including osteoporosis if used for more than 6 months), and a recurrence of endometriosis is possible after discontinuing GnRH agonists.

Another drawback is that drug-induced menopause can become costly when used for an extended duration, and danazol (Danocrine) can also cause weight gain. Using continuous hormonal contraceptive pills to treat endometriosis results in the lowest fertility rates of any medical treatment. Progestin is as effective as GnRH antagonists but may cause weight gain and symptoms of depression.

When ovarian masses are present, surgery is performed to rule out cancer. There are several types of conservative surgery: Endometrial implants can be removed laparoscopically with conventional or laser techniques (no benefit shown for laser laparoscopy over electrocautery or suture methods). A presacral neurectomy may be performed for central pelvic pain. It's effective in about 50% or fewer of appropriate candidates. Laparoscopic uterosacral nerve ablation (LUNA) is another method used to treat central pelvic pain, although definitive studies supporting the efficacy of LUNA are lacking.

The treatment of last resort for women who don't want to have children or for extensive disease is a total abdominal hysterectomy with or without bilateral salpingo-oophorectomy. It's unclear whether ovarian conservation is appropriate, and success rates vary.

NURSING CONSIDERATIONS

✦ Minor gynecologic procedures are contraindicated immediately before and during menstruation.

✦ Advise adolescents to use sanitary napkins instead of tampons; this can help prevent retrograde flow in girls with a narrow vagina or small introitus.

✦ Because infertility is a possible complication, advise the patient who wants children not to postpone childbearing.

✦ Recommend an annual pelvic examination and Papanicolaou test to all patients.

ERECTILE DISORDER

Erectile dysfunction, or impotence, refers to a male's inability to attain or maintain penile erection sufficient to complete intercourse. The patient with primary impotence has never achieved a sufficient erection. Secondary impotence is more common but no less disturbing than the primary form and implies that the patient has succeeded in completing intercourse in the past.

Treatment

✦ Varies according to stage of disease, patient's age, desire to have children

✦ Androgens

✦ Progestins and continuous combined hormonal contraceptives

✦ GnRH agonists

✦ Surgery

Key nursing actions

✦ Minor gynecologic procedures are contraindicated immediately before and during menstruation.

✦ Advise adolescents to use sanitary napkins instead of tampons.

✦ Because infertility is a possible complication, advise the patient who wants children not to postpone childbearing.

✦ Recommend annual pelvic examination and Pap test.

Characteristics of erectile disorder

✦ Refers to inability to attain and maintain penile erection sufficient to complete intercourse

✦ Primary: has never achieved sufficient erection

✦ Secondary: patient has previously succeeded in completing intercourse

✦ Transient periods of impotence not considered dysfunction

✦ Affects all age-groups; increases in frequency with age

Transient periods of impotence aren't considered dysfunction and probably occur in half of adult males. Erectile disorder affects all age-groups but increases in frequency with age. The prognosis for erectile dysfunction patients depends on the severity and duration of their impotence and the underlying causes.

CAUSES

Causes of erectile dysfunction include psychogenic factors (50% to 60% of cases), organic causes, or both psychogenic and organic factors in some patients. This complexity makes the isolation of the primary cause difficult.

Psychogenic causes of erectile dysfunction include intrapersonal causes that reflect personal sexual anxieties and generally involve guilt, fear, depression, or feelings of inadequacy resulting from previous traumatic sexual experience; rejection by parents or peers; exaggerated religious orthodoxy; abnormal mother-son intimacy; or homosexual experiences.

Other causes include psychogenic factors that reflect a disturbed sexual relationship — possibly stemming from differences in sexual preferences between partners, lack of communication, insufficient knowledge of sexual function, or nonsexual personal conflicts and situational impotence — or a temporary condition in response to stress.

Organic causes include chronic diseases that cause neurologic and vascular impairment, such as cardiopulmonary disease, diabetes, multiple sclerosis, or renal failure; liver cirrhosis causing increased circulating estrogen due to reduced hepatic inactivation; spinal cord trauma; complications of surgery, particularly radical prostatectomy; drug- or alcohol-induced dysfunction; and genital anomalies or central nervous system defects (rare).

PATHOPHYSIOLOGY

Neurologic dysfunction results in lack of the autonomic signal and, in combination with vascular disease, interferes with arteriolar dilation. The blood is shunted around the sacs of the corpus cavernosum into medium-sized veins, which prevents the sacs from filling completely. Also, perfusion of the corpus cavernosum is initially compromised because of partial obstruction of small arteries, leading to loss of erection before ejaculation.

Psychogenic causes may exacerbate emotional problems in a circular pattern; anxiety causes fear of erectile dysfunction, which causes further emotional problems.

SIGNS AND SYMPTOMS

There are three classifications of secondary erectile disorder: A *partial* erectile disorder is the inability to achieve or sustain a full erection. A man with an *intermittent* erectile disorder is sometimes potent with the same partner. A patient who is potent only with certain partners has a *selective* erectile disorder.

Some men lose erectile function suddenly, and others lose it gradually. If the cause isn't organic, erection may still be achieved through masturbation.

Immediately before a sexual encounter, patients with psychogenic impotence may feel anxious, perspire, have palpitations, and lose interest in sexual activity.

Causes
+ Psychogenic factors (50% to 60% of cases)
+ Organic causes
+ Combination

How it happens
+ Neurologic dysfunction results in lack of autonomic signal
+ In combination with vascular disease, interferes with arteriolar dilation
+ Psychogenic causes may exacerbate emotional problems in circular pattern
+ Anxiety causes fear of erectile dysfunction, which causes further emotional problems

Key signs and symptoms
+ Partial: inability to achieve or sustain full erection
+ Intermittent: sometimes potent with same partner
+ Selective: potent only with certain partners
+ If cause is not organic, erection may still be achieved through masturbation
+ Patients with psychogenic form may feel anxious, perspire, have palpitations, lose interest in sexual activity before intercourse

Complications
+ Severe depression
+ Strain on sexual relationships

Diagnosis
+ Detailed sexual history to differentiate between organic and psychogenic factors, primary and secondary form
+ Ruling out chronic diseases
+ Fulfilling diagnostic criteria for DSM-IV diagnosis

Treatment
+ Sex therapy including both partners
+ Reversal of organic cause, if possible
+ Psychological counseling
+ Exploring alternatives for sexual expression
+ Viagra or Levitra
+ Testosterone supplementation for hypogonadal men
+ Adrenergic antagonists

Key nursing actions
+ Help the patient feel comfortable about discussing his sexuality.
+ Assess his sexual health during your initial nursing history.
+ After penile implant surgery, instruct the patient to avoid intercourse until the incision heals, usually in 6 weeks.

To help prevent impotence
+ Provide information about resuming sexual activity.

COMPLICATIONS

A complication of erectile dysfunction is severe depression (patients with psychogenic or organic drug-induced erectile dysfunction), causing the impotence or resulting from it. It may also place a strain on sexual relationships.

DIAGNOSIS

A detailed sexual history helps differentiate between organic and psychogenic factors and primary and secondary impotence. Questions typically include:
+ Does the patient have intermittent, selective nocturnal, or early morning erections?
+ Can he achieve erections through other sexual activity?
+ When did his dysfunction begin, and what was his life situation at that time?
+ Did erectile problems occur suddenly or gradually?
+ What prescription or nonprescription drugs is he taking?
+ How often and how much alcohol does he drink?

A diagnosis of erectile disorder also includes ruling out such chronic diseases as diabetes and other vascular, neurologic, or urogenital problems. Additionally, such a diagnosis includes fulfilling the diagnostic criteria for the *Diagnostic and Statistical Manual of Mental Disorders*, 4th ed. (*DSM-IV*) diagnosis (when the disorder causes marked distress or interpersonal difficulty).

TREATMENT

Treatment for psychogenic impotence includes sex therapy including both partners (the course and content of therapy depend on the specific cause of dysfunction and the nature of the partner relationship) and teaching or helping the patient to improve verbal communication skills, eliminate unreasonable guilt, or reevaluate attitudes toward sex and sexual roles.

The cause of organic impotence is reversed, if possible. If reversing the cause isn't possible, psychological counseling will help the couple deal realistically with their situation and explore alternatives for sexual expression. In appropriate patients, sildenafil (Viagra) or vardenafil (Levitra) causes vasodilatation within the penis and may effectively manage erectile dysfunction.

Other treatments include testosterone supplementation for hypogonadal men (it isn't given to men with prostate cancer) and an adrenergic antagonist, yohimbine, to enhance parasympathetic neurotransmission. Prostaglandin E injected directly into the corpus cavernosum may induce an erection for 30 to 60 minutes in some men. An inflatable or noninflatable penile implant can be surgically inserted in some patients with organic impotence.

NURSING CONSIDERATIONS

+ When you identify a patient with impotence, help him feel comfortable about discussing his sexuality. Assess his sexual health during your initial nursing history. When appropriate, refer him for further evaluation or treatment.
+ After penile implant surgery, instruct the patient to avoid intercourse until the incision heals, usually in 6 weeks.

To help prevent impotence
+ Promote establishment of responsible health and sex education programs at primary, secondary, and college levels.
+ Provide information about resuming sexual activity as part of discharge instructions for any patient with a condition that requires modification of daily activities.

Such patients include those with cardiac disease, diabetes, hypertension, and chronic obstructive pulmonary disease and all postoperative patients.

HYDROCELE

A hydrocele is a collection of fluid between the visceral and parietal layers of the tunica vaginalis of the testicle or along the spermatic cord. It's the most common cause of scrotal swelling.

CAUSES

Possible causes of hydrocele include congenital malformation (infants), trauma to the testes or epididymis, infection of the testes or epididymis, and testicular tumor.

PATHOPHYSIOLOGY

Congenital hydrocele occurs because of a patency between the scrotal sac and the peritoneal cavity, allowing peritoneal fluids to collect in the scrotum. The exact mechanism of congenital hydrocele is unknown.

In adults, the fluid accumulation may be caused by infection, trauma, tumor, an imbalance between the secreting and absorptive capacities of scrotal tissue, or an obstruction of lymphatic or venous drainage in the spermatic cord. This leads to a displacement of fluid in the scrotum, outside the testes. Subsequent swelling results, leading to reduced blood flow to the testes.

SIGNS AND SYMPTOMS

A patient with hydrocele will complain of scrotal swelling and a feeling of heaviness. He may have an inguinal hernia (often present in congenital hydrocele). The size of the scrotum can range from slightly larger than the testes to the size of a grapefruit or larger, and the patient may have fluid collection with either a flaccid or a tense mass. With acute epididymal infection or testicular torsion, he will experience pain. Scrotal tenderness is the result of severe swelling.

COMPLICATIONS

Complications may include epididymitis and testicular atrophy.

DIAGNOSIS

When diagnosing a hydrocele, transillumination distinguishes a fluid-filled mass from a solid one (a tumor doesn't transilluminate). Ultrasound allows visualization of the testes and determination of the presence of a tumor. Fluid biopsy determines the cause and differentiates between normal cells and a malignancy.

TREATMENT

Usually, no treatment of congenital hydrocele is indicated, as this condition frequently resolves spontaneously by age 1. Otherwise, there are possible treatments for hydrocele. These include surgical repair to prevent strangulation of the bowel (inguinal hernia with bowel present in the sac). For a tense hydrocele that impedes blood circulation or causes pain, fluid is aspirated and a sclerosing drug is injected into the scrotal sac. For recurrent hydrocele, the tunica vaginalis may be excised,

Characteristics of hydrocele

✦ Collection of fluid between visceral and parietal layers of tunica vaginalis of testicle or spermatic cord

Causes

✦ Congenital malformation
✦ Trauma or infection to testes or epididymis

How it happens

✦ Occurs from patency between scrotal sac and peritoneal cavity
✦ Peritoneal fluids collect in scrotum
✦ May be caused by organic factors

Key signs and symptoms

✦ Scrotal swelling, feeling of heaviness or tenderness
✦ Inguinal hernia
✦ Enlarged scrotum
✦ Fluid collection with flaccid or tense mass

Complications

✦ Epididymitis
✦ Testicular atrophy

Diagnosis

✦ Transillumination distinguishes fluid-filled mass from solid
✦ Ultrasound allows visualization of testes, determination of presence of tumor

Treatment

✦ May resolve itself by age 1
✦ Surgical repair
✦ Fluid aspiration

Key nursing actions

✦ Place a rolled towel between the patient's legs and elevate the scrotum to reduce severe swelling.

✦ Advise the patient to wear a loose-fitting athletic supporter lined with soft cotton dressings.

Characteristics of polycystic ovarian syndrome

✦ Metabolic disorder characterized by multiple ovarian cysts
✦ Obesity in 50% to 80% of cases
✦ Prognosis good for ovulation and fertility with treatment

Causes

✦ Theory: abnormal enzyme activity triggers excess androgen secretion, endocrine abnormalities

How it happens

✦ Lack of pulsatile release of gonadotropin-releasing hormone
✦ Small follicles begin to accumulate because no selection of a dominant follicle
✦ Follicles may respond abnormally to hormonal stimulation
✦ Endocrine abnormalities may cause condition, or cystic abnormalities

Key signs and symptoms

✦ Mild pelvic discomfort
✦ Lower back pain
✦ Dyspareunia

Complications

✦ Malignancy
✦ Risk of cardiovascular disease
✦ Type 2 diabetes mellitus

---

and a suprainguinal excision may be performed for a testicular tumor detected by ultrasound.

NURSING CONSIDERATIONS

✦ Place a rolled towel between the patient's legs and elevate the scrotum to help reduce severe swelling. Or, if the patient has mild or moderate swelling, advise him to wear a loose-fitting athletic supporter lined with soft cotton dressings.
✦ Encourage sitz baths, and apply heat or ice packs to decrease inflammation.

POLYCYSTIC OVARIAN SYNDROME

Polycystic ovarian syndrome is a metabolic disorder characterized by multiple ovarian cysts. About 22% of the women in the United States have the disorder, and obesity is present in 50% to 80% of these women. Among those who seek treatment for infertility, more than 75% have some degree of polycystic ovarian syndrome, usually manifested by anovulation alone. Prognosis is good for ovulation and fertility with appropriate treatment.

CAUSES

The precise cause of polycystic ovarian syndrome is unknown. Theories include abnormal enzyme activity triggering excess androgen secretion from the ovaries and adrenal glands and endocrine abnormalities causing all of the signs and symptoms of polycystic ovarian disease (amenorrhea, polycystic ovaries on ultrasound, and hyperandrogenism [part of the Stein-Leventhal syndrome]).

PATHOPHYSIOLOGY

A general feature of all anovulation syndromes is a lack of pulsatile release of gonadotropin-releasing hormone. Initial ovarian follicle development is normal. Many small follicles begin to accumulate because no selection of a dominant follicle occurs. These follicles may respond abnormally to the hormonal stimulation, causing an abnormal pattern of estrogen secretion during the menstrual cycle. Endocrine abnormalities may cause polycystic ovarian syndrome or cystic abnormalities; muscle and adipose tissue are resistant to the effects of insulin, and lipid metabolism is abnormal.

SIGNS AND SYMPTOMS

Signs and symptoms of classic polycystic ovarian syndrome (Stein-Leventhal syndrome) include mild pelvic discomfort, lower back pain, dyspareunia, abnormal uterine bleeding secondary to disturbed ovulatory pattern, hirsutism, acne, and male-pattern hair loss.

COMPLICATIONS

Possible complications of polycystic ovarian syndrome include malignancy due to sustained estrogenic stimulation of the endometrium, increased risk of cardiovascular disease, and type 2 diabetes mellitus due to insulin resistance.

Polycystic ovarian disease may produce secondary amenorrhea, oligomenorrhea, and infertility.

DIAGNOSIS

Diagnosis of polycystic ovarian disease includes history and physical examination showing bilaterally enlarged polycystic ovaries and menstrual disturbance, usually dating back to menarche. Visualization of the ovary through ultrasound, laparoscopy, or surgery (often for another condition) may confirm ovarian cysts.

Diagnostic studies and procedures include basal body temperature graphs and endometrial biopsy that show slightly elevated urinary 17-ketosteroid levels and anovulation. The patient typically has an elevated ratio of luteinizing hormone to follicle-stimulating hormone (usually 3:1 or greater), and elevated levels of testosterone and androstenedione. Anovulation results in unopposed estrogen action during the menstrual cycle. Direct visualization by laparoscopy rules out paraovarian cysts of the broad ligament, salpingitis, endometriosis, and neoplastic cysts.

TREATMENT

Treatment of polycystic ovarian syndrome includes monitoring the patient's weight to maintain a normal body mass index in order to reduce risks associated with insulin resistance, which may cause spontaneous ovulation in some women.

Treatment of polycystic ovarian disease may include the administration of drugs. Clomiphene (Clomid) is prescribed to induce ovulation. The patient wanting to become pregnant can be given medroxyprogesterone (Provera) for 10 days each month. Low-dose hormonal contraceptives treat abnormal bleeding for the patient needing reliable contraception.

NURSING CONSIDERATIONS

✦ Preoperatively, watch for signs of cyst rupture, such as increasing abdominal pain, distention, and rigidity, and monitor vital signs for fever, tachypnea, or hypotension (possibly indicating peritonitis or intraperitoneal hemorrhage).
✦ Postoperatively, encourage frequent movement in bed and early ambulation as ordered to prevent pulmonary embolism.
✦ Provide emotional support, offering appropriate reassurance if the patient fears cancer or infertility.

PROSTATITIS

Prostatitis, or inflammation of the prostate gland, may be acute or chronic. Acute prostatitis most commonly results from gram-negative bacteria and is easy to recognize and treat. However, chronic prostatitis, the most common cause of recurrent urinary tract infections (UTIs) in men, is less easy to recognize. Up to 35% of men age 50 and older have chronic prostatitis. Granulomatous prostatitis (tuberculous prostatitis), nonbacterial prostatitis, and prostatodynia (painful prostate) are other classifications of the disease.

CAUSES

Escherichia coli cause 80% of cases of bacterial prostatitis; *Klebsiella, Enterobacter, Proteus, Pseudomonas, Streptococcus,* or *Staphylococcus* organisms cause 20% of cases.

These organisms probably spread to the prostate by an ascending urethral infection or through the bloodstream, invasion of rectal bacteria through lymphatics,

Diagnosis
✦ History, physical examination showing bilaterally enlarged polycystic ovaries, menstrual disturbance
✦ Visualization of ovary through ultrasound, laparoscopy, surgery
✦ Basal body temperature graphs
✦ Endometrial biopsy
✦ Elevated ratio of luteinizing hormone to follicle-stimulating hormone
✦ Elevated testosterone, androstenedione

Treatment
✦ Monitor patient's weight
✦ Clomiphene
✦ Medroxyprogesterone

Key nursing actions
✦ Preoperatively, watch for signs of cyst rupture.
✦ Postoperatively, encourage frequent movement in bed and early ambulation as ordered to prevent pulmonary embolism.

Characteristics of prostatitis
✦ Inflammation of prostate gland
✦ Acute form commonly result of gram-negative bacteria
✦ Chronic form commonly caused by recurrent UTIs
✦ Granulomatous prostatitis, nonbacterial prostatitis, prostatodynia other classifications

Causes
✦ *E. coli* cause 80% of bacterial prostatitis
✦ *Klebsiella, Enterobacter, Proteus, Pseudomonas, Streptococcus, or Staphylococcus* cause 20%

Alert!

✦ Acute prostatitis is associated with benign prostatic hyperplasia in older men.

How it happens

✦ Spasms in genitourinary tract or tension in pelvic floor muscles cause inflammation, nonbacterial prostatitis
✦ Bacterial infections result of previous or concurrent infection
✦ Bacteria ascend from infected urethra, bladder, lymphatics, blood through prostatic ducts into prostate
✦ Infection stimulates inflammatory response
✦ Prostate becomes larger, tender, firm
✦ Inflammation usually limited to gland's excretory ducts

Key signs and symptoms

✦ Chills
✦ Lower back pain
✦ Perineal fullness
✦ Suprapubic tenderness
✦ Frequent and urgent urination
✦ Dysuria
✦ Nocturia

Complications

✦ UTI
✦ Infected and abscessed testis

Diagnosis

✦ Tender, warm, enlarged prostate
✦ Firm, irregularly shaped, slightly enlarged prostate
✦ Prostatic calculi
✦ Identification of causative infectious organism

reflux of infected bladder urine into prostate ducts, infrequent or excessive sexual intercourse, such procedures as cystoscopy or catheterization (less commonly), and bacterial invasion from the urethra (chronic prostatitis).

Granulomatous prostatitis is caused by *Mycobacterium tuberculosis.* The cause of nonbacterial prostatitis is unknown, but possible causes include infection by a protozoa or virus. The cause of prostatodynia is also unknown.

 CLINICAL ALERT Acute prostatitis is associated with benign prostatic hyperplasia in older men.

PATHOPHYSIOLOGY

Spasms in the genitourinary tract or tension in the pelvic floor muscles may cause inflammation and nonbacterial prostatitis.

Bacterial prostatic infections can be the result of a previous or concurrent infection. The bacteria ascend from the infected urethra, bladder, lymphatics, or blood through the prostatic ducts and into the prostate. Infection stimulates an inflammatory response in which the prostate becomes larger, tender, and firm. Inflammation is usually limited to a few of the gland's excretory ducts.

SIGNS AND SYMPTOMS

Acute prostatitis begins with chills, lower back pain (especially when standing) caused by compression of the prostate gland, perineal fullness, suprapubic tenderness, frequent and urgent urination, dysuria, nocturia, urinary obstruction due to blocked urethra by enlarged prostate, and cloudy urine.

Signs of systemic infection include fever, myalgia, fatigue, and arthralgia. Signs and symptoms of chronic bacterial prostatitis may include the same urinary symptoms as the acute form but to a lesser degree, and recurrent symptomatic cystitis.

Other possible signs include evidence of UTI, such as urinary frequency, burning, cloudy urine, painful ejaculation, bloody semen, persistent urethral discharge, and sexual dysfunction.

COMPLICATIONS

Possible complications of prostatitis include UTI (common) and infected and abscessed testis (removed surgically).

DIAGNOSIS

Diagnosis of prostatitis may include a rectal examination that shows evidence of acute prostatitis, such as a very tender, warm, and enlarged prostate, and in chronic bacterial prostatis, the finding of a firm, irregularly shaped, and slightly enlarged prostate due to fibrosis. Palpation reveals a normal prostate gland by exclusion in nonbacterial prostatitis.

In addition, pelvic X-ray shows prostatic calculi. Urine culture identifies the causative infectious organism for bacterial prostatis. In nonbacterial prostatis, urine culture shows no evidence of UTI or a causative organism.

Firm diagnosis of prostatitis depends on a comparison of urine cultures of specimens obtained by the Meares-Stamey four-glass test. A significant increase in colony count in the prostatic specimens confirms prostatitis. This test requires four specimens: The first specimen is collected when the patient starts voiding (voided bladder one [VB1]). The second specimen is obtained midstream (VB2). The third specimen is taken after the patient stops voiding and the physician massages the prostate to produce secretions (expressed prostate secretions [EPS]). The fourth specimen is the final voided specimen (VB3).

TREATMENT

Systemic antibiotic therapy is the treatment of choice for acute prostatitis.

Co-trimoxazole (Bactrim) is given orally for 30 days (for culture showing sensitivity). I.V. co-trimoxazole or I.V. gentamicin (Garamycin) plus ampicillin (Unasyn) until sensitivity test results are known is administered. Parenteral therapy is instituted for 48 hours to 1 week; then an oral agent is prescribed for 30 more days. Generally, this combination has favorable test results and clinical response. Co-trimoxazole is given for at least 6 weeks for chronic prostatitis due to *E. coli.*

Supportive therapy includes bed rest, adequate hydration, analgesics, antipyretics, sitz baths, and stool softeners as necessary.

In symptomatic chronic prostatitis, the patient is advised to drink at least eight glasses of water daily. Regular careful massage of the prostate relieves discomfort, but vigorous massage may cause secondary epididymitis or septicemia. In addition, regular ejaculation helps promote drainage of prostatic secretions.

Other therapies include anticholinergics and analgesics to help relieve nonbacterial prostatitis symptoms. Alpha-adrenergic blockers and muscle relaxants may also be given to relieve pain, and continuous low-dose anabolic steroid therapy is effective in some men.

If drug therapy is unsuccessful, surgical treatment may be necessary. During transurethral resection of the prostate, all infected tissue is removed. This procedure isn't usually performed on young adults because it may cause retrograde ejaculation and sterility. A total prostatectomy can be curative but may cause impotence and incontinence.

NURSING CONSIDERATIONS

Patient care is primarily supportive.
+ Ensure bed rest and adequate hydration. Provide stool softeners and administer sitz baths, as ordered.
+ As necessary, prepare to assist with suprapubic needle aspiration of the bladder or a suprapubic cystostomy.
+ Emphasize the need for strict adherence to the prescribed drug regimen. Instruct the patient to drink at least eight glasses of water per day. Have him report adverse drug reactions (rash, nausea, vomiting, fever, chills, and GI irritation).

TESTICULAR TORSION

Testicular torsion is an abnormal twisting of the spermatic cord due to rotation of a testis or the mesorchium (a fold in the area between the testis and epididymis) that causes strangulation and, if left untreated, eventual infarction of the testis. Onset may be spontaneous or may follow physical exertion or trauma. This condition is almost always (90%) unilateral. The greatest risk occurs during the neonatal period and again between ages 12 and 18 (puberty), but it may occur at any age. Infants with torsion of one testis have a greater incidence of torsion of the other testis later in life than do males in the general population. The prognosis is good with early detection and prompt treatment.

Treatment
+ Systemic antibiotic
+ Bed rest
+ Adequate hydration
+ Analgesics
+ Antipyretics
+ Sitz baths
+ Stool softeners

Key nursing actions
+ Ensure bed rest and adequate hydration.
+ Provide stool softeners and administer sitz baths, as ordered.
+ As necessary, prepare to assist with suprapubic needle aspiration of the bladder or a suprapubic cystostomy.
+ Instruct the patient to drink at least eight glasses of water per day.
+ Instruct the patient to report adverse drug reactions.

Characteristics of testicular torsion
+ Abnormal twisting of spermatic cord
+ Due to rotation of testis or mesorchium
+ Causes strangulation, eventual infarction of testis
+ Onset spontaneous or may follow exertion, trauma
+ Almost always unilateral
+ Greatest risk during neonatal period and in puberty; may occur at any age
+ Prognosis good with early detection and prompt treatment

Extravaginal torsion

In extravaginal torsion, rotation of the spermatic cord above the testis causes strangulation and, eventually, infarction of the testis.

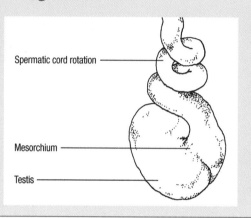

Causes

+ Intravaginal: testicular twisting from abnormality of coverings of testis, abnormally positioned testis, incomplete attachment of testis and spermatic fascia to scrotal wall
+ Extravaginal torsion: loose attachment of tunica vaginalis to scrotal lining causes spermatic cord rotation
+ Sudden forceful contraction of cremaster muscle may precipitate condition

How it happens

+ In testicular torsion, testis rotates on its vascular pedicle and twists arteries and vein in spermatic cord
+ Causes interruption of circulation to testis
+ Vascular engorgement, ischemia develop
+ Scrotal swelling, unrelieved by rest or elevation of scrotum

Key signs and symptoms

+ Excruciating pain in affected testis or iliac fossa of pelvis and edematous
+ Elevated, ecchymotic scrotum with loss of cremasteric reflex on affected side
+ Abdominal pain, nausea, vomiting

CAUSES

In intravaginal torsion (the most common type of testicular torsion in adolescents), testicular twisting may result from several conditions: abnormality of the coverings of the testis, abnormally positioned testis, and incomplete attachment of the testis and spermatic fascia to the scrotal wall, leaving the testis free to rotate around its vascular pedicle.

In extravaginal torsion (most common in neonates), loose attachment of the tunica vaginalis to the scrotal lining causes spermatic cord rotation above the testis. Sudden forceful contraction of the cremaster muscle may precipitate this condition.

PATHOPHYSIOLOGY

Normally, the tunica vaginalis envelops the testis and attaches to the epididymis and spermatic cord. Normal contraction of the cremaster muscle causes the left testis to rotate counterclockwise and the right testis to rotate clockwise. In testicular torsion, the testis rotates on its vascular pedicle and twists the arteries and vein in the spermatic cord, causing an interruption of circulation to the testis. Vascular engorgement and ischemia develop, causing scrotal swelling unrelieved by rest or elevation of the scrotum. If manual reduction is unsuccessful, the torsion must be surgically corrected within 6 hours after the onset of symptoms to preserve testicular function (70% salvage rate). After 12 hours, the testis becomes dysfunctional and necrotic. (See *Extravaginal torsion.*)

SIGNS AND SYMPTOMS

Signs and symptoms of testicular torsion include excruciating pain in the affected testis or iliac fossa of the pelvis and edematous, elevated, and ecchymotic scrotum with loss of the cremasteric reflex on the affected side (stimulation of the skin on the inner thigh retracts the testis on the same side). Associated symptoms include abdominal pain and nausea and vomiting.

COMPLICATIONS

Possible complications of testicular torsion include testicular infarction, necrosis, and infertility.

DIAGNOSIS

In testicular torsion, physical examination shows tense, tender swelling in the scrotum or inguinal canal, persistent reddening of the overlying skin and, possibly, palpable twisting of the spermatic cord (when examined before severe edema develops).

Doppler ultrasonography helps distinguish testicular torsion from strangulated hernia, undescended testes, or epididymitis. Absent blood flow and avascular testis are present in torsion.

TREATMENT

Treatment of testicular torsion consists of immediate surgical repair by orchiopexy (fixation of a viable testis to the scrotum and prophylactic fixation of the contralateral testis) or orchiectomy (excision of a nonviable testis) to decrease the risk of autoimmune response to a necrotic testis and its contents, damage to the unaffected testis, and subsequent infertility. Manual manipulation of the testis counterclockwise to improve blood flow before surgery may be done but isn't always possible.

NURSING CONSIDERATIONS

✦ Promote the patient's comfort before and after surgery.
✦ After surgery, administer pain medication as ordered. Monitor voiding, and apply an ice bag with a cover to reduce edema. Protect the wound from contamination. Otherwise, allow the patient to perform as many normal daily activities as possible.

Complications
✦ Testicular infarction
✦ Necrosis
✦ Infertility

Diagnosis
✦ Tense, tender swelling in scrotum or inguinal canal
✦ Persistent reddening of overlying skin
✦ Palpable twisting of spermatic cord

Treatment
✦ Immediate surgical repair by orchiopexy or orchiectomy
✦ Manual manipulation of testis counterclockwise to improve blood flow

Key nursing actions
✦ After surgery, administer pain medication as ordered.
✦ Monitor voiding, and apply an ice bag with a cover to reduce edema.
✦ Protect the wound from contamination.

Less common disorders
Selected references
Index

Less common disorders

DISEASE AND CAUSES	PATHOPHYSIOLOGY	SIGNS AND SYMPTOMS
Amyloidosis		
• Pressure caused by accumulation and infiltration of amyloid that leads to atrophy of nearby cells; abnormal immunoglobulin synthesis and reticuloendothelial cell dysfunction may occur • Familial inheritance in persons with Portuguese ancestry • May occur with tuberculosis, chronic infection, rheumatoid arthritis, multiple myeloma, Hodgkin's disease, paraplegia, brucellosis, and Alzheimer's disease	A rare, chronic disease of abnormal fibrillar scleroprotein accumulation that infiltrates body organs and soft tissues. Perireticular type affects the inner coats of blood vessels whereas pericollagen type affects the outer coats. Amyloidosis can result in permanent, even life-threatening, organ damage.	• Proteinuria, leading to nephrotic syndrome, eventually to renal failure • Heart failure caused by cardiomegaly, arrhythmias, and amyloid deposits in subendocardium, endocardium, and myocardium • Stiffness and enlargement of tongue, decreased intestinal motility, malabsorption, bleeding, abdominal pain, constipation, and diarrhea • Appearance of peripheral neuropathy • Liver enlargement, commonly with azotemia, anemia, albuminuria and, rarely, jaundice
Ankylosing spondylitis		
• No known cause; strongly associated with presence of human leukocyte antigen (HLA)-B27 • Familial inheritance	Fibrous tissue of the joint capsule is infiltrated by inflammatory cells that erode the bone and fibrocartilage. Repair of the cartilaginous structures begins with the proliferation of fibroblasts, which synthesize and secrete collagen. The collagen forms fibrous scar tissue that eventually undergoes calcification and ossification, causing the joint to fuse or lose flexibility.	• Intermittent lower back pain that's most severe after inactivity or in the morning • Stiffness, limited lumbar spine motion • Pain and limited expansion of chest • Peripheral arthritis in shoulders, hips, and knees • Kyphosis in advanced stages • Hip deformity and limited range of motion • Mild fatigue, fever, and anorexia or weight loss
Aspergillosis		
• Fungal infection caused by *Aspergillus* species; transmitted by inhalation of fungal spores or invasion of spores through wounds or injured tissue	*Aspergillus* species produce extracellular enzymes, such as proteases and peptidases, that contribute to tissue invasion, leading to hemorrhage and necrosis.	Incubation is a few days to weeks; may be asymptomatic or mimic tuberculosis, causing a productive cough and purulent or blood-tinged sputum, dyspnea, empyema, and lung abscesses • Allergic aspergillosis causes wheezing, dyspnea, pleural pain, and fever; aspergillosis endophthalmitis appears 2 to 3 weeks after eye surgery • Cloudy vision, eye pain, and reddened conjunctiva • Purulent exudate on exposure to anterior and posterior chambers of the eye

DISEASE AND CAUSES	PATHOPHYSIOLOGY	SIGNS AND SYMPTOMS
Bell's palsy		
• Considered an idiopathic facial paralysis; infectious cause suggested	Blockage of the seventh cranial nerve due to inflammation around the nerve where it leaves bony tissue leads to unilateral or bilateral facial weakness or paralysis. The blockage may result from hemorrhage, tumor, meningitis or local trauma.	• Unilateral facial weakness or paralysis, with aching at the jaw angle • Drooping mouth, causing salivation • Distorted taste • Impaired ability to fully close the eye on the affected side • Loss of taste and tinnitus
Bronchiectasis		
• Conditions associated with continued damage to bronchial walls and abnormal mucociliary clearance cause tissue breakdown to adjacent airways; such conditions include cystic fibrosis, immunologic disorders, and recurrent bacterial respiratory tract infections	Inflammation and destruction of the structural components of the bronchial wall leading to chronic abnormal dilatation.	*In early stages:* • Asymptomatic with complaints of frequent pneumonia or hemoptysis • Chronic cough producing foul-smelling, mucopurulent secretions • Coarse crackles during inspiration • Wheezing, dyspnea, sinusitis, fever, and chills *In advanced stage:* • Chronic malnutrition and right-sided heart failure caused by hypoxic pulmonary vasoconstriction
Bronchiolitis		
• No known cause; may be associated with specific diseases or conditions, such as bone marrow, heart or lung transplants, rheumatoid arthritis, lupus erythematosus, and Crohn's disease	Infection or other unknown factors cause necrosis of the bronchial epithelium and destruction of ciliated epithelial cells. As the submucosa becomes edematous, cellular debris and fibrin form plugs in the bronchioles.	*Subacute symptoms:* • Fever, persistent nonproductive cough, dyspnea, malaise, and anorexia • Physical assessment reveals dry crackles *Less common:* • Productive cough, hemoptysis, chest pain, general aches, and night sweats
Celiac disease		
• Results from a complex interaction involving dietary, genetic, and immunologic factors	Ingestion of gluten causes injury to the villi in the upper small intestine, leading to a decreased surface area and malabsorption of most nutrients. Inflammatory enteritis also results, leading to osmotic diarrhea and secretory diarrhea.	• Recurrent diarrhea, abdominal distention, stomach cramps, weakness, or increased appetite without weight gain • Normochromic, hypochromic, or macrocytic anemia • Osteomalacia, osteoporosis, tetany, and bone pain in lower back, rib cage, and pelvis • Peripheral neuropathy, paresthesia, or seizures • Dry skin, eczema, psoriasis, dermatitis herpetiformis, and acne rosacea • Amenorrhea, hypometabolism, and adrenocortical insufficiency • Mood changes and irritability

DISEASE AND CAUSES	PATHOPHYSIOLOGY	SIGNS AND SYMPTOMS
Cholera		
• Acute enterotoxin-mediated GI infection caused by gram-negative bacillus, which is transmitted through water and food that's contaminated with fecal material from carriers or people with active infections	Following ingestion of a significant inoculum, colonization of the small intestine occurs. The secretion of a potent enterotoxin results in a massive outpouring of isotonic fluid from the mucosal surface of the small intestine. Profuse diarrhea, vomiting, fluid and electrolyte loss occurs and may lead to hypovolemic shock, metabolic acidosis, and death.	Incubation period is several hours to 5 days • Acute, painless, profuse watery diarrhea, and vomiting • Intense thirst, weakness, and loss of skin tone • Muscle cramps • Cyanosis • Oliguria • Tachycardia • Falling blood pressure, fever, and hypoactive bowel sounds
Endocarditis		
• Infection caused by bacteria, viruses, fungi, rickettsiae, and parasites	Endothelial damage allows microorganisms to adhere to the surface where they proliferate and promote the propagation of endocardial vegetation.	• Weakness and fatigue • Weight loss, fever, night sweats, and anorexia • Arthralgia, splenomegaly, and new systolic murmur
Esophageal varices		
• Portal hypertension	Shunting of blood to the venae cavae caused by portal hypertension, leads to dilatation of esophageal veins.	• Hemorrhage and subsequent hypotension • Compromised oxygen supply • Altered level of consciousness
Fanconi's syndrome		
• Inherited renal tubular transport disorder	Changes in the proximal renal tubules caused by atrophy of epithelial cells and loss of proximal tube volume results in a shortened connection to glomeruli by an unusually narrow segment. Malfunction of the proximal renal tubules leads to hyperkalemia, hypernatremia, glycosuria, phosphaturia, aminoaciduria, uricosuria, retarded growth, and rickets.	• Mostly normal appearance at birth with slightly lower birth weights • After 6 months: weakness, failure to thrive, dehydration, cystine crystals in the corners of the eye, and retinal pigment degeneration • Yellow skin with little pigmentation • Slow linear growth
Hypersplenism		
• Increased activity of the spleen, where all types of blood cells are removed from circulation due to chronic myelogenous leukemia, lymphomas, Gaucher's disease, hairy cell leukemia, and sarcoidosis	Spleen growth may be stimulated by an increase in its workload, such as the trapping and destroying of abnormal red blood cells (RBCs).	• Enlarged spleen • Cytopenia

DISEASE AND CAUSES	PATHOPHYSIOLOGY	SIGNS AND SYMPTOMS
Idiopathic pulmonary fibrosis		
• Chronic progressive lung disease associated with inflammation and fibrosis • No known cause	Interstitial inflammation made up of an alveolar septal infiltrate of lymphocytes, plasma cells, and histiocytes. Fibrotic areas are composed of dense acellular collagen. Areas of honeycombing that form are composed of cystic fibrotic air spaces, commonly lined with bronchiolar epithelium and filled with mucus. Smooth muscle hyperplasia may occur in areas of fibrosis and honeycombing.	• Dyspnea • Nonproductive cough • Chest heaviness • Wheezing • Anorexia • Weight loss
Kaposi's sarcoma		
• Acquired immunodeficiency syndrome-related cancer	A malignant cancer arising from vascular endothelial cells, Kaposi's sarcoma affects endothelial tissue, which compromises all blood vessels.	• Red-purple circular lesions, slightly raised on the face, arms, neck, and legs • Internal lesions, especially in GI tract, identified by biopsy
Keratitis		
• Inflammation of cornea caused by microorganisms, trauma, or autoimmune disorders	Bacterial infection leading to ulceration of the cornea.	• Decreased visual acuity • Pain • Photophobia
Kyphosis		
• An excessive curvature of the spine with convexity backward caused by a congenital anomaly, tuberculosis (TB), syphilis, malignant or compression fracture, arthritis, or rickets	Pathophysiology is related to causative factor.	• Abnormally rounded thoracic curve
Legionnaires' disease		
• Infection caused by gram-negative bacillus, *Legionella pneumophila*	Transmission of disease occurs with inhalation of organism carried in aerosols produced by air-conditioning units, water faucets, shower heads, humidifiers, and contaminated respiratory equipment.	• Dry cough • Myalgia • GI distress • Pneumonia • Cardiovascular collapse
Leprosy		
• Infection caused by *Mycobacterium leprae*	Chronic, systemic infection with progressive cutaneous lesions that attacks the peripheral nervous system.	• Skin lesions • Anesthesia • Muscle weakness • Paralysis

DISEASE AND CAUSES	PATHOPHYSIOLOGY	SIGNS AND SYMPTOMS
Medullary sponge kidney		
• Genetic disorder	Collecting ducts in the renal pyramids dilate, forming cavities, clefts, and cysts that produce complications of calcium oxalate calculi and infections.	• Renal calculi • Hematuria • Infection (fever, chills, and malaise)
Myocarditis		
• Inflammation of the myocardium caused by bacterial, fungal, viral, or protozoal infections; heat stroke; ionizing radiation; rheumatic fever; and diphtheria	Initial infection triggers an autoimmune, cellular, and possibly humoral response resulting in myocardial inflammation and necrosis.	• Rapid, irregular, and weak pulse • Chest tenderness • First heart sound resembles second heart sound • Fatigue
Neurofibromatosis		
• Inherited disorder	Group of developmental disorders of the nervous system, muscles, bones, and skin that affects the cell growth of neural tissue.	• Café-au-lait spots • Multiple, pediculated, soft tumors • Hearing loss
Osgood-Schlatter disease		
• No known cause	Osteochondrosis of the tibia, disease of the growth or ossification centers in children.	• Frequent fractures • Pain at inferior aspect of patella
Pediculosis		
• Infestation by the lice parasite	Ectoparasite that attaches itself to the hair shaft with claws, and feeds on blood several times daily; resides close to the scalp to maintain its body temperature. Itching may be caused by an allergic reaction to louse saliva or irritability.	• Itching • Eczematous dermatitis • Inflammation • Tiredness • Irritability • Weakness • Lice present in hair (head, axilla, and pubic)
Pheochromocytoma		
• Polyglandular multiple endocrine neoplasia	Tumor of the chromaffin cells of the adrenal medulla that causes an increased production of catecholamines.	• Hypertension • High blood sugar • High lipid levels • Headache • Palpitations • Sweating • Dizziness • Constipation • Anxiety

DISEASE AND CAUSES	PATHOPHYSIOLOGY	SIGNS AND SYMPTOMS
Pleurisy		
• Several causes including lupus, rheumatoid arthritis, and TB	Inflammation of the pleura with exudation into the cavity and lung surface.	• Chilliness • Stabbing chest pain • Fever • Suppressed cough • Pallor • Dyspnea
Pyloric stenosis		
• Congenital; no known cause	Pyloric sphincter muscle fibers thicken and become inelastic, leading to a narrowed opening. The extra peristaltic effort that's necessary leads to hypertrophied muscle layers of the stomach.	• Progressive nonbilious vomiting, leading to projectile vomiting at ages 2 to 4 weeks
Retinal detachment		
• Caused by trauma, after cataract surgery, severe uveitis, and primary or metastatic choroidal tumors	The neural retina separates from the underlying retinal pigment epithelium.	• Floaters, flashing lights, scotoma in peripheral visual field (painless) and, eventually, a curtain or veil occurs in the field of vision
Retinitis pigmentosa		
• Autosomal recessive disorder in 80% of affected children • Less commonly transmitted as an X-linked trait	Slow, degenerative changes in the rods cause the retina and pigment epithelium to atrophy. Irregular black deposits of clumped pigment are in equatorial region of retina and eventually in the macular and peripheral areas.	• Progressive night blindness, visual field constriction with ring scotoma, and loss of acuity progressing to blindness
Rocky Mountain spotted fever		
• Infection caused by *Rickettsia rickettsii* carried by several tick species	*R. rickettsii* multiplies within endothelial cells and spreads through the bloodstream. Focal areas of infiltration lead to thrombosis and leakage of RBCs into surrounding tissue.	• Fever, headache, mental confusion, and myalgia • Rash develops as small macules progress to maculopapules and petechiae (Initially, rash starts on wrists and ankles and spreads to trunk. A rash noted on palms and soles is especially diagnostic.)
Sarcoidosis		
• No known cause • Evidence suggests that the disease is the result of exaggerated cellular immune response to a limited class of antigens	Organ dysfunction results from an accumulation of T lymphocytes, mononuclear phagocytes, and nonsecreting epithelial granulomas, which distort normal tissue architecture.	• Mainly generalized, most commonly involving the lung with resulting respiratory symptoms • Fever, fatigue, and malaise

DISEASE AND CAUSES	PATHOPHYSIOLOGY	SIGNS AND SYMPTOMS
Scabies		
• Human itch mite (*Sarcoptes scabiei* var. *hominis*)	Mite burrows superficially beneath stratum corneum depositing eggs that hatch, mature, and reinvade the skin.	Occur from sensitization reaction against excreta that mites deposit • Intense itching, worsens at night; threadlike lesions on wrists, between fingers, and on elbows, axillae, belt line, buttocks, and male genitalia
Sjögren's syndrome		
• Autoimmune rheumatic disorder with no known cause; genetic and environmental factors may be involved	Lymphocytic infiltration of exocrine glands causes tissue damage that results in xerostomia and dry eyes.	*In xerostomia:* • Dry mouth; difficulty swallowing and speaking; ulcers on the tongue, buccal mucosa and lips; severe dental caries *In ocular involvement:* • Dry eyes; gritty, sandy feeling; decreased tearing; burning, itching, redness, and photosensitivity *Extraglandular:* • Arthralgias, Raynaud's phenomenon, lymphadenopathy, and lung involvement
Strabismus		
• Eye malalignment that's frequently inherited; controversy exists whether amblyopia is caused by or results from strabismus	In paralytic (nonconcomitant) strabismus, paralysis of one or more ocular muscles may be caused by an oculomotor nerve lesion. In nonparalytic (concomitant) strabismus, unequal ocular muscle tone is caused by supranuclear abnormality within the CNS.	• Noticeable eye malalignment by external eye examination, ophthalmoscopic observation of the corneal light reflex in center of pupils, diplopia, and other vision disturbances
Thrombophlebitis		
• Caused by endothelial damage, accelerated blood clotting, and reduced blood flow	Alteration in epithelial lining causes platelet aggregation and fibrin entrapment of RBCs, white blood cells, and additional platelets; the thrombus initiates a chemical inflammatory process in the vessel epithelium that leads to fibrosis, which may occlude the vessel lumen or embolize.	• Varies with site and length of affected vein • Affected area usually extremely tender, swollen, and red
Trigeminal neuralgia		
• No known cause; possibly a compression neuropathy • At surgery or autopsy, the intracranial arterial and venous loops are found to compress the trigeminal nerve root at the brain stem	Painful disorder that's located along the distribution of one or more of the trigeminal nerve's sensory divisions, most commonly the maxillary.	• Searing or burning pain lasting seconds to 2 minutes at the trigeminal nerve distribution • Touching a trigger point typically elicits pain

DISEASE AND CAUSES	PATHOPHYSIOLOGY	SIGNS AND SYMPTOMS
Vitiligo		
• No known cause; usually acquired but may be familial (autosomal dominant) • Possible immunologic and neurochemical basis suggested	Destruction of melanocytes (humoral or cellular) and circulating antibodies against melanocytes results in hypopigmented areas.	• Progressive, symmetric areas of complete pigment loss with sharp borders, generally appearing in periorifical areas, flexor wrists, and extensor distal extremities
Wilson's disease		
• Inherited copper toxicosis	Defective mobilization of copper from hepatocellular lysosomes for excretion by way of bile allows excessive copper retention in the liver, brain, kidneys, and corneas, leading to tissue necrosis and subsequent hepatic and neurologic disorders.	*Kayser-Fleischer ring:* • Rusty brown ring of pigment at periphery of corneas • Signs of hepatitis leading to cirrhosis • Tremors, unsteady gait, muscular rigidity, inappropriate behavior, and psychosis • Hematuria, proteinuria, and uricosuria

Selected references

Atlas of Pathophysiology. Springhouse, Pa.: Springhouse Corp., 2002.

Bender, K. "West Nile Virus: A Growing Challenge," *AJN* 103(6):32-39; quiz 40; June 2003.

Cameron, B.L. "Making Diabetes Management Routine," *AJN* 102(2): 26-32; quiz 33, February 2002.

Davis, S.L. "How the Heart Failure Picture Has Changed," *Nursing2002* 32(11 Pt 1): 36-44; quiz N221-22, November 2002.

Funnell, M.M. "Diabetes Update from the American Diabetes Association: Preventing Type 2 Diabetes with Weight Loss and Exercise," *Nursing Management* 34(7 Suppl):10, June 2003.

Gould, B.E. *Pathophysiology for the Health Professions,* 2nd ed. Philadelphia: W.B. Saunders Co., 2002.

Groer, M. *Advanced Pathophysiology: Application to Clinical Practice.* Philadelphia: Lippincott Williams & Wil-kins, 2001.

Herlihy, B., and Maebius, N.K. *The Human Body in Health and Illness,* 2nd ed. Philadelphia: W.B. Saunders Co., 2003.

Holcomb, S.S. "Stopping the Cascade of Diabetes Insipidus," *Nursing2002* 32(3):32cc1-32cc6, March 2002.

Lea, D.H. "Ahead to the Past: How Genetics Is Changing Your Practice," *Nursing2002* 32(6):48-51, June 2002.

Pathophysiology Made Incredibly Easy, 2nd ed. Springhouse, Pa.: Lippincott Williams & Wilkins, 2002.

Porth, C. *Pathophysiology: Concepts of Altered Health States,* 6th ed. Philadelphia: Lippincott Williams & Wilkins, 2002.

Prezbindowski, K.S. *Study Guide to Accompany Porth's Pathophysiology: Concepts of Altered Health States.* Philadelphia: Lippincott Williams & Wilkins, 2002.

Professional Guide to Signs and Symptoms, 4th ed. Springhouse, Pa.: Lippincott Williams & Wilkins, 2004.

Sargent, C. and Murphy D. "What You Need to Know about Colorectal Cancer," *Nursing2003* 33(2):36-41, February 2003.

"The Seventh Report of the Joint National Committee on Prevention, Detection, Evaluation, and Treatment of High Blood Pressure: The JNC 7 Report," *JAMA* 289(19): 2560-72, Epub May 2003. Erratum in: *JAMA* 290(2):197, July 2003.

Watson, A.C. "Recognizing the Faces of Cancer Pain," *Nursing2003* 33(4):32hn1-32hn8, April 2003.

Whetstone, G., and Boswell, S. "The Geriatric Heart," *AJN* 102(9 Suppl):22-24, September 2002.

Workman, M.L. "Breast Cancer: New Strategies to Beat an Old Enemy," *Nursing2002* 32(10):58-63; quiz 64, October 2002.

Zimmerman, V.L. "BRCA Gene Mutations and Cancer," *AJN* 102(8):28-36, August 2002. Erratum in: *AJN* 102(11):13, November 2002.

Index

t refers to a table; i refers to an illustration; **boldface** refers to a full-color illustration.

t refers to a table; i refers to an illustration; **boldface** refers to a full-color illustration.

t refers to a table; i refers to an illustration; **boldface** refers to a full-color illustration.

t refers to a table; i refers to an illustration; **boldface** refers to full-color illustration

t refers to a table; i refers to an illustration; **boldface** refers to a full-color illustration.

t refers to a table; i refers to an illustration; **boldface** refers to a full-color illustration.

t refers to a table; i refers to an illustration; **boldface** refers to a full-color illustration.

t refers to a table; i refers to an illustration; **boldface** refers to a full-color illustration.

t refers to a table; i refers to an illustration; **boldface** refers to a full-color illustration.